AMERICAN PSYCHIATRIC PRESS

REVIEW
OF
PSYCHIATRY

VOLUME

16

AMERICAN PSYCHIATRIC PRESS

REVIEW
OF
PSYCHIATRY

VOLUME

16

EDITED BY

LEAH J. DICKSTEIN, M.D.,
MICHELLE B. RIBA, M.D., and
JOHN M. OLDHAM, M.D.

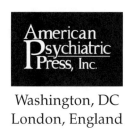

Washington, DC
London, England

Copyright © 1997 American Psychiatric Press, Inc.
00 99 98 97   4 3 2 1
ALL RIGHTS RESERVED
Manufactured in the United States of America on acid-free paper

American Psychiatric Press, Inc.
1400 K Street, N.W.
Washington, DC   20005

American Psychiatric Press Review of Psychiatry, Volume 16
ISSN 1041-5882
ISBN 0-88048-443-8

The correct citation for this book is *American Psychiatric Press Review of Psychiatry*, Volume 16. Edited by Dickstein LJ, Riba MB, Oldham JM. Washington, DC, American Psychiatric Press, 1997.

**AMERICAN PSYCHIATRIC PRESS REVIEW OF PSYCHIATRY,
VOLUME 10** (1991)

Allan Tasman, M.D., and Stephen M. Goldfinger, M.D., Editors

Schizophrenia
Daniel R. Weinberger, M.D., Section Editor

Dissociative Disorders
David Spiegel, M.D., Section Editor

Sexual Abuse of Children and Adolescents
Elissa P. Benedek, M.D., Section Editor

Neuroscience
Joseph T. Coyle, M.D., Section Editor

New Perspectives on Human Development
Leah J. Dickstein, M.D., Section Editor

**AMERICAN PSYCHIATRIC PRESS REVIEW OF PSYCHIATRY,
VOLUME 11** (1992)

Allan Tasman, M.D., and Michelle B. Riba, M.D., Editors

Severe Personality Disorders
Thomas A. Widiger, Ph.D., and John G. Gunderson, M.D., Section Editors

Brain, Behavior, and the Immune System
Marvin Stein, M.D., and Andrew H. Miller, M.D., Section Editors

Anxiety Disorders
Jack M. Gorman, M.D., and Laszlo A. Papp, M.D., Section Editors

Concurrent Diagnoses
Joel Yager, M.D., Section Editor

Hospital Psychiatry
Richard L. Munich, M.D., and Glen O. Gabbard, M.D., Section Editors

AMERICAN PSYCHIATRIC PRESS REVIEW OF PSYCHIATRY,
VOLUME 12 (1993)

John M. Oldham, M.D., Michelle B. Riba, M.D.,
and Allan Tasman, M.D., Editors

Changing Perspectives on Homosexuality
Terry S. Stein, M.D., Section Editor

Posttraumatic Stress Disorder
Robert S. Pynoos, M.D., M.P.H., Section Editor

Brain Imaging
Nancy C. Andreasen, M.D., Ph.D., Section Editor

Combined Treatments
Bernard D. Beitman, M.D., Section Editor

The Neuropsychiatry of Memory
Stuart C. Yudofsky, M.D., and Robert E. Hales, M.D., Section Editors

AMERICAN PSYCHIATRIC PRESS REVIEW OF PSYCHIATRY,
VOLUME 13 (1994)

John M. Oldham, M.D., and Michelle B. Riba, M.D., Editors

History of Psychiatry in America
Michael J. Vergare, M.D., and John S. McIntyre, M.D., Section Editors

Biological Markers
Jack M. Gorman, M.D., and Laszlo A. Papp, M.D., Section Editors

Ethics
Jeremy A. Lazarus, M.D., Section Editor

Psychotherapy With Children and Adolescents
Clarice J. Kestenbaum, M.D., and Owen Lewis, M.D., Section Editors

Sleep Disorders
Charles F. Reynolds III, M.D., and David J. Kupfer, M.D., Section Editors

Dedicated to all psychiatric and other clinicians who want to be maximally informed of the latest scientific knowledge related to psychiatric disorders so that they can offer their patients the highest quality medical and psychological treatments currently available.

Contents

Section

II

Section

III

Obsessive-Compulsive Disorder Across the Life Cycle

Section

IV

Psychopharmacology Across the Life Span

Section

**Psychological and Biological Assessment
at the Turn of the Century**

Section

VI

Computers, the Patient, and the Psychiatrist

Contributors

Norman Alessi, M.D.
Division Director, Child and Adolescent Psychiatry; Chief Information Officer; Director, Psychiatric Informatics Program, University of Michigan Medical Center, Ann Arbor, Michigan

Victoria L. Banyard, Ph.D.
Department of Psychology, University of New Hampshire, Durham, New Hampshire

Judith S. Beck, Ph.D.
Director, Beck Institute for Cognitive Therapy and Research, Bala Cynwyd, Pennsylvania; Clinical Assistant Professor of Psychology in Psychiatry, University of Pennsylvania, Philadelphia, Pennsylvania

Joseph Biederman, M.D.
Chief, Pediatric Psychopharmacology Unit, Massachusetts General Hospital; Professor of Psychiatry, Harvard Medical School, Boston, Massachusetts

Elizabeth S. Bowman, M.D.
Associate Professor, Department of Psychiatry, Indiana University School of Medicine, Indianapolis, Indiana

Lisa D. Butler, Ph.D.
Postdoctoral Fellow, Department of Psychiatry and Behavioral Sciences, Stanford University School of Medicine, Stanford, California

Cheryl N. Carmin, Ph.D.
Associate Professor of Clinical Psychology in Psychiatry, The University of Illinois at Chicago

Daniel Carpenter, Ph.D.
Instructor of Psychology in Psychiatry, Cornell University Medical College, New York, New York

David M. Clark, D.Phil.
Professor of Psychiatry and Wellcome Principal Research Fellow, Department of Psychiatry, University of Oxford, Warneford Hospital, Oxford, United Kingdom

John F. Clarkin, Ph.D.
Professor of Clinical Psychology in Psychiatry, Cornell University
Medical College; Director of Psychology, New York
Hospital—Westchester Division, White Plains, New York, and Payne
Whitney Clinic, New York, New York

Lee S. Cohen, M.D.
Director, Perinatal and Reproductive Psychiatry Clinical Research
Program, Massachusetts General Hospital; Assistant Professor of
Psychiatry, Department of Psychiatry, Harvard Medical School,
Boston, Massachusetts

Philip M. Coons, M.D.
Professor, Department of Psychiatry, Indiana University School of
Medicine, Indianapolis, Indiana

Naakesh A. Dewan, M.D.
Director of Information and CQM Services, New York
Hospital—Cornell University Medical Center, Westchester Division,
White Plains; Assistant Professor, Department of Psychiatry, Cornell
University Medical College, New York, New York

Susan F. Diaz, M.D.
Department of Obstetrical Medicine, Division of Behavioral Health,
Women and Infants Hospital, Providence, Rhode Island

Leah J. Dickstein, M.D.
Professor, Associate Chair for Academic Affairs, and Director,
Division of Attitudinal and Behavioral Medicine, Department of
Psychiatry and Behavioral Sciences; Associate Dean for Faculty and
Student Advocacy, University of Louisville School of Medicine,
Louisville, Kentucky

John P. Docherty, M.D.
Professor and Vice Chair, Department of Psychiatry, Cornell
University Medical College; Deputy Medical Director, The New York
Hospital—Cornell Medical Center, New York, New York

Jane Eisen, M.D.
Department of Psychiatry and Human Behavior, Brown University
School of Medicine, Providence, Rhode Island

Lynn R. Grush, M.D.
Associate Director, Perinatal and Reproductive Psychiatry Clinical Research Program, Massachusetts General Hospital; Instructor, Department of Psychiatry, Harvard Medical School, Boston, Massachusetts

Milton Huang, M.D.
Assistant Director, Psychiatric Informatics Program, University of Michigan Medical Center, Ann Arbor, Michigan

Steven E. Hyler, M.D.
Associate Professor of Clinical Psychiatry, Columbia University College of Physicians and Surgeons, and New York State Psychiatric Institute, New York, New York

Philip G. Janicak, M.D.
Professor and Medical Director, Psychiatric Institute, Department of Psychiatry, University of Illinois at Chicago, Chicago, Illinois

Paul E. Keck, Jr., M.D.
Associate Professor of Psychiatry and Pharmacology, Biological Psychiatry Program, Department of Psychiatry, University of Cincinnati College of Medicine, Cincinnati, Ohio

Robert Kennedy, M.A.
Department of Psychiatry, Albert Einstein College of Medicine, Bronx, New York

Wilma Koutstaal, Ph.D.
Postdoctoral Fellow, Department of Psychology, Harvard University, Cambridge, Massachusetts

Thomas Kramer, M.D., F.A.P.A.
Coordinator of Training, Arkansas Mental Health Research and Training Institute; Assistant Professor of Psychiatry, University of Arkansas for Medical Sciences, Little Rock, Arkansas

Henrietta L. Leonard, M.D.
Professor, Department of Psychiatry and Human Behavior, Brown University School of Medicine, Providence, Rhode Island

John March, M.D., M.P.H.
Assistant Professor, Department of Psychiatry and Behavioral Sciences and Department of Psychology, Social and Health Sciences, Duke University Medical Center, Durham, North Carolina

Steven Mattis, Ph.D.
Director, Psychological Services, Hillside Hospital–Long Island Jewish Medical Center; Professor of Psychiatry, Albert Einstein College of Medicine, Bronx, New York

Kevin M. McConkey, Ph.D.
Professor of Psychology and Head, School of Psychology, University of New South Wales, Sydney, New South Wales, Australia

Susan L. McElroy, M.D.
Codirector, Biological Psychiatry Program; Associate Professor of Psychiatry, University of Cincinnati College of Medicine, Cincinnati, Ohio

Marvin Miller, M.D.
Assistant Professor of Psychiatry, University of Indiana School of Medicine, Indianapolis, Indiana

Victor Milstein, Ph.D.
Research Psychologist, Larue D. Carter Memorial Hospital; Professor, Department of Psychiatry, Indiana University School of Medicine, Indianapolis, Indiana

James E. Mitchell, M.D.
Professor and Chairman, Department of Neuroscience, University of North Dakota, Fargo, North Dakota

Frederick L. Newman, Ph.D.
Professor, Health Services Administration, Florida International University; Adjunct Professor of Psychiatry, Center for Family Studies, University of Miami, Miami, Florida

John M. Oldham, M.D.
Director, New York State Psychiatric Institute; Professor and Vice Chairman, Department of Psychiatry, Columbia University College of Physicians and Surgeons, New York, New York

Raymond Ownby, M.D., Ph.D.
Associate Professor, Department of Psychiatry, University of Miami School of Medicine, Miami, Florida

Carlos N. Pato, M.D.
Associate Professor, Department of Psychiatry, State University of New York at Buffalo

Michele T. Pato, M.D.
Associate Professor, Department of Psychiatry, State University of
New York at Buffalo

Joseph V. Penn, M.D.
Child Psychiatry Fellow, Department of Psychiatry and Human
Behavior, Brown University School of Medicine, Providence, Rhode
Island

Carol B. Peterson, Ph.D.
Research Associate, Department of Psychiatry, University of
Minnesota, Minneapolis, Minnesota

C. Alec Pollard, Ph.D.
Professor, Department of Community and Family Medicine, St. Louis
University School of Medicine, St. Louis, Missouri

Paul Quinlan, D.O.
Fellow, Psychiatric Informatics Program, University of Michigan
Medical Center, Ann Arbor, Michigan

Michelle B. Riba, M.D.
Associate Clinical Professor of Psychiatry and Associate Chair for
Education and Academic Affairs, Department of Psychiatry,
University of Michigan Medical Center, Ann Arbor, Michigan

Andrew Satlin, M.D.
Director of Geriatric Psychiatry, Department of Psychiatry, McLean
Hospital, Belmont; Assistant Professor of Psychiatry, Harvard
Medical School, Boston, Massachusetts

Daniel L. Schacter, Ph.D.
Professor of Psychology, Department of Psychology, Harvard
University, Cambridge, Massachusetts

Marc Schwartz, M.D.
Research Associate, Yale University; President, HealthCalls America,
New Haven, Connecticut

Jan Scott, M.D., F.R.C.Psych.
Professor, University Department of Psychiatry, Royal Victoria
Infirmary, Newcastle upon Tyne, United Kingdom

Deborah A. Sichel, M.D.
Center for Women and Families, Hestia Institute, Wellesley, Massachusetts; Instructor, Department of Psychiatry, Harvard Medical School, Boston, Massachusetts

Thomas Spencer, M.D.
Assistant Chief, Pediatric Psychopharmacology Unit, Massachusetts General Hospital; Assistant Professor of Psychiatry, Harvard Medical School, Boston, Massachusetts

David Spiegel, M.D.
Professor, Department of Psychiatry and Behavioral Sciences, Stanford University School of Medicine, Stanford, California

Gail Steketee, Ph.D.
Professor, Boston University, School of Social Work, Boston, Massachusetts

Stephen M. Strakowski, M.D.
Associate Professor of Psychiatry, Psychotic Disorders Research Program, Department of Psychiatry, University of Cincinnati College of Medicine, Cincinnati, Ohio

Zebulon Taintor, M.D.
Professor and Vice Chairman of Psychiatry, New York University Medical Center; and Chief of Staff, Manhattan Psychiatric Center, New York, New York

Michael E. Thase, M.D.
Professor of Psychiatry, Western Psychiatric Institute and Clinic, Department of Psychiatry, University of Pittsburgh School of Medicine, Pittsburgh, Pennsylvania

Bertram Warren, M.D., F.A.P.A.
Chair, American Psychiatric Association Committee on Information Systems; Clinical Director, Union County Psychiatric Clinic, Fanwood, New Jersey

Charles Wasserman, M.D.
Psychiatrist-in-Charge, Nursing Home Consultation Service, Department of Psychiatry, McLean Hospital, Belmont; Instructor in Psychiatry, Harvard Medical School, Boston, Massachusetts

Elizabeth Weller, M.D.
Frederick H. Allen Chair, Department of Psychiatry, Children's
Hospital of Philadelphia; Vice Chair, Department of Psychiatry,
University of Pennsylvania School of Medicine; Medical Director,
The Child Guidance Center, Children's Hospital of Philadelphia,
Philadelphia, Pennsylvania

Adrian Wells, Ph.D.
Senior Lecturer in Clinical Psychology, Department of Clinical
Psychology, School of Psychiatry and Behavioural Sciences,
Manchester Royal Infirmary, Manchester, United Kingdom

Scott A. West, M.D.
Codirector, Psychopharmacology Research Program, Psychiatric
Institute of Florida, Orlando, Florida

Timothy Wilens, M.D.
Staff Member, Pediatric Psychopharmacology Unit, Massachusetts
General Hospital; Associate Professor of Psychiatry, Harvard Medical
School, Boston, Massachusetts

Linda M. Williams, Ph.D.
Family Research Laboratory, University of New Hampshire,
Durham; Research Director, Stone Center, Wellesley College,
Wellesley, Massachusetts

Barbara C. Wilson, Ph.D.
Director, Center for Neuropsychological Services, North Shore
University Hospital, Manhasset, New York; Associate Professor, New
York University Medical Center

Elizabeth A. Winans, Pharm.D.
Clinical Assistant Professor, Department of Pharmacy Practice;
Psychiatric Institute, University of Illinois at Chicago, Chicago,
Illinois

Jesse H. Wright, M.D., Ph.D.
Professor, Department of Psychiatry and Behavioral Sciences,
University of Louisville School of Medicine; Medical Director,
Norton Psychiatric Clinic, Louisville, Kentucky

Foreword to Volume 16

Leah J. Dickstein, M.D., Michelle B. Riba, M.D., and John M. Oldham, M.D.

As the 21st century approaches, psychiatrists and all other physicians, as well as other mental health and general health professionals, want access to the latest scientific research affecting the care of patients with mental illness. As with the first 15 volumes in the Review of Psychiatry series, Volume 16 brings professionals the latest and most important scientific knowledge to ensure correct diagnosis and the most effective treatment for their patients.

Section I coeditors Jesse H. Wright, M.D., Ph.D., and Michael E. Thase, M.D., invited international leaders in the field of cognitive therapy to describe its clearly effective uses in the treatment of major Axis I and II psychiatric disorders, including anxiety, substance abuse, personality, and eating disorders and other chronic and severe mental disorders such as depressive and bipolar disorders and schizophrenia. The clearly written and detailed chapters include excellent descriptions of symptoms, diagnostic criteria, treatment procedures and worksheets, interactions with pharmacotherapy, comorbidity concerns, and outcome expectations. Recognized as an effective treatment modality for more than two decades, cognitive-behavioral treatment, with its use of structured time, can unquestionably be of clinical importance to all professionals faced with time limitations in patient care.

David Spiegel, M.D., editor of Section II, focused his expert authors on the medically (and legally) sensitive and important topic of trauma and memories across the life cycle. The chapters span topics from the experimental cognitive psychology literature and other research-based studies of child trauma, to recovered and repressed memories, to intentional forgetting and voluntary thought suppression. The clear and detailed information presented should enable professionals to treat patients who have experienced trauma more appropriately and to use patients' memories with an understanding of how trauma may have affected these memories.

Section III editors Michele T. Pato, M.D., and Gail Steketee, Ph.D., have brought chapters covering the emerging data on obsessive-compulsive disorder, including important considerations across the life cycle and by gender. Chapter topics include a separate focus on children, adolescents, and adults; the perinatal period; and the longitudinal course of obsessive-compulsive disorder.

The enormity of the problem for patients who have these often unrecognized and, consequently, untreated disorders is increasingly being identified. For example, because of new treatment guidelines, ob-sessive-compulsive disorder in pregnant women is identified more often and, with increased patient education, is treated appropriately in a variety of ways.

Susan L. McElroy, M.D., Section IV editor, has selected critical topics in psychopharmacology that are of important practical relevance to clinicians. Chapters cover child and adolescent psychopharmacology; geriatric psychopharmacology; and psychopharmacological treat-ment of psychotic, bipolar, and attention-deficit/hyperactivity disor-ders across the life cycle. The chapters on psychotic disorders and ADHD, with their emphasis on life cycle differences, are of extreme importance to decreasing morbidity and needless human suffering. Chaper authors denote the emerging knowledge about unique differ-ences in physiology and pathophysiology, interactions of comorbid diseases and side effects, and toxicity and pharmacological interac-tions that should be known in order for clinicians to appropriately as-sess and correctly prescribe psychotropics. Differences in diagnosis and treatment across the life span, particularly with the increasing numbers of psychopharmacological agents available and their unique indications and effects with similarities and differences across the life cycle, are clearly described.

Section V editors John F. Clarkin, Ph.D., and John P. Docherty, M.D., have brought together contributions that survey the importance of biological and psychological assessment for psychiatrists in their clini-cal practice. Topics include the use of laboratory tests to ensure and further excellent clinical care. Biological factors associated with specific psychiatric disorders and their role in treatment selection, as well as monitoring of clinical efficacy and toxicity, are reviewed. Also re-viewed are the role of neuropsychological assessment in improving diagnosis, and therefore treatment, and the use of neuropsychological assessment in an era of managed systems of care. For example, the common dilemma facing the clinician when making the differential diagnosis between delirium, dementia, and depression is outlined. The neuropsychological assessment, including lesser known tests of executive motor function and skills and perceptual and conceptual functions, is reviewed. Reasons for referral of children, including the differential diagnosis of autism, communication disorders, and mental retardation (which involves assessment for often undetected audi-ological problems) and diagnosis of attention-deficit/hyperactivity dis-order are discussed. Eleven guidelines for psychological instrument selection for assessment of treatment outcome are offered. These guidelines, which address issues ranging from relevance to target group to cost to clinical utility, are intended to help the clinician and program of services with diagnosis and treatment planning. A detailed discussion of performance measurement in healthcare delivery systems brings to a close this extremely useful section.

Finally, Zebulon Taintor, M.D., editor of Section VI, has enlisted several colleagues who are experienced in the use of computers in work with psychiatric patients. The authors' descriptions of the unquestionable assistance of computers in effective psychiatric care should challenge all to incorporate their use into patient care.

We want to express our gratitude to the section editors, chapter authors, and their staffs who have worked to bring this volume to completion. Furthermore, we want to acknowledge the excellent knowledge, skills, and commitment of the American Psychiatric Press editorial staff, under the leadership of Carol C. Nadelson, M.D., Editor-in-Chief, Claire Reinburg, Editorial Director, and Pamela Harley, Managing Editor, Books, and Dr. Dickstein's assistants, Cheryl R. Garrison and Carolyn Childress.

I

Cognitive Therapy

Contents

Section I

Cognitive Therapy

Foreword

Jesse H. Wright, M.D., Ph.D., and
Michael E. Thase, M.D., Section Editors

Cognitive therapy has developed over the last 30 years into one of the predominate psychotherapeutic approaches to mental disorders. When Beck first proposed the basic theories of cognitive therapy in the early 1960s, there had been little research on cognitive and behavioral pathology in depression, anxiety disorders, or other common psychiatric conditions. Empirical study of the outcome of psychotherapy was at a rudimentary stage. However, Beck's pioneering observations helped to spark an intensive research effort that has proliferated into a broad and intensive series of fundamental investigations on cognitive and behavioral therapies.

This section of the *American Psychiatric Press Review of Psychiatry* focuses on several of the more important applications of cognitive therapy. In some cases (i.e., anxiety disorders and eating disorders), substantial research evidence has been collected for the efficacy of cognitive therapy. Chapters on some of the newer uses for cognitive therapy (i.e., for personality disorders, substance abuse, and chronic and severe psychiatric disorders) have also been included. Cognitive therapy is best known for the extensive research that has documented it as an effective treatment for depression (Dobson 1989; Thase 1995). Methods for using cognitive therapy with complicated or treatment-resistant cases of depression are detailed in Chapter 5 of this volume, on chronic and severe mental disorders. A full description of cognitive therapy procedures for depression can be found in Volume 7 of this series and in a number of more recent reviews on this topic (see, e.g., Wright and Beck 1994; Thase and Wright 1996; Beck and Rush 1995).

The overall direction of research and clinical development of cognitive therapy has been toward fulfilling the criteria for a system of psychotherapy: 1) a comprehensive theory, 2) a body of research to support this theory, 3) an operationalized therapy that is directly linked to theoretical concepts, and 4) established efficacy of the treatment (see A. T. Beck 1993; J. Beck, Chapter 3). The chapter authors in this section present basic theories, demonstrate how treatment interventions are guided by both theory and empirical data, and review available outcome studies.

In Chapter 1, Clark and Wells describe the formidable array of cognitive and behavioral procedures for use in the treatment of anxiety disorders. The cognitive model for anxiety is based on findings that patients with anxiety disorders misinterpret signals of physical or personal danger. Such individuals often come to catastrophic conclusions and/or underestimate their ability to cope with situations. Specific formulations and treatment procedures are offered for each of the anxiety disorders. The authors note that cognitive and behavioral interventions are usually combined in clinical practice in the treatment of anxiety disorders. For example, a patient with panic might benefit from revision of erroneous beliefs about bodily sensations (cognitive restructuring) and response prevention or breathing training. Cognitive therapy has been shown to be an effective treatment for panic disorder, social phobia, and generalized anxiety disorder. Behavioral interventions coupled with cognitive therapy also have been found to be helpful for obsessive-compulsive disorder (OCD). Research on hypochondriasis, a condition that cognitive-behavioral therapy theorists link closely with the DSM-IV anxiety disorders, and posttraumatic stress disorder (PTSD) has been limited but has yielded promising results.

Because of the close interplay between cognitive and behavioral factors, some therapists prefer to use the term *cognitive-behavioral therapy* to describe their treatment approach. Often, authors who use the term *cognitive therapy* are communicating their interest in the more specific model of treatment developed by Beck and associates, whereas those who use the term cognitive-behavioral therapy embrace a broader array of theoretically based interventions. However, this convention is hardly uniform, and we consider the designations of cognitive therapy and cognitive-behavioral therapy to be essentially interchangeable. In this volume, we have accepted the authors' choice of names for therapies that are directed at both cognitive and behavioral change.

In Chapter 2, Thase reviews the development of cognitive-behavioral therapy for substance abuse and substance use disorders. He notes that more traditional models of psychotherapy and counseling have yielded unacceptably low success rates for these common, yet disabling conditions. Thase describes the cognitive and behavioral factors known to perpetuate substance abuse and substance use disorders and illustrates therapeutic techniques used to help patients to better cope with attitudes, beliefs, cravings, and symptoms of withdrawal. Although extensive research on cognitive-behavioral treatments of substance abuse and substance use disorders is not yet available, relevant data are reviewed that point to the powerful potential of these approaches.

Personality disorders are among the most common and most vexing conditions seen by mental health professionals. The traditional approach to characterological disturbances has been psychodynamically oriented psychotherapy. Judith Beck details a new conceptualization and treatment method for personality disorders in Chapter 3. Cognitive therapy for personality disorders is directed at modifying underlying dysfunctional beliefs and associated maladaptive behavioral strategies. Beck describes characteristic patterns of pathological beliefs and compensatory strategies for each type of personality disorder. The chapter on personality disorders contains a wide variety of innovative strategies that should be of considerable interest to clinicians who treat these challenging patients.

The fourth chapter of this section, by Mitchell and Peterson, provides a concise description of cognitive-behavioral treatment of eating disorders. Because all available epidemiologic evidence suggests that the incidence of eating disorders continues to increase, the availability of empirically validated treatments such as those described by Mitchell and Peterson has profound public health significance, particularly when the potential long-term value of relapse prevention strategies is taken into account.

The final chapter of this section is devoted to the treatment of chronic and severe psychiatric disorders. Scott and Wright observe that conditions such as chronic depression, bipolar disorder, and schizophrenia can be approached with a combined treatment model of pharmacotherapy and cognitive-behavioral interventions. The rationale for adding cognitive-behavioral therapy to medication management for patients with these conditions includes lack of full response of many of these patients to pharmacotherapy; hopelessness; impaired social skills; underlying dysfunctional attitudes; negative symptoms; and treatment noncompliance. The authors present detailed descriptions and case illustrations of cognitive-behavioral therapy for severely ill patients. Significant modifications in therapy techniques may be required to meet the needs of these individuals. However, preliminary research has indicated that cognitive-behavioral therapy may have considerable utility in the treatment of chronic and severe conditions.

This review section on cognitive therapy comprises a status report on some of the major and newer applications for this treatment approach. Continued research is needed to clarify the effectiveness, indications, and limitations of cognitive and behavioral methods. Nevertheless, there is a strong rationale for applying cognitive therapy in the treatment of anxiety disorders, substance abuse, characterological disturbances, eating disorders, and chronic and severe mental illnesses. A cognitive-behavioral model has been described for each of these conditions, specific therapeutic interventions have been developed, and in most cases the therapy has been tested in outcome studies. The strong empirical tradition of cognitive therapy suggests that there will be further development of cognitive theories and procedures for a wide range of disorders. Moreover, the procedurally specific nature of these treatments makes them well suited for training and ongoing assessment of fidelity/quality assurance. It is approaches such as the these that help to ensure the future of psychotherapy and, ultimately, positive outcomes for our patients.

References

Beck AT: Cognitive therapy: past, present, and future. J Consult Clin Psychol 61:194–198, 1993

Beck AT, Rush AJ: Cognitive therapy, in Comprehensive Textbook of Psychiatry/VI, 6th Edition. Edited by Kaplan HI, Sadock BJ. Baltimore, MD, Williams & Wilkins, 1995, pp 1847–1857

Dobson KS: A meta-analysis of the efficacy of cognitive therapy for depression. J Consult Clin Psychol 57:414–419, 1989

Thase ME: Reeducative psychotherapies, in Treatments of Psychiatric Disorders, 2nd Edition, Vol 1. Gabbard GO, Editor-in-Chief. Washington, DC, American Psychiatric Press, 1995, pp 1169–1204

Thase ME, Wright JH: in Psychiatry, Vol 2. Edited by Tasman A, Kay J, Lieberman JA. Philadelphia, PA, WB Saunders, 1996, pp 1418–1438

Wright JH, Beck AT: Cognitive therapy, in The American Psychiatric Press Textbook of Psychiatry, 2nd Edition. Edited by Hales RE, Yudofsky SC, Talbott JA. Washington, DC, American Psychiatric Association, 1994, pp 1083–1114

Chapter 1

Cognitive Therapy for Anxiety Disorders

David M. Clark, D.Phil., and Adrian Wells, Ph.D.

Considerable progress has been made in developing effective pharmacological interventions for anxiety disorders. Alprazolam, imipramine, phenelzine, and certain selective serotonin reuptake inhibitors (SSRIs) have all been shown to be effective in certain anxiety disorders. However, not all patients are responsive to, or willing to, take these medications, and there are doubts about the long-term efficacy of pharmacological interventions. For example, studies published so far suggest that between 25% and 80% of patients relapse after discontinuation of drug treatment for panic disorder (Clark et al. 1994; Fyer 1988; Sheehan 1986). Clearly, there is a need for additional interventions. In recent years, a nonpharmacological treatment that has received considerable research support is cognitive therapy (CT). In the present chapter we provide an overview of the cognitive approach to the conceptualization and treatment of anxiety disorders and hypochondriasis and review controlled trials evaluating the effectiveness of CT.

The Cognitive Approach to Understanding Anxiety Disorders

Cognitive therapy is a brief (8–16 sessions) psychological treatment based on the cognitive model of emotional disorders (Beck 1976). The cognitive model assumes that it is not events per se, but rather people's expectations and interpretations of events, that are responsible for the production of negative emotions such as anxiety, anger, or sadness. Each negative emotion is associated with a characteristic set of interpretations. In anxiety, the important interpretations, or cognitions, relate to perceived physical or psychosocial danger. Once an individual perceives a situation or sensation as dangerous, an "anxiety program"

This chapter is an expanded and updated version of a paper delivered at the 7th Congress of the Association of European Psychiatrists in Copenhagen, September 22, 1994.

David M. Clark is a Wellcome Trust Principal Research Fellow. The authors are grateful to Anke Ehlers and Paul Salkovskis for helpful comments on an early draft and to Hester Barrington-Ward for her invaluable help in preparing the manuscript.

becomes activated. The anxiety program is a complex constellation of somatic, cognitive, and behavioral changes, many of which are probably inherited from our evolutionary past and originally served to protect us from harm in objectively dangerous primitive environments. However, when, as in anxiety disorders, the danger is more imagined than real, these anxiety responses are largely inappropriate. Instead of serving a useful function, they contribute to a series of vicious circles that tend to maintain or exacerbate the anxiety disorder.

Two types of vicious circle are common in anxiety disorders. First, the reflexively elicited somatic and cognitive symptoms of anxiety become further sources of perceived danger. For example, blushing may be taken as an indication that one has made a fool of oneself, and this may lead to further embarrassment and blushing; a shaking hand may be taken as an indication of impending loss of control, and this may trigger more anxiety and shaking; or a racing heart may be taken as evidence of an impending heart attack, and this may produce further anxiety and cardiac symptoms. Second, patients often engage in cognitive and behavioral strategies that are intended to prevent the feared events from occurring. However, because the fears are unrealistic, the main effect of these strategies is that patients are prevented from disconfirming their negative beliefs. For example, patients who are concerned that the unusual and racing thoughts they experience during anxiety attacks indicate that they are in danger of going mad often make strenuous efforts to control their thoughts and (erroneously) believe that if they had not done so, they would have gone "crazy."

Having outlined the cognitive approach to anxiety disorders in general terms, we will now describe the specific cognitive models that are used to understand different anxiety disorders. Each model contains not only the key features outlined above but also certain disorder-specific elements that are crucial for treatment. The models for two common, yet contrasting anxiety disorders—panic disorder and social phobia—are described in detail. Models for other disorders are outlined more briefly. After describing each model, we assess the empirical status of the model.

Panic Disorder

Panic disorder is a severe condition characterized by sudden attacks of physical symptoms such as breathlessness, palpitations, chest pain, and dizziness. Individuals with panic disorder often think they are dying, and for this reason they may initially seek help at an emergency room. Because many of the attacks appear to come "out of the blue," it was initially thought that the central problem might be a neurochemical disturbance. In contrast to this point of view, a number of theorists (Beck et al. 1985; Clark 1986, 1988; Ehlers and Margraf 1989; Margraf et al. 1986; Salkovskis 1988) have suggested that panic might be best understood from a cognitive perspective.

According to the cognitive model of panic disorder,

individuals who experience recurrent panic attacks do so because they have a relatively enduring tendency to interpret certain bodily sensations in a catastrophic fashion. The sensations that are misinterpreted are mainly those involved in normal anxiety responses (e.g., palpitations, breathlessness, dizziness, paresthesias) but also include some other sensations. The catastrophic misinterpretation involves perceiving these sensations as much more dangerous than they really are and, in particular, interpreting the sensations as indicative of *immediately* impending physical or mental disaster—for example, perceiving a slight feeling of breathlessness as evidence of impending cessation of breathing and consequent death, perceiving palpitations as evidence of an impending heart attack, perceiving a pulsing sensation in the forehead as evidence of a brain haemorrhage, or perceiving a shaky feeling as evidence of impending loss of control and insanity. (Clark 1988, p. 149)

The sequence of events that, it is suggested, occurs in panic attacks is shown in Figure 1–1. External stimuli (e.g., a department store for an agoraphobic individual) and internal stimuli (i.e., body sensations, thoughts, images) can both provoke panic attacks. The sequence that culminates in an attack starts with the stimuli being interpreted as a sign of impending danger. This interpretation produces a state of apprehension that is associated with a wide range of bodily sensations. If these anxiety-produced sensations are interpreted in a catastrophic fashion (e.g., impending insanity, death, loss of control), a further increase in apprehension occurs and produces more bodily sensations, leading to a vicious circle that culminates in a panic attack.

Once an individual has developed a tendency to catastrophically interpret bodily sensations, two further processes contribute to the maintenance of panic disorder. First, because the individual is frightened of certain sensations, he or she becomes hypervigilant and repeatedly scans his or her body for cues or warning signs of another attack. This internal focus of attention allows the individual to notice sensations that many other people would not be aware of. Once noticed, these sensations are taken as further evidence of the presence of some serious physical or mental disorder. Second, various "safety behaviors" tend to maintain the individual's negative interpretations (Salkovskis 1988, 1991). For example, an individual with panic disorder who is preoccupied with the idea that he may be suffering from cardiac disease might avoid exercise and believe that this avoidance helps prevent him from having a heart attack. However, because he has no cardiac disease, the real effect of the avoidance would be to prevent him from learning that his symptoms are not dangerous.

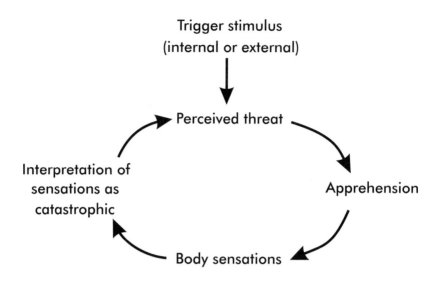

Figure 1–1. Suggested sequence of events in a panic attack.
Source.   Reprinted from Clark DM: "A Cognitive Approach to Panic." *Behaviour Research and Therapy* 24:461–470, 1986. Used with permission.

The cognitive model accounts both for panic attacks that are preceded by elevated anxiety and for panic attacks that are not and, instead, appear out of the blue. For both types of attack, it is argued that the critical event is the misinterpretation of certain bodily sensations. In attacks preceded by heightened anxiety, the sensations are often a consequence of the preceding anxiety, which in turn results from anticipating an attack or some other anxiety-evoking event that is unrelated to panic. In attacks that are not preceded by heightened anxiety, the misinterpreted sensations are initially caused by a different emotional state (anger, excitement, disgust) or by innocuous events such as exercising (breathlessness, palpitations), drinking too much coffee (palpitations), or standing up too quickly after sitting (dizziness). In such attacks, the individual frequently fails to distinguish between the triggering bodily sensations and the subsequent panic and thus perceives the attack as coming out of the blue.

When the cognitive model is being applied to individual patients, it is often useful to distinguish between the first panic attack and the subsequent development of repeated attacks and panic disorder. Community surveys (Brown and Cash 1990; Norton et al. 1986; Margraf and Ehlers 1988; Wilson et al. 1991) indicate that between 7% and 28% of the general adult population will experience an occasional, unexpected panic attack. It is unlikely that there is a single explanation for these relatively common autonomic events. Stressful life events, hormonal changes, illness, caffeine, drugs, and a variety of transient medical conditions could all produce occasional perceived autonomic changes. However, the cognitive theory assumes that individuals go on to develop the rarer condition of repeated panic attacks and panic disorder (approximately 3%–5% of the general population [Wittchen and Essau 1991]) only if they develop a tendency to interpret these perceived autonomic events in a catastrophic fashion. Such a tendency could either be a consequence of learning experiences that predate the first attack (e.g., observing parents panicking or modeling illness-related behavior [Ehlers 1993]) or arise as a consequence of the way the patient, physicians, and significant others respond to the first attack.

Recent experimental studies (see Clark 1996; McNally 1994 for detailed reviews) have provided considerable support for the cognitive theory of panic. In particular, the following has been shown:

1. Panic disorder patients are more likely to interpret bodily sensations in a catastrophic fashion than are other anxiety disorder patients and nonpatients (Clark et al., in press; Harvey et al. 1993; McNally and Foa 1987).
2. Conditions that activate catastrophic interpretations of bodily sensations lead to greater anxiety in panic disorder patients than in control subjects (Clark et al. 1988; Ehlers et al. 1988).
3. Panic attacks induced by pharmacological challenge tests (e.g., inhalation of CO_2 or infusion of sodium lactate) and naturally occurring attacks can both be prevented by reducing panic disorder patients' tendency to interpret bodily sensations in a catastrophic fashion (Clark 1993; Rapee et al. 1986; Salkovskis et al. 1991; Sanderson et al. 1989).
4. Panic disorder patients engage in safety behaviors that prevent disconfirmation of their fears (Salkovskis et al. 1996)
5. Panic disorder patients show enhanced autonomic awareness (Ehlers and Breuer 1992), and this finding predicts the persistence of the disorder in untreated patients (Ehlers 1995).

Social Phobia

Social phobia, like panic disorder, is a common and potentially disabling anxiety disorder. Individuals with social phobia fear, and whenever possible avoid, social and performance situations (e.g., meeting people, eating in restaurants, public speaking, signing checks in public). This fear often leads these individuals to underperform at work or school and makes it difficult for them to make and maintain close relationships. Complications include alcoholism, depression, and, ultimately, suicide.

When in social situations, individuals with social phobia fear that they are in danger of behaving in an inept and unacceptable fashion and that such behavior will have disastrous consequences in terms of loss of status, loss of worth, and rejection. These fears persist despite numerous social interactions in which the individuals do not receive negative feedback from others. Why? Answers to this question are likely to be of considerable help in planning effective treatment. For this reason, a number of authors (Beck et al. 1985; Butler 1985; Hartman 1983; Heimberg and Barlow 1988; Leary 1983; Trower and Gilbert 1989) have proposed cognitive-behavioral models of social phobia that include consideration of this issue. The most recent model, which builds on preceding models, is that proposed by Clark and Wells (1995). The processes that, this model suggests, occur when an individual with social phobia is in a feared social situation are illustrated in Figure 1–2. On the basis of early experience, individuals with social phobia are said to develop a series of assumptions about themselves and social situations. For example, "Unless someone shows that they like me, they dislike me." "Unless I am liked by everyone, I am worthless." "If I show I am anxious, people will think I am odd and will reject me." These assumptions lead them to interpret normal social interactions in a negative way and to view them as signs of danger. For example, if an individual with social phobia is talking to someone at a party and the other person briefly looks out of the window, the social phobic individual may think, I'm being boring. This interpretation makes the patient anxious and triggers two processes that have a crucial role in maintaining the anxiety.

First, a shift in attention takes place. When individuals with social phobia believe they are in danger of negative evaluation by others, they shift their attention to detailed monitoring and observation of themselves. They then use the interoceptive information produced by self-monitoring to infer what other people think of them. In this way, they become trapped in a closed system in which most of the evidence for their fears is self-generated and disconfirmatory information is ignored. Common examples of using interoceptive information to infer how one appears include equating *feeling* out of control with *being* observably out of control and thinking one *looks* as anxious as one *feels*. These inferences can lead to marked distortions. For example, an individual may have a strong shaky feeling and assume that others must be able to see his or her hand shaking violently, when all that can be observed by others is a mild tremor or nothing at all. Often, the negative impression that individuals with social phobia construct of their observable self is best described as a compelling feeling. However, sometimes this impression is also accompanied by images in which the phobic individuals see themselves as if viewed from an observer's perspective. Such images contain visible exaggerations (e.g., shaking hands, humiliated posture).

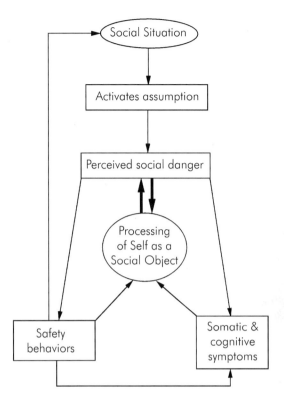

Figure 1–2.   Processes that are hypothesized to occur when an individual with social phobia enters a feared situation.
Source.   Adapted from Clark and Wells 1995.

Second, individuals with social phobia engage in safety behaviors that are intended to improve their social performance but actually prevent disconfirmation of their fears and make them appear more distant to other people. For example, a social phobic individual who is worried that she may say something stupid will try to prevent this by comparing what she is about to say with everything she has said in the last few minutes. This process will make her appear less involved in the conversation and help maintain her belief that she is in danger of being seen as stupid.

Individuals with social phobia also use maladaptive information processing strategies when anticipating entering a feared social situation and after leaving such situations. When anticipating a social interaction, they review in detail what they think might happen. As they start to do this, they become anxious and their thoughts tend to be dominated by recollections of past failures, by negative images of themselves in the situation, and by predictions of poor performance and humiliation. Sometimes these ruminations lead the phobic individual to completely avoid the situation. If this does not happen and the phobic individual enters the situation, he or she is likely to already be in a self-focused processing mode, expect failure, and be less likely to notice any signs of being accepted by other people.

After leaving a social event, individuals with social phobia often go over the event in their mind. During this "postmortem," the individual's anxious feelings and negative self-perceptions are likely to figure particularly prominently because they were processed in detail while the individual was in the situation and hence they have been strongly encoded in memory. The unfortunate consequence of this is that the individual's review is likely to be dominated by his or her negative self-perception, and the interaction is likely to be seen as much more negative than it really was.

Research on patients with social phobia and highly socially anxious individuals has provided support for several key aspects of Clark and Wells's model. In particular, it has been shown that

1. Social phobic patients underestimate their social performance (Rapee and Lim 1992; Stopa and Clark 1993) and overestimate how anxious they appear to others (Bruch et al. 1989; McEwan and Devins 1983).
2. Highly socially anxious individuals, compared with individuals with low levels of social anxiety, have poorer memory for the details of social interactions (Daly et al. 1989; Hope et al. 1990; Kimble and Zehr 1982).
3. Among highly socially anxious individuals, overestimation of how anxious they think they appear to others is strongly correlated with how anxious they feel (W. Mansell, D. M. Clark, "How Do I Appear to Others? Biased Processing of the Observable Self in Social Anxiety," manuscript submitted for publication 1996).
4. When anticipating a social interaction, highly socially anxious individuals show a relative bias toward recall of negative information about the way they appear to others (W. Mansell, D. M. Clark, "How Do I Appear to Others? Biased Processing of the Observable Self in Social Anxiety," manuscript submitted for publication 1996).
5. Social phobic patients who are encouraged to drop their safety behaviors during a social interaction show greater improvements in negative beliefs and anxiety during a subsequent behavior test than social phobic patients who are asked to continue using their normal safety behaviors (Wells et al. 1995).

Hypochondriasis

Individuals with primary hypochondriasis persistently believe they have a physical illness despite medical reassurance that they are well.

Warwick and Salkovskis (1989, 1990) have outlined a cognitive model of the development and maintenance of this disabling condition. It is suggested that previous learning experiences (e.g., family sayings, stories in the media, or direct experience of medical mismanagement) lead potential patients to develop a series of negative beliefs about symptoms, diagnosis, and the medical profession. Examples are "Bodily changes are usually a sign of serious illness," "If medication doesn't take away a pain, it is a serious disease," "If a doctor sends you for tests, she is convinced there is something wrong," and "Tests are the only way to rule out a serious illness." These assumptions lie dormant and have no major effect on the potential patient until a critical incident occurs. For example, an individual has been overworking and experiences unfamilar symptoms. The assumptions lead the individual to interpret the new symptoms as signs of a serious illness. A variety of processes then contribute to the maintenance of this negative interpretation. First, as in panic, patients become hypervigilant for symptoms and as a consequence notice symptoms of which they were not previously aware. Second, anxiety about health produces physiological changes that patients take as further signs of disease. For example, a fast pulse may be taken as a sign of progressive cardiac disease. Third, checking behaviors become prominent. For example, a patient who was worried he might have throat cancer frequently checked that his throat was "clear" by intentionally and repeatedly swallowing when there was nothing in his mouth. He erroneously interpreted the fact that it was difficult to swallow under these circumstances as evidence that there was something wrong with his throat. Fourth, patients repeatedly seek reassurance that they are well from friends and doctors. However, their assumptions ("Doctors often miss serious illness" or "It is impossible to know with absolute certainty that one is not ill") mean that the responses they get from others rarely seem convincing. Thus, the act of seeking reassurance simply maintains their somatic preoccupation. Finally, patients seem to operate a confirmatory bias under which information that could be viewed as consistent with their beliefs is given precedence, while information inconsistent with the idea they have a serious disease is ignored.

Research studies have provided support for several aspects of Warwick and Salkovskis's model, but further investigations are required. To date, hypochondriacal patients have been shown 1) to have an increased ability to detect normal somatic changes (Tyrer et al. 1980); 2) to differ from other anxiety disorder patients and nonpatient control subjects in their beliefs about symptoms, diagnosis, and the medical profession (Salkovskis and Clark 1993); and 3) to differ from panic disorder patients in misinterpreting a wider range of signs and symptoms (panic disorder patients' misinterpretations mainly focus on autonomic symptoms) and in interpreting autonomic symptoms as signs of more delayed catastrophe, such as developing heart disease rather than currently having a heart attack (Salkovskis and Clark 1993).

Obsessive-Compulsive Disorder

The cognitive approach to understanding obsessive-compulsive disorder (OCD) takes as its starting point Rachman and De Silva's (1978) finding that healthy subjects and obsessive-compulsive patients cannot be distinguished in terms of the content of their intrusive thoughts, but that obsessive-compulsive patients find the thoughts more distressing and have more of them. Salkovskis (1985) proposed a cognitive model that builds on this finding. He argued that what is abnormal in OCD is not the intrusive thoughts themselves, but rather the individuals' interpretations of these thoughts. In particular, he proposed that obsessional individuals interpret the occurrence and content of their intrusive thoughts as "an indication that they might be responsible for harm to themselves or others unless they take action to prevent it" (Salkovskis and Kirk 1996, p. 185). This interpretation is said to be responsible for the discomfort and anxiety experienced when the intrusive thought occurs. It also motivates two types of behavior that have the effect of maintaining the disorder. First, the individual attempts to *neutralize* the intrusive thought, image, or impulse by performing an overt or covert act that is intended to prevent harm from occurring. Examples are hand washing in compulsive washers, checking electrical outlets in obsessional checkers, and "putting right" thoughts in compulsive ruminators. As harm is not in fact likely to follow the occurrence of an intrusive thought, the main function of these neutralizing behaviors is to prevent the individual from discovering this point. Second, because of the meaning of intrusive thoughts, the obsessive-compulsive individual tries to supress such thoughts, and it is hypothesized that attempts at suppression have the paradoxical effect of increasing the frequency of intrusive thoughts.

Research studies have provided support for the hypothesis that perceived responsibility for the consequences of having an intrusive thought plays a role in OCD. Salkovskis and Kirk (1996) reported that obsessive-compulsive patients scored higher than both other anxiety disorder patients and nonpatients on a measure of perceived responsibility for the consequences of intrusive thoughts. Lopatka and Rachman (1995) experimentally manipulated perceived responsibilty and found that obsessive-compulsive patients' discomfort and urge to check declined when responsibilty was reduced. The hypothesis that neutralizing maintains OCD was supported by Foa and co-workers (1984), who found that repeatedly provoking obsessions and preventing patients from compulsive checking/washing produced greater improvements in OCD than repeated provocation alone. No studies have investigated the effects of thought suppression in obsessional patients. However, Trinder and Salkovskis (1994), in a nonclinical study of naturally occurring intrusive thoughts, found that suppression produced an increase in thought frequency.

Generalized Anxiety Disorder

Currently, there is no generally agreed-on cognitive model of generalized anxiety disorder (GAD). This is partly because the definition of GAD has changed significantly in recent years. When first introduced in DSM-III in 1980 (American Psychiatric Association 1980), GAD was a residual category: it was the diagnosis for individuals with symptoms that were regarded as manifestations of anxiety but that did not meet the diagnostic criteria for any other anxiety disorder. It was not until 1987 and the advent of DSM-III-R (American Psychiatric Association 1987) that GAD acquired its own specific defining feature: worry about several different life circumstances. This change was retained in DSM-IV (American Psychiatric Association 1994), and most researchers now agree that the key feature of GAD is difficulty controlling worry about a variety of topics (Moras et al. 1996).

One of the first attempts to explain the diffuse nature of worries in GAD was the model outlined by Beck and colleagues (1985). This model proposed that individuals are anxious about many topics because their beliefs about themselves and the world make them prone to interpret a wide range of situations or circumstances in a threatening fashion. The beliefs, or dysfunctional assumptions, were seen as highly varied. However, most were assumed to revolve around issues of acceptance, competence, responsibility, and control, as well as the symptoms of anxiety. In a series of elegant experiments, Mathews and colleagues (see Mathews 1990 for a review) showed that GAD patients have an information-processing bias that serves to maintain high levels of vigilance for personal danger. The bias involves selectively attending to threatening information and interpreting a wide range of ambiguous events in a threatening fashion. Borkovec and colleagues (see Borkovec 1994 for a review) reported a series of experiments that showed that when GAD patients worry, they have less imagery and more verbal thought than control subjects. Imagery elicited more physiological arousal, so it was suggested that in patients with GAD, worry might also serve as a form of cognitive avoidance. That is, worrying is a way of thinking about a distressing topic without considering the worst aspects of it in detail. If this is what GAD patients are doing, the persistence of their worries becomes more understandable. A behavioral equivalent of this type of avoidance is procrastination, which also appears to be particularly common in GAD (Borkovec 1994).

More recently, Wells (1995) proposed a meta-cognitive model of

GAD. This model focuses less on the specific topics that GAD patients worry about and more on patients' appraisal of worry itself, which in the model is viewed as the main problem. In particular, it is suggested that GAD patients hold certain positive and negative beliefs about worry that would have the effect of making worry more likely and more protracted. The positive beliefs concern the idea that worrying is the best way of avoiding future catastrophes. For example, "If I worry, I will be prepared to deal with problems in the future." Borkovec and Roemer (1995) found that GAD patients are more likely to think that worry is an effective problem-solving method than are individuals without GAD. An individual who holds this belief should be more likely to worry.

The negative beliefs center on themes of mental or physical harm resulting from worry and general beliefs about the uncontrollability of intrusive thoughts. Examples are "Worrying will send me crazy or damage my health"; "I am losing control"; and "Not being able to control my thoughts is a sign of weakness." These beliefs lead individuals with GAD to worry about their worry and to attempt to suppress the worrying thoughts once they have started. Unfortunately, active attempts at suppression are likely to transiently increase the frequency of the worrying thoughts (Clark et al. 1991; Trinder and Salkovskis 1994; Wegner 1989), reinforcing patients' beliefs in the uncontrollability and dangers of worrying. Negative beliefs about worrying will also lead patients to try to avoid stimuli that would normally trigger worry. The problem with this strategy is that patients are prevented from discovering that worry is controllable and harmless.

Posttraumatic Stress Disorder

Several authors (Creamer et al. 1992; Ehlers and Steil 1995; Foa and Riggs 1993; Foa et al. 1989; Janoff-Bulman 1985) have proposed cognitive models of the development and maintenance of posttraumatic stress disorder (PTSD). Although differing in detail, these models have in common the assumption that PTSD is persistent if individuals appraise the trauma and/or its sequelae in a way that leads to an ongoing sense of threat, as opposed to being able to see the event as an isolated incident from the past. Janoff-Bulman (1985) focuses on the way in which a traumatic event might shatter previously positive views that individuals held about themselves and their world. Foa and Riggs (1993) also highlight the shattering of positive views but, in addition, point out that in some cases of persistent PTSD, the traumatic event may confirm preexisting negative beliefs about oneself consistent with these suggestions. Frazier and Schauben (1994) found that postrape symptomatology was postively associated with blaming one's actions and with blaming aspects of one's personality. Keane and colleagues

(1985) also found that PTSD was particularly severe in Vietnam War veterans who perceived other people to have failed to react in a positive or supportive manner. Finally, Foa and Riggs (1993) and Ehlers and Steil (1995) have focused on individuals' appraisal of PTSD symptoms during the first few weeks after a trauma. For example, Ehlers and Steil (1995) proposed that negative interpretations of intrusive recollections that most people experience in the immediate aftermath of a traumatic event will increase the likelihood that an individual will engage in strategies to control the intrusions. These strategies would then act to maintain or even exacerbate the intrusions. Ehlers and Steil reported findings from two studies with victims of road traffic accidents that are consistent with this hypothesis.

Links Between Cognitive and Biological Processes

Cognitive models of anxiety disorders are sometimes presented as incompatible with biological models of pathophysiology. This is unfortunate. There are many ways in which cognitive and biological processes are likely to interact in the development and maintenance of anxiety disorders. Panic disorder is a good example. Cognitive theory claims that misinterpretation of body sensations is a necessary condition for the development of panic disorder, but it seems likely that biological factors may also play a role in triggering attacks. For example, some individuals appear to have more labile or reactive autonomic nervous systems than do others. As we tend to notice bodily sensations when there is a change in autonomic processes, such individuals are likely to experience more sensations that could be misinterpreted. Consistent with this suggestion, Anastasiades and co-workers (1990) found that panic disorder patients showed more cardiac variabilty than control subjects even when not panicking.

Treatment Procedures

In the cognitive therapy of anxiety disorders, the aim is to help patients to identify and modify the negative thoughts that accompany anxious episodes and the beliefs on which these thoughts are based. As we have seen, each anxiety disorder is characterized by a distinctinve set of negative thoughts. Although there is some overlap in the processes involved in maintaining these thoughts, the detailed way in which cognitive and behavioral processes interact to maintain anxiety differs from disorder to disorder. For this reason, specialized forms of cognitive therapy have been developed for each anxiety disorder. In this section, we describe in detail specialized forms of CT for the treatment of panic disorder and social phobia. For other anxiety disorders, a briefer description of the distinctive features of therapy is given, along with sources that provide more detailed descriptions for the interested reader. Many psychological treatments for anxiety disorders include a component of direct modification of negative thinking. We consider a treatment to be a form of CT only if its main aim is the explicit identification and modification of distorted thinking. Most treatments that have this aim use a complex mixture of cognitive and behavioral procedures to change thinking, as will be evident from the descriptions below.

Panic Disorder

Clark, Salkovskis, Beck, and colleagues have devised a treatment for panic disorder that is based on the cognitive model of panic. Treatment starts by reviewing with the patient a recent panic attack and identifying the main sensations and the negative thoughts associated with the sensations. Careful questioning about the sequence of events is used to derive an individual version of the panic vicious circle. An example of such a sequence is presented in Figure 1–3. Once therapist and patient agree that the panic attacks involve an interaction between bodily

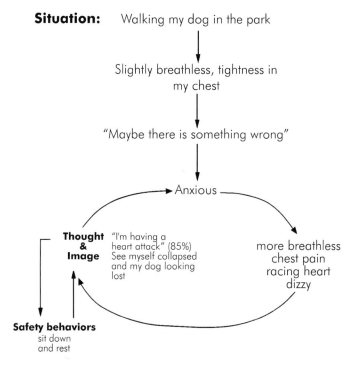

Figure 1–3. A specific panic attack.

sensations and negative thoughts about the sensations, therapy focuses on teaching the patient to challenge his or her misinterpretations of the sensations.

Identification of the triggers of an attack.   Many patients interpret the unexpected nature of some of their panic attacks as an indication that they are suffering from cardiac disease or some other physical abnormality. For these patients, it is often helpful to identify the triggers of the unexpected attacks. Diary records and discussion usually reveal that the trigger of their unexpected attacks is a slight bodily change caused by a different emotional state (e.g., excitement, anger, or disgust) or by some innocuous event, such as exercise (breathlessness or palpitations), suddenly standing up after sitting (dizziness), rapid eye movement (i.e., the world seems to move), or drinking too much coffee (palpitations).

Cognitive procedures.   One of the most useful cognitive procedures involves helping patients to understand the significance of past events that are inconsistent with their negative beliefs. For example, the telephone may have rung while a patient was sitting at home experiencing palpitations, breathlessness, and a tight chest and thinking he or she was having a heart attack. Answering the telephone momentarily distracted the patient from the negative thoughts, and, as a consequence, the physical symptoms and panic ceased. Questions such as "Do you think answering the telephone is a good treatment for heart attacks?" and "If answering the telephone isn't stopping a heart attack, what is it doing?" can be used to help the patient see the significance of this observation.

Education about the nature of anxiety can also be helpful, especially if it is tailored to patients' idiosyncratic concerns. For example, patients who are concerned that they might faint during a panic attack are often helped by being told that blood pressure increases during a panic attack but that fainting is associated with a drop in blood pressure (see Clark 1989, p. 76, for an illustrative transcript). Similarly, patients who report predominantly left-sided pain and take this as evidence of a cardiac abnormality often benefit from being shown the results of an investigation (Beunderman et al. 1988) that compared the location of chest pain in patients referred to a cardiology clinic. Predominantly left-sided pain was more characteristic of anxious patients *without* cardiac abnormalities than of patients who had experienced myocardial infarctions or had angina pectoris.

Images of feared outcomes (e.g., fainting, dying, or going mad) often accompany panic attacks. Usually, these images can be treated as equivalent to a negative thought (e.g., "I'm about to faint") and dealt with in the same way. However, it is sometimes necessary to directly modify the image by transforming it into a less threatening and more realistic image. It is particularly likely that such an approach will be needed when the intrusive image is repetitive and stereotyped. The images that accompany a panic attack invariably stop at the worst moment. Encouraging the patient to visualize what in reality would happen next can therefore be helpful. For example, a patient who saw herself collapsed on the floor after fainting was encouraged to visualize slowly coming round, getting to her feet, and leaving.

Behavioral experiments. Most of the behavioral experiments used with panic disorder patients fall into one of two categories: 1) inducing feared sensations to demonstrate possible innocuous causes of the patients' symptoms, and 2) stopping safety behaviors to help patients disconfirm their negative beliefs about the consequences of the sensations. Some of the most commonly used procedures for inducing feared sensations include focusing attention on the body, reading and dwelling on pairs of words representing feared sensations and catastrophes (e.g., palpitations–dying, breathless–suffocate, numbness–stroke, racing thoughts–insanity), and reproducing the way patients breathe in a panic attack, if it seems likely that they normally overbreathe. For patients who interpret the dizziness that accompanies attacks as a sign that they might faint, the maneuver of dropping safety behaviors may involve inducing dizziness (by entering a feared situation and/or overbreathing) and then not holding on to a solid object or tensing one's legs. For patients who are concerned that they might have something wrong with their heart and who avoid exercise because of this concern, the safety behaviors maneuver might involve encouraging the patient to exercise, particularly when feared sensations are present. Usually, this maneuver would first be practiced in a therapy session and then assigned as homework.

Social Phobia

Several cognitive-behavioral treatment programs have been developed for social phobia. All involve identifying and challenging negative social-evaluative thoughts and exposing patients to feared and avoided social situations. The exact details of treatment vary from program to program. For illustrative purposes, we outline the CT program that is currently in use in Oxford and is based on the Clark and Wells's (1995) model described earlier in this chapter.

Treatment starts by reviewing recent episodes of social anxiety. As in the treatment of panic, careful questioning is used to develop an individual version of the cognitive model. An example of this process is presented in Figure 1–4. The model should include the patient's safety behaviors and a description of the interoceptive information that the patient is aware of when he or she is self-focused. This information typically includes bodily sensations and a felt sense of how the person might appear to others. Sometimes the felt sense is also accompanied by an image in which the patient sees himself or herself as if viewed from an observer's perspective. The image contains visible (or audible) distortions that are derived from the interoceptive cues. For example, the patient shown in Figure 1–4 felt that the muscles around her mouth tensed when she was the focus of attention. This feeling was transformed in the image into a contorted mouth, which she thought everyone must be able to see. Similarly, a warm forehead and a slight sweating sensation can be transformed into a picture of rivulets of sweat running down the forehead.

Safety behaviors experiment. Once patient and therapist have agreed on a working version of the cognitive model, key elements of the model are manipulated. We found that changing safety behaviors is often the best way to start. During a treatment session, patients are asked to role-play a feared social interaction under two conditions. In one condition, they are asked to use all their normal safety behaviors. In the other condition, they are asked to drop their safety behaviors and focus attention on the other person(s), rather than on themselves. After the role-plays, patients rate how anxious they felt, how anxious they thought they appeared, and how well they thought they per-

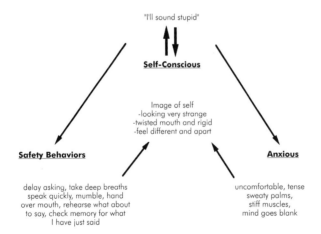

Figure 1–4. Elements of the cognitive model for an individual with social phobia.
Source. Reprinted from Clark DM: "Panic Disorder and Social Phobia," in *The Science and Practice of Cognitive-Behaviour Therapy.* Edited by Clark DM, Fairburn CG. Oxford, UK, Oxford University Press, 1996. Copyright 1996, Oxford University Press. Used with permission.

formed. By comparing these ratings, several points can be established. First, to patients' considerable surprise, the habitual safety behaviors often make the patient feel *more* anxious, not less anxious. Second, ratings of how anxious patients think they appear and how well they think they performed closely follow the ratings of how they felt, suggesting that they are using their feelings to infer how they appear to others.

Video and audio feedback. Once it is established that patients are using interoceptive cues to infer how they appear to others, the next step is to obtain realistic information about how they actually appear. One way of doing this is to ask the actors in the safety behaviors experiment to give the patient feedback. The feedback usually indicates that the patient appeared less anxious than he or she estimated, again establishing that feelings are not a good indicator of how one appears. Video and audio feedback are another particularly good way of making this point. We routinely videotape the safety behaviors experiment and show the patient the video during the next session. Before viewing the video, the patients are asked to visualize how they think they will appear. This constructed image is then compared with how they actually appear. The actual appearance is invariably better than patients expect.

To maximize the amount of cognitive change produced by each treatment session, we audiotape sessions and ask patients to listen to the tape as part of their homework. In this way they can consolidate and develop further the answers to their negative thoughts that were identified in the session. The audio record also gives patients invaluable information about how they sound, and this again corrects their distorted impressions. For example, a professional woman talked quietly in meetings. She did this so that she would not attract attention. The consequence was that other people had to strain to hear what she was saying and hence stared at her more. It was agreed that she would experiment with speaking louder in meetings. While she was practicing this in the session, it became evident that she overestimated the volume of her own voice, thinking she was shouting when she was not. This was corrected by playing back the audiotape and comparing the volume of the patient's "shout" with the therapist's normal speech. To the patient's surprise, her "shout" was quieter than the therapist's normal voice. Further discussion revealed a probable basis for the misperception. Because the patient normally spoke very quietly, speaking up initially seemed to require considerable effort, and this was mistaken for volume.

At this point in therapy, homework assignments typically involve dropping safety behaviors and shifting to an external focus of attention during social interactions. The rationale for this maneuver is that the evidence patients normally use to infer how they appear to others (i.e., the contents of their self-awareness) is inaccurate and thus it is necessary to focus more on the interaction and other people's responses to obtain a more accurate impression of how one appears.

Testing of predictions about negative evaluation by others. Normal social interactions provide only limited opportunities to test patients' distorted beliefs about the consequences of behaving in ways that they perceive as inept. This problem can be partly overcome by asking patients to intentionally perform behaviors that they falsely believe will lead to negative evaluation. For example, a secretary feared that if she spilt her drink in a local bar, people she knew would think that she was an alcoholic and would reject her. The first step in challenging this belief was to ask her how she thought the other people would react if they thought spilling her drink meant she was an alcoholic. She said that they would stare at her and start whispering. This was then tested by intentionally spilling a drink in a conspicuous fashion. To her amazement no one showed interest, except the barman, who briefly glanced in her direction but hardly paused in his conversation. Similarly, patients can be asked to experiment with introducing boring topics into conversations, pausing while speaking, stammering, or expressing opinions that they know others will disagree with. Surveys are another useful way of collecting information about how others respond. For example, a social phobic individual who stuttered and was concerned other people would think she was stupid was reassured by a survey in which 15 people were asked what they thought of someone who stutters. To her surprise, nobody thought it was a sign of stupidity, and respondents provided a wide range of nonthreatening explanations for why someone might stutter.

Dealing with the postmortem. Because normal social interactions rarely provide patients with unambiguous feedback on how well they have performed and how others have perceived them, individuals with social phobia often conduct a "postmortem" after a social interaction. In the postmortem, the social phobic individual's anxious feelings and negative self-perceptions figure particularly prominently, and so the postmortem provides further, incorrect evidence of social failure. In cognitive therapy, this point is established with the patient and then the postmortem is banned.

Modification of assumptions. The assumptions that lead social phobic individuals to interpret social situations in a threatening fashion can be modified by the use of Socratic questioning. For example, the assumption "If someone doesn't like me, it means I am inadequate" can be modified by questions such as "How do you know that someone does not like you?"; "Are there any reasons why someone might not respond well to you other than your adequacy, for example, their mood, your reminding them of someone else, their mind being elsewhere, etc.?"; "Can you think of any examples of where someone was not liked yet he or she was not inadequate, for example, Jesus and the Pharisees?"; "If one person doesn't like you and another does, who is right?"; and "If one person doesn't like you, does that write you off as a person?"

Hypochondriasis

Like individuals with panic disorder, individuals with hypochondriasis misinterpret bodily sensations as signs of severe illness. However, the range of signs and symptoms misinterpreted by hypchondriacal individuals is broader, the time course of the feared catastrophe tends to be longer, checking and reassurance seeking are more prominent, and dysfunctional beliefs about the medical profession are also present.

Salkovskis, Warwick, and colleagues (Salkovskis 1989; Salkovskis and Bass 1996; Salkovskis and Warwick 1986; Warwick and Salkovskis 1989) have devised a cognitive therapy program that draws on the procedures used for panic disorder but is specifically tailored to deal with hypochondriasis. First, because many hypochondriacal patients are skeptical about the relevance of psychological treatment, particular emphasis is placed on engaging patients in therapy. This is done not by reiterating the fact that medical tests have proved negative, but by using careful assessment and monitoring to identify some positive evidence that psychological factors may play a role in patients' complaints. Second, the role that symptom checking and reassurance seeking plays in maintaining somatic preoccupation is identified, and attempts are made to cut down, and ideally eliminate, both processes. At this point, patients are often surprised to find that their checking was causing some of the symptoms they took as evidence of a physical disease. For example, a patient who was concerned that she might have bowel cancer discovered that the blood she saw in her feces was a consequence of anal lacerations caused by frequent rubbing with toilet paper in order to detect bloody discharges. Third, dysfunctional assumptions about bodily symptoms and medical diagnostic procedures are identified and challenged.

Obsessive-Compulsive Disorder

The CT approach to the treatment of OCD focuses on identifying and modifying obsessional patients' appraisals of their obsessional thoughts, images, and impulses and on reversing maintaining factors. One of the main maintaining factors is neutralization. For this reason, the behavioral procedures of exposure and response prevention figure prominently. In addition, cognitive procedures are used to directly challenge patients' beliefs about the consequences of their obsessions. For example, some patients believe that having a thought about something can make it happen. This belief can be treated as a general hypothesis, and the therapist can get the patient to entertain a series of scenarios unrelated to his or her obsessions to examine whether it is true. For example, "If you close your eyes and try very hard to imagine that you are rich, do you have more money in your bank account? If imagining does not work in this case, why should it work for obsessional thoughts?" Another common procedure is to ask patients to keep records of the frequency of obsessional intrusions on days when they make an effort to suppress the intrusions and on days when, for the sake of experiment, they do not. Patients usually discover from these recordings that their normal strategy of suppression increases intrusions. Readers interested in a fuller account of treatment are referred to Salkovskis and Kirk (1996).

Generalized Anxiety Disorder

Cognitive-behavioral therapy for GAD usually involves helping patients to challenge the negative content of their worries by their writing down their thoughts and looking at the evidence for and against them. For many of the patients' real-life concerns, standard problem-solving strategies are also helpful. Patients are also made more aware of the way in which avoidance of making decisions and other forms of procrastination maintain the worry cycle. Strategies such as Borkovec and co-workers' (1983) stimulus control procedure, in which patients agree to postpone worrying until a particular agreed-on time of day, are useful for helping patients to get distance from their worries. Often, they find that when the "worry period" arrives, the concerns seem much less pressing. In addition to these commonly used procedures, Wells's (1995) recently proposed meta-cognitive model of GAD suggests that focusing on patients' beliefs about worry itself is likely to be particularly helpful. Patients would first be socialized in a model in which worry about worry and attempts to control their thoughts are seen as the main reasons for the persistence of their anxiety. They would then be encouraged to abandon control and conduct behavioral experiments to challenge negative beliefs about worry. For example, patients who are concerned that they might lose mental control by worrying are encouraged to test this out by trying to worry more. In the later stages of treatment, positive beliefs about worry are also tackled. Readers interested in further details of this approach are referred to Wells 1995, in press; Wells and Butler 1996.

Posttraumatic Stress Disorder

The most commonly used psychological treatment for PTSD is the behavior therapy technique of exposure, which involves repeated imaginal reliving of the event and reversing avoidance of situations that serve as reminders of the event. This intervention is based on the assumption that avoidance of thinking about the event normally prevents its assimilation. Unfortunately, although exposure has been shown to be an effective treatment (Foa et al. 1991), a sizeable proportion of patients continue to have residual PTSD symptomatology. Cognitive therapists argue that this is because exposure alone fails to address some of the key cognitive variables involved in maintaining PTSD. For this reason, CT adds to exposure a detailed assessment of cognitive distortions in the way patients think about how they behaved during the event, the implications of the event for their present and future, the way others responded after the event, and the patients' interpretation of the symptoms that most people experience shortly after a traumatic event. When distortions are evident and they appear to be associated with strong affect, CT techniques are used to help patients challenge their thoughts and beliefs.

Outcome Studies

Panic Disorder

Controlled trials of the full CT program. Five controlled trials have investigated the effectiveness of the full CT program outlined above in panic disorder patients. Beck and co-workers (1992) allocated panic disorder patients to 12 weeks of CT or 8 weeks of supportive therapy. When assessed at comparable time points (4 and 8 weeks), patients given CT had improved significantly more than those given supportive therapy, a finding which indicates that the effectiveness of CT is not entirely attributable to nonspecific therapy factors. In addition, the gains achieved in treatment were maintained at 1-year follow-up.

Clark and co-workers (1994) compared CT with an alternative active psychological treatment and with a pharmacological intervention. Panic disorder patients were randomly allocated to CT, applied relaxation, imipramine (mean dose = 233 mg/day), or a 3-month waiting list followed by allocation to treatment. During treatment, patients had up to 12 sessions in the first 3 months and up to 3 booster sessions in the next 3 months. Imipramine was gradually withdrawn after 6 months. All treatments included homework assignments involving self-exposure to feared situations. Comparisons with the waiting-list group showed that all three treatments were more effective than the waiting-list condition. Comparisons between treatments showed that at 3 months, CT was superior to both applied relaxation and imipramine. Between 3 and 6 months, imipramine-treated patients continued to improve, whereas those who had received CT or applied relaxation showed little change. As a consequence, at 6 months, CT did not differ from imipramine, and both were superior to applied relaxation. Imipramine was gradually withdrawn after the 6-month assessment. Between 6 and 15 months, 40% of imipramine patients relapsed, compared with only 5% of CT patients. At 15 months, CT was again superior to both applied relaxation and imipramine.

Öst, the originator of applied relaxation, has also compared CT and applied relaxation (Öst and Westling 1995). CT and applied relaxation were both associated with substantial improvements. In the initial report (Öst and Westling 1995), there were no significant differences between the treatments. However, Öst (personal communication, December 1995) has pointed out that each of the four therapists' initial training cases in CT had been included in the analysis. Only 1 of the 4 training case patients (25%) became free of panic, but 13 of the 15 subsequent CT patients (87%) became panic free and achieved high endstate function at the end of treatment. When the data are reanalyzed excluding the four CT training cases, a significant difference is found between CT and applied relaxation in terms of the percentage of patients achieving high end-state function at post-treatment (87% [13/15] for CT vs. 47% [8/17] for applied relaxation), but the two treatments do not differ significantly in the percentage of patients who became panic free. For both treatments, the gains made during therapy were maintained at the 1-year follow-up.

Arntz and van den Hout (1996) have recently reported an independent evaluation of CT and applied relaxation. Their group was not involved in the development of either treatment. Therapists were given specialist training in CT from Clark and Salkovskis and specialist training in applied relaxation from Öst. A significantly greater proportion of CT patients achieved panic-free status at the end of treatment, and this difference was maintained at follow-up.

Finally, Margraf and Schneider (1991) conducted a component analysis of CT. The full cognitive treatment (which combined cognitive and behavioral procedures) was compared with an intervention involving cognitive procedures alone and an intervention involving situational and interoceptive exposure without explicit cognitive restructuring. Comparison with a waiting-list control group indicated that all three treatments were highly effective. On most measures, there were no significant differences, though combined treatment was superior to exposure on an intention-to-treat analysis of the percentage of patients who became panic free. In all three groups, treatment gains were fully maintained at 1-year follow-up. Change in panic-related cognitions was a significant predictor of immediate improvement in all three treatments, suggesting that the cognitive and the behavioral procedures both have their effects through the common mechanism of cognitive change.

Results from the five trials reviewed above are summarized in Table 1–1. In each trial the therapists were given some training by the Oxford group. Taken together, the trials indicate that properly conducted CT is a highly effective treatment for panic disorder, with intention-to-treat analyses indicating that 74%–94% of patients become panic free and that these gains are maintained at follow-up. It is also clear that the effects of the treatment are not entirely due to nonspecific therapy factors, as three studies (Arntz and van den Hout 1996; Beck et al. 1992; Clark et al. 1994) found cognitive therapy to be superior to an equally credible alternative psychological treatment. One study (Clark et al. 1994) compared CT with imipramine in adequate dose. CT was superior to imipramine early in treatment and again at 1-year follow-up. Finally, CT seems to travel well, as the results obtained with CT are remarkably consistent across five countries (England, Germany, The Netherlands, Sweden, and United States).

Briefer forms of the CT program.   The excellent results obtained with the full CT package have encouraged researchers to investigate whether it might be possible to obtain similar results with a briefer form of the treatment. If so, more patients could potentially benefit from the treatment. The studies of full treatment described above had a total of 12–16 sessions. The first group to report an evaluation of a briefer version was Black, Wesner, Bowers, and Gabel (1993). These investigators devised their own brief (8-session) version of cognitive therapy that included additional psychological procedures also specifically devised by the investigators. Panic disorder patients were randomly allocated to brief CT, fluvoxamine, or placebo medication. Main assessments were at pretreatment and 8 weeks later. No follow-up was reported. Response to fluvoxamine was superior to the response to brief cognitive therapy on a number of measures in a completers analysis. However, the unusually high dropout rate[1] (40% for brief CT compared with between 0% and 5% in the studies of full CT reviewed above) suggests that the investigators' modifications affected the treatment's acceptability.

Clark and associates (1995) have recently reported a more successful attempt to produce a brief version of CT. The total number of sessions

---

[1]The dropout rate reported here is slightly higher (40% vs. 36%) than that given in the original paper, which contains a typographic error (D. W. Black, personal communication, October 1994).

Table 1–1. Controlled trials of (full) cognitive therapy for panic disorder: intention-to-treat analyses

| Study | Treatments | Percentage (number) of patients panic-free | |
		Post-treatment	Follow-up
Beck et al. (1992)	CT	94 (16/17)	77 (13/17)[a]
	ST	25 (4/16)[b]	—
Clark et al. (1994)	CT	86 (18/21)	76 (16/21)[c]
	AR	48 (10/21)	43 (9/21)[c]
	IMIP	52 (11/21)	48 (10/21)[c]
	WL	7 (1/16)	—
Öst and Westling (1995)[d]	CT	74 (14/19)	89 (17/19)[c]
	AR	58 (11/19)	74 (14/19)[c]
Arntz and van den Hout (1996)	CT	78 (14/18)	78 (14/18)
	AR	47 (9/19)	47 (9/19)
	WL	28 (5/18)	—
Margraf and Schneider (1991)	Combined CT	91 (20/22)[e]	—
	Pure cognitive	73 (16/22)[e]	—
	Pure EXP	52 (11/21)[e]	—
	WL	5 (1/20)	—
Total across all studies for CT		85 (82/97)	80 (60/75)

Note. Intention-to-treat analysis includes dropouts as well as completers. Dropouts are coded as still panicking. CT = cognitive therapy; ST = supportive therapy; AR = applied relaxation; IMIP = imipramine; EXP = interoceptive and situational exposure; WL = waiting list.
[a]One-year follow-up.
[b]At 8 weeks, which is the end of supportive therapy. At this time 71% of CT patients were panic free.
[c]Percentage of patients who were panic free at follow-up and who received no additional treatment during the follow-up period.
[d]The figures for CT are conservative because they include the therapists' four training cases.
[e]Four-week follow-up.
Source. Reprinted from Clark DM: "Panic Disorder: From Theory to Therapy," in *Frontiers of Cognitive Therapy: The State of the Art and Beyond.* Edited by Salkovskis PM. New York, Guilford, 1996. Copyright 1996, Guilford Press. Used with permission.

was reduced to seven by devising a series of self-study modules covering the main stages in therapy. Patients read the self-study modules and completed the homework outlined in the modules before discussing an area with their therapist. In this way, the therapist was able to devote more attention to misunderstandings and problems. Panic disorder patients were randomly allocated to brief CT, full CT, or waiting list. Brief and full CT were both superior to no treatment and did not differ from each other in efficacy. In addition, the substantial improvement observed with both treatments was as large as that obtained in the Oxford group's previous trial (Clark et al. 1994), in which the same selection criteria were used.

Barlow's panic control treatment. At the same time that CT for panic was being developed, Barlow and colleagues were independently developing another cognitive-behavioral therapy (CBT), *panic control treatment* (PCT), which also focuses on patients' fears of bodily sensations. Although differing in some respects, CT and PCT share many common procedures. Five studies have investigated the effectiveness of PCT. As one might expect from the similarity in procedures, these studies have established that it is also a highly effective treatment for panic disorder. Barlow and co-workers (1989) compared PCT with another cognitive treatment, with progressive muscle relaxation, and with a waiting-list control. Both cognitive treatments were consistently superior to the waiting-list condition and were more effective than relaxation at reducing panic frequency. Klosko and co-workers (1990) compared PCT with alprazolam, placebo, and a waiting-list control. PCT was superior to alprazolam, placebo, and the waiting-list control.[2] The percentages of patients who became panic free on alprazolam and placebo were similar to those found in the Cross-National Collaborative Panic Study (1992), but alprazolam was not significantly different from placebo, probably because of the very small sample size in the latter condition.

Shear and co-workers (1994) compared PCT with a specially devised nonprescriptive treatment. PCT appeared to be slightly less successful than in the preceding two studies and did not differ significantly from nonprescriptive treatment. In discussing the study, the authors pointed out that PCT may not have been delivered optimally, as therapist adherence ratings were lower than expected. An additional possible explanation for a lack of difference between treatments was a design confound. The first three sessions in the nonprescriptive treatment were identical to those in the PCT and may have accounted for much of the common outcome variance. Unfortunately, it is not possible to examine this suggestion because the investigators did not conduct an assessment after the third session.

Finally, Craske and co-workers (1995) investigated a brief (four-session) version of PCT. Panic disorder patients were randomly allocated to four

---

[2]In the original paper, the authors did not report that PCT was superior to alprazolam; however, in a subsequent correction (*Journal of Consulting and Clinical Psychology* 63:830, 1995), they pointed out that significantly more patients achieved panic-free status with PCT than with alprazolam.

---

sessions of PCT or four sessions of nondirective supportive therapy. Brief PCT was more effective than nondirective supportive therapy in reducing panic and phobic fear, suggesting that it has a specific effect. However, the overall panic-free rate at the end of treatment (53%) was relatively low, suggesting that a number of patients would have benefited from more sessions of treatment.

Social Phobia

Several investigators have devised and evaluated cognitive-behavioral treatments for social phobia. Although the specific treatment programs differ in emphasis, all use a mixture of cognitive and behavioral procedures to help patients modify their negative beliefs about their performance in social situations and about the way their behavior is evaluated by others. Heimberg and co-workers (1990) found that a group CBT was superior to an equally credible psychological control intervention. A follow-up study (Heimberg et al. 1993) suggested that differences between the treatments were still evident 5 years after treatment termination. Lucas and Telch (1993) replicated Heimberg et al.'s (1990) finding that group CBT was superior to a credible psychological control intervention. Mattick and Peters (1988) compared cognitive restructuring and exposure with exposure alone and found that the combined condition was more effective than exposure alone on measures of end-state functioning and avoidance. In addition, correlational analysis showed that treatment-induced changes in a cognitive variable (fear of negative evaluation) were a significant predictor of improvement in both treatments. A subsequent study (Mattick et al. 1989) replicated these results and also found that cognitive restructuring alone (without exposure) was somewhat less effective than combined treatment. In both studies, the gains that patients made during combined treatment were maintained or enhanced at 3-month follow-up. However, some other studies have found that CBT and exposure alone are both effective and do not differ from each other (see Feske and Chambless 1995; Heimberg and Juster 1995 for reviews). Finally, Heimberg and associates (1994) recently reported preliminary results of a multisite comparison between group CBT, phenelzine, placebo medication, and a psychological control treatment. Phenelzine produced a more rapid response than group CBT. However, at the end of active treatment (12 weeks), group CBT and phenelzine were both superior to the two placebo conditions, and the proportion of patients who were classified as improved was similar in the two active treatments. Patients who responded were monitored during an untreated follow-up period. During this period, CBT patients maintained their gains, but a number of the patients in the phenelzine group relapsed.

Taken together, these studies indicate that current CBT programs are effective and specific interventions for social phobia. Immediate response to phenelzine is similar, or may be slightly better, than that to CBT, but CBT may be superior to phenelzine in the long term. However, inspection of the percentage responder data suggests that there is still room for improvement in treatment effectiveness. Heimberg and co-workers (1990) found that 65% of group CBT patients were improved at the end of treatment. Mattick and Peters (1988) used a more stringent improvement criterion and found that only 38% of the combined exposure and cognitive restructuring treatment group achieved "high end-state function." It has been suggested that the more detailed analysis of maintenance processes provided by more recent cognitive models of social phobia may help therapists to focus treatment more precisely, but this remains to be demonstrated.

Hypochondriasis

One study has investigated the effectiveness of CT in hypochondriasis. Warwick and co-workers (1996) compared 16 sessions of CT with a waiting-list control. CT was significantly more effective in reducing disease conviction, bodily checking, reassurance seeking, and assessor-rated health anxiety. At the end of treatment, CT patients showed 76% improvement in assessor health anxiety ratings, compared with 5% improvement for the patients on the waiting list. This finding is important because it is the first time that a treatment for hypochondriasis has been shown to be effective in a controlled trial. However, the study had several limitations that need to be addressed in future research. In particular, there was only one therapist, and no follow-up was reported.

Obsessive-Compulsive Disorder

The best-validated psychological treatment for obsessive-compulsive patients with overt rituals is the behavior therapy technique of exposure and response prevention. Van Oppen and co-workers (1995) compared CT that was conducted along the lines advocated by Salkovskis with exposure and response prevention. Both treatments were effective, but significantly more patients were rated as recovered in CT. There is no generally established psychological treatment for obsessional ruminators. Encouragingly, Freeston (1994) showed that ruminators treated with CT showed significantly greater improvement than a waiting-list control group.

Generalized Anxiety Disorder

Five studies have investigated the effectiveness of detailed CT interventions in GAD. Durham and Turvey (1987) found that CT and a combination of relaxation plus graded exposure both were effective, but the former therapy produced more stable gains across a 6-month post-treatment follow-up. Butler and co-workers (1991) found that CT was superior to behavior therapy alone (graded exposure and relaxation training) and that both were superior to a no-treatment control. Treatment gains were maintained at 6-month follow-up, when 42% of CT and 5% of behavior therapy patients were rated as having high end-state function (defined as within the normal range on the Hamilton Anxiety Scale and the Beck Anxiety Inventory). Durham and co-workers (1994) found that CT was more effective than psychodynamic psychotherapy. Power and collaborators found that cognitive therapy combined with brief relaxation training was superior to pharmacotherapy in two studies. In the first (Power et al. 1989), CT was superior to both diazepam and placebo at both post-treatment and 12-month follow-up. In the second (Power et al. 1990), CT was superior to placebo and enhanced the efficacy of diazepam alone, and showed better maintenance of gains with less frequent return to treatment during a six-month follow-up.

Taken together, these studies suggest that CT is a specific and effective treatment for GAD and that it may be more effective than pharmacotherapy, both immediately and in the long term. However, inspection of the percentage responder data (presented in preceding paragraph) suggests that there is room for further improvement. Wells (1995) has suggested that further gains could be achieved by focusing therapy more on patients' beliefs about worry itself, but this remains to be demonstrated.

Posttraumatic Stress Disorder

To date, there are no major published evaluations of CT in PTSD. Foa and colleagues have reported two evaluations of treatments that mainly focus on exposure but also contain a small amount of cognitive restructuring. In the first study (Foa et al. 1991), a treatment that included cognitive restructuring—*stress inoculation training* (SIT)—was compared with prolonged exposure, supportive counseling, and a waiting-list control. At the end of treatment, SIT was superior to supportive counseling and the waiting-list control. Prolonged exposure was intermediate and did not differ from any of the other conditions. However, patients treated with SIT showed some loss of gains after treatment, whereas patients treated with prolonged exposure continued to improve, although differences were not significant. In the second study (Foa et al. 1995), women who had been raped in the last month and were suffering from PTSD were allocated to a brief (five-session) cognitive-behavioral prevention program or to a no-treatment control group. The prevention program significantly accelerated recovery from PTSD. Resick and Schnicke (1992) evaluated a treatment program that has a much more extensive cognitive component but differs from a typical CT program in following a rigid, session-by-session protocol in terms of the particular beliefs that are addressed. Rape victims suffering from PTSD who received this group therapy showed significantly greater improvements than those allocated to a waiting-list control condition. Taken together, these studies suggest that CT is a promising approach to PTSD, but further research is clearly required.

Conclusions

Comparisons with other psychological interventions and waiting-list control groups indicate that cognitive therapy is an effective and specific treatment for panic disorder, social phobia, and generalized anxiety disorder. Results comparing immediate response to CT and pharmacotherapy have been mixed. In some trials, CT has been more effective, but in one trial there was no difference, and in another trial pharmacotherapy was slightly more effective. In contrast to the immediate response data, follow-up analyses after medication discontinuation that are currently available consistently favor CT. Preliminary data suggest that CT may also be an effective treatment for hypochondriasis, obsessive-compulsive disorder, and posttraumatic stress disorder. These conclusions are, of course, based on evaluations of current versions of CT. However, there is a dynamic interplay between basic research on cognitive models and treatment procedures. In the last 10 years, theoretical advances have led to changes in the content of CT protocols that have improved efficacy. It seems likely that a similar evolution will occur in the next 10 years.

References

American Psychiatric Association: Diagnostic and Statistical Manual of Mental Disorders, 3rd Edition. Washington, DC, American Psychiatric Association, 1980

American Psychiatric Association: Diagnostic and Statistical Manual of Mental Disorders, 3rd Edition, Revised. Washington, DC, American Psychiatric Association, 1987

American Psychiatric Association: Diagnostic and Statistical Manual of Mental Disorders, 4th Edition. Washington, DC, American Psychiatric Association, 1994

Anastasiades P, Clark DM, Salkovskis PM, et al: Psychophysiological responses to panic and stress. Journal of Psychophysiology 4:331–338, 1990

Arntz A, van den Hout M: Psychological treatments of panic disorder without agoraphobia: cognitive therapy versus applied relaxation. Behav Res Ther 34:113–121, 1996

Barlow DH, Craske MG, Czerny JA, et al: Behavioral treatment of panic disorder. Behavior Therapy 20:261–282, 1989

Beck AT: Cognitive Therapy and the Emotional Disorders. New York, International Universities Press, 1976

Beck AT, Emery G, Greenberg RL: Anxiety Disorders and Phobias: A Cognitive Perspective. New York, Basic Books, 1985

Beck AT, Sokol L, Clark DA, et al: Focused cognitive therapy for panic disorder: a crossover design and one-year follow-up. Am J Psychiatry 147:778–783, 1992

Beunderman R, Van Dis H, Koster RW, et al: Differentiation in prodromal and acute symptoms of patients with cardiac and non-cardiac chest pain, in Advances in Theory and Practice in Behaviour Therapy. Edited by Emmelkamp PMG, Everaerd WTAM, Kraaimaat F, et al. Amsterdam, Swets & Zeitlinger, 1988, pp 231–240

Black DW, Wesner R, Bowers W, et al: A comparison of fluvoxamine, cognitive therapy, and placebo in the treatment of panic disorder. Arch Gen Psychiatry 50:44-50, 1993

Borkovec TD: The nature, functions, and origins of worry, in Worrying: Perspectives on Theory, Assessment and Treatment. Edited by Davey GCL, Tallis F. Chichester, UK, Wiley, 1994, pp 5–34

Borkovec TD, Roemer L: Perceived functions of worry among generalised anxiety disorder subjects: distraction from more emotionally distressing topics? Journal of Behaviour Therapy and Experimental Psychiatry 26:25–30, 1995

Borkovec TD, Wilkinson L, Folensbee R, et al: Stimulus control applications to the treatment of worry. Behav Res Ther 21:247–251, 1983

Brown TA, Cash TF: The phenomenon of nonclinical panic: parameters of panic, fear, and avoidance. Journal of Anxiety Disorders 4:15–29, 1990

Bruch BA, Gorsky JM, Collins TM, et al: Shyness and sociability reexamined: a multicomponent analysis. J Pers Soc Psychol 57:904–915, 1989

Butler G: Exposure as a treatment for social phobia: some instructive difficulties. Behav Res Ther 23:651–657, 1985

Butler G, Fennell M, Robson P, et al: A comparison of behavior therapy and cognitive behavior therapy in the treatment of generalized anxiety disorder. J Consult Clin Psychol 59:167–175, 1991

Clark DM: A cognitive approach to panic. Behav Res Ther 24:461–470, 1986

Clark DM: A cognitive model of panic, in Panic: Psychological Perspectives. Edited by Rachman SJ, Maser J. Hillsdale, NJ, Erlbaum, 1988, pp 71–89

Clark DM: Anxiety states: panic and generalized anxiety disorder, in Cognitive Behaviour Therapy for Psychiatric Problems: A Practical Guide. Edited by Hawton K, Salkovskis PM, Kirk J, et al. Oxford, UK, Oxford University Press, 1989, pp 52–96

Clark DM: Cognitive mediation of panic attacks induced by biological challenge tests. Behav Res Ther 15:75–84, 1993

Clark DM: Panic disorder: from theory to therapy, in Frontiers of Cognitive Therapy: The State of the Art and Beyond. Edited by Salkovskis PM. New York, Guilford, 1996, pp 318–344

Clark DM, Wells A: A cognitive model of social phobia, in Social Phobia: Diagnosis, Assessment, and Treatment. Edited by Heimberg R, Liebowitz M, Hope DA, et al. New York, Guilford, 1995, pp 69–93

Clark DM, Salkovskis PM, Gelder MG, et al: Tests of a cognitive theory of panic, in Panic and Phobias 2. Edited by Hand I, Wittchen HU. Berlin, Springer-Verlag, 1988, pp 149–158

Clark DM, Ball S, Pape DT: An experimental investigation of thought suppression. Behav Res Ther 29:253–258, 1991

Clark DM, Salkovskis PM, Hackmann A, et al: A comparison of cognitive therapy, applied relaxation and imipramine in the treatment of panic disorder. Br J Psychiatry 164:759–769, 1994

Clark DM, Salkovskis PM, Hackmann A, et al: A comparison of standard and brief cognitive therapy for panic disorder. Paper presented at the World Congress of Behavioural and Cognitive Therapies, Copenhagen, Denmark, July 1995

Clark DM, Salkovskis PM, Öst LG, et al: Misinterpretation of body sensations in panic disorder. J Consult Clin Psychol (in press)

Craske MG, Maidenberg E, Brystritsky A: Brief cognitive-behavioural versus nondirective therapy for panic disorder. Journal of Behaviour Therapy and Experimental Psychiatry 26:113–120, 1995

Creamer M, Burgess P, Pattison P: Reaction to trauma: a cognitive processing model. J Abnorm Psychol 101:452–459, 1992

Cross-National Collaborative Panic Study Study Panel: Drug treatment of panic disorder: comparative efficacy of alprazolam, imipramine and placebo. Br J Psychiatry 160:191–222, 1992

Daly JA, Vangelisti AL, Lawrence SG: Self-focused attention and public speaking anxiety. Personality and Individual Differences 10:903–913, 1989

Durham R, Murphy T, Allan T, et al: Cognitive therapy, analytic psychotherapy and anxiety management training for generalised anxiety disorder. Br J Psychiatry 165:315–323, 1994

Durham RC, Turvey AA: Cognitive therapy versus behaviour therapy in the treatment of chronic general anxiety: outcome at discharge and at six-month follow-up. Behav Res Ther 25:229–234, 1987

Ehlers A: Interoception and panic disorder. Advances in Behaviour Research and Therapy 15:3–21, 1993

Ehlers A: A one-year prospective study of panic attacks: clinical course and factors associated with maintenance. J Abnorm Psychol 104:164–172, 1995

Ehlers A, Breuer P: Increased cardiac awareness in panic disorder. J Abnorm Psychol 101:371–382, 1992

Ehlers A, Margraf J: The psychophysiological model of panic attacks, in Fresh Perspectives on Anxiety Disorders. Edited by Emmelkamp PMG, Everaerd WTAM, Kraaimaat F, et al. Amsterdam, Swets & Zeitlinger, 1989, pp 1–29

Ehlers A, Steil R: Maintenance of intrusive memories in posttraumatic stress disorder: a cognitive approach. Behavioural and Cognitive Psychotherapy 23:217–250, 1995

Ehlers A, Margraf J, Roth WT, et al: Anxiety induced by false heart rate feedback in patients with panic disorder. Behav Res Ther 26:1–11, 1988

Feske U, Chambless DL: Cognitive-behavioral versus exposure only treatment for social phobia: a meta-analysis. Behavior Therapy 26:695–720, 1995

Foa EB, Riggs DS: Posttraumatic stress disorder and rape, in American Psychiatric Press Review of Psychiatry, Vol 12. Edited by Oldham JM, Riba MB, Tasman A. Washington, American Psychiatric Press, 1993, pp 273–303

Foa EB, Steketee G, Graspar JB, et al: Deliberate exposure and blocking of obsessive-compulsive rituals: immediate and long-term effects. Behavior Therapy 15:450–472, 1984

Foa EB, Steketee G, Rothbaum BO: Behavioral/cognitive conceptualizations of posttraumatic stress disorder. Behavior Therapy 20:155–176, 1989

Foa EB, Rothbaum BO, Riggs DS, et al: Treatment of posttraumatic stress disorder in rape victims: a comparison between cognitive-behavioral procedures and counseling. J Consult Clin Psychol 59:715–723, 1991

Foa EB, Hearst-Ikeda D, Perry KJ: Evaluation of a brief cognitive-behavioral program for the prevention of chronic PTSD in recent assault victims. J Consult Clin Psychol 63:948–955, 1995

Frazier P, Schauben L: Causal attributions and recovery from rape and other stressful life events. J Soc Clin Psychol 13:1–14, 1994

Freeston MH: Characteristics and treatment of obsessions without overt compulsions. Unpublished doctoral thesis, School of Psychology, University of Laval, Quebec, Canada, 1994

Fyer AJ: Effects of discontinuation of antipanic medication, in Panic and Phobias 2. Edited by Hand I, Wittchen HU. Berlin, Springer-Verlag, 1988, pp 47–53

Hartman LM: A metacognitive model of social anxiety: implications for treatment. Clin Psychol Rev 3:435–456, 1983

Harvey JM, Richards JC, Dziadosz T, et al: Misinterpretation of ambiguous stimuli in panic disorder. Cognitive Therapy and Research 17:235–248, 1993

Heimberg RG, Barlow DH: Psychosocial treatments for social phobia. Psychosomatics 29:27–37, 1988

Heimberg RG, Juster HR: Cognitive-behavioral treatments: a review, in Social Phobia: Diagnosis, Assessment, and Treatment. Edited by Heimberg R, Liebowitz M, Hope DA, et al. New York, Guilford, 1995

Heimberg RG, Dodge CS, Hope DA, et al: Cognitive-behavioural group treatment for social phobia: comparison with a credible placebo control. Cognitive Therapy and Research 14:1–23, 1990

Heimberg RG, Salzman DG, Holt CS, et al: Cognitive-behavioural group treatment for social phobia: effectiveness at 5-year follow-up. Cognitive Therapy and Research 14:1–23, 1993

Heimberg RG, Juster HR, Brown EJ, et al: Cognitive-behavioural versus pharmacological treatment of social phobia: posttreatment and follow-up effects. Paper presented at the annual meeting of the Association for Advancement of Behavior Therapy, San Diego, CA, November 1994

Hope DA, Heimberg RG, Klein JF: Social anxiety and the recall of interpersonal information. Journal of Cognitive Psychotherapy 4:185–195, 1990

Janoff-Bulman R: The aftermath of victimization: rebuilding shattered assumptions, in Trauma and Its Wake: The Study and Treatment of Posttraumatic Stress Disorder. Edited by Figley CR. New York, Brunner/Mazel, 1985, pp 15–35

Keane TM, Scott WO, Chavoga GA, et al: Social support in Vietnam veterans with posttraumatic stress disorder: a comparative analysis. J Consult Clin Psychol 53:95–102, 1985

Kimble CE, Zehr HD: Self-consciousness, information load, self-presentation, amd memory in a social situation. Journal of Social Psychology 118:39–46, 1982

Klosko JS, Barlow DH, Tassinari R, et al: A comparison of alprazolam and behavior therapy in the treatment of panic disorder. J Consult Clin Psychol 58:77–84, 1990

Leary MR: Understanding Social Anxiety. Beverly Hills, CA, Sage, 1983

Lopatka C, Rachman SJ: Perceived responsibility and compulsive checking: an experimental analysis. Behav Res Ther 33:673–684, 1995

Lucas RA, Telch MJ: Group versus individual treatment of social phobia. Paper presented at the annual meeting of the Association for Advancement of Behavior Therapy, Atlanta, GA, November 1993

Margraf J, Ehlers A: Panic attacks in nonclinical subjects, in Panic and Phobias 2. Edited by Hand I, Wittchen HU. Berlin, Springer-Verlag, 1988, pp 103–116

Margraf J, Schneider S: Outcome and active ingredients of cognitive-behavioral treatments for panic disorder. Paper presented at the annual meeting of the Association for Advancement of Behavior Therapy, New York, November 1991

Margraf J, Ehlers A, Roth WT: Biological models of panic disorder and agoraphobia: a review. Behav Res Ther 24:553–567, 1986

Mathews M: Why worry? The cognitive function of anxiety. Behav Res Ther 28:455–468, 1990

Mattick RP, Peters L: Treatment of severe social phobia: effects of guided exposure with and without cognitive restructuring. J Consult Clin Psychol 56:251–260, 1988

Mattick RP, Peters L, Clarke JC: Exposure and cognitive restructuring for social phobia: a controlled study. Behavior Therapy 20:3–23, 1989

McEwan KL, Devins GM: Is increased arousal in social anxiety noticed by others? J Abnorm Psychol 92:417–421, 1983

McNally RJ: Panic Disorder: A Critical Analysis. New York, Guilford, 1994

McNally RJ, Foa EB: Cognition and agoraphobia: bias in the interpretation of threat. Cognitive Therapy and Research 11:567–581, 1987

Moras K, Borkovec TD, DiNardo PA, et al: Generalized anxiety disorder, in DSM-IV Sourcebook, Vol 2. Edited by Widiger TW, Frances AJ, Pincus HA, et al. Washington, DC, American Psychiatric Press, 1996, pp 607–621

Norton GR, Dorward J, Cox BJ: Factors associated with panic attacks in nonclinical subjects. Behavior Therapy 17:239–252, 1986

Öst LG, Westling B: Applied relaxation vs cognitive therapy in the treatment of panic disorder. Behav Res Ther 33:145–158, 1995

Power KG, Jerrom DWA, Simpson RJ, et al: A controlled comparison of cognitive-behaviour therapy, diazepam and placebo in the management of generalised anxiety. Behavioural Psychotherapy 17:1–14, 1989

Power KG, Simpson RJ, Swanson V, et al: A controlled comparison of cognitive behavior therapy, diazepam, and placebo, alone and in combination, for the treatment of generalized anxiety disorder. Journal of Anxiety Disorders 4:267–292, 1990

Rachman SJ, De Silva P: Abnormal and normal obsessions. Behav Res Ther 16:101–110, 1978

Rapee RM, Lim L: Discrepancy between self- and observer ratings of performance in social phobics. J Abnorm Psychol 101:728–731, 1992

Rapee RM, Mattick RP, Murrell E: Cognitive mediation in the affective component of spontaneous panic attacks. Journal of Behaviour Therapy and Experimental Psychiatry 17:245–253, 1986

Resick PA, Schnicke MK: Cognitive processing therapy for sexual assault victims. J Consult Clin Psychol 60:748–756, 1992

Salkovskis PM: Obsessional-compulsive problems: a cognitive-behavioural analysis. Behav Res Ther 23:571–583, 1985

Salkovskis PM: Phenomenology, assessment, and the cognitive model of panic, in Panic: Psychological Perspectives. Edited by Rachman SJ, Maser J. Hillsdale, NJ, Erlbaum, 1988, pp 111–137

Salkovskis PM: Somatic problems, in Cognitive Behaviour Therapy for Psychiatric Problems: A Practical Guide. Edited by Hawton K, Salkovskis PM, Kirk J, et al. Oxford, UK, Oxford University Press, 1989, pp 235–276

Salkovskis PM: The importance of behaviour in the maintenance of anxiety and panic: a cognitive account. Behavioural Psychotherapy 19:6–19, 1991

Salkovskis PM, Bass C: Hypochondriasis, in The Science and Practice of Cognitive-Behaviour Therapy. Edited by Clark DM, Fairburn CG. Oxford, UK, Oxford University Press, 1996, pp 313–340

Salkovskis PM, Clark DM: Panic disorder and hypochondriasis. Advances in Behaviour Research and Therapy 15:23–48, 1993

Salkovskis PM, Kirk J: Obsessive-compulsive disorder, in The Science and Practice of Cognitive-Behaviour Therapy. Edited by Clark DM, Fairburn CG. Oxford, UK, Oxford University Press, 1996, pp 179–208

Salkovskis PM, Warwick HMC: Morbid preoccupations, health anxiety and reassurance: a cognitive-behavioural approach to hypochondriasis. Behav Res Ther 24:597–602, 1986

Salkovskis PM, Clark DM, Hackmann A: Treatment of panic attacks using cognitive therapy without exposure or breathing retraining. Behav Res Ther 29:161–166, 1991

Salkovskis PM, Clark DM, Gelder MG: Cognition-behaviour links in the persistence of panic. Behav Res Ther 34:453–458, 1996

Sanderson WC, Rapee RM, Barlow DH: The influence of an illusion of control of panic attacks induced via inhalation of 5.5% carbon dioxide–enriched air. Arch Gen Psychiatry 46:157–162, 1989

Shear MK, Pilkonis PA, Cloitre M, et al: Cognitive-behavioural treatment compared with nonprescriptive treatment of panic disorder. Arch Gen Psychiatry 51:395–401, 1994

Sheehan DV: Tricyclic antidepressants in the treatment of panic and anxiety disorders. Psychosomatics 27:10–16, 1986

Stopa L, Clark DM: Cognitive processes in social phobia. Behav Res Ther 31:255–267, 1993

Trinder H, Salkovskis PM: Personally relevant intrusions outside the laboratory: long-term suppression increases intrusion. Behav Res Ther 32:833–842, 1994

Trower P, Gilbert P: New theoretical conceptions of social anxiety and social phobia. Clin Psychol Rev 9:19–35, 1989

Tyrer PJ, Lee I, Alexander J: Awareness of cardiac function in anxious, phobic and hypochondriacal patients. Psychol Med 10:171–174, 1980

Van Oppen P, de Haan E, van Balkom AJ, et al: Cognitive therapy and exposure in vivo in the treatment of obsessive-compulsive disorder. Behav Res Ther 33:379–390, 1995

Warwick HMC, Salkovskis PM: Hypochondriasis, in Cognitive Therapy: A Clinical Casebook. Edited by Scott J, Williams JMG, Beck AT. London, Routledge, 1989, pp 78–102

Warwick HMC, Salkovskis PM: Hypochondriasis. Behav Res Ther 28:105–117, 1990

Warwick HMC, Clark DM, Cobb A, et al: A controlled trial of cognitive-behavioural treatment of hypochondriasis. Br J Psychiatry 169:189–195, 1996

Wegner DM: White Bears and Other Unwanted Thoughts: Suppression, Obsession, and the Psychology of Mental Control. New York, Viking, 1989

Wells A: Meta-cognition and worry: a cognitive model of generalised anxiety disorder. Behavioural and Cognitive Psychotherapy 23:265–280, 1995

Wells A: Cognitive Therapy of Anxiety: A Practical Guide. Chichester, UK, Wiley (in press)

Wells A, Butler G: Generalised anxiety disorder, in The Science and Practice of Cognitive-Behaviour Therapy. Edited by Clark DM, Fairburn CG. Oxford, UK, Oxford University Press, 1996, pp 155–178

Wells A, Clark DM, Salkovskis PM, et al: Social phobia: the role of in-situation safety behaviors in maintaining anxiety and negative beliefs. Behavior Therapy 26:153–161, 1995

Wilson KG, Sandler LS, Asmundson GJG, et al: Effects of instructional sets on self-reports of panic attacks. Journal of Anxiety Disorders 5:43–63, 1991

Wittchen HA, Essau CA: The epidemiology of panic attacks, panic disorder and agoraphobia, in Panic Disorder and Agoraphobia. Edited by Walker JR, Norton GR, Ross CA. Pacific Grove, CA, Brooks-Cole, 1991, pp 103–149

Chapter 2

Cognitive-Behavioral Therapy for Substance Abuse Disorders

Michael E. Thase, M.D.

Substance abuse disorders, including alcoholism and addictions involving either prescription medications, tobacco, or illicit drugs, are the most common mental disorders affecting adults in the United States (Kessler et al. 1994; Regier et al. 1990). Indeed, even after excluding nicotine dependence, at least 15% of the adult population of the United States suffer from one or more DSM-IV (American Psychiatric Association 1994) substance abuse disorders. These disorders cost society hundreds of billions of dollars and are a major factor in homicide, suicide, fatal automobile accidents, property crimes (e.g., theft), and the spread of the human immunodeficiency virus (HIV). Most individuals with substance abuse disorders express the desire to quit and have tried numerous times to do so, unsuccessfully. New treatments for these vexing disorders are sorely needed; reviews of the efficacy of treatments clearly document the limitations of standard interventions (Institute of Medicine 1990; McLellan et al. 1982, 1993; Woody et al. 1995). This chapter describes a relatively new application of cognitive-behaviorial therapy for the treatment of substance abuse disorders.

Overview of Cognitive-Behavioral Therapy

The system of therapy known as cognitive-behavioral therapy (CBT), developed by Beck and colleagues, has been evolving since the mid-1970s (Beck 1976; Beck et al. 1979, 1985, 1990, 1993). CBT is a structured, time-limited model of treatment that is suitable for both individual and group formats. A typical course of therapy lasts from 12 to 20 sessions;

This work was supported in part by Grants DA-07673 and DA-08541 from the National Institute on Drug Abuse. The author wishes to thank Ms. JoAnn Penick for help in the preparation of this chapter.

twice-weekly sessions are often used early in the course of treatment. Longer-term models are sometimes recommended for treatment of patients with serious Axis II pathology (e.g., Beck et al. 1990). After completion of acute-phase therapy, periodic "booster" sessions are sometimes recommended to foster relapse prevention skills (e.g., Thase 1992).

The cognitive-behavioral model of treatment emphasizes an active, collaborative therapeutic relationship, in which therapist and patient work together to identify the cognitive and behavioral antecedents of the targeted problems and to implement various strategies to ameliorate the problems, improve coping, and lessen the risk of relapse. Sessions are structured such that they begin with the setting of an agenda or work list, progress to include attention to several agenda items, and conclude with a summary of what has been accomplished and assignment of relevant homework or self-help activities. Such assignments, which are considered critical to the success of CBT, further distinguish this model of therapy from other, more traditional forms of psychotherapy and counseling.

The strategies used in CBT involve a seamless integration of a wide range of cognitive and behavioral techniques. The therapist's choice and timing of selection of particular techniques should follow logically from the case formulation (e.g., Beck et al. 1993; Persons 1989). Cognitive interventions are typically introduced with a series of open-ended questions, referred to as Socratic questioning or guided discovery. Guided discovery is used to reveal the patient's logical errors, automatic negative thoughts, and/or dysfunctional attitudes. Rather than bluntly pointing out the errors revealed in the patient's thinking, the effective therapist guides discovery in a manner analogous to that used by a skilled teacher or coach. Once identified, cognitive errors or dysfunctional attitudes may be challenged by the use of interventions such as "examining the evidence," generating "pros and cons," and "considering the alternatives." Throughout this process, the effective therapist is attentive to the patient's demeanor and nonverbal behavior in order to elicit feedback, answer questions, and deal with the patient's unspoken resistance.

Behavioral methods include activity scheduling, graded task assignments, role playing, behavioral rehearsal, guided exposure (to fearful stimuli), contingency contracting, and deep muscle relaxation or related strategies to aid management of insomnia, cravings, and other symptoms of autonomic arousal. These interventions are principally designed to improve coping skills, decrease the impact of aversive emotional states, and increase the availability of socially sanctioned reinforcers. Behavioral strategies also serve as a medium to elicit negative automatic thoughts and other types of cognitive symptomatology.

The Cognitive Model of Substance Abuse

Vulnerability Factors

Cognitive-behavioral therapy case formulations emphasize a *stress-diathesis* model of vulnerability. Thus, the addictive disorder is viewed as developing in a person with certain liabilities or risk factors at a critical or stressful period in the life cycle. Said another way, stress may activate or uncover a particular vulnerability. Most people initially ingest addictive substances to obtain the pleasure or excitement of being "high," particularly when the experience is shared with peers. Others learn that particular substances can relieve pain, quiet anxiety, counteract boredom, or dampen dysphoria. As a result, substance use has both powerful primary and secondary reinforcer properties. However, only a minority of those who use a potentially habit-forming substance subsequently develop a substance abuse disorder.

At the neurobiological level, most drugs of abuse share at least partially overlapping effects on the brain regions responsible for hedonic or pleasurable responses. Moreover, there are phenomenologic differences in responses to psychostimulants (e.g., cocaine and amphetamine), marijuana, opiates, sedatives, and alcohol that suggest that some individuals may be predisposed to prefer substances with more activating or "sharpening" effects, whereas others find calming or soporific effects to be more desirable. In some cases, such as when a depressed person first begins to use cocaine or an anxious person begins to drink excessively, the substance abuse disorder may be understood as a form of self-medication (e.g., Khantzian 1985). Indeed, evidence indicates that people with Axis I mental disorders have a nearly threefold increase in risk of development of a substance abuse disorder (Regier et al. 1990). The association between psychopathology and predisposition to substance abuse is less straightforward for the majority of people who abuse substances. Further, even when the self-medication diathesis is well justified, treatment of the primary mental disorder often does not result in amelioration of the substance abuse disorder.

Other relevant risk factors for development of an addictive disorder include lower socioeconomic status, increased life stress and other adversities, and a family history of a substance abuse disorder (American Psychiatric Association 1995; Glantz and Pickens 1992). Although one or more genetic risk factors are likely, specific genes have not yet been identified (American Psychiatric Association 1995). Men are at greater risk for opiate, cocaine, and alcohol addictions, whereas women are at greater risk for sedative-hypnotic dependence. Individual vulnerability traits may include impulsivity, increased novelty seeking, low frustration tolerance, low self-esteem, and decreased assertiveness. Individuals with Cluster B Axis II disorders, such as antisocial or borderline personality disorders, are also at particularly high risk, perhaps because these characterological disorders are associated with manifold other risk factors (Glantz and Pickens 1992; Nace et al. 1991; Poldrugo and Forti 1988).

The Role of Cognitive Factors

Although substance use begins as a voluntary or volitional process, people have great difficulty stopping the pattern once abuse or dependence has developed. Typically, during the transitional period spanning the interval between onset of drug use and development of dependence, the individual ignores evidence indicating that drug or alcohol use is becoming problematic and often exaggerates his or her ability to quit. The addict "in progress" also may overemphasize the positive aspects of getting high, including hedonistic effects and pragmatic factors (e.g., "All my friends do it!"). Thus, both denial/minimization of the hazards and magnitude of the addiction and a developing system of interdependent beliefs about the benefits of drug or alcohol use serve to reinforce and maintain the addictive behavior (Beck et al. 1993). Of course, the unpleasant physiological cues associated with various withdrawal syndromes provide substantial incentives for continued substance use, as nothing remedies withdrawal symptoms better than resumed usage of the addictive substance.

The substance-abusing individual's beliefs about drinking or drug taking are considered dysfunctional because they are relatively rigid and associated with pathological behavior, and persist despite evidence that refutes such beliefs (Beck et al. 1993). Relevant dysfunctional beliefs include statements such as "I'll be miserable without getting high" and "I'm not really addicted—I can always stop later" (Table 2–1). Moreover, there is a shift in focus toward beliefs that emphasize the positive expectancies of substance use (e.g., "If only I can score, I'll feel a lot better"

Table 2–1.   Beliefs about substance abuse: examples

- I don't have any control over craving.
- Once it starts, the only way to cope with craving is to use.
- I've passed the point of no return—I'll never be able to stop drinking.
- You need willpower not to drink, and I don't have it.
- I can't have fun without getting high.
- It doesn't matter if I stop using—no one cares.
- I can't cope without drinking.
- My life is already ruined—I might as well get high.
- No one can push me around—I'll quit when I'm ready.

or "I'll need to get high in order to handle this"). Over time, there also tends to be a devaluation of more traditional reinforcers and social contingencies, such as those provided by family, employers, and "straight" (i.e., nonusing) friends.

For the addicted individual trying to abstain from drug or alcohol abuse, there is typically an internal conflict between more "mainstream" beliefs about the wisdom of not using and those in support of continued substance abuse (Beck et al. 1993). Such conflicted internal "dialogues" may elicit anxiety or dysphoria, which, in turn, tend to amplify the noxiousness of cravings or withdrawal symptoms.

The behavioral inclination or response predisposition to settle this unpleasant state of affairs by drinking or using drugs is referred to as an *urge*. As is the case with other operant behaviors, the reinforcement resulting from terminating an urge with consumption of drugs or alcohol is powerful, and with repetition, the individual becomes quite adept at the various instrumental behaviors necessary to maintain the pattern (Figure 2–1). The intense frustration that accompanies nonreward of a highly reinforced behavioral pattern such as an urge is often accompanied by emotional outbursts and aggressive behavior, which, in turn, may also yield reinforcing results. For example, a financially strapped person in opiate withdrawal may bully and coerce money from a family member. Whereas the addicted individual had not previously exploited his or her relatives, thereafter the probability of further impositions is increased.

Urges are usually either accompanied or preceded by a mixed cognitive-affective experience known as *craving*. Cravings may arise spontaneously or may be triggered by seeing or thinking about something related to the addiction. Anxiety, anger, boredom, or dysphoria similarly may trigger cravings. Laboratory studies document that cue-induced cravings are associated with instantaneous autonomic arousal, indicating that classical conditioning of responses has occurred (O'Brien 1992). Cognitions accompanying cravings include those that serve as permissive for substance abuse ("I've got to get high *just this one last time* in order to deal with these feelings"), in addition to more instrumental thoughts about how to obtain drugs or alcohol.

The thoughts that accompany urges and cravings are examples of a class of cognitive disturbance referred to as *automatic negative thoughts*. Automatic thoughts are more superficial or accessible than beliefs and constitute the individual's moment-by-moment mental dialogue or "running commentary" about one's self, world, and future. Automatic negative thoughts, which may be experienced in words or visual images, are intrusive and repetitive; they are also usually perceived as accurate or true.

A wave of automatic negative thoughts is typically associated with emotional arousal. In fact, the strength of the affective distress is cor-

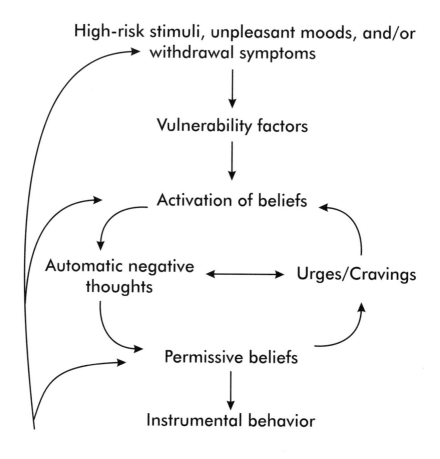

Figure 2–1. Cognitive model of substance abuse.

related with the perceived veracity of the automatic negative thoughts (Thase and Beck 1993). This association serves as the basis for a type of logical distortion known as *emotional reasoning*. An example of emotional reasoning is found in the following statement: "I feel this way, therefore it must be true." The content of automatic thoughts thus provides a barometer of one's mood states. In both spontaneous and chemically induced euphorias, a positive monologue is found, and at least 90% of automatic thoughts are positively valenced (e.g., Schwartz and Garamoni 1986; Thase and Beck 1993). During periods of well-being, the normal balance between positive and negative cognitions typically conforms to a ratio of 2 or 3 to 1, a so-called "golden zone" (Schwartz and Garamoni 1986). In states of severe distress, the normal "balanced" mental dialogue between negative and positive or neutral thoughts shifts into an imbalanced negative monologue. Disruption of such negative monologues via distraction or more complex cognitive techniques is a standard therapeutic strategy that often delivers a significant shift in mood (e.g., Beck et al. 1979, 1993).

In addition to emotional reasoning, a number of other errors in logic and information processing are revealed in automatic negative thoughts. These errors include personalization, catastrophization, "black/white" (dichotomous) thinking, selective abstraction, mind reading, selective recall, and minimization of the positive (see, e.g., Beck et al., 1979). Such logical errors seem to help "bend" perception so that it is consistent with an activated or prevailing belief. For example, when you have the misfortune of being stuck in an extremely slow line at the grocery, you might feel frustrated or angry and have the automatic negative thought "This *always* happens to me." At that moment, there is a distortion of recall such that you do not remember the hundreds (or thousands) of times that you have had the good fortune to pick fast-moving lines.

Repetitive automatic negative thoughts may be collated by themes to reveal salient underlying dysfunctional attitudes or beliefs. In Beck's (1976) original model, the term *cognitive triad* is used to describe a collation of automatic negative thoughts into themes about self, world, and future. The triadic thoughts of a person in drug withdrawal might include "I'm so miserable I can't stand it another moment" (self), "My wife doesn't understand me" (world), and "I'll never be able to kick this habit" (future). Obviously, from the outsider's perspective, each of these statements involves some degree of logical distortion. However, the sufferer typically does not challenge these cognitions, which serve only to intensify the urge to get high.

As the severity of the addiction worsens, cravings are perceived as imperative and irresistible. Thus, the individual's belief about his or her substance abuse problem may transform into a "need"—that is, an essential, life-sustaining ingredient. There may also be a broader generalization of the stimuli that trigger cravings and urges. For example, abstinent cocaine-abusing individuals experience cravings not only when they see paraphernalia or people with whom they have used drugs, but also in response to more neutral stimuli such as a $10 bill (i.e., the cost of a "rock" of crack cocaine) or a bus (i.e., a means of transportation to the crack house). Thus, the cravings and urges occur more frequently. Again, the experience of craving is reinforced by consumption. Once this pattern of repetitive indulgence is established, most addicted individuals also develop permissive beliefs: "I am powerless to stop this!" and "If I don't use (drink), I will die!" Conversely, there is a loss of self-efficacy—that is, the subjective appraisal of competence—to cope with problems in a substance-free state. This state of perceived helplessness is well recognized in the Alcoholics Anonymous (AA) credo that the alcoholic is powerless in the face of the addiction.

Antecedent Beliefs

The cognitive patterns described above pertain to the mental life of people who have begun to have problems involving drugs or alcohol. In the cognitive model of substance abuse, a deeper set of core beliefs or schemas is posited as an additional predisposing factor (e.g., Beck et al. 1993). Schemas are the "silent" cognitive structures that serve as fundamental guides or templates against which experience is evaluated. Relatively simplistic examples of schemas include the mental structure responsible for the ability to conserve volume (i.e., 6 ounces of water is the same whether or not the container is tall or wide) or the stored memory of how to tie a knot. In terms of psychological well-being, relevant schemas include one's basic impressions about his or her competence, romantic desirability, capacity to handle adversity, trustworthiness of others, and so forth. Schemas also serve as "filters" for information processing. For example, a person with a problematic schema about competence ("I just don't have what it takes to succeed") will have a lower threshold for perceiving criticism or negative feedback. Similarly, a schema about the untrustworthiness of caregivers might result in perceiving a therapist's distraction and interpreting it in a highly personalized way ("She's like all the others—she just doesn't care").

Problematic schemas are developmentally acquired but, fortunately, are modifiable throughout adult life. For example, the schema "I'm incompetent" might result from the combination of harsh parental expectations coupled with some specific problem in learning, such as attention-deficit disorder. In therapy, the patient is helped to collect evidence from as many sources as possible in order to reevaluate the schema. In the example described above, competence would be assessed across situations, and when evidence of specific examples of poor performance is unearthed, the attributions for the cause of the problem are explored. Therapy aims to help the patient shift attributions of causality from the global to the specific and from the fixed (irreversible) to the modifiable. In some cases, excessive self-blame (internality) is problematic, whereas other patients may have problems as a result of attributing causality to external factors too often.

Cognitive Aspects of Relapse

Another relevant cognitive construct is the *abstinence violation effect* (Curry et al. 1987). This refers to the perception of loss of control that many alcoholic or drug-addicted individuals experience following ingestion of only a single drink or "hit." The abstinence violation effect involves both dichotomous, or black/white, thinking (i.e., any drug or alcohol use constitutes a full relapse, and, therefore, use should continue to full intoxication because the damage is already done) and self-medication of the resultant painful cognitions and affects (i.e., "I feel miserable about using, but at least I know how to sooth my pain").

Specific Components of Cognitive-Behavioral Therapy

Cognitive-behavioral therapy is typically conducted on an outpatient basis, but it may be modified for use with inpatients (e.g., Thase and Wright 1991). Similarly, CBT may be used as the principal prescriptive therapy or, when indicated, in combination with pharmacotherapy. Examples of the latter application include the concomitant use of CBT and methadone substitution therapy, disulfiram, or naltrexone. Like other prescriptive therapies, CBT neither negates the value of nor contraindicates the patient's participation in self-help activities such as AA or Narcotics Anonymous (NA). To the contrary, simultaneous participation in self-help activities is strongly encouraged (e.g., Beck at al. 1993). For people who find the spiritual foundation of AA or NA to be unacceptable, alternatives such as Rational Recovery are sometimes available.

Pretherapy Considerations

Individuals with substance abuse disorders typically enter treatment with a complex set of problems. Some are mandated to treatment by court order or an employee assistance program, whereas others are influenced or even coerced by ultimatums from frustrated family members. Still others must face the need for treatment in the wake of an auto accident or hospitalization for a medical complication of substance abuse (e.g., pancreatitis or subacute bacterial endocarditis). Of course, comorbid psychiatric disorders, particularly mood and anxiety disorders, may be manifest in more acute or symptomatically florid presentations that necessitate emergent entry into treatment.

Initial clinical considerations include assessment of the need for inpatient or outpatient medical detoxification. Alcohol and sedative-hypnotic withdrawal can have potentially lethal medical sequelae. Thus, careful medical monitoring and appropriate treatment with benzodiazepines or phenobarbital are warranted. Conversely, although opiate withdrawal is not nearly as medically hazardous, the first 48 to 96 hours of abstinence may be so subjectively uncomfortable that detoxification with methadone or clonidine may be required. Cocaine withdrawal syndromes are generally not medically dangerous, aside from psychiatric complications such as onset of suicidality or paranoia.

Withdrawal syndromes of patients with mixed addictions, such as alcohol-cocaine or opiate-alcohol dependence, can be particularly vexing. Changes in healthcare financing and reevaluation of the cost-effectiveness of standard medical practices have led to a decreasing use of inpatient detoxification strategies. In the 1990s, extended 21- or 28-day hospitalizations for detoxification and initiation of psychosocial interventions are increasingly rare. Nevertheless, a short inpatient stay for detoxification still may be necessary to initiate the treatment of patients with severe addictive disorders.

Some treatment programs prefer to defer engagement in formal psychotherapy or other treatments until abstinence is achieved or until an individual has demonstrated motivation for therapy by attending a specified number of self-help sessions. These policies surely protect scarce therapeutic resources: they limit treatment to a more accessible subset of more highly motivated patients. However, such tests of motivation ultimately may be counterproductive because they systematically deny services to those who need them the most. There is no empirical support for the adage that the addicted individual must "bottom out" before he or she is accessible to treatment.

Therapeutic Relationship

Substance-abusing individuals are traditionally considered to be difficult to work with in psychotherapy. They are at high risk to withdraw from therapy prematurely, and the productivity of the working alliance may be compromised by poor attendance, dishonesty, and the patient's dysfunctional beliefs about therapy. Substance abuse and alcoholism are socially proscribed activities (i.e., bad behavior), and one habitual way of coping with shame is to conceal or hide the problem. Moreover, some addicted persons, particularly those with serious Axis II pathology, derive a sense of mastery or power from the successful lie (i.e., "getting one over" on the professional). Obviously, such behaviors are counterproductive in therapy, and their successful management requires a high level of professional skill. Therapists need to be objective and direct in response to dishonest or disingenuous behavior without taking confrontation to an adversarial level. In fact, blunt confrontations about the patient's use of denial, long a staple of some traditionally oriented counseling approaches, may actually serve to further alienate the patient from the treatment alliance (Miller and Rollnick 1991).

Most people with substance abuse problems have mixed feelings about entering therapy and, on more than a few occasions, have entered treatment under the coercion of family members ("If you don't get help, I'm leaving!") or legal authorities ("If you don't get help, you'll go to jail!"). Also, socioeconomic and cultural differences may heighten patients' expectations that their therapists will not be able to understand their problems. The astute therapist usually will initiate an open discussion of these roadblocks in order to help clarify the patient's motivations for, and reservations against, therapy.

Effective therapy follows a number of "ground rules" that also apply to more traditional treatment approaches. For example, the therapist should schedule regular sessions and make every effort to begin and end them on time. Conversely, flexibility in scheduling is desirable. Similarly, some form of emergency or crisis intervention contact should be available. The therapist must also work hard to establish and maintain rapport, balancing between the postures of an overly detached professionalism and an overly solicitous "enabler." Most therapists follow the policy that sessions will not take place when the patient is inebriated or intoxicated. It is sometimes necessary to set other limits, but this needs to be done in a gentle and empathic manner. The patient's affective "storms" should be met with quiet confidence and honest concern for the patient's well-being. Even highly experienced therapists working with people who abuse substances often benefit from professional or peer supervision to help manage more demanding or difficult patients.

The therapeutic relationship also is fostered by recognition of the patient's motivation for treatment or readiness for change (Prochaska et al. 1992). Following this paradigm, readiness for change is understood as a continuum, ranging from precontemplation to contemplation, preparation, action, and maintenance stages. Thus, an intervention geared for use with a patient in the action phase (e.g., using a relaxation exercise to lessen craving) is less likely to be successful for someone contemplating change than a strategy better suited for this earlier stage (e.g., listing the advantages and disadvantages of stopping drinking).

Case Formulation

The essential components of case conceptualization are summarized in Table 2–2. Although much of the relevant "database" is collected during the initial sessions, case conceptualization continues to evolve throughout the therapy.

In our work at the Center for Psychiatric and Chemical Dependency Services at the University of Pittsburgh School of Medicine, we have found that it is often helpful to defer some of the information-gathering activities traditionally included in the initial session in order to attend more to nurturing the patient's motivation for engaging in therapy. For example, when we modified our intake procedures to include an initial session of motivational interviewing (Miller and Rollnick 1991), we

Table 2–2.   Information included in the case formulation

- Current nature and severity of addiction(s)
- Current symptomatology/comorbidity
- Beliefs about substance abuse
- Past treatment history
- Personal experiences with quitting
- Assessment of readiness for change
- Social support for abstinence
- Living, employment, and legal circumstances
- Medical status
- Relevant childhood experiences
- Antecedent "core" beliefs or schemas
- Implications for therapy

observed a 20% increase in treatment retention during the critical first month of therapy.

Assessment of Outcome

One fundamental tenet of CBT is that the impact of therapy on targeted problems should be measured. To this end, a measure of the frequency and amount of substance use should be obtained at baseline and repeated periodically. The Addiction Severity Index (ASI; McLellan et al. 1992) is well suited for this purpose. Patient self-report is clearly an imperfect means of gathering such data, and frequently assessment may be supplemented by more objective parameters (e.g., the alcohol breathalyzer or qualitative urine drug screens). Cognitively oriented assessment inventories include the Beliefs About Substance Use Inventory, the Relapse Prediction Scale, and the Cravings Beliefs Questionnaire (see Beck et al. 1993). Other commonly used assessments, such as the Hopkins Symptom Checklist, Beck Anxiety and Depression Inventories, and the Hamilton Rating Scale for Depression, may be obtained periodically to monitor comorbid symptomatology. It should be kept in mind, however, that elevations of such symptom ratings are common both during detoxification and shortly thereafter and do not necessarily indicate the need for concomitant psychotropic medication.

Educating Patients About Cognitive-Behavioral Therapy

The collaborative-empirical framework of CBT necessitates that patients gain a working understanding of the important concepts of the model and the key ingredients of therapy. Education about the cognitive-behavioral model of addiction and its treatment thus typically begins in the initial sessions, hand in hand with development of the case formulation. This process may be facilitated by eliciting the patient's understanding about his or her drug problem and what changes might be necessary in order to overcome the problem. Introducing a process to be used subsequently, the therapist may ask the patient to rate the strength (i.e., accuracy or certainty) of these beliefs on an 0-to-100 scale, using 100 to represent absolute certainty. A standard goal of CBT is to construct interventions that help the patient revise highly believable dysfunctional beliefs in the direction of more rational and balanced alternatives.

Next, the cognitive-behavioral model is introduced, often with diagrams or drawings to illustrate the relationships between beliefs, automatic thoughts, cravings, and behaviors (see, for example, Figure 2–1). It is helpful for the therapist to illustrate how therapy techniques are used to help people cope with problematic thoughts, beliefs, and behaviors. Examples drawn from the patient's experience help to make the illustration more personal and salient. This is particularly true for beliefs and automatic negative thoughts, which can be confusing concepts in abstraction, yet crystal clear when the patient is asked to speak his or her thoughts "out loud." In the initial session, for example, the therapist may ask the patient how he or she felt in the waiting room, just before the session began. The automatic negative thoughts that accompany these feelings are next elicited by the question "What thoughts were running through your mind at the time?" Usually, with some encouragement, the patient will verbalize some distorted or exaggerated cognition that was associated with an apprehensive or anxious mood. Next, the therapist may juxtapose the patient's expected outcome with his or her own assessment of how the session has gone so far. Pairing a distorted cognition with a disconfirmatory experience is a powerful introductory exercise.

Beliefs about substance use are usually more difficult to uncover than automatic negative thoughts. Some patients readily grasp the concept of underlying beliefs by following the "downward arrow" from an automatic thought to a belief revealed by inductive questioning (Figure 2–2). For others, the homework task of completing the Beliefs About Substance Abuse Inventory (see Beck et al. 1993) is illuminative. In yet other cases, the therapist may "prime the pump" by describing relevant beliefs that other patients have associated with certain automatic thoughts or behaviors. In any case, it is important for the therapist to convey that recognition of beliefs is a skill that can be mastered with proper coaching and practice. One example of an initial homework assignment directly linked to this educational exercise is to have the patient record his or her thoughts associated with feelings of boredom, anxiety, or depression. These self-help interventions, like all subsequent homework assignments, are reviewed at the beginning of the next session.

Identification of the Pros and Cons

A standard cognitive strategy, weighing the "pros and cons," is commonly used to help patients contemplate the advantages and disadvantages of an anticipated change. In an early session, this method may be applied to help to enhance motivation to quit substance use (Table 2–3). It is important for the therapist not to let the patient underestimate the disadvantages of stopping, a process that typically includes withdrawal symptoms or cravings, increased depressive or anxiety symptoms, loss of the substance's desirable effects, loss of friendships and social relationships, and facing the often considerable consequences of the addictive disorder. Nevertheless, the "pros"—the aspects in support of quitting—nearly always outweigh the "cons," and

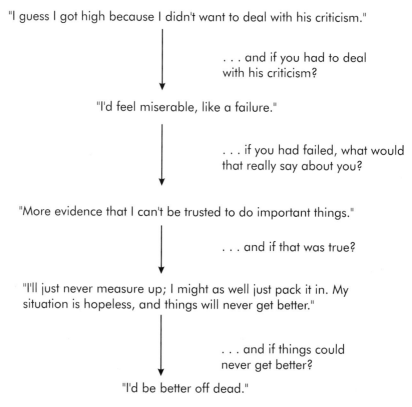

"I guess I got high because I didn't want to deal with his criticism."

. . . and if you had to deal with his criticism?

"I'd feel miserable, like a failure."

. . . if you had failed, what would that really say about you?

"More evidence that I can't be trusted to do important things."

. . . and if that was true?

"I'll just never measure up; I might as well just pack it in. My situation is hopeless, and things will never get better."

. . . and if things could never get better?

"I'd be better off dead."

Figure 2–2. Downward arrow approach to eliciting core beliefs.

Table 2–3. A "pros and cons" exercise about abstinence

	Advantages	Disadvantages
Abstinence	More money Approval of mother Less paranoia about cops More time to do other things Healthier lifestyle	Withdrawal symptoms Will feel like a wimp Miss the high Will feel overwhelmed Might not succeed Loss of excitement
Continued use	Doesn't rock the boat Keep friends who use No health problems yet No withdrawal symptoms Exciting times when high	Money spent on dope Potential trouble Might catch HIV Feel like a junkie Criticism from mother

this fact, made obvious, helps to galvanize the patient's willingness to take action.

Identification and Alteration of Beliefs

The following vignette illustrates the use of Socratic questioning and "examining the evidence" technique to begin to modify dysfunctional beliefs about substance abuse.

Patient: I'm really bummed out about drinking last night. I had been sober since our last session [5 days previously], and I'd even gone to two AA meetings.

Therapist: I agree that you're making progress . . . Before this past week, how long had it been since you had abstained for 5 days?

Patient: At least 6 months . . .

Therapist: So 5 consecutive sober days is an accomplishment. Why don't you fill me in on what led to your decision to drink last night. Maybe we can learn something from it.

Patient: Well, it's not that interesting. I'm just not sure . . .

Therapist: What time did you begin drinking?

Patient: About 7 P.M. I bought a six-pack and drank it while I watched the basketball game.

Therapist: And where did the six-pack come from?

Patient: I picked it up on the way home from work, at about 5:30 P.M.

Therapist: So, at some point before 5:30 P.M. you must have been thinking about the pros and cons of drinking.

Patient: Well, I guess that happened in the car on the way home from work. I had a really stressful day. My boss was on me all day to get my productivity up, and it really didn't seem fair.

Therapist: And how did that make you feel?

Patient: I was stressed out . . . kind of like mad and nervous at the same time.

Therapist: You mentioned one automatic negative thought, "This isn't fair!" Can you recall what else ran through your mind?

Patient: Variations on the same theme. Don't get me wrong—it's a good job, but sometimes management can be such complete jerks. They make things difficult and demanding when it doesn't have to be that way. The boss's poor planning becomes my big headache!

Therapist: I've jotted down a couple of those statements because they are excellent examples of the kinds of automatic thoughts that might trigger an uncomfortable feeling state. So, you're thinking that your boss is a jerk and that you have to suffer because of his mismanagement and you're feeling angry and tense?

Patient: Right!

Therapist: So let's look for the cognitive connection between those thoughts and feelings and your subsequent actions—buying and drinking beer.

Patient: Stress at work is certainly one of my triggers—I've got a long track record of drinking after work, and so do a lot of my co-workers.

Therapist: So, can you put those beliefs into words?

Patient: It's like this: "Drinking is a good way to unwind."

Therapist: How certain are you that this belief is true? And what about the belief involving your co-workers?

Patient: I'm certain that when I'm uptight, drinking helps, at least temporarily. The fact that my buddies all do it is further proof. It's like our way of life.

Therapist: So are you saying "Drinking is the best way that I know of to unwind after work?"

Patient: Yes . . . but I also know that my drinking was causing trouble. That's why I'm in therapy.

Therapist: Okay, so let's look at yesterday to get a handle on the beliefs that helped you get around that fact.

Patient: I know that when I left work I wanted to go drinking, but I still had some willpower. Several of my buddies stopped at our regular "watering hole," and I was able to say no. But, traffic was bad and I just couldn't calm down. I guess I resented that they could drink and I couldn't. So, I got off the next exit and bought the six-pack.

Therapist: Do you recall a specific self-statement running through your mind that gave you permission to buy the beer?

Patient: I thought something like "Just a couple of beers won't hurt that much." After the day I had, I felt like I deserved it!

Therapist: So here's the conflict—you felt like you deserved to do something that would make you feel better in the short run, but is hurting you in the long run. Let's examine the evidence about your belief that drinking is the best way to unwind after work. Yesterday you were uptight and you drank some beer. Are you certain today that you were correct in your assessment?

Patient: No, not at all. I should have tried another way of handling it.

Therapist: "Should" statements usually reflect somebody else's standard or rules. What evidence do you have that it would be advantageous to find other ways of coping?

Patient: Well . . . one more DUI and I won't be driving. Also, my last two relationships ended partly because my girlfriends said that I drank too much. Last month I got written up at work for having too many absences.

Therapist: Okay, that sounds like a strong basis for working on strengthening alternative beliefs, such as "Drinking is harmful to me" and "I can find other ways to cope with stress without drinking." How does that sound?

Patient: It sounds great, but it's easier said than done.

Therapist: You're right. That's why I'd like to recommend that we revise our agenda so that we spend the next 30 minutes today brainstorming and beginning to practice other ways to cope with stress. And after that, we'll spend as much time as we need to until you've mastered these alternative ways. Does this make sense to you?

Patient: It sure does!

Lifestyle Changes

The role of "persons, places, and things" as discriminative stimuli for substance use has been long recognized. The effective therapist thus must introduce the possibility that changes in lifestyle confer a powerful advantage for the recently detoxified individual who is attempting to remain abstinent. This is particularly true early in the course of treatment, before the patient has gained mastery of strategies to cope with cravings or to address effectively permissive attitudes and beliefs.

Potential lifestyle changes include, but are not limited to, finding "sober" housing, avoiding contact with people who still use drugs or alcohol, increasing contact with people who do not use, and developing healthier leisure-time activities. Not uncommonly, the decision to begin a healthy, sober lifestyle creates a void in a person's friendship and peer network. If sustained, this state of social deprivation is incompatible with well-being. In such cases, peers met at AA or NA meetings, estranged family members, or friends from the past might be called on to broaden social support. Role playing and behavioral rehearsal strategies are often used to help the patient face anxieties about contacting someone and fears of possible rejection.

Other lifestyle changes can be encouraged with standard behavioral strategies such as activity scheduling and graded task assignments (see Beck et al. 1993). A healthy alternative activity, such as a daily exercise period, may be scheduled into a block of time previously used for substance-related activity. In graded task assignments, a more complex or overwhelming, but ultimately desirable, activity is broken down into a series of more manageable steps. The stepwise completion of these tasks may be planned with an activity schedule. Patients are encouraged to complement the more intrinsic rewards of completing assigned "healthy" tasks with self-reinforcing statements. Similarly, contingency contracts, including specified rewarding activities with a spouse or significant other (e.g., McCrady et al. 1986), can be incorporated to help increase the likelihood that the patient will engage in the targeted behaviors.

For some individuals, desirable lifestyle changes, such as securing sober housing or separating from a substance-abusing spouse, are not readily feasible. Although these circumstances may make treatment more difficult, they do not contraindicate therapy. It is important for the therapist not to engage in self-fulfilling prophecies ("If only Bill could get better housing, he could make it") that undermine the chances for success.

Management of Life Problems

Problems with employment, relationships, health, and legal circumstances are endemic to substance-abusing populations and serve as critical stimuli for cravings and instrumental drug-seeking behaviors. In addition, chronic stressors such as unemployment serve to maintain low self-esteem and helpless/hopeless attributional styles, which, in turn, increase the likelihood of selecting more immediately rewarding substance-related behaviors, as opposed to longer-term strategies such as schooling or job training.

Whether the stressor is chronic or acute, it may serve to activate the patient's beliefs about the "benefits" of drug or alcohol use. Specifically, intoxication delivers a welcomed, albeit short-lived, relief from dysphoric affects and/or enhancement of self-esteem, as well a numbing escape from the reality of the problem at hand. In the case of interpersonal conflicts, the addicted individual may also experience a sense of mastery or control by defiantly asserting his or her autonomy.

Therapy addresses these manifold problems in several ways. First, the patient's problems may be enumerated and prioritized. A relatively straightforward approach to problem-solving strategies (Nezu et al. 1989) may be introduced. This approach centers on 1) formulation of a clear definition of the problem and its likely implications, 2) exploration of all possible solutions, 3) consideration of the pros and cons of each solution, and 4) implementation of the most feasible solution.

Second, the therapist may respond to anticipated problems by providing education and more practical assistance. This includes education about reduction of high-risk behaviors (e.g., needle sharing, unsafe sex, or driving while intoxicated), referral for appropriate medical evaluation and treatment, and referral for vocational rehabilitation, housing, or other social services. For many seriously addicted individuals, hopelessness is maintained by a dearth of options for socially sanctioned reinforcers. The value of the therapist as an ombudsman or case manager for social service interventions should not be discounted.

Involvement of Significant Others

Most severely chemically dependent individuals have alienated a large number (if not all) of their sober friends and significant others. Nevertheless, the support provided by a "straight" (i.e., nonchemically abusing) loved one is an important positive prognostic factor (e.g., Booth et al. 1992; Cawthra et al. 1991; Rae 1972). It stands to reason that therapeutic efforts to engage significant others in the treatment process may hold particular promise. Not surprisingly, however, chemically dependent individuals are often reluctant to include significant others in the treatment plan; this reluctance may reflect avoidance of shameful affects or the use of secrecy in order to maintain the option of renewed substance abuse.

In most treatment settings, involvement of significant others cannot be mandated, although methadone maintenance clinics are sometimes an exception to this rule. Therefore, the therapist needs to seek voluntary collaboration and must be prepared to explore, via Socratic questioning, the patient's typically negative reaction. The following example is illustrative:

Therapist: We've found that the chances of success in therapy are better when we can involve a spouse or significant other in the therapy. What are your thoughts about that?

Patient: I don't think it's a good idea. My wife's pretty mad at me, and I don't think she'd really want to come.

Therapist: I understand your reluctance. A lot of people have been in a similar position at the beginning of treatment. Have you talked with her about this?

Patient: Not really . . . it's just that she's so critical . . . [Posture stiffens, arms crossed]

Therapist: You look kind of distressed by this. What thoughts are on your mind, right now?

Patient: Not much . . . Maybe I'm mad at her too. Complain, complain, complain! Maybe I don't want her to be part of my therapy!

Therapist: What if she came to one of the sessions?

Patient: I might feel ganged up on . . . picked on.

Therapist: And what would that say about you and me?

Patient: What do you mean?

Therapist: If I was to join in with your wife and gang up on you?

Patient: You'd be working for her, like trying to make me "be good."

Therapist: And if that was true?

Patient: I'd hate it, I'd rebel. It would make me want to use . . . just to show you that I couldn't be pushed around!

Therapist: Let me summarize, to make sure that I understand your position. You're concerned that if your wife attends a session that she'll complain about you and your behavior and that I'll "buy in" to her view of things. This will trigger kind of a defensive posture on your part, you'll feel picked on . . . alone . . . angry . . . and might deal with this by getting high?

Patient: Exactly!

Therapist: Okay, we've been working together for 4 weeks, and although that's not a long time, you must have formed some opinions about me. Based on this, what do you think the chances are that I'll turn my back on you and your interests and join in with your wife to criticize you?

Patient: Well, when you say it that way, I don't think it's very likely. But, in my guts, I still feel it might happen.

Therapist: Yes, although its unlikely that it would happen, I guess I can't give you absolute assurance that you won't feel ganged up on if we got together with your wife. But, honestly, if this happened, would you have any alternative ways of coping with these thoughts and feelings other than storming out of the session and getting high?

Patient: Yeah . . . I could say "I don't like this, I want this couples session to stop!"

Therapist: That's a great start. Any other alternatives?

Patient: I could say "This isn't working—I'm feeling ganged up on," *or* I could ask you directly to help us communicate.

Therapist: I agree that you've got several alternative ways of coping if the session is going poorly. We should also be certain that the potential advantages or benefits of involving your wife outweigh the disadvantages or risks. Do you feel up to working on a "pros and cons" exercise?

Patient: Sure.

In the case vignette described above, the therapist initially used the downward arrow technique. Midway through the intervention, at the point that the patient became visibly angry and verbalized the affectively charged, "hot" thought ("I'll show you I can't be pushed around"), the therapist switched to clarification of the cognitive-affective-behavioral relationship. Several appropriate interventions were possible, and in this case, the therapist chose one intended to 1) foster the therapeutic alliance and 2) bring the focus of the session back to the task at hand (i.e., involving the spouse in the treatment team). In this manner, the patient's veiled threat to use drugs if the spouse is included was defused, and the advantages and disadvantages of her participation could be considered more rationally.

Contingency Management

Recognition and implementation of response-contingent reinforcers is a hallmark of behavioral approaches to psychopathology. Although contingency management has shown promise for treatment of substance abuse problems for several decades (e.g., Azrin 1976), the recent work of Higgins and associates (1991, 1993, 1994) has rekindled enthusiasm for this strategy. Specifically, this group incorporates a monetary-based point system with which cocaine-dependent patients earn a progressively greater number of points for each consecutive negative urine specimen. Points that are earned are used for purchase of retail items; at no point does cash change hands. In one study (Higgins et al. 1994), a maximum of $997.50 could be earned during 12 weeks of treatment. Although some professionals have concerns about "paying" chemically dependent patients to remain abstinent, the fact remains that such contingency-management interventions consistently increase the success of treatment programs. Alternative contingency-management interventions have used desired interpersonal activities (McCrady et al. 1986) or liberalization of methadone dosing policies (Stitzer et al. 1992) as reinforcers.

Relapse-Prevention Strategies

Helping patients achieve abstinence or sobriety is only half the work: virtually all recently abstinent individuals are at incredibly high risk for relapse (Daley 1989; Marlatt and Gordon 1985). Most cognitive-behavioral strategies incorporate explicit relapse-prevention strategies. A significant amount of therapy thus is spent 1) helping patients learn to recognize high-risk stimuli (including the classic triad of persons, places, and things, as well as relevant thoughts and images) that activate automatic thoughts and cravings/urges, and 2) practicing alternative ways of coping. Intervention may be targeted at a number of levels. For example, activity scheduling of "healthy" lifestyle activities may serve to decrease the probability of exposure to high-risk stimuli. Self-directed relaxation or some other distraction strategy may be used to help patients dampen uncomfortable urges. Relaxation-based counterconditioning strategies may also be used to help desensitize patients to exposure to high-risk stimuli (e.g., O'Brien et al. 1990). A cognitive approach may be used to enhance recognition of facilitative or permissive beliefs and to practice alternative coping self-statements. Conversely, role playing and behavioral rehearsal strategies may be used to help patients gain greater self-efficacy about being able to refuse partaking (Monti et al. 1989). Cognitive and behavioral strategies also may be taught, proactively, to help patients who have lapsed disengage from a downward spiral before entering into a full-blown relapse. No single intervention typically suffices, and, as in other skill-based approaches to complex human problems, the patient is well served by learning several different relapse-prevention strategies and practicing them extensively.

A hallmark of cognitive-behavioral therapies is that skills learned by the patient during sessions are viewed as strategies that can be used for a lifetime. Thus, it is the therapist's job to encourage patients to "adopt" these activities as their own, to practice them frequently, and to elaborate upon them through development of a personalized coping or self-help plan. Although confirmatory empirical data are not yet available, clinical experience suggests that patients who continue to use such a self-help program after termination may have the best chance for long-term abstinence.

Management of Psychiatric Comorbidity

A major potential advantage for the model of CBT developed by Beck and colleagues (1993) is its adaptability for use with patients suffering from comorbid depression and anxiety. Modules for management of dysphoria, anhedonia, inactivity, insomnia, generalized anxiety, procrastination, panic attacks, and symptoms associated with posttraumatic stress syndromes may be drawn from extant treatment manuals (e.g., Beck and Emery 1985; Beck et al. 1979) and implemented as needed for comorbid Axis I and II symptomatology. It is important to keep in mind that such patients typically require more frequent and/or longer sessions, specifically because the "curriculum" of therapy needs to be more encompassing. When the severity of psychiatric symptomatology is marked or when the proper treatment of an Axis I disorder mandates it, concomitant pharmacotherapy is added to the treatment plan. Populations for whom the combination of CBT and pharmacotherapy could be considered include all patients with bipolar disorder and schizophrenia, most patients with obsessive-compulsive disorder, and many patients with depressive symptoms in the upper half of the severity continuum.

Research Findings

Cognitive-behavioral therapy and related therapeutic strategies are gaining increasing credibility for treatment of alcoholism, heroin addiction, and cocaine addiction (Beck et al. 1993; Woody et al. 1995). However, much work remains to be done, and a majority of substance-abusing patients enrolled in clinical trials either drop out of therapy or fail to achieve sobriety or abstinence. Nevertheless, a fairly consistent pattern of results has emerged: a substantial portion of patients with substance abuse disorders improve significantly as a result of cognitive and behavioral therapies, and these effects are often over and above those attributable to nonspecific supportive interventions or attention-placebo conditions (Carroll et al. 1994a; Higgins et al. 1993; Kadden et al. 1989; Monti et al. 1993; Woody et al. 1983). Moreover, although the results of contingency-based behavioral treatments may lessen after reinforcements for abstinence have been faded (e.g., Higgins et al. 1994), treatment programs that emphasize development of coping skills or cognitively oriented relapse-prevention techniques may have additional, late-emerging benefits after termination of therapy (Carroll et al. 1994a, 1994b; Cooney et al. 1991).

At this time, several lines of evidence indicate that cognitive-behavioral therapies may provide incremental benefit for at least a subset of chemically dependent patients vis-à-vis conventional models of counseling. In an early randomized clinical trial conducted by Woody and colleagues (1984), professional psychotherapy, as operationalized by Beck et al.'s model of CBT and the psychodynamically oriented supportive expressive psychotherapy (SEP), were specifically more effective than drug counseling in a subset of opiate-addicted individuals characterized by higher levels of pretreatment "psychiatric symptomatology." Heroin-addicted individuals with low levels of pretreatment anxiety and depression benefited as much from the less expensive counseling intervention. Preliminary analyses of a recently completed multicenter clinical trial sponsored by the National Institute on Alcoholism and Alcohol Abuse (Project MATCH 1993) also reportedly show a slight advantage for CBT (relative to counseling and a briefer motivational intervention) in alcoholic patients with higher levels of pretreatment symptomatology.

Although the presence of more severe psychiatric symptoms may predict a greater benefit for patients with professional psychotherapy (i.e., either cognitive-behavioral or psychodynamically oriented psychotherapy), the work of Beutler (1979) suggests that a second variable, *coping style,* may identify which patients are most likely to respond to these very different professional psychotherapies. Beutler marshaled evidence to suggest that patients with more externalizing (i.e., sociopathic) coping styles fared better with more behaviorally oriented treatments, whereas patients with more internalizing coping styles were more likely to benefit from verbal-expressive therapies. Consistent with this, Kadden and co-workers (1989) found that alcoholic patients with high scores on a self-report measure of sociopathy responded better to coping skills therapy than to an interactional model of treatment. This finding is particularly salient because sociopathy is an important predictor of poor therapy outcomes (e.g., Woody et al. 1985).

An ongoing multicenter clinical trial sponsored by the National Institute on Drug Abuse is examining treatments of cocaine addiction. CBT is being compared with a psychodynamically based intervention, SEP, individual drug counseling (IDC), and a low-contact control condition consisting of group drug counseling (Crits-Christoph et al., in press). Final results of the full-scale clinical trial will not be available until 1998. However, a glimpse of the anticipated results may be obtained from analyses of outcomes from the pilot, or training, phase of the project. Overall, the treatments were not significantly different with respect to effects on cocaine intake and related difficulties. However, in the subset of patients with a higher pretreatment level of psychiatric severity, those treated with CBT and SEP benefited more than those who received drug counseling. Further, as was suggested by Beutler (1979), there was a trend for patients with comorbid antisocial personality disorder to respond better to CBT than to SEP. Interpretation of these very preliminary findings from the pilot phase of an ongoing trial warrant caution, particularly because all therapists were still receiving training.

To date, the model of CBT developed by Beck and colleagues (1993) has not been formally paired with the contingency-management approach of Higgins and colleagues (1993, 1994). This combined approach may hold particular promise in that contingency management may foster enhanced retention and offer a greater chance of achieving abstinence, whereas CBT may offer improved coping and relapse-prevention skills for use after the contingencies have been faded.

Conclusions

Cognitive-behavioral therapy offers a comprehensive model of understanding addictive behavior and a coherent, active approach to treatment. It is used for both inpatients and outpatients, with individuals and groups, and singly and in combination with appropriate pharmacotherapies. Moreover, CBT is fully compatible with self-help interventions such as AA. Cognitive-behavioral models of treatment of substance abuse disorders are still in relatively early stages of development. Available evidence indicates that a significant number of patients who enter substance abuse treatment with CBT will benefit from therapy and that those with more marked psychopathology may derive greater benefit from CBT than from other more traditional models of counseling or therapy. As expertise mounts and further refinements are implemented, it is likely that even more promising models of CBT will help an even greater number of chemically dependent individuals.

References

American Psychiatric Association: Diagnostic and Statistical Manual of Mental Disorders, 4th Edition. Washington, DC, American Psychiatric Association, 1994

American Psychiatric Association: Practice guideline for the treatment of patients with substance use disorders: alcohol, cocaine, opioids. Am J Psychiatry 152(suppl):1–59, 1995

Azrin NH: Improvements in the community-reinforcement approach to alcoholism. Behav Res Ther 14:339–348, 1976

Beck AT: Cognitive Therapy and the Emotional Disorders. New York, International Universities Press, 1976

Beck AT, Rush AJ, Shaw BF, et al: Cognitive Therapy of Depression. New York, Guilford, 1979

Beck AT, Emery G, Greenberg RL: Anxiety Disorders and Phobias: A Cognitive Perspective. New York, Basic Books, 1985

Beck AT, Freeman A, and Associates: Cognitive Therapy of Personality Disorders. New York, Guilford, 1990

Beck AT, Wright FD, Newman CF, et al: Cognitive Therapy of Substance Abuse. New York, Guilford, 1993

Beutler LE: Toward specific psychological therapies for specific conditions. J Consult Clin Psychol 47:882–897, 1979

Booth BM, Russell DW, Soucek S, et al: Social support and outcome of alcoholism treatment: an exploratory analysis. Am J Drug Alcohol Abuse 18:87–101, 1992

Carroll KM, Rounsaville BJ, Gordon LT, et al: Psychotherapy and pharmacotherapy for ambulatory cocaine abusers. Arch Gen Psychiatry 51:177–187, 1994a

Carroll KM, Rounsaville BJ, Nich C, et al: One-year follow-up of psychotherapy and pharmacotherapy for cocaine dependence. Arch Gen Psychiatry 51:989–997, 1994b

Cawthra E, Borrego N, Emrick C: Involving family members in the prevention of relapse: an innovative approach. Alcoholism Treatment Quarterly 8:101–112, 1991

Cooney NL, Kadden RM, Litt MD, et al: Matching alcoholics to coping skills or interactional therapies: two-year follow-up results. J Consult Clin Psychol 59:598–601, 1991

Crits-Christoph P, Siqueland L, Blaine J, et al: The NIDA Cocaine Collaborative: rationale and methods. Arch Gen Psychiatry (in press)

Curry S, Marlatt GA, Gordon JR: Abstinence violation effect: validation of an attributional construct with smoking cessation. J Consult Clin Psychol 55:145–149, 1987

Daley DC: Relapse: Conceptual, Research, and Clinical Perspectives. New York, Haworth Press, 1989

Glantz M, Pickens R: Vulnerability of Drug Abuse. Washington, DC, American Psychological Association, 1992

Higgins ST, Delaney DD, Budney AJ, et al: A behavioral approach to achieving initial cocaine abstinence. Am J Psychiatry 148:1218–1224, 1991

Higgins ST, Budney AJ, Bickel WK, et al: Achieving cocaine abstinence with a behavioral approach. Am J Psychiatry 150:763–769, 1993

Higgins ST, Budney AJ, Bickel WK, et al: Incentives improve outcome in outpatient behavioral treatment of cocaine dependence. Arch Gen Psychiatry 51:568–576, 1994

Institute of Medicine: Broadening the Base of Treatment for Alcohol Problems. Washington, DC, National Academy Press, 1990

Kadden RM, Getter H, Cooney HL, et al: Matching alcoholics to coping skills or interactional therapies: posttreatment results. J Consult Clin Psychol 57:698–704, 1989

Kessler RC, McGonagle KA, Zhao S, et al: Lifetime and 12-month prevalence of DSM-III-R psychiatric disorders in the United States: results from the National Comorbidity Survey. Arch Gen Psychiatry 51:8–19, 1994

Khantzian EJ: The self-medication hypothesis of addictive disorders: focus on heroin and cocaine dependence. Am J Psychiatry 142:1259–1264, 1985

Marlatt GA, Gordon JR: Relapse Prevention: Maintenance Strategies in the Treatment of Addictive Behaviors. New York, Guilford, 1985

McCrady BS, Noel NE, Abrams DB, et al: Comparative effectiveness of three types of spouse involvement in outpatient behavioral alcoholism treatment. J Stud Alcohol 47:459–467, 1986

McLellan AT, Luborsky L, O'Brien CP, et al: Is treatment for substance abuse effective? JAMA 247:1423–1428, 1982

McLellan AT, Kushner H, Metzger D, et al: The fifth edition of the Addiction Severity Index. J Subst Abuse Treat 9:199–212, 1992

McLellan AT, Arndt IO, Metzger DS, et al: The effects of psychosocial services in substance abuse treatment. JAMA 269:1953–1959, 1993

Miller WR, Rollnick S: Motivational Interviewing, New York, Guilford, 1991

Monti PM, Abrams DB, Kadden RM: Treating alcohol dependence. New York, Guilford, 1989

Monti PM, Rohsenow DJ, Rubonis AV, et al: Cue exposure with coping skills treatment for male alcoholics: a preliminary investigation. J Consult Clin Psychol 61:1011–1019, 1993

Nace EP, Davis CW, Gaspari JP: Axis-II comorbidity in substance abusers. Am J Psychiatry 148:118–120, 1991

Nezu AM, Nezu CM, Perri MG: Problem-Solving Therapy for Depression: Theory, Research, and Clinical Guidelines. New York, Wiley, 1989

O'Brien CP: Conditioned responses, craving, relapse, and addiction. Facts About Drugs and Alcohol 1:1–3, 1992

O'Brien CP, Childress AR, McLellan T, et al: Integrating systemic cue exposure with standard treatment in recovering drug-dependent patients. Addict Behav 15:355–365, 1990

Persons JB: Cognitive Therapy in Practice: A Case Formulation Approach. New York, WW Norton, 1989

Poldrugo F, Forti B: Personality disorders and alcoholism treatment outcome. Drug Alcohol Depend 21:171–176, 1988

Prochaska JO, DiClemente CC, Norcross JC: In search of how people change: applications to addictive behaviors. Am Psychol 47:1102–1114, 1992

Project MATCH (Matching Alcoholism Treatment to Client Heterogeneity): Rationale and methods for a multisite clinical trial matching patients to alcoholism treatment. Alcohol Clin Exp Res 17:1130–1145, 1993

Rae JB: The influence of the wives on the treatment outcome of alcoholics: a follow-up study at two years. Br J Psychiatry 120:601–613, 1972

Regier DA, Farmer ME, Rae DS, et al: Comorbidity of mental disorders with alcohol and other drug abuse: results from the Epidemiologic Catchment Area (ECA) Study. JAMA 264:2511–2518, 1990

Schwartz RM, Garamoni GL: A structural model of positive and negative states of mind: asymmetry in the internal dialogue, in Advances in Cognitive-Behavioral Research and Therapy, Vol 5. Edited by Kendall PC. New York, Academic Press, 1986, pp 1–62

Stitzer ML, Iguchi MY, Felch LJ: Contingent take-home incentive: effects on drug use of methadone maintenance patients. J Consult Clin Psychol 60:927–934 [B], 1992

Thase ME: Transition and aftercare, in Cognitive Therapy With Inpatients: Developing a Cognitive Milieu. Edited by Wright JH, Thase ME, Beck AT, et al. New York, Guilford, 1992, pp 414–435

Thase ME, Beck AT: An overview of cognitive therapy, in Cognitive Therapy With Inpatients: Developing a Cognitive Milieu. Edited by Wright JH, Thase ME, Beck AT, et al. New York, Guilford, 1992, pp 3–34

Thase ME, Wright JH: Cognitive behavior therapy manual for depressed inpatients: a treatment protocol outline. Behavior Therapy 22:579–595, 1991

Woody GE, Luborsky L, McLellan AT, et al: Psychotherapy for opiate addicts: does it help? Arch Gen Psychiatry 40:639–645, 1983

Woody GE, McLellan AT, Luborsky L, et al: Severity of psychiatric symptoms as a predictor of benefits from psychotherapy: the Veterans Administration–Penn Study. Am J Psychiatry 141:1172–1177, 1984

Woody GE, McLellan AT, Luborsky L, et al: Sociopathy and psychotherapy outcome. Arch Gen Psychiatry 42:1081–1086, 1985

Woody GE, Mercer DE, Luborsky L: Individual psychotherapy for substance use disorders, in Treatments of Psychiatric Disorders, Vol 1. Gabbard GO, Editor-in-Chief. Washington, DC, American Psychiatric Press, 1995, pp 801–811

Chapter 3

Cognitive Approaches to Personality Disorders

Judith S. Beck, Ph.D.

Patients with personality disorders can be complex, perplexing, and challenging to the clinician. They often have difficulty forming a therapeutic alliance, being goal directed, and following through with assignments. At times they seem purposely to thwart the clinician's attempts to ameliorate their distress, with the clinician being left to ponder why these patients behave so nonadaptively.

A. T. Beck (in press) theorizes that the kind of behavioral strategies observed in patients with personality disorders may at some point have been evolutionarily adaptive. Some individuals undoubtedly would not have survived in prehistoric times had they not been overly endowed with traits of aggressiveness, competitiveness, suspiciousness, avoidance, dependence, or compulsiveness. The exaggerated and inflexible representation of these traits, whether due to genetic overendowment, learning, or both, may be disadvantageous to many people in our current society.

Personality disorders are, according to DSM-IV (American Psychiatric Association 1994), characterized by "an enduring pattern of inner experience and behavior that deviates markedly from the expectations of the individual's culture, is pervasive and inflexible, has an onset in adolescence or early adulthood, is stable over time, and leads to distress or impairment" (p. 629). This "enduring pattern of inner experience and behavior" may be considered to consist of the beliefs, the characteristic thinking and emotional reactions across situations, and the behavioral repertoire acquired during the developmental period. Personality traits, as defined in DSM-IV, are "enduring patterns of perceiving, relating to, and thinking about the environment and oneself that are exhibited in a wide range of social and personal contexts" (p. 630). Individuals with better-adjusted personalities have personality traits that are not rigidly fixed; they process information more adaptively and can utilize a broader set of behavioral strategies according to the demands of the situation and their own personal goals.

A careful diagnostic evaluation and history aids the clinician in differentiating Axis I and Axis II disorders. During severe depression, for example, patients may display maladaptive strategies, such as relying heavily on others, avoiding many activities, or resisting the therapist's attempts to mobilize them. They may also hold global, negative beliefs, characterizing themselves as helpless, unlovable, or both. If, however, their dysfunctional behavior and beliefs were not present to a significant degree in the premorbid period, the diagnosis of a comorbid Axis II disorder should not be made. Further, it is expected that once the Axis I disorder remits, the patient will return to his or her previous, relatively adaptive manner of functioning. Axis II disorders are marked by pervasive, chronic, enduring dysfunction across situations and time, whereas Axis I disorders are usually more acute and episodic.

Pretzer and A. T. Beck (1996) note that a concurrent Axis II disorder can have a significant impact on the clinical presentation, development, and course of an Axis I disorder. Millon (1996) suggests that an Axis II disorder "creates, by definition, a psychic vulnerability that not only disposes the individual to the development of an Axis I disorder, but also complicates the course of that disorder once it, in fact, exists" (p. 173).

A significant number of patients in clinical samples are diagnosed with personality disorders. Turkat and Maisto (1985) found that up to half of the patients seen at some clinical centers have personality disorders. A study examining both inpatients and outpatients who were treated for psychiatric problems at a large medical center showed that about one-third had one or more personality disorders (Koenigsberg et al. 1985). More recent surveys confirm such high Axis I–Axis II comorbidity (see, e.g., Millon 1996).

Patients with Axis I disorder and comorbid personality disorder usually experience a poorer response to treatment than patients with Axis I disorder alone. According to Reich and Green (1991), the literature on outcome studies for both inpatients and outpatients with Axis I disorders using many different treatment approaches indicates that patients with personality pathology show significantly poorer outcome with pharmacotherapy, psychotherapy, or both, as compared with patients without Axis II pathology. Gunderson and Phillips (1995) reported that the use of medication for patients with Axis II disorders, while widespread, has not been demonstrated to have "extensive or predictable effects" (p. 1433). Similarly, Mays and Franks (1985) found the presence of a concurrent personality disorder to be a major factor in ineffective or negative outcomes for traditional psychotherapy.

Only a few controlled research studies have been conducted investigating the efficacy of cognitive therapy for personality disorders, and most of these have looked at the effect of an Axis II diagnosis on the outcome of treatment for an Axis I disorder. Some investigators have found that Axis I patients with comorbid personality disorders do not respond to cognitive-behavioral treatment as well as patients without a concurrent Axis II diagnosis (Stiles 1991; Turner 1987). Persons and co-workers (1988) found a higher dropout rate in patients with Axis II disorders when compared with patients with no Axis II diagnosis.

In contrast, Shea and co-workers (1990), in examining the results of the National Institute of Mental Health Treatment of Depression Collaborative Research Program, found that personality disorder patients in the cognitive-behavioral therapy modality did not have a worse outcome than those without a personality disorder (though they did in the other treatment conditions). Stuart and colleagues (1992) similarly found equal responses to cognitive therapy in depressed patients with or without Axis II comorbidity. Woody and co-workers (1985) found that patients with concurrent diagnoses of opiate dependence, depression, and antisocial personality disorder improved significantly with a combined short-term course of cognitive therapy and methadone maintenance program (though patients without a comorbid depressive diagnosis had a poorer outcome). Other investigators have found that anxious patients with concurrent Axis II diagnoses who completed cognitive-behavioral treatment showed significant improvement (Arntz and Dreessen 1990; Sanderson et al. 1994).

A few controlled outcome studies on cognitive or cognitive-behavioral therapy for patients with personality disorder have been reported. Linehan (1991) found a favorable response for borderline personality disorder (BPD). Stravynski and co-workers (1982) found social skills training alone to be as effective for avoidant personality patients as social skills training with the addition of one cognitive strategy (i.e., disputing beliefs). Pretzer (1994), in a review of the literature on behavior therapy for personality disorders, describes the findings as encouraging but notes that there have not yet been sufficient studies to draw firm conclusions.

There have also been a small number of uncontrolled clinical reports and single-case design studies investigating the efficacy of cognitive therapy for personality disorders. Pretzer and A. T. Beck (1996) reported that in general these studies indicate a positive trend and that cognitive therapy is a promising approach. A. T. Beck and associates (1990) concluded that "standard" cognitive therapy for depression and anxiety has limited effectiveness for patients with Axis II disorders and that a modified, more comprehensive approach is required for this difficult population. Young (1990) describes common difficulties in using standard cognitive therapy for patients with personality disorders. Patients with Axis II disorders may not have easy access to their feelings, thoughts, or images; they may have difficulty focusing on specific problems or collaborating with the therapist in working on their problems; they may be unmotivated to do homework; and they certainly demonstrate great difficulty in modifying their very strong, rigid beliefs.

Patients with Axis II pathology often hold beliefs that interfere with therapy when they first enter treatment. Patients with Axis I disorders uncomplicated by Axis II pathology often display a positive, adaptive bias, holding beliefs such as "My therapist will probably help," "I can make changes," and "I will get better." In contrast, patients with Axis II pathology, with or without Axis I disorder, usually hold a less adaptive set of beliefs. Obsessive-compulsive personality disorder patients, for example, may believe that their therapist will try to control them, thereby making them too vulnerable. Narcissistic patients may respond to their therapist's failure to grant them special favors with a sense of being treated as unspecial, as "a nobody." Schizotypal patients may fear their therapist is "out to get them." Thus, patients with Axis II disorders who may engage in therapy for treatment of an Axis I disorder pose special challenges to the therapist when their characteristically dysfunctional ways of reacting to others appear in the therapeutic relationship.

Behavioral Strategies

Perhaps the most striking feature of patients with personality disorders is the relatively impoverished set of behavioral strategies from which they can draw. They consistently and compulsively overutilize certain behaviors even when these modes of functioning are clearly disadvantageous and lead to significant distress to themselves and/or others.

Avoidant patients, for example, may refrain from revealing their dysfunctional thoughts and beliefs in therapy. Dependent patients may rely too heavily on the therapist and fail to take steps to get better on their own. Antisocial patients may turn away the therapist's genuine attempts to help and instead exploit the therapist in some way. Histrionic patients may regale the therapist with interesting tales instead of collaborating to solve their difficulties. The same characteristic patterns of functioning that these patients display inside the office are utilized repeatedly and disadvantageously across situations and across time, with resultant distress to themselves or others.

It should be noted that an individual with a healthy personality uses identical behavioral strategies at times (e.g., avoidance, dependence, dramatics, suspiciousness) when it is adaptive to do so. Personality disorder patients, however, locked into a more narrow set of behaviors, do not have free reign to select from a larger repertoire.

A. T. Beck and associates (1990) have identified both the overutilized set of behavioral strategies of personality disorder patients and the strategies in which these patients are deficient. Histrionic patients are relatively unskilled at moderating their responses. Avoidant patients have a deficiency in sociability. Schizoid patients find it difficult to develop intimacy and to experience warm feelings toward others. Antisocial patients lack empathy and a desire to help others altruistically. Obsessive-compulsive personality disorder patients are underdeveloped in impulsivity. Dependent patients lack self-sufficiency. Paranoid patients and schizotypal patients have a deficiency in trusting others. Narcissistic patients are intolerant of being regarded as equal to others instead of special. Finally, patients with borderline personality disorder (BPD) lack several of the behavioral patterns listed above or use them maladaptively.

Core Beliefs

Patients with Axis II pathology characteristically have globally negative beliefs about themselves, their worlds, and other people. Individuals with a healthy personality, in contrast, have stable, adaptive, relativistic beliefs ("I am reasonably competent and lovable," "My world has some danger and some safety in it," "Other people may be beneficent, neutral, or malevolent"). When their global, negative beliefs ("I am incapable," "The world is out of my control," "Other people will hurt me") are triggered, personality disorder patients view situations in a negative, extreme manner even if circumstances do not warrant such a view. Even when there is strong evidence to the contrary, they act and react as if their perceptions are accurate, because of a perceptual bias that interferes with adaptive information processing (Pretzer and A. T. Beck 1996).

A paranoid patient, for example, became highly anxious when his doctor proposed he receive a certain medical test and rejected the suggestion out-of-hand because his beliefs "I am vulnerable" and "Others may hurt me" became activated. A dependent patient in a similar situation failed to ask her doctor questions to ascertain the reasonableness of a major medical procedure because of her belief "I am inadequate." In situations that impinge on their vulnerabilities, personality disorder patients often fail to assess and process information correctly and to respond adaptively. They usually selectively attend to, distort, store, and retrieve information in a dysfunctional way.

The rigidity and inflexibility of beliefs are maintained by the patients' failure to accommodate new data in an adaptive manner. An avoidant patient, for example, discounted his neighbor's kind remarks, believing he must have fooled her into viewing him in a positive way. A narcissistic patient did not recognize that co-workers were regarding her positively when they treated her as "one of the gang." Individuals with relatively healthier personalities assimilate new information more appropriately, adjusting their core beliefs to match reality more closely, and develop a wider range of behavioral patterns, varying their behavior when it is beneficial for them to do so.

Although individuals have innumerable beliefs, A. T. Beck (in press) proposes that pinpointing the core beliefs about the self is crucial in conceptualizing personality disorder patients. These negative beliefs may be categorized in two realms: beliefs associated with helplessness (e.g., "I am incompetent," "I am vulnerable," "I am weak") and beliefs associated with unlovability ("I'm bad," "I'm defective," "I'm not good enough to be loved"). Because these beliefs are distressing to patients, they develop strategies to help them cope with or prevent the activation of these painful ideas.

Interaction of Beliefs and Behavioral Strategies

When the very rigid, negative core beliefs of personality disorder patients are activated, these patients experience intense emotional pain. As a result, they develop a series of assumptions to guide their behavior in an effort to forestall core belief activation. Antisocial personality disorder patients, for example, have core beliefs that they are weak or vulnerable and that others are hostile, demeaning, or exploitative. They develop guidelines for themselves to avoid exposure to their own weakness: "If I exploit others first, I'll make out okay" and "If I don't [exploit first], others will harm me." A major behavioral strategy for these patients, therefore, is to seek opportunities to take advantage of others. Dependent patients view themselves as fundamentally incapable and see other people as their lifeline. Their typical assumptions are "If I rely on others, I'll be okay" and "If I try to rely on myself, I'll fail." Understanding the beliefs patients hold about themselves and others and the assumptions they develop to get along in the world helps to explain why these patients act so dysfunctionally at times. A simplified description of the core beliefs, assumptions, and compensatory strategies for each personality disorder is presented in Table 3–1.

Schemas

Beliefs and strategies are embedded in mental structures, *schemas*, that allow the individual to process information, derive meaning from their experiences, and select behavioral responses (A. T. Beck 1964). Because the schemas of patients with personality disorders are dysfunctionally broad, rigid, and prominent, they become activated in a wide range of circumstances, and this leads patients to misinterpret information, become disproportionately emotionally aroused, and act maladaptively. A schizotypal patient entering a benign social situation, for example, had an activation of a dysfunctional schema in which he perceived threat, began to believe (inaccurately) that others were viewing him as defective, had an emotional (and physiological) reaction of anxiety, felt an intense desire to avoid, and mobilized himself to flee. When a BPD patient's therapist began to set limits in a therapy session, a dysfunctional schema became activated. The patient interpreted the therapist's behavior as punishment, began to view herself as "bad," had an emotional reaction of hurt and then anger, became physiologically aroused, experienced a desire to lash out, and then verbally assaulted the therapist.

Young (1990) describes three characteristic processes of schemas in personality disorder patients. In *schema maintenance*, the individual processes information in such a way as to reinforce the schema. (Every time the dependent patient relies on someone else, his belief about being helpless is strengthened.) In *schema avoidance*, the individual avoids thinking about or engaging in activities that might trigger the schema. (The avoidant patient avoids participating in or even thinking about situations that evoke her fears of rejection.) In *schema compensation*, the patient consistently acts in a way contrary to what might be expected from the schema. (The narcissistic patient continually attempts to get others to treat him in a special way.)

Layden and co-workers (1993) describe an additional characteristic of schemas in some BPD patients. Antagonistic beliefs (e.g., about dependence and mistrust) may be simultaneously activated. The BPD patient may strongly believe she or he needs another person to survive and yet at the same time believe that it is dangerous to trust the other person. Understanding conflicting beliefs helps therapist and patient grasp more clearly the strong ambivalence and seemingly contradictory behavior of the BPD patient in certain situations.

Often personality disorder patients seek to create a niche where the hidden fears they hold about themselves will not come true. Narcissistic patients invite flattery and demand entitlement to avoid feeling unspecial. Schizoid patients seek solitary living and work environments. Dependent patients seek out significant others who will take care of them. Obsessive-compulsive personality disorder patients organize and structure their environment and exert as much control over themselves and others as they can. However, these compensatory strategies often fail, activating the schema and evoking stress. Failure of these behavioral patterns to avoid activation of the negative beliefs may then contribute to the development of an Axis I (syndromal) disorder.

Developmental Contributions

The dysfunctional beliefs of patients with personality disorders usually originate in childhood experiences. As the child develops and starts to organize his or her experience, he or she begins to form basic understandings of self, world, and others. Children who grow up without personality disorders are able to assimilate both positive and negative data and develop balanced, stable views. In contrast, personality disorder patients usually have had traumatic childhoods, during which

Table 3–1. Personality disorders: beliefs and strategies

Personality disorder	Core belief about self	Belief about others	Assumptions	Behavioral strategy
Avoidant	I'm undesirable.	Other people will reject me.	If people know the real me, they'll reject me. If I put on a facade, they may accept me.	Avoid intimacy.
Dependent	I'm helpless.	Other people should take care of me.	If I rely on myself, I'll fail. If I depend on others, I'll survive.	Rely on other people.
Obsessive-compulsive	My world can go out of control.	Other people can be irresponsible.	If I'm not totally responsible, my world could fall apart. If I impose rigid rules and structure, things will turn out okay.	Control others rigidly.
Paranoid	I'm vulnerable.	Other people are malicious.	If I trust other people, they will harm me. If I am on my guard, I can protect myself.	Be overly suspicious.
Antisocial	I'm vulnerable.	Other people are potentially exploitative.	If I don't act first, I can be hurt. If I can exploit first, I can be on top.	Exploit others.

Disorder	View of self	View of others	Conditional beliefs	Strategy
Narcissistic	I'm inferior. (The manifest compensatory belief is I'm superior.)	Other people are superior. (The manifest compensatory belief is others are inferior.)	If others regard me in a nonspecial way, it means they consider me inferior. If I achieve my entitlements, it shows I'm special.	Demand special treatment.
Histrionic	I'm nothing.	Other people may not value me for myself alone.	If I am not entertaining, others won't be attracted to me. If I am dramatic, I'll get others' attention and approval.	Entertain.
Schizoid	I'm a social misfit.	Other people have nothing to offer me.	If I keep my distance from others, I'll make out better. If I try to have relationships, they won't work out.	Distance self from others.
Schizotypal	I am defective.	Other people are threatening.	If I sense that others are feeling negatively toward me, it must be true. If I'm wary of others, I can divine their true intentions.	Assume hidden motives.
Borderline personality disorder	I'm defective. I'm helpless. I'm vulnerable. I'm bad.	Other people will abandon me. People can't be trusted.	If I depend on myself, I won't survive. If I trust others, they'll abandon me. If I depend on others, I'll survive but ultimately be abandoned.	Vacillate in extremes of behavior.

Source. Adapted from Beck AT, Freeman A, and Associates: *Cognitive Therapy of Personality Disorders*. New York, Guilford, 1990.

they developed distinctly negative views of themselves and others. These views may or may not have been valid to some degree at the time. However, the beliefs persist into adult life, when they are generally not realistic or accurate and lead patients to perceive situations in a distorted way. These distorted perceptions, in turn, result in dysfunctional emotional and behavioral reactions (J. S. Beck 1996).

The trauma that children who later develop personality disorders experience may be blatant (e.g., sexual, physical, verbal abuse). It also can be more subtle but persistent and chronic (e.g., punitive caregivers; highly critical family members, teachers, or peers; demeaning or harsh people to whom the child is continually exposed). Many adults who experienced early trauma, however, do not develop personality disorders. A. T. Beck (in press) has theorized that some children may be genetically predisposed to developing characterological difficulties and/or lack strong, supportive adults to buffer their negative childhood experiences.

As children process these negative experiences, their negative views become more solidified and their tendency to distort information increases. They begin to interpret smaller negative events as broad, global confirmation of their core beliefs. For example, a child who fails a school test overgeneralizes that she is a failure as a person. Another child interprets mistreatment by a few peers as evidence that he is a wholly defective person. In addition, these children either fail to recognize positive events contrary to the core belief or discount these data. For example, the child who tends to view himself as unlovable may not notice that some children are friendly to him or may discount their actions ("Jon is nice to me, but that's only because he's my neighbor"; "Louise probably asked me to come to her house because she couldn't find anyone else to play with"). Negative core beliefs become solidified over time as the child continues to assimilate negatively perceived data quite readily while failing to incorporate positive data in a straightforward way.

Dysfunctional beliefs and strategies are idiosyncratic to the individual. Two children in a similar situation may, therefore, react in very different ways. A child with a learning disability, for example, may begin to believe strongly that he is incapable; he may then develop a pattern of giving up whenever tasks are even a little difficult and relying too heavily on others for help. If these beliefs and behavioral patterns persist into adulthood without counterbalancing positive beliefs and more functional strategies, this child may develop a dependent personality disorder. Another child with a similar learning disability may overcompensate for feelings of inadequacy and drive himself very hard to succeed. Padesky (1986) notes that some patients' beliefs and compensatory strategies may have been adaptive when they were first developed, but bring considerable distress later on.

Reactions to Current Situations

The beliefs of personality disorder patients lead them to perceive and interpret situations in extreme ways. Their interpretations, in turn, influence how they react emotionally, physiologically, and behaviorally.

When their core beliefs are activated, personality disorder patients react with a great deal of emotion. Their thinking style becomes much more primitive, polarized, and global. Seemingly small events can trigger a great deal of anguish because of the meanings these patients attach to them. The kind of reaction varies according to the patients' construction of situations.

An avoidant patient, for example, perceives that he is being ignored by a sales clerk in a clothing store. He thinks, "She doesn't want to wait on me"; has an activation of his core belief "I'm worthless"; feels deeply humiliated; turns red; droops his head; and leaves the store, promising himself he will shop for clothes only through a catalog from now on. A narcissistic patient derives a different meaning from the same situation. She has an activation of her core belief "I'm unimportant"; thinks, "Who does that sales clerk think she is, treating me this way"; feels extremely hurt and angry; clenches her fists; experiences tightness in her arms, shoulders, and chest; loudly lambastes the clerk; and demands to see the manager in order to get the clerk fired. When the manager tells the personality disorder patient that she is overreacting, her core belief gets increasingly activated, and her dysfunctional overreaction increases. The sales clerk, it should be noted, may or may not have actually or purposely ignored these patients. Personality disorder patients are acutely sensitive to situations relevant to their vulnerabilities. They are hypervigilant for signs that could possibly confirm their beliefs and thus tend at times to misread nonthreatening or neutral situations as quite negative or potentially harmful.

Other people in personality disorder patients' milieus usually perceive this characteristic overreaction, and many personality disorder patients, too, recognize that their cognitive, emotional, and behavioral reactions are more extreme than those of others. This realization further reinforces their notion that there is something wrong with them. Their core belief gets strengthened by their initial interpretation of events and by a secondary interpretation of their own reaction.

A *cognitive conceptualization diagram* (see Figure 3–1 for form with instructions and Figure 3–2 for an example of completed form) helps clinician and patient understand the connection between reactions to current situations and underlying beliefs and compensatory strategies (J. S. Beck 1995). Using data directly received from the patient about currently distressing situations, the clinician can question further to determine the meaning of the patient's thoughts in order to identify

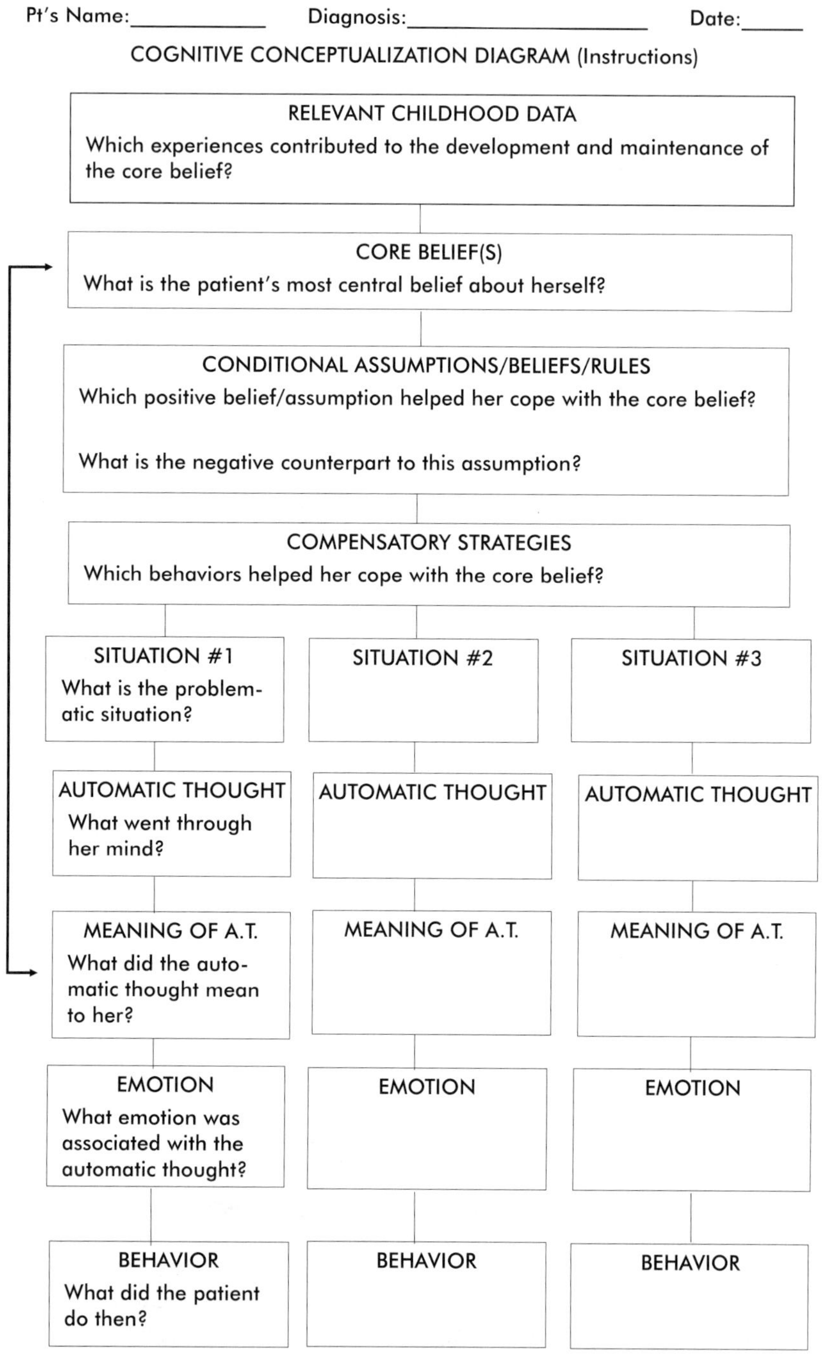

Pt's Name:____________ Diagnosis:____________________ Date:_____
COGNITIVE CONCEPTUALIZATION DIAGRAM (Instructions)
RELEVANT CHILDHOOD DATA
Which experiences contributed to the development and maintenance of the core belief?
CORE BELIEF(S)
What is the patient's most central belief about herself?
CONDITIONAL ASSUMPTIONS/BELIEFS/RULES
Which positive belief/assumption helped her cope with the core belief?
What is the negative counterpart to this assumption?
COMPENSATORY STRATEGIES
Which behaviors helped her cope with the core belief?
SITUATION #1
What is the problematic situation?
SITUATION #2
SITUATION #3
AUTOMATIC THOUGHT
What went through her mind?
AUTOMATIC THOUGHT
AUTOMATIC THOUGHT
MEANING OF A.T.
What did the automatic thought mean to her?
MEANING OF A.T.
MEANING OF A.T.
EMOTION
What emotion was associated with the automatic thought?
EMOTION
EMOTION
BEHAVIOR
What did the patient do then?
BEHAVIOR
BEHAVIOR

Figure 3–1. Cognitive conceptualization diagram (with instructions).
Source. Copyright 1996, J. S. Beck, Ph.D.

COGNITIVE CONCEPTUALIZATION DIAGRAM (Example)

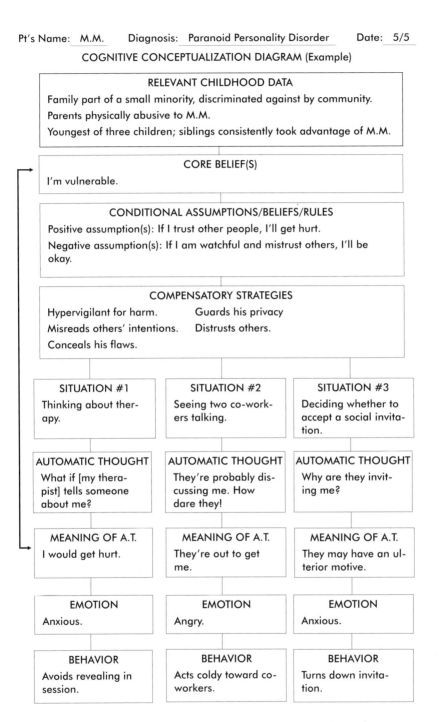

RELEVANT CHILDHOOD DATA
Family part of a small minority, discriminated against by community.
Parents physically abusive to M.M.
Youngest of three children; siblings consistently took advantage of M.M.

CORE BELIEF(S)
I'm vulnerable.

CONDITIONAL ASSUMPTIONS/BELIEFS/RULES
Positive assumption(s): If I trust other people, I'll get hurt.
Negative assumption(s): If I am watchful and mistrust others, I'll be okay.

COMPENSATORY STRATEGIES
Hypervigilant for harm.   Guards his privacy
Misreads others' intentions.   Distrusts others.
Conceals his flaws.

SITUATION #1	SITUATION #2	SITUATION #3
Thinking about therapy.	Seeing two co-workers talking.	Deciding whether to accept a social invitation.
AUTOMATIC THOUGHT	**AUTOMATIC THOUGHT**	**AUTOMATIC THOUGHT**
What if [my therapist] tells someone about me?	They're probably discussing me. How dare they!	Why are they inviting me?
MEANING OF A.T.	**MEANING OF A.T.**	**MEANING OF A.T.**
I would get hurt.	They're out to get me.	They may have an ulterior motive.
EMOTION	**EMOTION**	**EMOTION**
Anxious.	Angry.	Anxious.
BEHAVIOR	**BEHAVIOR**	**BEHAVIOR**
Avoids revealing in session.	Acts coldly toward co-workers.	Turns down invitation.

Figure 3–2. Cognitive conceptualization diagram (example).
Source. Copyright 1996, J. S. Beck, Ph.D.

beliefs that the patient may not have previously articulated. The diagram, properly completed, helps explain why the patient has specific, characteristic reactions.

Treatment

The cognitive therapy approach to patients with personality disorders shares some features with the approach to patients with relatively straightforward Axis I disorders such as depression and anxiety. Sessions tend to be quite structured, unless the patient cannot tolerate such structure. (A histrionic patient, for example, perceived a session as too tightly organized and protested that the therapist did not give her sufficient time to express herself.) Cognitive therapists are usually quite active, though they may initially have to decrease their activity for certain personality disorder patients who negatively interpret their therapists' level of activity as attempts to control them.

In addition, the treatments for both Axis I and Axis II patients share an emphasis on education: instructing patients about the nature of their disorder, about the process of therapy, about the cognitive model, and about their specific cognitive profile. Patients are also taught new techniques to alleviate dysphoria and improve the life skills, social skills, and problem-solving skills in which they have a deficiency. Patient and therapist collaboratively determine how the patient can practice these new skills as homework daily. Guided discovery, in which the therapist questions the patient to identify underlying beliefs, and Socratic questioning, through which the therapist helps the patient examine the validity and utility of the patient's thoughts and assumptions, are standard techniques. Collaboration and a strong therapeutic alliance are essential (though often much more difficult to achieve with personality disorder patients). Finally, relapse prevention is emphasized, as the clinician teaches patients strategies to use both during treatment and after the course of therapy is over).

When patients with personality disorders present for treatment with a comorbid Axis I disorder, the initial focus is on gaining remission of the more acute syndrome. With some patients, only slight variations in treatment are necessary initially. When the Axis I disorder remits, often in 12 sessions or fewer, some patients terminate therapy without having resolved their Axis II issues. Others remain in therapy for a longer period to modify their underlying beliefs and compensatory strategies. A third group of patients generally proves to be more difficult to treat: those whose personality disorder interferes with the standard treatment of their Axis I disorder. They may remain in therapy for many months. For these patients, the treatment itself activates their core beliefs, and modifications of standard cognitive therapy are necessary

(A. T. Beck et al. 1990; J. S. Beck 1996; Freeman et al. 1990; Pretzer and Fleming 1989).

Using the Therapeutic Relationship

Although it is often more difficult to establish a strong therapeutic alliance with personality disorder patients, this challenge can become an opportunity for the clinician. Because it is usually not clear to the clinician at the first interview whether treatment will need to be varied, it is advisable to initiate "standard" cognitive therapy (J. S. Beck 1995) that facilitates symptom reduction as efficiently as possible. However, if the standard approach becomes discomfiting to the patient, the clinician can turn this outcome to an advantage.

First, if the patient becomes distressed by the process of therapy, the clinician can negotiate with him or her to vary the treatment (at least initially). The clinician's flexibility usually strengthens the therapeutic alliance when the patient recognizes that the therapist is on his or her side and genuinely wants to seek ways that therapy can be most helpful. Second, the patient's distress can be used as an opportunity to identify and evaluate automatic thoughts on the spot ("hot" cognitions) and help the patient realize that not all his or her perceptions are accurate. Third, conceptualizing the patient's distress in the therapy session provides an opportunity for the clinician to generate hypotheses (to be tested later) about the patient's reactions to people outside of therapy. Thus, difficulties in the initial use of standard cognitive therapy, as well as any problems that arise in session, afford the clinician the opportunity to conceptualize why the patient is reacting the way he or she is in order to forge a stronger alliance and to gain insight into how the patient may characteristically react outside the therapy session. In addition, the therapeutic relationship can be used to get a sense of how other people may emotionally react to the patient (as the clinician monitors his or her own reaction to the patient).

A patient with BPD, for example, reacted quite angrily in the initial session when his therapist interrupted him to summarize her understanding of the patient's presenting problem. By apologizing and promising to allow the patient to continue his story uninterrupted, the clinician demonstrated that she did care and was willing to be flexible. Later in the session, the clinician used this situation as an opportunity to reinforce the cognitive model. She asked the patient what had gone through his mind when she had interrupted him, and he reported that he had had the thought "She doesn't want to hear what's important to me." Then he felt hurt and angry, became physiologically aroused, and acted in a hostile manner. Evaluation of this dysfunctional thought with standard Socratic questioning helped the patient to recognize that an alternative explanation was more valid: the therapist actually wanted to make sure that she did accurately understand what was important to him. Finally, they brainstormed how, in future sessions, the patient could let the clinician know he was distressed in a more moderate way. By handling the patient's distress in this manner, the clinician had an opportunity to reinforce the patient's understanding of the cognitive model, provide an experience in which the patient discovered his thinking can be distorted, demonstrate her desire to vary the therapy to help him, teach the patient a more socially appropriate behavioral strategy, and conceptualize the patient's experience more fully. In short, the therapist turned a situation that could have damaged the therapeutic alliance into one that strengthened it and deepened her understanding of the patient.

Thus, in treatment of patients with Axis II disorders, the clinician generally needs to spend considerable time in developing and maintaining a therapeutic alliance. As with all patients, the clinician elicits feedback from the patient at the end of each therapy session. With personality disorder patients, the therapist takes special care to monitor patients' verbal and nonverbal reactions during the session, to problem-solve interpersonal difficulties that arise on the spot, to use the therapeutic relationship as a vehicle for identifying and modifying patients' characteristic beliefs about others, and to teach patients new interpersonal strategies.

Enhancing Treatment Compliance

Treatment compliance is often much more difficult to achieve with patients who have Axis II disorders. The clinician's first task is to conceptualize, in cognitive terms, why a problem has arisen. For example, a paranoid patient held the broad assumption "If I trust other people, I'll be vulnerable to harm." The clinician hypothesized that a subset of this assumption had been activated in the therapy session ("If I trust my therapist, open up to her, and do as she suggests, I could get hurt"). The patient, indeed, did avoid revealing much about himself in the session, resisted the clinician's suggestion of a homework assignment to call friends he had lost touch with, and failed to report his unease when she asked for feedback at the end of the session. An antisocial patient had a different dysfunctional assumption: "If I listen to others, I won't get what I want." This belief hindered his ability to engage in therapy. He superficially complied, appearing to agree with the clinician, but failed to follow through with assignments or make significant changes in his thinking, belief structure, or behavior.

To enhance his or her understanding of patients' resistance, the clinician questions them to identify their underlying beliefs. One method is to ask them for the meaning of their thoughts when resistance is encountered, as in the following interchange with an obsessive-compulsive personality disorder patient:

Clinician: What went through your mind this morning as you thought about taking your medication?
Patient: I hate this stuff. It's artificial.
Clinician: What does it mean to you, to take something artificial?
Patient: It's not me. It's like something else is controlling me. I should be able to get over this by myself.
Clinician: What does it mean that you can't or haven't gotten over this yourself?
Patient: That I'm weak. If I have to take pills to control my moods, I'm not in control of myself. I'm weak.

The clinician and patient then evaluated this idea about weakness and were able to reframe the meaning of taking medication (i.e., that doing something that goes against one's grain but is helpful is a sign of strength, not of weakness).

A second method is to provide patients with the first part of a conditional assumption, specifying the desired behavior, as in the following interchange with a schizoid personality disorder patient:

Patient: I know I was supposed to make conversation with people at work, but I don't know. I just didn't.
Clinician: What assumption were you making? "If I talk to people then . . ."?
Patient: It won't lead to anything. It's not worth the bother.

The clinician and patient then conceptualized how this specific assumption was part of a broader assumption (i.e., "If people get to know me, they'll find out I'm nothing").

Overcoming resistance and gaining compliance starts with a cognitive formulation of the problem. As with any difficulty in therapy, the clinician seeks to understand why the problem has arisen and how the situation fits into the clinician's overall conceptualization of the case. He or she identifies what specific assumptions and broader beliefs became activated and which compensatory strategy the patient used. The therapist then devises interventions to ameliorate the difficulty, including evaluation of these beliefs and cognitive and behavioral strategies to increase the likelihood that the patient will comply in treatment sessions and follow through with homework assignments.

A dependent personality disorder patient, for example, had agreed to organize his desk at home but reported at several succeeding sessions that he had failed to do so. He overgeneralized this specific failure, labeling himself as "completely incompetent." His therapist elicited the patient's perception that he was too incapable and overwhelmed to do the task. She helped him to recall previous times he had strongly believed that he was incompetent but had proceeded to do a task that seemed overwhelming. They explored the possibility that he may have felt overwhelmed because of an activation of his core belief and that his strong belief of incompetence might not be true, or not completely true, in this situation. They uncovered and evaluated his fear that if he succeeded in this task, his therapist would impose ever-increasing demands on him that he would ultimately be unable to fulfill.

Having modified the patient's beliefs of incompetence and decreased his fears, the clinician next asked the patient to imagine taking the first step to do the task and had him rehearse what he could say to himself when he became anxious. Based on this imaginal rehearsal, she helped him to compose a coping card (a statement they jointly composed on an index card) to read immediately before tackling the job again. This card was used to remind him that the evidence showed that he most likely *was* competent enough to do the first step (i.e., simply separating into two piles the items that belonged on the desk and the items that belonged elsewhere).

To minimize the chance of procrastination, they agreed that the patient would try the assignment as an "experiment" immediately after the therapy session and that he would leave a message on the clinician's voice mail, telling her how the task had gone. Reducing the intensity of how much he believed the core belief, changing the assignment to taking just the first step, eliciting the patient's agreement to do the task immediately after the session, labeling the task as an "experiment" instead of an "assignment," and reading a coping card decreased the patient's anxiety. Allowing him the opportunity to leave her a voice-mail message demonstrated to the patient that his therapist cared and wanted to help. In fact, he went beyond the agreed-on assignment and finished organizing the whole desk. In later sessions, the therapist taught the patient how to give credit to himself and how to decrease his reliance on the therapist and others to motivate him.

Varying Session Structure

A recommended format for many cognitive therapy patients includes a mood check, provision of a bridge between sessions, setting of an agenda, review of homework, discussion of agenda items, final summary, and feedback (J. S. Beck 1995). Some patients with Axis II pathology, however, feel uncomfortable with this format and have a host of automatic thoughts when the clinician suggests this organization of topics at the first session. A narcissistic patient, for example, had the thought, "She's treating me like all her other patients. Doesn't she realize I need *special* treatment?" A histrionic patient had the thought, "When will she give me time to express myself? I can't give her the flavor of my life in just 2 minutes!" An antisocial patient thought, "She's going to try to get me to do something I don't want to do."

The clinician elicits the patient's concerns when he or she displays a negative affect shift as they are discussing how therapy might proceed. If the patient's unease is not alleviated by additional provision of a rationale for the proposed structure, the clinician proposes a different format or invites the patient to suggest changes.

Clinician: What if we spend the first 15 minutes or so having you tell me whatever is on your mind, without following any agenda. Then I can tell you what themes I heard, to make sure I really understood. Then perhaps we can catch up on some of these other things [mood check, homework review, etc.] if we haven't already covered them. How does that sound?

Some patients with Axis II pathology have difficulty collecting their thoughts and expressing themselves succinctly, and this inhibits efficient use of therapy time. A worksheet, "Preparing for a Therapy Session" (Figure 3–3), is useful for many personality disorder patients. An avoidant patient, for example, found that the worksheet forced her to think about therapy issues between sessions. An obsessive-compulsive personality disorder patient was helped to provide broader answers about his experiences in the previous week instead of minutely detailed ones. A BPD patient was able to organize her thinking better and more quickly express the issues that were of greatest concern to her. A dependent patient found the worksheet encouraged her to make her own decisions about how to spend the time in session, rather than relying on the clinician. One narcissistic patient, it should be noted, reacted angrily to the suggestion he try to fill out the worksheet: "You're trivializing my problems, expecting me to fit myself into a bunch of questions. My problems are way too complex for that!" Variations in session structure and process must take into account patients' potential idiosyncratic reactions.

Developing Treatment Goals

Specifying how they would like to be different by the end of therapy is difficult for some patients with Axis II pathology who cannot imagine how they would like to change, who do not believe change is possible, or who primarily want *others* to change. Specialized strategies can aid them in identifying specific, achievable behavioral goals.

One difficulty arises when patients say they want "to be happier" but are unable to be more specific. A follow-up question—"What will

---

Preparing for a Therapy Session

1. What problem do I want to work on today?
   Relationship with Pam.
2. How have I been feeling this week compared with other weeks?
   A little less depressed.
3. What happened this week that my therapist should know about?
   Fight with Pam.
4. What did we cover during the last session?
   Disagreement doesn't necessarily mean disrespect.
5. Anything that bothered me about last session? Any unfinished business?
   No.
6. Anything I'm reluctant to tell my therapist?
   No.
7. What did I do for homework?
   Dysfunctional Thought Record when I was upset.
   Read therapy notes.

Figure 3–3. "Preparing for a Therapy Session": a worksheet useful for many personality disorder patients.
Source. Adapted from Thomas Ellis, Ph.D. Copyright 1996, J. S. Beck, Ph.D.

you be doing differently when you *are* happier?"—can elicit more targeted objectives. Inquiring about individual components of their lives is also useful. "If you were happier, what would you be doing differently at work?" "with friends and family?" "in your leisure time?" "in your household management?" "in regard to your physical health?" "in nurturing your intellectual/spiritual/cultural side?" (The next step involves helping patients understand that people feel better *after* they start doing these things and that it is therefore disadvantageous to put off making changes.)

Another technique invites patients to envision, in detail, the way they would like their life to be several years hence. Doing so helps patients think concretely about the changes they need to strive for.

Clinician: Can you imagine a typical day, say 5 years from now? Imagine that you feel much better about yourself; what does your life look like, from the time you wake up to the time you go to sleep? When do you want to imagine getting up, getting out of bed? What do you do next? (Or, what do you want to imagine you do next?) What next?

Certain ideas may interfere with the process of goal setting. Patients with Axis II pathology may profoundly believe, "I can't change," or "Change is dangerous," or "Change won't help me feel better," or "Change may lead others to expect too much from me." Some patients (especially eager-to-please dependent patients) are willing to suspend judgment while they do small behavioral experiments to test their ideas. Many personality disorder patients, though, need to evaluate and modify their beliefs before they are willing to put much effort into achieving their goals. Dysfunctional beliefs about change can be evaluated using the same strategies outlined later in this chapter in the discussion of belief change.

Patients who set goals for other people can easily become frustrated or angry if the therapist fails to use delicacy in helping them see that they have direct control only over *themselves*, not others. The following interchange illustrates how a clinician refocused goal setting to elicit achievable objectives for a histrionic patient:

Clinician: How would you like to be different by the end of therapy?

Patient [laughs]: I'd like *everything* to be different.

Therapist: Can you tell me more specifically which things?

Patient: Well, I'd like my husband to be nicer to me, my kids to listen to me more, my boss not to heap so much work on me, my mother not to nag me and make me feel so guilty.

Clinician: These sound important. Could we take them one by one to see what we can accomplish that would be reasonable?

Patient [hesitates]: Okay.

Therapist [giving patient the choice]: Which one should we start with?

Patient: Umm . . . My husband! He's so inconsiderate. He's always coming home late, never shows me any appreciation. He's so serious. He needs to lighten up, have some fun, go back to the way he used to be.

Clinician: I can see you'd really like him to be different. If he's willing to come in for couples counseling and if he wants to change in these ways, too, then I could work with him directly on these things. Do you think he'd want to come in?

Patient [glumly]: No. He's not that unhappy. But he's making *me* unhappy.

Clinician: Then would you want to work on how *you* can make *you* happier?

Patient: I guess.

Clinician: Would you like to learn different ways of asking your husband for some of these things? Or would you like help in identifying friends who could provide some of these things? Would you like to react less strongly when your husband disappoints you?

Patient [thinks for a moment]:   I still want to change *him*. It's not fair that *I* have to change.

Clinician: I wish we could get you what you want. But I don't want to mislead you into thinking that just by our working together we can make big changes in him. We may be able to influence him though, by focusing on what you say to him and how you react to him. . . . What do you think?

Patient: I'm not sure. I *guess* it makes sense.

Clinician [sensing the patient needs time to have this alternative viewpoint sink in]:   How would you feel about giving this some more thought during the week? Then we can talk more about it at our next session.

Patient: Okay.

Goal setting with personality disorder patients, as in the examples above, may require modification of beliefs and expectations before these patients are prepared to set specific behavioral goals for themselves.

Implementing Skills Training

Before embarking on skills training, it is important to ascertain whether patients have a deficiency in a particular skill or hold beliefs that interfere with their ability to use skills they already possess. A dependent patient intellectually knew how to assert herself with a co-worker and so did not require traditional assertiveness training to deal with him. The cognitive therapist assessed her level of skill by asking, "If you knew for sure your co-worker would react okay in this situation, what would you say to him? What would you *like* to be able to say to him?" The patient was readily able to formulate a reasonable response, and this indicated that, instead of skills training, she needed to work on identifying and modifying an interfering belief, "If I assert myself, others will be unwilling to help me when I need them."

However, as mentioned previously in the section on compensatory strategies, many patients *do* have a deficiency in various strategies and skills. Paranoid patients need to learn appropriate ways of checking out their suspicions; obsessive-compulsive personality disorder patients need to learn to be more spontaneous, flexible, and imperfect; and histrionic patients need to learn methods to moderate their emotional displays. Many personality disorder patients need to learn straightforward problem-solving skills. Most are successful in learning and practicing these skills through role playing in session, using specific persons as role models, imagining themselves behaving differently in specific situations, trying out new behaviors in session with the therapist and outside of session with others, practicing repeatedly with the therapist and trusted friends, and following a graded hierarchy of increasingly difficult situations in which they use their newly acquired skills.

Implementing Cognitive Interventions

The initial phase of implementing cognitive interventions with patients involves helping them accept the cognitive model: first, that their thinking in specific situations influences their emotional, physiological, and behavioral reactions; second, that their thinking is often dysfunctional and/or distorted when they are distressed; and third, that they can experience relief by evaluating, testing, and modifying their thinking. Many patients with Axis II pathology readily agree with the first part of the model but do not initially accept the second or third part. The clinician should acknowledge that he or she does not know for sure that patients' thinking is inaccurate or that they can learn to change their thinking and lessen their dysphoria. Such an acknowledgment often makes patients more amenable to experiments in which, as a team, clinician and patient discover what happens following various cognitive interventions.

A number of cognitive interventions at the automatic-thought level have been extensively described (A. T. Beck et al. 1979, 1985; J. S. Beck 1995; McMullin 1986), including the following:

- Identifying automatic thoughts
- Labeling cognitive errors
- Using Socratic questioning to ascertain the validity of automatic thoughts
- Restructuring images at the automatic-thought level
- Using the Dysfunctional Thought Record
- Examining advantages and disadvantages of believing automatic thoughts
- Decatastrophizing
- Seeking alternative explanations
- Applying to oneself advice one would give to others
- Performing behavioral experiments to test ideas

Modification of some of these techniques is often needed for personality disorder patients.

- *Avoidant patients* may resist the clinician's attempt to elicit automatic thoughts because of the underlying belief "If I start to feel a little bad, I'll get totally overwhelmed." The clinician often must help patients modify this belief before they are willing to think about distressing situations and identify their distress-provoking thoughts.

- *Paranoid and schizotypal patients* may be loath to uncover their thoughts for fear the clinician will somehow use this information against them. Helping these patients specify criteria for relatively trustworthy people versus definitely untrustworthy people increases their willingness to reveal their thinking. Decatastrophizing their fears also increases the likelihood of compliance.
- *Patients with BPD* may feel invalidated when the clinician attempts to determine the validity of their thoughts. The clinician needs to repair their alliance by explaining that the objective is to decrease patients' distress by helping them evaluate their *thinking,* not to invalidate their emotions.
- *Antisocial patients* may superficially agree with a restructuring of their automatic thoughts, providing falsely high ratings of the strength of their belief in an alternative response. The clinician may gently probe whether they may be responding in such a way as to get the therapist "off their back."
- *Schizoid patients* may be unmotivated to evaluate their thoughts, because they often do not feel a good sense of mastery or pride when they accomplish a task. Trying such an evaluation in session with the goal of seeing if this intervention helps, even a small amount, can be sufficient to gain compliance.
- *Dependent patients* may fear that learning to change their thinking, and therefore feeling better, may lead to the therapist's demanding that they become more independent. Uncovering and decatastrophizing this fear usually motivates these patients to act more autonomously.
- *Obsessive-compulsive personality disorder patients* may overuse tools such as the Dysfunctional Thought Record, sometimes spending hours at a time, striving to do as complete and thorough a job as humanly possible. Use of such a record may be counterproductive because it may strengthen, not reduce, their dysfunctional compensatory strategies.
- *Narcissistic patients* may discount the process of identifying and evaluating their automatic thoughts, labeling such interventions as too simplistic to ameliorate their complex difficulties. Appealing to their narcissism, the clinician can sympathize that such a special person with so much potential does not deserve to suffer and that it would be a shame if the patient failed to try any strategy that could possibly help.
- *Histrionic patients* may have difficulty accepting an alternative response because of the belief "If something 'feels' true, it must be true." Identifying patients' previously strongly held ideas, which were later discovered to be invalid, may help these patients understand that "feeling" true and "being" true are not always synonymous.

Thus, the clinician will usually need to vary strategies, strengthen the therapeutic alliance, and/or modify interfering beliefs before using more straightforward cognitive interventions at the automatic-thought level with personality disorder patients.

Effecting Belief Change

Modification of personality disorder patients' core beliefs and of their characteristic pattern of processing information involves focusing on both the present and the past and using both intellectual and experiential methods. The process takes considerable, consistent effort over time.

Explaining Patients' Cognitive Profile

The first step involves helping patients understand the connections between their early experiences, underlying beliefs and compensatory strategies, and reactions to current situations. These connections can be made clearer by use of the cognitive conceptualization diagram (see Figure 3–1), which the clinician can complete between sessions. The clinician may at some point present to the patient a blank diagram to be completed jointly in a session or a simplified diagrammatic or verbal version. The major objective of presenting data in this fashion is for patients to gain an understanding of how their most basic negative beliefs about themselves (i.e., core beliefs) influence the development of dysfunctional behavioral patterns (i.e., compensatory strategies) and currently affect their interpretation of and reactions across situations.

The next step is to help patients realize that these global, rigid, deeply held beliefs are "ideas" (which likely originated with the patients' interpretations of adverse developmental experiences), not necessarily "truths." Presentation of an information-processing model helps explain to patients how a core belief can "feel" true and yet not be wholly true, as in the following interchange with a BPD patient:

Therapist: I have a hypothesis about why it is that you "feel" so worthless. It's as if you have a screen around your head and on it is imprinted "I'm worthless" millions of times. Whenever something happens to you that could possibly be interpreted as confirming that idea, that information easily passes through the screen and you process it right away. Can you remember some examples of when you felt worthless this week?

Patient: Sure, there were lots of times, like yesterday when I took a 3-hour nap and didn't get my work done . . . this morning when I realized I hadn't gotten my laundry done . . . last night when I stayed up late watching a movie and eating too much . . .

Therapist: And when all these things happened did you immediately think you were worthless?

Patient: Yes.

Therapist: Now a second part of my hypothesis is that whenever you do something or something happens to you that might show that you're *not* worthless, I don't think you process that information in a straightforward way. I think it may bounce off the screen, and so you ignore it. Or it has to get distorted to fit through the screen. Now were there any things you did this week that someone *else* might say showed you *weren't* worthless, that you were actually an okay person?

Patient: Uh, not really.

Therapist: Let's see, you told me a few minutes ago that you had volunteered to stay late at work to finish a project. At the time did you think, "Volunteering shows I'm worthwhile or okay"?

Patient: No.

Therapist: What did you make of it?

Patient: That it was my responsibility to stay.

Therapist: So might this be an example of how you *discount* positive information? Can you give me any more examples?

[Patient provides, with prompting by therapist, other examples of discounting or ignoring positive data.]

Therapist: Do you think the hypothesis could be right? That you tend to interpret negative data as confirming your idea that you're worthless? That you also tend to screen out or discount positive data? What if this way of processing information has been going on since childhood? Now do you see how this idea that you're worthless could "feel" so true and yet not be true?

An explanation such as the one presented above is the first step in getting patients to start questioning the validity of their core belief. Such questioning, however, may engender a great deal of anxiety, because patients are really questioning their sense of self. Listing advantages of modifying the core belief and the disadvantages (with an adaptive response to each disadvantage) usually motivates patients to tolerate time-limited anxiety in exchange for concrete long-term gains.

Modifying Core Beliefs

The clinician needs a variety of interventions that can be aimed at changing core beliefs.

Core Belief Worksheet. The Core Belief Worksheet (Figure 3–4) is helpful when patients acknowledge that they may be distorting information and then become willing to do the hard work involved in restructuring their beliefs (J. S. Beck 1995). The worksheet helps patients to monitor, on an ongoing basis, how much progress they are making in reducing the strength of their old core belief and increasing the strength of a new core belief, jointly developed in treatment sessions. Clinicians and patients can assess the strengths of the beliefs at the beginning of each session by filling out the top portion of the worksheet. Patients fill out the bottom portion of the worksheet at each session and between sessions to learn a new way of processing information relevant to their belief.

CORE BELIEF WORKSHEET

NAME: S.   **DATE:** 3/21

OLD CORE BELIEF: I'm a failure.

    How much do you believe the old core belief right now? (0–100) 70%
    *What's the most you've believed it this week? (0–100) 90%
    *What's the least you believed it this week? (0–100) 50%

NEW BELIEF: *I'm competent, though with both strengths and weaknesses.*

    How much do you believe the new belief right now? (0–100) 50%

EVIDENCE THAT CONTRADICTS OLD CORE BELIEF AND SUPPORTS NEW BELIEF	EVIDENCE THAT SEEMS TO SUPPORT OLD CORE BELIEF WITH REFRAME
Worked out a new contract with Mr. R.	*Business still has significant problems, BUT I'm doing all I can to solve problems now.*
Got an extension from S	
Writing letters and phoning daily to try to resolve problem with "A company."	*I can't get my mother to take her medication, BUT this isn't really under my control.*
Continuing in the ABC project [charitable volunteer activity].	*Dad blames me for potential bankruptcy, BUT (1) the business had problems when I took over, (2) I share the responsibility for continued problems with several other people, and (3) even if this business fails, it doesn't mean I'm a failure as a person.*

*Should situations related to an increase or decrease in the strength of the belief be topics for the session agenda?

Figure 3–4. Core Belief Worksheet.
Source. Copyright 1996, J. S. Beck, Ph.D.

Extreme contrasts.   Such contrasts help patients compare themselves with someone they believe has an even greater degree of the quality embodied in the core belief than they do. For example, a BPD patient believed that he was completely bad. His therapist guided him in comparing himself with a mass murderer, a child molester, and a rapist (all in the news), whom he considered to have more "badness" than he. Together, therapist and patient did a careful analysis of each of these villains, and the patient learned to recall them and compare himself when his self-belief of badness became activated.

"Yardsticks."   "Yardsticks," jointly developed in session, help patients evaluate themselves or other people more reasonably. The therapist of a paranoid personality disorder patient, for example, helped the patient learn to discriminate among people who were in the range of reasonably trustworthy (including several friends, many family members, many co-workers), those who were (by objective criteria) marginally trustworthy (including a brother and a neighbor who sometimes took slight advantage of the patient), and those who were definitely untrustworthy (an uncle who had molested him as a child, a former co-worker who spread a rumor about the patient). This yardstick helped him decrease his sense of vulnerability around people who he came to realize belonged in the first category of reasonable trustworthiness.

Behavioral experiments.   Cognitive therapists often suggest behavioral experiments to patients to encourage them to test their beliefs. After assessing data that indicated the reasonableness of a schizotypal patient's new supervisor at work, a clinician encouraged the patient to tell his supervisor directly that he could not complete a task as requested and ask for assistance. After practicing skills of negotiation through role playing, the patient also began to change his response to his parents' unreasonable requests at home. Doing these things helped modify his belief that relationships are threatening and that he is helpless to improve them.

Cognitive continua.   Cognitive continua help break down polarized thinking. A dependent patient believed he was completely inadequate. His therapist guided him in describing people who were more inadequate than he. For example, they decided that a man the patient's age who had good potential and no psychiatric or physical disorder, but who sat around the house all day and night being completely unproductive, was displaying 0% adequacy. The therapist next asked the patient to describe people at the 25%, 50%, and 75% mark of adequacy. The patient then realized that his usual range of functioning was roughly 60%–80%. Previously he had viewed himself as 100% inadequate.

Metaphors. The use of metaphors can help patients to see the possible invalidity of their core belief. Recalling the story of Cinderella, for example, helped an avoidant patient entertain the possibility that she had been mistreated as a child not because of her inherent "badness," but because her parents had problems of their own.

Acting as if. Encouraging patients to "act as if" they do not believe their beliefs may help lead them to behave more functionally and erode the dysfunctional beliefs when negative outcomes fail to occur. A mother with obsessive-compulsive personality disorder, for example, was counseled to "act as if" she believed that being flexible, more lenient, and positive with her adolescent daughter was desirable. Imagining precisely how she would respond to her daughter in specific situations and then carrying through in real life led her to conclude that she did not have to be completely responsible for her daughter's behavior and that loosening her strict demands gained better compliance in the long run.

. . .

The above interventions are primarily present-oriented (i.e., they deal primarily with helping the patient address present issues, and use current material). With most personality disorder patients, it is necessary to help them reassess the data they have interpreted as supporting the development and maintenance of the core belief over time.

Historical review of the evidence. Through a historical review of the evidence (J. S. Beck 1995; Young 1990), the clinician can help patients recall these data, look for alternative explanations for these events, identify contrary data, and reassess the overall validity of this belief in the past. A dependent patient, for example, who grew up believing she was incapable and unable to cope concluded, after a careful historical review of the evidence, that she had overprotective parents who did not give her many opportunities to conquer challenges on her own. However, she actually did cope reasonably well in many instances when she could not rely on her parents.

Rational/emotional role-play. Sometimes the interventions described above lead patients to change their view of themselves "intellectually" but not "emotionally" or at a "gut" level. As a narcissistic patient explained, "I know in my head that it's okay to be one of the crowd; I don't have to be the best; but in my gut I still feel if I'm not treated like a prince, I'm a nobody." These patients require additional interventions before they are fully able to use cognitive restructuring to change underlying beliefs.

In a rational/emotional role-play, the therapist and patient role-play different parts of the patient's mind. Initially, the therapist takes the "intellectual" side, while the patient role-plays his or her emotional, or gut-level, side. Such a role-play helps the patient express the emotional reasoning supporting the core belief, and the therapist can then counter that reasoning with a more realistic viewpoint. When the patient, after role-playing in this manner, can no longer think of any more reasons for the validity of the core belief, patient and therapist switch parts so that the patient has the opportunity to respond on a rational basis to the emotional arguments.

Restructuring of early memories.   Another strategy for patients who still "feel" their core belief is true even after repeated interventions at the intellectual level is restructuring of early memories (J. S. Beck 1995; Edwards 1989). One such intervention involves having the patient reexperience in imagery form, with emotional intensity, a traumatic event during which his or her negative core belief originated. The therapist interviews the "younger self" to assess what meaning the child derived from the incident and helps the patient reinterpret this event by having the patient imagine his or her current self or another person carrying on a dialogue with the younger self.

Imaginary dialogues.   Another experiential technique involves having patients create imaginary dialogues in which they tell their parents or other significant people what they want or feel (Young 1990). Patients can alternately play both roles, or the therapist can take a part. These dialogues often help patients better understand why the other person reacted toward them in a way that proved traumatic and gives them an alternative explanation for the event, thereby helping to erode their core belief.

Relapse Prevention

A number of specific strategies for relapse prevention of Axis I disorders have been outlined (J. S. Beck 1995; Ludgate 1995). These strategies are equally applicable to patients with personality disorders. First, patients are encouraged to start spacing out their therapy sessions when they have gained sufficient symptom relief and mastery of cognitive therapy tools and when they are likely to do "self-therapy" between sessions. Every-other-week sessions allow patients to begin to solve problems, practice new behaviors, and respond to dysfunctional thoughts and beliefs more independently. Before moving to less-frequent sessions, however, the therapist addresses certain key issues, described below, with patients.

While still in weekly or every-other-week therapy, patients identify typical situations that tend to trigger their schemas and then list the early warning signs that a core belief has been activated. These signs may include significant emotional arousal, extreme negative thinking, and increased desire to use compensatory strategies that could have a negative outcome. The therapist asks patients to predict problems that are likely to occur in the coming days, weeks, and months. Together they do advance problem solving and record desirable adaptive responses to predicted automatic thoughts and beliefs that may arise. Finally, patients can be directly taught how to conduct a self-therapy session (J. S. Beck 1995) and encouraged to experiment with doing so during alternate weeks when they do not have a therapy session.

Countertransference

When patients with personality disorders bring to the therapeutic relationship the same dysfunctional beliefs and compensatory strategies that are present in their other relationships, therapists may experience dysfunctional reactions themselves. The therapist of a schizoid patient, for example, felt slightly angry when the patient failed to display any warmth toward him, despite his thoughtful and caring responses toward her. A therapist who had extended herself significantly in an attempt to build the therapeutic alliance experienced a sense of being unappreciated by her narcissistic patient. A therapist with a BPD patient was fearful of the emotional displays of the patient in treatment sessions.

Therapists who work with personality disorder patients need to attend to their own emotional reactions during therapy (Pretzer and Fleming 1989). This practice can lead to significant insight into the effect of these patients on others in their environment and help the therapists to refine their conceptualization of the patient. If such insight fails to reduce their distress and to increase their empathy, therapists may consider evaluating their own automatic thoughts, assessing how realistic their expectations are for themselves and for the patient, examining appropriate limit setting with the patient, and/or consulting with other professionals.

Summary and Conclusions

The treatment of patients with personality disorders is often complex and challenging. A sound cognitive conceptualization is essential so that both clinicians and patients can understand in a nonpejorative way patients' propensity for extreme emotional reactions and behavior and recognize that their responses are usually influenced by very painful, global negative beliefs about the self and others. Modifying underlying beliefs requires consistent, careful analysis of current situations, learning to process information related to the self and others differently, and restructuring the meaning of childhood trauma during which core beliefs originated and became more strongly held and entrenched. Changes in the belief system can motivate patients to learn new behavioral strategies that were previously underdeveloped and to reduce their reliance on the dysfunctional strategies that may have contributed to the development of the disorder for which they originally sought therapy.

Cognitive therapy for patients with Axis II disorders shares many features with the approach for patients with Axis I conditions, such as a focus on solving current problems, changing distorted thinking, and implementing behavioral change. Patients with Axis II disorders, however, usually need to spend additional time and energy on forging and cementing the therapeutic alliance, on learning new behavioral strategies, and on modifying, through intellectual and experiential methods, their rigid negative beliefs about the self.

With a greater appreciation of why personality disorder patients of each Axis II diagnosis act and react as they do, and with an accurate cognitive conceptualization of the individual patient, the clinician may find that a patient's personality pathology, while complex, is not perplexing. Use of the specialized interventions described in this chapter can make treatment more effective. Further work is needed to design more efficient and efficacious treatments for personality disorder patients with various comorbid Axis I disorders, for those without a concomitant acute disorder, and for those with dual diagnosis. Research on the cognitive approach is still quite limited, though promising, and future investigations are imperative to establish the efficacy of treatment for this significant segment of the psychiatric population.

References

American Psychiatric Association: Diagnostic and Statistical Manual of Mental Disorders, 4th Edition. Washington, DC, American Psychiatric Association, 1994

Arntz A, Dreessen L: Do personality disorders influence the results of cognitive behavioral therapies? International Cognitive Therapy Newsletter No 6, 1990, pp 3–6

Beck AT: Thinking and depression, II: theory and therapy. Arch Gen Psychiatry 10:561–571, 1964

Beck AT: Cognitive aspects of personality disorders and their relation to syndromal disorders: a psychoevolutionary approach, in Personality and Psychopathology. Edited by Cloninger CR. Washington, DC, American Psychiatric Press (in press)

Beck AT, Rush AJ, Shaw BF, et al: Cognitive Therapy of Depression. New York, Guilford, 1979

Beck AT, Emery G, Greenberg RL: Anxiety Disorders and Phobias: A Cognitive Perspective. New York, Basic Books, 1985

Beck AT, Freeman A, and Associates: Cognitive Therapy of Personality Disorders. New York, Guilford, 1990

Beck JS: Cognitive Therapy: Basics and Beyond. New York, Guilford, 1995

Beck JS: Cognitive therapy of personality disorders, in Frontiers of Cognitive Therapy: The State of the Art and Beyond. Edited by Salkovskis PM, Clark DM. New York, Guilford, 1996, pp 165–181

Edwards DJ: Cognitive restructuring through guided imagery: lessons from Gestalt therapy, in Comprehensive Handbook of Cognitive Therapy. Edited by Freeman A, Simon K, Beutler L, et al. New York, Plenum, 1989, pp 283–297

Freeman A, Pretzer J, Fleming B, et al: Clinical Applications of Cognitive Therapy. New York, Plenum, 1990

Gunderson JG, Phillips KA: Personality disorders, in Comprehensive Textbook of Psychiatry/VI, 6th Edition, Vol 2. Edited by Kaplan HI, Sadock BJ. Baltimore, MD, Williams & Wilkins, 1995, pp 1425–1461

Koenigsberg HW, Kaplan RD, Gilmore MM, et al: The relationship between syndrome and personality disorder in DSM-III: experience with 2,462 patients. Am J Psychiatry 142:207–217, 1985

Layden MA, Newman CF, Freeman A, et al: Cognitive Therapy of Borderline Personality Disorders. Boston, Allyn & Bacon, 1993

Linehan MM, Armstrong HE, Suarez A, et al: Cognitive-behavioral treatment of chronically suicidal borderline patients. Arch Gen Psychiatry 48:1060–1064, 1991

Ludgate JW: Maximizing Psychotherapeutic Gains and Preventing Relapse in Emotionally Distressed Clients. Sarasota, FL, Professional Resources Press, 1995

Mays DT, Franks CM: Negative outcome: what to do about it, in Negative Outcome in Psychotherapy and What to Do About It. Edited by Mays DT, Franks CM. New York, Springer, 1985, pp 281–301

McMullin RE: Handbook of Cognitive Therapy. New York, WW Norton, 1986

Millon T: Disorders of Personality: DSM-IV and Beyond. New York, Wiley, 1996

Padesky CA: Personality disorders: cognitive therapy into the 90's. Paper presented at the Second International Conference on Cognitive Psychotherapy, Umea, Sweden, September 1986

Persons JB, Burns BD, Perloff JM: Predictors of drop-out and outcome in cognitive therapy for depression in a private practice setting. Cognitive Therapy and Research 12:557–575, 1988

Pretzer JL: Cognitive therapy of personality disorders: the state of the art. Clinical Psychology and Psychotherapy 1(5):257–266, 1994

Pretzer JL, Beck AT: A cognitive theory of personality disorders, in Major Theories of Personality Disorder. Edited by Clarkin JF, Lenzenweger MF. New York, Guilford, 1996, pp

Pretzer JL, Fleming B: Cognitive-behavioral treatment of personality disorders. Behavior Therapist 12:105–109, 1989

Reich JH, Green AI: Effect of personality disorders on outcome and treatment. J Nerv Ment Dis 179(2):74–82, 1991

Sanderson WC, Beck AT, McGinn LK: Cognitive therapy for generalized anxiety disorder: significance of comorbid personality disorders. Journal of Cognitive Psychotherapy 8:13–18, 1994

Shea MT, Pilkonis PA, Beckman E, et al: Personality disorders and treatment outcome in the NIMH Treatment of Depression Collaborative Research Program. Am J Psychiatry 147:711–717, 1990

Stiles TC: The effects of standard cognitive therapy for unipolar major depressed patients with or without a personality disorder. Paper presented at the Society for Psychotherapy Research, Lyon, France, 1991

Stravynski A, Marks IM, Yule W: Social skills problems in neurotic outpatients: social skills training with and without cognitive modification. Arch Gen Psychiatry 39:1378–1385, 1982

Stuart S, Simons AD, Thase ME, et al: Are personality assessments valid in acute major depression? J Affect Disord 24:281–290, 1992

Turkat ID, Maisto SA: Personality disorders: application of the experimental method to the formulation and modification of personality disorders, in Clinical Handbook of Psychological Disorders: A Step-by-Step Treatment Manual. Edited by Barlow DH. New York, Guilford, 1985, pp 503–570

Turner RM: The effects of personality diagnosis on the outcome of social anxiety symptom reduction. Journal of Personality Disorders 1:136–143, 1987

Woody GE, McLellan AT, Luborsky L, et al: Sociopathy and psychotherapy outcome. Arch Gen Psychiatry 42:1081–1086, 1985

Young J: Cognitive Therapy for Personality Disorders: A Schema-Focused Approach. Sarasota, FL, Professional Resource Exchange, 1990

Chapter 4

Cognitive-Behavioral Treatment of Eating Disorders

James E. Mitchell, M.D., and Carol B. Peterson, Ph.D.

Psychotherapy utilizing cognitive-behavioral techniques is widely regarded by experts in the field as the treatment of choice for *bulimia nervosa* (BN), and there is a large controlled treatment literature supporting its efficacy (e.g., Agras 1991; Fairburn 1988; Wilson and Fairburn 1993). Although studied less intensively thus far, cognitive-behavioral strategies are also widely used in the treatment of *anorexia nervosa* (AN) (Garner 1992), and early reports also suggest that these techniques are also very useful in the treatment of *binge-eating disorder* (BED), the term for the newly defined eating disorder whose criteria are provided in the appendix of the DSM-IV (American Psychiatric Association 1994) for further study (Agras et al. 1995).

In this chapter we first review some of the underlying theoretical principles that have guided the development of cognitive behavioral interventions for eating disorders. We then describe specific treatment procedures in detail, including information on treatment procedures that can be used across all three groups of patients—BN, AN, and BED patients—while also discussing strategies most appropriate for subgroups of such patients. We then, before offering some final comments, review the controlled treatment literature in this area and consider some of the more important questions that both remain unanswered and provide important directions for future research.

Theoretical Model

The theoretical model for use of cognitive-behavioral therapy (CBT) for the treatment of BN was first advocated by Fairburn in 1981. This formulation followed closely on the heels of the first in-depth clinical description of this disorder by Russell in 1979. As will be made clear, and as was stressed by Wilson and Fairburn in a review in 1993, one must bear in mind that both the "cognitive" and the "behavioral" need to be emphasized when using this terminology, because both are incorporated into important parts of many treatment programs for patients with eating disorders.

First, the specific behavioral abnormalities represent very important features of the eating disorders (Mitchell 1990). Not uncommonly, these behavioral abnormalities are numerous and, at times, potentially medically dangerous (Pomeroy and Mitchell 1989). These include episodic binge eating (present in all individuals with BN and BED and in a subgroup of patients with AN), self-induced vomiting (present in approximately 90% of patients presenting for treatment of BN and, again, in a subgroup of AN patients), and, less commonly, abuse of laxatives, diuretics, and over-the-counter diet pills. Patients occasionally exhibit other abnormal eating-related behaviors, such as rumination, misuse of ipecac to induce vomiting, and chewing and spitting out of food. Although perhaps less dramatic behaviorally, but equally important theoretically and therapeutically, is the dietary restriction that seems to underlie both AN and BN and whose role in BED remains to be determined. Most patients with BN tend to restrict their food intake at times when they are not binge eating, whereas dietary restrictions are particularly onerous for patients with AN, and for some this is the primary problem behavior.

Second, cognitive issues center on the extreme importance placed on slimness as a model of attractiveness, and the accompanying dissatisfaction with body weight and shape. This cognitive set is often accompanied by an inability to adequately perceive one's own body realistically and, particularly in AN patients, by overestimation of the size of the body or specific body parts. The body dissatisfaction, desire for weight loss, and preoccupation with thinness at times assume delusional severity among patients with AN. Also, as pointed out by Garner and Bemis (1985), the drive for thinness accompanying body dissatisfaction appears to be ego syntonic for many patients with AN, and they actively resist the notion of changing their attitudes and behaviors. Thus, illness becomes a "way of life." The approach then is to attempt to interrupt and change the pattern of abnormal behaviors early in treatment, and in particular to encourage the patient to begin to eat regular balanced meals and, in the case of AN patients, to gain weight. As treatment progresses using the cognitive-behavioral model, the emphasis gradually shifts to changing the underlying cognitions concerning shape and weight that contribute to the extreme dietary restriction and any residual episodes of binge eating.

Cognitive-behavioral therapy of eating disorders is unusual among the cognitive-behavioral treatments for psychiatric disorders in that a strong emphasis is placed on the nutritional counseling aspects of the intervention. Most programs emphasize the need for improvement in patterning of meals early into the treatment, and not uncommonly dietitians are incorporated into treatment activities of outpatient clinics, on inpatient units, and in day treatment programs.

Although not a major focus of this chapter, many patients with eating disorders have associated comorbid psychiatric conditions, and several of these conditions are also amenable to CBT. Therefore, additional treatment programming to address these associated problems is at times indicated. Associated comorbid psychiatric conditions amenable to CBT include mood disorders (which have a very high lifetime comorbidity in both AN and BN and which also would appear to be increased in prevalence among individuals with BED and obesity), anxiety disorders, personality disorders, and substance use disorders (Mitchell et al. 1991). Indeed, these comorbid conditions at times dominate the clinical picture and may dictate alternative interventions before the eating disorder can be treated effectively. This is especially true for patients with comorbid substance use disorders, with whom some degree of behavioral control over the alcohol and/or drug use is necessary before the eating disorder can be effectively addressed. Another example is patients who are severely depressed and potentially suicidal, for whom treatment of the mood disturbance and the need for safety are paramount.

Specific Strategies in the Cognitive-Behavioral Treatment of Eating Disorders

Although CBT is more didactic and structured than most other types of psychotherapy, basic clinical skills are still essential, particularly those related to formation of a strong therapeutic alliance. Therapeutic rapport is especially important in the treatment of AN, because individuals with this disorder are often quite reluctant to change behavioral patterns (Garner and Bemis 1985). Maintaining such rapport can be challenging, because CBT usually requires the therapist to cover a large amount of information in an efficient, time-limited fashion. However, results from research studies on psychotherapy outcome in which manual-based therapies are used highlight the importance of nonspecific factors, including the therapeutic alliance (e.g., Horvath and Luborsky 1993; Rounsaville et al. 1987).

Nutritional Counseling

This type of intervention is important both for individuals who are consuming inadequate amounts of food, as with AN patients, and for those whose eating patterns are chaotic, as with BN and BED patients. Nutritional counseling can be conducted by any clinician who has adequate experience, although it is often helpful to enlist the assistance of a dietitian, especially in formulating meal plans.

Because patients are often fearful initially about implementing changes, an early focus on psychoeducation can help to establish rapport and introduce the importance of altering nutritional intake. The clinician may start by explaining the psychological and biological effects of semistarvation, referring to the Keys experiment (Keys et al. 1950) on healthy men to illustrate these phenomena. In this study, Keys and colleagues found that normal young men, when they were placed on a calorically restricted diet and subsequently experienced significant weight loss, began to exhibit many symptoms commonly observed in individuals with eating disorders, including mood lability, preoccupation with food, concentration impairment, sleep disturbance, cold intolerance, and diminished libido. When allowed to refeed, some of the subjects exhibited disturbance in hunger and satiety cues and began to engage in binge-eating behavior. Although the subjects' body weights initially increased after refeeding, their overeating eventually ceased, and they eventually returned to their premorbid body weights.

It is important for individuals with eating disorders to understand the Keys study in order to learn about the sequelae of excessive dietary restriction and weight loss and, in particular, to link what they are experiencing to the known symptoms of semistarvation. Often, insight into the relationship between starvation and its physical and emotional sequelae provides the first occasion during which individuals with AN become aware of the negative consequences of their excessive dietary restriction. Such awareness can help to make the eating disorder symptoms more ego dystonic and can enhance motivation in treatment. The Keys study is also helpful for individuals with problems with binge eating to develop an understanding that their excessive food restriction between eating episodes can precipitate or exacerbate overeating behavior. For all individuals with eating disorders, the Keys study highlights that mood lability and other psychological features can be ameliorated with nutritional rehabilitation.

A second focus of nutritional counseling is to establish a target weight range and meal plan. Standardized weight charts (e.g., Metropolitan Life Insurance Company 1983) can be used as guidelines, although additional factors, such as premorbid weight status, age, and the weight necessary to maintain menses, are also important to consider. Patients will often become quite upset when informed of their "standard" weight range, usually because they perceive it as too high, and may initially express an unwillingness to gain the amount of weight necessary to ensure medical stability. Also, patients with BN may be distressed because they are intent on losing weight, and when encouraged to accept their current weight, which is often in a normal weight range, they may become quite fearful. Further, most are convinced that they will gain weight if they refrain from engaging in self-induced vomiting or laxative abuse.

When patients are upset when informed of their "standard" weight range, it is important for the clinician to validate their concerns and to inform them that their discomfort will be a focus of treatment. Simultaneously, the clinician must be firm that the goal weight will not be changed and that it is set with the intention of correcting the effects of starvation and maintaining a stable medical status. Through psychoeducation, the ineffectiveness of purging techniques in preventing weight gain can be emphasized (Fairburn et al. 1993). The clinician may also find it useful to review the results of the treatment outcome studies that indicate that the majority of individuals treated with CBT for BN and BED do not gain weight (Agras et al. 1992; Mitchell et al. 1990; Wilfley et al. 1993). For individuals who are overweight, the clinician can suggest that the patients try to establish better control over their binge-eating behavior before making efforts to lose weight, emphasizing that dietary restriction may exacerbate overeating symptoms (see Fairburn et al. 1993 for further discussion).

Different strategies can be utilized for meal planning, although the general goal is to establish a pattern of regular intake of meals and snacks that incorporate a variety of foods. For some individuals, it is sufficient to instruct them to eat three meals and two or three snacks per day (Fairburn et al. 1993). In other cases, patients need to plan specific times, types, and amounts of foods to eat (Mitchell 1990). This strategy is especially useful in eliminating the spontaneous decision making that is often problematic early in treatment. We find it useful to provide general guidelines such as the American Dietetic Association diet with instructions for consuming certain amounts of different types of food (e.g., grains, fruits), rather than specific guidelines for calorie and fat intake, which can intensify preoccupations. In general, a focus early in outpatient treatment on drastically increasing food intake is not usually realistic.

Instead, it is more appropriate to start with limited expectations when working with both AN and BN patients and to address the problems that arise systematically. Because food consumption is often so restrictive or chaotic at the beginning of treatment, an initial emphasis can be placed on the timing of meals and snacks, followed by an increasing focus on appropriate food selection and meal content as patterning improves. Patients are usually quite reluctant to increase the frequency of food consumption and expand the variety of content, fearing immediate weight gain. This issue must be addressed differently depending on the nature of the eating disorder. For individuals with BN and BED, psychoeducation about the increase in metabolism associated with more regular eating can alleviate some anxiety. For individuals with AN who need to gain weight, cognitions that interfere with improved intake can be addressed using the cognitive restructuring techniques described later in this chapter.

Finally, nutritional counseling should attempt to challenge patients' rigid conceptions of foods as "good" or "bad." Patients are encouraged to eat all types of food in moderation, including fats, which are essential for certain physiological processes, including reproductive health.

Early in treatment, however, many individuals who have difficulty with binge eating may appropriately decide that certain "trigger" foods are too high risk to consume, even in small amounts. These types of foods (which are usually high in fat) can be gradually reintroduced later in treatment when the patient feels more in control of her or his eating. In vivo exposure assignments, in which the patient creates a hierarchy of high risk or feared foods and gradually begins to consume them in order from least to most feared, comprise a technique that is useful for many patients. This technique can be used during sessions (in individual therapy or in a group-meal format) or as a homework assignment between sessions.

Self-Monitoring

An essential component of the CBT treatment of eating disorders is use of written self-monitoring assignments. This procedure must be introduced as early in treatment as possible, so that both patient and clinician can become aware of the patterns in eating, cognitions, and mood, as well as monitor changes as therapy progresses. Because many patients find this procedure tedious, the clinician should emphasize its importance from the outset. Self-monitoring can be introduced as a technique to gain a clearer picture of patterns and an essential step for making subsequent changes. In fact, many patients are quite surprised when they become aware of the amounts and patterns of their eating. Also, self-monitoring allows for the extension of therapy outside of sessions and enables the patient to maintain a consistent focus on improvement. Finally, research has indicated that self-monitoring alone can be helpful in symptom reduction (Agras et al. 1989).

The content of the self-monitoring usually evolves over the course of treatment. Early on, the focus of self-monitoring is on the timing and content of meals and snacks, as well as the frequency of problematic eating and eating-related behaviors, such as binge eating, vomiting, and laxative use. The pattern of dietary restriction also usually becomes apparent with the review of food records. As treatment progresses, more emphasis is placed on the examination of behavioral cues and consequences, and, subsequently, self-monitoring can focus on cognitions associated with eating behaviors, as well as underlying beliefs and schemas (Vitousek and Hollon 1988). It is important fairly early on in therapy for patients to begin to monitor thoughts and feelings as well as behaviors and symptoms to become familiar with the cognitive-behavioral model. An example of self-monitoring is shown in Figure 4–1.

Cues and Consequences

Behavioral principles of stimulus control can be useful in interrupting and altering behavioral patterns. One method of explaining these prin-

Female patient—22 years of age

Date	Time	Place	Food consumed	ED	Thoughts	Feelings
Monday	8:00 A.M.	Home	1 container of nonfat yogurt	R	"I ate too much last night. I have to cut back today so I don't gain weight."	Anxious
	2:00 P.M.	Work	1 medium-size apple	R	"I've done well so far—I haven't eaten any fat. I'll try to keep myself from eating until tonight."	Happy
	4:00 P.M.		6 pretzels	R	"I'm getting hungry, but I can't let myself eat more. Otherwise, I'll never lose weight."	Anxious, irritable
	8:00 P.M.		1 bowl chocolate ice cream	R	"I blew it. I can't believe my roommate brought home ice cream. Now I'm going to gain weight."	Anxious, sad, angry
	8:30 P.M.		3/4 carton of ice cream	B/V	"I blew it for today anyway, so I might as well finish the container, get rid of it by vomiting so I don't gain weight, and start over again tomorrow. I have no self-control."	Anxious, sad, relieved, disgusted

Figure 4–1. Self-monitoring: an example. ED = eating disorder. *Symptoms:* R = dietary restriction; B = binge eating; V = vomiting.

ciples to patients is to use the terms *cues* and *consequences*. Specifically, cues, or "triggers," precede symptoms and become conditioned stimuli to elicit such behaviors. Examples of common cues of eating disorder symptoms include experiencing interpersonal conflict, experiencing strong affective states, eating while watching television, seeing a picture of a thin person, and consuming food high in fat or calories. Interestingly, one of the most common cues for BN patients is boredom (Mitchell 1990).

Various techniques can be used to avoid or change responses to cues. Patients can develop strategies to avoid cues—for instance, driving a different route home from work, leaving the house after eating, or refraining from reading fashion magazines. We also suggest that patients develop their own list of alternative behaviors to use when confronted with the urge to engage in unhealthy behaviors. An example of such a list is shown in Table 4–1. When such a list is being prepared, emphasis is placed on choosing practical alternatives, especially those that have been effective for the individual in previous situations.

Another powerful behavioral technique involves teaching patients to build in a pause following a cue to binge-eat, purge, or restrict. To build in a pause, patients may be encouraged to start by introducing a very brief interval between the stimulus and the response—for instance, deciding to wait 2 minutes after the onset of the urge to binge-eat before actually engaging in the behavior. After successfully pausing for 2 minutes, the patient can increase the interval to 3 minutes, and so on. It is important to emphasize to patients that pausing even momentarily can be a significant step in breaking the conditioned relationship between the cue and the response and in establishing control over the eating behavior.

Other stimulus-control techniques include restricting high-risk behavior to certain settings (e.g., eating only at the dining-room table and not in any other part of the house or in the car) and exposure to cues

Table 4–1. Alternative behaviors for patient with an eating disorder to use when confronted with the urge to engage in unhealthy behaviors

Social	Multisensory	Cognitive
Visiting a friend	Listening to music	Reading a book
Calling someone on the phone	Taking a bubble bath	Watching a movie
Writing a letter	Having a massage	Doing a puzzle
Attending a support meeting	Petting a dog or cat	Writing in a journal; going to a museum

that do not elicit symptoms (e.g., studying in the school library if binge eating is less likely to occur there; remaining with friends after meals to prevent vomiting). Patients can also be taught to use exposure-response prevention techniques—for instance, exposing themselves to a high-risk situation, such as going to a movie, but carrying only enough money for admission to make the purchase of binge food impossible. "Scheduling" bulimic symptoms is an alternative approach in which the aim is also to separate cues from symptoms (Steel et al. 1995).

In addition to stimulus control, it is important to emphasize the consequences of behaviors, especially the rewards associated with maintaining healthier behavioral patterns. In the context of operant conditioning, the first step is to examine whether existing consequences are actually reinforcing maladaptive behavior patterns. For example, excessive exercise can be reinforced by positive feedback from the individual's peer group. The second step is to implement new rewards to reinforce healthier behavior patterns, as well as to minimize rewards of problematic behavior.

Patients should identify rewards that are powerful for them and that can be administered proximally to the time a goal is attained. These can be *material* rewards (e.g., the purchase of a desired object), *symbolic* rewards (e.g., gold stars on a chart for increased weight each week or day abstinent from binge eating), or *verbal* rewards (e.g., positive self-statements, such as "I did a good job meeting my goal"). Verbal rewards are also a useful way to improve self-esteem.

Discussing rewards can be a valuable lead-in to the topic of goal setting. It is important to emphasize goals from the beginning of treatment and to inform patients that setting even moderate goals is a useful step forward. This principle is especially important in work with individuals with AN, who often have difficulty making initial changes in behavior patterns. For example, an initial goal of eating one-half rather than one-quarter of a bagel as part of breakfast may be quite reasonable for some AN patients.

In the context of examining and trying to understand cues and consequences, patients often find it helpful to evaluate the positive and negative effects of their eating disorder. Most find that the immediate consequences are positive (e.g., stress reduction from binge eating; relief from fear of weight gain after vomiting; a sense of self-control from excessive exercise), whereas the longer-term effects are negative, albeit more easily ignored in the short term (e.g., dental problems from vomiting; emergency-room visits for dehydration; stress fractures resulting from excessive exercise). This pattern is consistent with basic behavioral principles, in that the immediate positive rewards are more likely to maintain behavior patterns than the longer-term negative effects are to discontinue them (much as the way a hangover does little to discourage heavy drinkers from consuming alcohol).

Cognitive Restructuring

After patients develop a clear understanding of cues and consequences of their symptoms, the model can be expanded to include cognitions, emotions/feelings, and behaviors as an introduction to cognitive restructuring (Figure 4–2). Specifically, it is helpful to explain to patients that thought patterns or cognitions (illustrated as an ongoing internal [unspoken] dialogue or monologue) can directly influence feelings and behaviors. For example, an individual with an eating disorder is likely to have different cognitions when viewing a buffet dinner (e.g.,"I can't eat in front of other people!"; "What if I overeat?"; "Look how many high-fat foods there are!"; "I know I'm going to gain weight if I eat anything") than is an individual without food or weight concerns (e.g., "This food looks great!"; "What should I eat first?"). Consequently, these cognitions lead to different emotional responses: anxiety and distress in the individual with an eating disorder; excitement and pleasure for the individual without an eating disorder. Subsequent behaviors differ as well, with the individual with the eating disorder being more likely to restrict and not eat anything, or to binge and purge in response to the cue.

To help familiarize the patient with this model, the clinician can ask him or her to identify specific examples in which thought patterns have contributed to eating disorder symptoms. With BN, for example, binge eating and vomiting can be triggered by the consumption of high-fat food followed by the cognitions "I've blown it! Now I'll definitely gain weight . . . I might as well eat everything, then vomit." An individual with AN might restrict intake after stepping on a scale, observing a slight weight gain, and thinking "I've gained weight! This means I'm getting fat. This is terrible! I'll have to fast all day tomorrow."

Once the patient recognizes the importance of these thoughts in influencing emotions and behavior, the clinician can begin to introduce specific strategies to help modify cognitions. The first step in changing

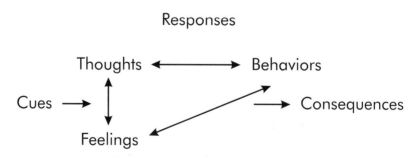

Figure 4–2. Model linking cues, response set, and consequences.

thought patterns, however, is to identify specific maladaptive thoughts, and self-monitoring is essential in determining problematic thinking patterns. These types of "cognitive errors" have been described in detail elsewhere (e.g., Beck et al. 1979; Garner and Bemis 1985; Peterson and Mitchell 1996). It can be helpful to provide patients with specific categories and examples of maladaptive thoughts, some of which are listed in Table 4–2.

After patients begin to become aware of their thought patterns and are able to articulate specific cognitions, the next step is to help them change cognitions with two methods: testing the thought and/or examining the evidence for and against the thoughts. Testing thoughts in CBT was first described by Beck in the context of collaborative empiricism (Beck et al. 1979). Specifically, the patient and clinician work together to devise "experiments" to test cognitions. For example, an individual with BN might state, "If I eat breakfast each day, I will immediately gain weight." This thought can be tested systematically by having the patient consume breakfast each day for a week, monitor her weight, and observe her binge-eating pattern. It is likely that she will discover that in addition to not gaining weight, she is less likely to binge-eat from extreme hunger later in the day.

Table 4–2.   Maladaptive cognitions in eating disorders

Type	Example
Overgeneralization	"I ate too much: I can never control my eating." "I ate a cookie: I have no self-control."
Catastrophizing	"I gained weight: I'll never stop gaining weight." "I had a binge-eating episode; this ruins all the progress I've made in treatment."
Dichotomous	"Vegetables are good foods; all foods with fats are bad foods." "My eating is either completely in control or completely out of control."
Minimization	"I may have made it the whole day without binge eating, but I should be able to make it through the whole weekend." "My eyes are pretty, but it doesn't matter because my legs are fat."
Mind reading	"That woman looked at me: she thinks I'm fat." "The people at work all admire how thin I am."
Self-fulfilling prophecy	"I can never keep an entire box of chocolate in my house." "I won't be able to eat according to my meal plan today."

After a cognition is identified, the patient and clinician evaluate its validity in the following manner. First, the *evidence* in support of and against the thought or belief is reviewed. Next, the *implications* of the cognition are examined. Finally, *alternative explanations* are generated. Not all of these steps will be appropriate for all cognitions requiring revision, but the sequence provides a systematic approach for both patient and clinician. Not uncommonly, the clinician will find it necessary to model this sequence several times while providing significant suggestions and prompts until the patient is comfortable with conducting the procedure independently.

Example

Patient: I know that people won't like me if I gain weight.

Clinician: Really? Well, let's evaluate the accuracy of that thought. First of all, what's the *evidence* in *support* of that belief?

Patient: Well, look around you at the TV and magazines: people who are thin are more popular; people who are fat are outcasts.

Clinician: I agree. That's an unfortunate prejudice that exists in our culture to some extent, so I'm glad you raised it. But what about the people you interact with more directly? What other evidence can you think of in support of your belief?

Patient: I guess I assume that one of the reasons people like me is that they admire my willpower. If I gain weight, they won't admire me or like me anymore.

Clinician: How do you know? Has anyone ever said that to you?

Patient: Not really.

Clinician: Well, that's helpful in understanding your original belief. We should also talk later about your view of others' admiration for you. But let's get back to your original statement, that people won't like you if you gain weight. What *evidence* can you think of that *contradicts* that belief?

Patient: None.

Clinician: Are you sure? I was just thinking about how it works when the situation is reversed. Are your feelings for your friends changed when they gain or lose weight?

Patient: Sometimes I'm jealous if they lose weight.

Clinician: Do you *actually* like them less?

Patient: Of course not. I like my friends for who they are, not because of how they look.

Clinician: So what's the evidence that the "rules," so to speak, are different for you? Why would others like you more or less based on your weight?

Patient: I don't know . . . It just feels that way. Probably because I would feel worse about myself. My friends are always telling me to eat more.

Clinician: Given how we've identified that you feel your self-worth is directly associated with your body weight, I can understand that you feel that way. We can continue to evaluate and understand that underlying belief about yourself. But as far as your original statement about other people goes, what are the implications of your belief? I mean, what if people did like you less when you reach a healthier body weight?

Patient: That's what I'm afraid of.

Clinician: Yes, I understand. But what would be the implications if they did?

Patient: It would be kind of shallow of them, I guess. My close friends have actually been encouraging me to gain weight because they're so worried about me.

Clinician: So what if some people didn't like you as much as you became healthier?

Patient: I probably don't want them as friends.

One of the most difficult tasks for the clinician conducting cognitive restructuring is to remain Socratic rather than to adopt a persuasive stance. This type of therapeutic posture can be challenging, but restructuring proceeds optimally through the process of the patient's challenging her or his own beliefs, rather than being "instructed" to change her or his thoughts. However, individuals with AN may benefit early in treatment from the use of "parroting" standard coping phrases (e.g., "Food is my medicine: I have to eat to get better") (Garner and Bemis 1985).

The final step in cognitive restructuring is to revise maladaptive cognitions. After the evidence, implications, and alternative explanations have been examined, the patient is encouraged to attempt to revise his or her initial thought by incorporating new-found information. It is important for the patient to avoid revising thoughts to be overly optimistic; instead, the goal of revision is to be as accurate as possible. In addition, thought revisions are most useful when stated in the patient's own words.

Example *(continued)*

Clinician: Now that you have evaluated the accuracy of your thought that others won't like you if you gained weight, how would you revise it?

Patient: I guess that since I don't base my own feelings for my friends on their weight, and since my friends have even told me they hope

I gain weight, it's probably more accurate to say that among the people who care about me as a person, it's not likely that they will like me less for gaining weight; and if someone did like me less, they wouldn't be a very supportive friend.

When eating and weight symptoms have stabilized, patients with eating disorders often require additional work using the cognitive-restructuring technique to enhance self-esteem and challenge maladaptive beliefs about self-worth (Baird and Sights 1986; Garner and Bemis 1985; McKay and Fanning 1987).

Sociocultural Issues and Body Image

One of the most difficult aspects of cognitive restructuring with eating disorder patients is the fact that their maladaptive beliefs, especially about weight and shape, are often validated in the current sociocultural context (Garner et al. 1985; Striegel-Moore et al. 1986). For this reason, it is usually necessary to address these issues directly with patients, especially when conducting cognitive restructuring focused on weight and shape issues (Peterson and Mitchell 1995).

Psychoeducational materials are a beneficial way to help patients become more aware of societal factors involved in eating disorders (Garner et al. 1985; Orbach 1978, 1982). Although the overvaluation of thinness and the stigma against obesity that exist in our society are clearly not the sole "cause" of eating disorders, cross-cultural research indicates that eating disorders cluster in societies that value thinness as an aesthetic ideal; in other societies, these disorders are extremely rare (Dolan 1991; Striegel-Moore et al. 1986). One stance to take is that as members of society, every individual can make a "choice" to what extent she or he wants to endorse widely held beliefs, and that awareness of these beliefs (and how they are dispersed) can help in making this decision. The notion that the media are unbiased purveyors of "truth" can also be challenged by providing information about profit motives inherent in advertising and marketing (Wolf 1991).

Because of the "normative discontent" among women in society about their weight and shape (Rodin et al. 1985), along with the extreme degree of body dissatisfaction reported by individuals with eating disorders (Cash and Brown 1987; Cooper et al. 1987), the clinician must work with the patient to set realistic goals in addressing body image issues. In general, one should encourage patients to progress on the "spectrum" from unmitigated body hatred to gradual acceptance, rather than promoting "affection" for one's body and body parts, which is often unrealistic early in treatment. Instead, the patient is asked to work on identifying aspects of her or his appearance that she or he feels neutral or even positive about and emphasizing these strengths, both outwardly and in the form of affirmations. For parts of the body disliked, the patient should attempt to revise self-statements to be as accurate as possible by eliminating denigrating language (e.g., "thirty-eight–inch hips" rather than "fat rear end"). The multidimensional construct of "body image" can also be expanded to include other forms of sensory experiences (e.g., tactile, spatial). Finally, many individuals with eating disorders can learn to substitute the goal of "strength," with an emphasis on the *function* of body parts (e.g. "My legs enable me to walk"), instead of striving for an unrealistic degree of thinness.

Most important, individuals with eating disorders should be encouraged to expand their self-definition beyond weight and shape, which are often primary determinants of self-evaluation (Fairburn and Garner 1988). Decentering techniques are effective in helping patients recognize their own value by focusing on qualities they value in others (Garner and Bemis 1985). Patients can then work to identify other aspects of themselves that can be sources of pride and enjoyment. Challenging underlying beliefs about the reliance of self-worth strictly on external attributes can help facilitate this process.

Problem-Solving Skills, Stress Management, Social Skills, and Assertiveness

Although initial sessions of CBT usually target problems related to eating, weight, and shape, other issues often arise that may serve to precipitate and maintain these symptoms. In addition, many patients with eating disorders have deficits in stress management, assertiveness, problem-solving, and social skills (Cattanach and Rodin 1988; Nowell 1989; Pillay and Crisp 1981). For this reason, it is often useful to introduce these related skills as separate treatment modules or to incorporate these techniques in the context of relapse prevention. In general, cognitive restructuring is a useful tool in addressing deficits in these areas. Later in treatment, patients are more comfortable with cognitive restructuring procedures and are willing to expand topic areas to include assertiveness and stress management.

More in-depth work in these areas may be required by patients with more marked skills deficits. For example, graded task assignments, role playing, and modeling can be utilized to facilitate assertiveness and social skills (Becker and Heimberg 1985; Pillay and Crisp 1981; Schroeder and Black 1985). Relaxation training, psychoeducation, systematic approaches to identifying solutions, and strategies for time management may be useful for patients who complain of stress and difficulties with problem solving (Fairburn et al. 1993; Woolfolk and Lehrer 1985).

Relapse Prevention

Because of the high relapse rate for all types of eating disorders (Herzog et al. 1988), it is crucial to address this possibility directly before termination of treatment. One useful way to explain the process of relapse to patients is to describe the abstinence violation effect (AVE) (Marlatt and Gordon 1985), in which relapse results when a "slip" is misinterpreted as "evidence" of a full-blown relapse. For this reason, patients are informed that they are likely to experience "slips" (e.g., urges to binge eat or restrict) and that the risk lies not in the slip, but in whether cognitive distortions (especially dichotomous thinking) lead to the exacerbation of symptoms.

It is also useful for patients to have a written relapse-prevention plan. First, the patient, with the clinician's help, identifies "signals" that would indicate problematic behavior (e.g., skipping meals, occasional overeating, weight loss, increased preoccupation with weight and shape). Second, the patient identifies specific plans to address each of these symptoms (e.g., to reinitiate self-monitoring, attend a self-help group, practice cognitive restructuring exercises, or contact his or her clinician). Finally, the patient undertakes gradual reexposure to high-risk foods (usually those high in fat or sugar) and situations (e.g., a buffet meal, eating in front of the television) before the termination of treatment.

Outcome Research

Since the original description of the use of cognitive-behavioral techniques in the treatment of BN by Fairburn in 1981, a fairly large and impressive treatment literature has accumulated in this area. As would be expected, initial treatment studies tended to focus on the use of waiting-list or minimal-intervention controls. More recently, investigators have begun to compare active treatments, to undertake dismantling studies, and to compare psychotherapy approaches with medication in the treatment of BN. The treatment literature on AN involving CBT techniques remains quite limited, with some systematic research developing in the area during the past few years, although the results of most studies are not yet available. BED, although only recently described, has begun to be targeted for controlled CBT intervention trials, with positive results (Telch et al. 1990; Wilfley et al. 1993).

The literature of BN is examined in detail in the present section. Results of studies that compared an active treatment that included a CBT treatment component with a waiting-list, minimal intervention, or briefer form of therapy as a control group are summarized in Table 4–3. As is evident, some studies used individual therapy, others used groups, and a few used a mixture of both approaches. Most of these studies

Table 4-3. Controlled trials of the treatment of bulimia nervosa that compared an active treatment that included a cognitive-behavioral therapy (CBT) treatment component with waiting-list/minimal intervention controls

Investigator(s)	Treatment format	Treatment cells	N (at start)	Complete (%)	Short-term outcome	
					% Reduction in binge-eating frequency	% Abstinent at end of treatment
Lacey 1983	Individual + group	Individual + group (Waiting list)	30	100	95	80
Connors et al. 1984	Group	Psychoeducational (Waiting list)	26	77	70	
Kirkley et al. 1985	Group	CBT	14	93	97	
		Nondirective	14	64	64	
Ordman and Kirschenbaum 1985	Individual	Full	10	100		20
		Brief	10	100		20
Lee and Rush 1986	Group	CBT (Waiting list)	15	73	70	29
Wolchik et al. 1986	Individual + group	Psychoeducational (Waiting list)	13	85	58	9
Laessle et al. 1987	Group	Behavior therapy (Waiting list)	8	100		38

Note. Data shown for all active treatment cells, not waiting-list controls. Empty cell indicates that measure was not reported.

were quite modest in terms of sample size, with the largest sample being that in the early study by Lacey (1983) ($N = 30$). The Lacey study is also an outlier in terms of the dramatic rate of abstinence from bulimic symptoms at the end of treatment.

Results of second-generation studies, which utilized modifications in the primary treatment or alternative treatments, are summarized in Table 4–4. Again, the sample sizes of most of these studies were relatively modest, with the exceptions being those in the two-cell comparison by Fairburn and colleagues (1986), the four-cell comparison by Freeman and co-workers (1988), and the four-cell group therapy study reported by Agras and colleagues (1989). The last-mentioned study included a self-monitoring control group in addition to a waiting-list control group, a very interesting strategy that established that self-monitoring in itself appears to have therapeutic benefit. More recent, the comparison of CBT and psychodynamic psychotherapy by Garner and colleagues (1993) and a group psychotherapy model comparison study reported by our group (Crosby et al. 1993; Mitchell et al. 1993) can be added to this list.

Several aspects of these studies merit special consideration. One issue concerns the use of exposure and response prevention (ERP). Leitenberg and colleagues (1984, 1988) have advocated a model that focuses on the use of exposure to binge eating and the uncoupling of this phenomenon from the vomiting response by preventing vomiting. The first study specifically examining this technique in a randomized trial was reported by Wilson and co-workers (1986). Two groups were compared, both utilizing cognitive restructuring, but only one including an ERP module. Although the percent reductions in binge-eating frequency and the percentage of subjects abstinent at the end of treatment were numerically higher for those also receiving ERP, the results failed to reach statistical significance, perhaps because of the relatively small sample sizes (i.e., $n = 9$ and 8 for the ERP and no-ERP cognitive restructuring groups, respectively). Leitenberg and colleagues subsequently reported their own randomized trial in 1988. As can be seen, subjects were assigned to receive CBT with or without ERP, and ERP was administered either in single settings or in multiple settings. Again, the results suggested superiority for the use of the ERP in combination with CBT, delivered in either single or multiple formats; however, the response rate in those receiving CBT alone was modest, raising questions about the comparability of this form of CBT to some other CBT approaches. Also, again, the sample sizes were small. The third and largest study to examine ERP systematically was conducted by Agras and colleagues (1989). In this study, the addition of ERP seemed actually to detract from or to interfere with the effectiveness of the CBT intervention. Although the methodological differences among these studies have been discussed by Leitenberg and Rosen (1989), the findings of

Table 4–4. Controlled trials comparing active treatments utilizing modifications in the primary treatment or alternative treatments

Investigators	Treatment format	Treatment cells	N (at start)	Complete (%)	% Reduction in binge-eating frequency	% Abstinent at end of treatment
Yates and Sambrailo 1984	Group	CBT + BT	24[a]	67[a]		13
		CBT				71
Wilson et al. 1986	Group	Cognitive restructuring + ERP	9	85	82	71
		Cognitive restructuring	8	67	51	33
Fairburn et al. 1986	Individual	CBT	12	92	87	27
		Short-term focal	12	92	82	36
Leitenberg et al. 1988	Group	CBT + ERP (ms)	13	92	67[b]	42
		CBT + ERP (ss)	13	85	73	36
		CBT	12	100	40	8
		(Waiting list)				
Freeman et al. 1988	Individual + group	Individual CBT	32	66	79	
		Individual BT	30	83	87	
		Group	30	63	87	
		(Waiting list)				
Agras et al. 1989	Group	Self-monitoring	19	86	63	24
		CBT	22	77	75	56
		CBT + ERP	17	94	52	31
		(Waiting list)				

(continued)

Table 4–4. Controlled trials comparing active treatments utilizing modifications in the primary treatment or alternative treatments *(continued)*

Investigators	Treatment format	Treatment cells	N (at start)	Complete (%)	% Reduction in binge-eating frequency	% Abstinent at end of treatment
Fairburn et al. 1991	Individual	CBT	25	84	96.7	71
		IPT	25	88	89.0	62
		BT	25	76	91.3	62
Mitchell et al. 1993	Group	CBT: High emphasis on abstinence/High intensity	33	88	76.9	96.7
		High/Low	41	88	77.9	73.2
		Low/High	35	86	87.5	70.6
		Low/Low	34	82	61.8	32.4
Thackwray et al. 1993	Individual	CBT	47[a]	83[a]	88.9	92
		BT			100.0	100
		Attention placebo			82.1	60
Garner et al. 1993	Individual	Psychodynamic	30	83	69	40
		CBT	30	83	73	11

Note. Data shown for all active treatment cells, not waiting-list controls. Empty cell indicates that measure was not reported. CBT = cognitive-behavioral therapy; BT = behavior therapy; ERP = exposure and response prevention; ms = multiple settings; ss = single setting; IPT = interpersonal psychotherapy.
[a]Only aggregate data presented. [b]Reduction in vomiting.

the Agras et al. study do raise questions concerning the use of ERP, and further study is indicated before ERP becomes a routine component of treatment.

The two studies by Fairburn and co-workers (1986, 1991) also deserve special consideration. The earlier one, which included a modest number of subjects, compared individual CBT with a short-term psychotherapy that focused on interpersonal relationships. The more recent study directly compared CBT with behavior therapy that did not include cognitive restructuring and with interpersonal psychotherapy (IPT), a therapy initially developed for depression (Klerman et al. 1984). IPT was a particularly interesting choice for a control condition, because it does not address issues related to weight and shape or encourage changes in the eating patterns, but instead maintains a focus on interpersonal issues. As noted, all therapies seemed to have powerful effects on eating behavior in the short term, although there were some advantages for CBT on some of the measures of core psychopathology as measured by the Eating Disorder Examination. However, at long-term follow-up, which combined the CBT cells and the two interpersonal therapy cells, those who had been treated with IPT eventually "caught up" to those who had been treated with CBT (Fairburn et al. 1995). This is a particularly important observation and suggests that a therapy directed toward interpersonal functioning that does not address behavior and cognitions may in the long run result in a comparable degree of improvement in both the behavioral and the cognitive components of eating disorders.

The investigation by Garner and co-workers (1993) is the only study specifically to compare CBT with a manual-based psychodynamic approach. The results indicated significantly higher remission rates among those receiving CBT at the end of treatment and at follow-up, although both groups experienced a significant improvement in the frequency of binge-eating behavior during treatment. Recently, a study by Thackwray and colleagues (1993) suggested that a behavioral approach that does not emphasize cognitive restructuring can be effective in the short term compared with both an attention placebo condition and CBT in terms of remission rates, although at follow-up the CBT cell had a higher remission rate.

Relative to the method of delivery of psychotherapy, several investigators have advocated the use of clustered therapy sessions more often than weekly, at least initially in treatment. Fairburn (1981; Fairburn et al. 1986) has long been an advocate of this approach, as has our group at Minnesota (Crosby et al. 1993; Mitchell et al. 1990, 1993). Using a group CBT model, our group tested four different methods of delivery of the therapy by manipulating two variables: 1) whether or not there was an emphasis on early interruption of bulimic symptoms and an attendant clustering of visits early in treatment, and 2) the overall amount of time spent in treatment (22.5 vs. 45 hours total) (Mitchell et al. 1993). This resulted in a two-by-two, four-cell design. An emphasis on early interruption with clustered visits early in treatment, or use of a twice-weekly intensive approach, or use of a combination of high intensity with clustered visits resulted in much higher abstinence rates than the use of weekly therapy, despite the use of the same therapists and the same manuals. These results support the idea of seeing patients more frequently than weekly early in the course of treatment.

Several investigators have also attempted to compare CBT with antidepressant medication therapy, a strategy that has developed in parallel to the psychotherapy literature and that has been increasingly popular over the last 10 to 15 years (Table 4–5; see also Abbott and Mitchell 1993; Crow and Mitchell 1994).

In 1990, our group reported that the percent reduction in binge-eating frequency and the percentage of subjects free of symptoms at the end of treatment were significantly higher for subjects who had been treated with group CBT, whether they also received active medication treatment with imipramine or with placebo; it was also found that the active drug alone was significantly less effective than group therapy but was superior to placebo alone (Mitchell et al. 1990). However, on certain variables, including level of depression and anxiety, the addition of active drug to group therapy improved outcome, suggesting that a combination might be particularly useful in patients with significant problems with comorbid depression and anxiety. Agras and co-workers (1992) conducted a similar study, demonstrating that CBT was superior to treatment with desipramine alone, although the combination of CBT and the antidepressant did improve outcome on certain variables.

A second study comparing CBT with desipramine, by Leitenberg and colleagues (1994), was terminated prematurely because of a high drop-out rate among those taking desipramine, and the results therefore cannot be compared with those of the above study. A German study by Fichter and co-workers (1991), which evaluated the effectiveness of adding fluoxetine or placebo to a structured inpatient behavioral treatment program for BN, indicated a greater reduction in frequency of binge eating for those patients receiving fluoxetine. However, the use of the treatment on an inpatient sample limits generalization of these results to ambulatory studies from the United States. Additional studies comparing drugs and psychotherapy in the treatment of bulimia nervosa are indicated.

Conclusions

There is a large and growing treatment literature suggesting that CBT for BN, delivered in either a group or an individual format, is clearly

Table 4–5. Trials comparing CBT with antidepressant medication therapy in the treatment of bulimia nervosa

Investigators	Treatment format	Treatment cells	N (at start)	Complete (%)	Short-term treatment outcome	
					% Reduction in binge-eating frequency	% Abstinent at end of treatment
Mitchell et al. 1990	Group	CBT + placebo	34	85	89	45
		CBT + imipramine	52	75	92	56
		Imipramine	54	67	49	16
		Placebo	31	84	3	0
Agras et al. 1992	Individual	Desipramine, 16 weeks	12	83[a]	−12.7[b]	35
		Desipramine, 24 weeks	12		44.1	42
		CBT + desipramine, 16 weeks	12		57.3	65
		CBT + desipramine, 24 weeks	12		89.2	70
		CBT	12		71.3	50

Note. Empty cell indicates that measure was not reported.
[a]Percentage reported was for all four groups combined. [b]Reduction in vomiting.

superior to waiting-list or minimal-intervention control conditions. Moreover, in most studies, CBT also has been shown to be superior to other active treatments, although the results on this last point are not yet definitive. There is also one large study suggesting that IPT, over time, "catches up" to the effects of CBT. Examining remission rates in the published studies, it is reasonable to conclude that strategies that use clustered visits early in treatment may lead to higher remission rates, with the one group-therapy study that specifically addressed this issue demonstrating a clear advantage in terms of remission rates. The results also suggest that one-quarter to one-half of patients fail to achieve remission with CBT. Whether such patients can be treated more successfully with other interventions is not clear and is the subject of a multicenter study in which CBT nonresponders are randomized to receive IPT or a series of medication trials.

The available studies also suggest that antidepressants are highly effective in reducing the frequency of targeted eating behaviors and in improving mood in patients with eating disorders. However, on most outcome variables, antidepressants appear to be less effective than CBT and, in particular, result in lower rates of remission.

There are a number of obvious omissions in this treatment literature, summarized as follows:

1. Although many people with BN are adolescents, only adults have been the subjects in most of the available treatment studies, and we know little about the treatment of this younger group of patients.
2. Many treatment studies exclude those individuals with certain forms of comorbid psychopathology, particularly those with active alcohol and drug abuse problems and, at times, those with comorbid affective disorders. Therefore, the patients accepted into the treatment protocols may be somewhat atypical and may have a better prognosis than the overall population of people with eating disorders.
3. Because of the expense and other difficulties involved, the number of long-term follow-up studies is still very small, and considerable work needs to be done on the longitudinal course of this disorder.
4. Very little is known about the natural course of BN (Herzog et al. 1988). It appears that many individuals with this disorder never seek treatment, and the available data suggest that many individuals probably recover on their own. Far more information about the natural course of this disorder in both treated and untreated samples is needed.

References

Abbott DW, Mitchell JE: Antidepressants vs psychotherapy in the treatment of bulimia nervosa. Psychopharmacol Bull 29:115–119, 1993

Agras WS: Nonpharmacologic treatment of bulimia nervosa. J Clin Psychiatry 52 (No 10, suppl):29–32, 1991

Agras WS, Schneider JA, Arnow B, et al: Cognitive-behavioral and response-prevention treatment for bulimia nervosa. J Consult Clin Psychol 57:215–221, 1989

Agras WS, Rossiter EM, Arnow B, et al: Pharmacologic and cognitive-behavioral treatment for bulimia nervosa: a controlled comparison. Am J Psychiatry 149:82–87, 1992

Agras WS, Telch CF, Arnow B, et al: Does interpersonal therapy help patients with binge eating disorder who fail to respond to cognitive-behavioral therapy? J Consult Clin Psychol 63:356–360, 1995

American Psychiatric Association: Diagnostic and Statistical Manual of Mental Disorders, 4th Edition. Washington, DC, American Psychiatric Association, 1994

Baird P, Sights JR: Low self-esteem as a treatment issue in the psychotherapy of anorexia and bulimia. Journal of Counseling and Development 64:449–451, 1986

Beck AT, Rush AJ, Shaw BF, et al: Cognitive Therapy of Depression. New York, Guilford, 1979

Becker RE, Heimberg RG: Social skills training approaches, in Handbook of Clinical Behavior Therapy With Adults. Edited by Hersen H, Bellack AS. New York, Plenum, 1985, pp 201–226

Cash TF, Brown TA: Body image in anorexia nervosa and bulimia nervosa. Behav Modif 2:487–521, 1987

Cattanach L, Rodin J: Psychosocial components of the stress process in bulimia. Int J Eat Disord 7:75–88, 1988

Connors ME, Johnson CL, Stuckey MK: Treatment of bulimia with brief psychoeducational group therapy. Am J Psychiatry 141:1512–1516, 1984

Cooper PJ, Taylor MJ, Cooper Z, et al: The development and validation of the Body Shape Questionnaire. Int J Eat Disord 6:485–494, 1987

Crosby RD, Mitchell JE, Raymond N, et al: Survival analysis of response to group psychotherapy in bulimia nervosa. Int J Eat Disord 13:359–368, 1993

Crow SJ, Mitchell JE: Rational therapy of eating disorders. Drugs 48:372–379, 1994

Dolan B: Cross-cultural aspects of anorexia nervosa and bulimia: a review. Int J Eat Disord 10:67–78, 1991

Fairburn CG: A cognitive behavioural approach to the management of bulimia. Psychol Med 11:707–711, 1981

Fairburn CG: The current status of the psychological treatments for bulimia nervosa. J Psychosom Res 32:635–645, 1988

Fairburn CG, Garner DM: Diagnostic criteria for anorexia nervosa and bulimia nervosa: the importance of attitudes to shape and weight, in Diagnostic Issues in Anorexia Nervosa and Bulimia Nervosa. Edited by Garner DM, Garfinkel PE. New York, Brunner/Mazel, 1988, pp 36–55

Fairburn CG, Kirk J, O'Connor M, et al: A comparison of two psychological treatments for bulimia nervosa. Behav Res Ther 24:629–643, 1986

Fairburn CG, Jones R, Peveler RC, et al: Three psychological treatments for bulimia nervosa: a comparative trial. Arch Gen Psychiatry 48:463–469, 1991

Fairburn CG, Marcus MD, Wilson GT: Cognitive-behavioral therapy for binge eating and bulimia nervosa: a comprehensive treatment manual, in Binge Eating: Nature, Assessment, and Treatment. Edited by Fairburn CG, Wilson GT. New York, Guilford, 1993, pp 301–404

Fairburn CG, Jones R, Peveler RC et al: Psychotherapy and bulimia nervosa: the long-term effects of interpersonal psychotherapy, behavior therapy, and cognitive-behavior therapy for bulimia nervosa. Arch Gen Psychiatry 50:419–428, 1995

Fichter MM, Leibl K, Rief W, et al: Fluoxetine versus placebo: a double-blind study with bulimic inpatients undergoing intensive psychotherapy. Pharmacopsychiatry 24:1–7, 1991

Freeman CPL, Barry F, Dunkeld-Turnbell J, et al: Controlled trial of psychotherapy for bulimia nervosa. BMJ 296:521–525, 1988

Garner DM: Psychotherapy for eating disorders. Current Opinion in Psychiatry 5:391–395, 1992

Garner DM, Bemis KM: Cognitive therapy for anorexia nervosa, in Handbook of Psychotherapy for Anorexia Nervosa and Bulimia. Edited by Garner DM, Garfinkel PE. New York, Guilford, 1985, pp 107–146

Garner DM, Rockert W, Olmsted MP, et al: Psychoeducational principles in the treatment of bulimia and anorexia nervosa, in Handbook of Psychotherapy for Anorexia Nervosa and Bulimia. Edited by Garner DM, Garfinkel PE. New York, Guilford, 1985, pp 513–572

Garner DM, Rockert W, Davis R, et al: Comparison of cognitive-behavioral and supportive-expressive therapy for bulimia nervosa. Am J Psychiatry 150:37–46, 1993

Herzog DB, Keller MB, Lavori PW: Outcome in anorexia nervosa and bulimia nervosa: a review of the literature. J Nerv Ment Dis 176:131–143, 1988

Horvath AO, Luborsky L: The role of the therapeutic alliance in psychotherapy. J Consult Clin Psychol 61:561–573, 1993

Keys A, Brozek J, Henschel AJ, et al: The Biology of Human Starvation. Minneapolis, University of Minnesota Press, 1950

Kirkley BG, Schneider JA, Agras WS, et al: Comparison of two group treatments for bulimia. J Consult Clin Psychol 53:43–48, 1985

Klerman GL, Weissman MM, Rounsaville BJ, et al: Interpersonal Psychotherapy of Depression. New York, Basic Books, 1984

Lacey JH: Bulimia nervosa, binge-eating and psychogenic vomiting: a controlled treatment study and long-term outcome. BMJ 286:1609–1613, 1983

Laessle RG, Waadt S, Pirke KM: A structured behaviorally oriented group treatment for bulimia nervosa. Psychother Psychosom 48:141–145, 1987

Lee NF, Rush AJ: Cognitive-behavioral group therapy for bulimia. Int J Eating Disord 5:599–615, 1986

Leitenberg H, Rosen J: Cognitive-behavioral therapy with and without exposure plus response prevention in treatment of bulimia nervosa: comment on Agras, Schneider, Arnow, Raeburn, and Telch. J Consult Clin Psychol 57:776–777, 1989

Leitenberg H, Gross J, Peterson J, et al: Analysis of an anxiety model and the process of change during exposure plus response prevention treatment of bulimia nervosa. Behavior Therapy 15:3–20, 1984

Leitenberg H, Rosen JC, Gross J, et al: Exposure plus response-prevention treatment of bulimia nervosa. J Consult Clin Psychol 56:535–541, 1988

Leitenberg J, Rosen JC, Wolf J, et al: Comparison of cognitive-behavior therapy and desipramine in the treatment of bulimia nervosa. Behav Res Ther 32:37–45, 1994

Marlatt GA, Gordon JR: Relapse Prevention: Maintenance Strategies in the Treatment of Addictive Behaviors. New York, Guilford, 1985

McKay M, Fanning P: Self-Esteem. Oakland, CA, New Harbinger Publications, 1987

Metropolitan Life Insurance Company: 1983 Metropolitan Height and Weight Tables. New York, Metropolitan Life Insurance Company, 1983

Mitchell JE: Bulimia Nervosa. Minneapolis, University of Minnesota Press, 1990

Mitchell JE, Pyle RL, Eckert ED, et al: A comparison study of antidepressants and structured intensive group psychotherapy in the treatment of bulimia nervosa. Arch Gen Psychiatry 47:149–157, 1990

Mitchell JE, Specker S, Seim H: Comorbidity and medical complications of bulimia nervosa. J Clin Psychiatry 52 (No 10, suppl):13–20, 1991

Mitchell JE, Pyle RL, Pomeroy C, et al: Cognitive-behavioral group psychotherapy of bulimia nervosa: importance of logistical variables. Int J Eat Disord 14:277–287, 1993

Nowell R: The role of therapeutic recreation with eating disorder patients. Psychiatric Medicine 7:285–292, 1989

Orbach S: Fat Is a Feminist Issue. New York, Berkeley Books, 1978

Orbach S: Fat Is a Feminist Issue II. New York, Berkeley Books, 1982

Ordman AM, Kirschenbaum DS: Cognitive-behavioral therapy for bulimia: an initial outcome study. J Consult Clin Psychol 53:305–313, 1985

Peterson CB, Mitchell JE: Cognitive behavior therapy, in Treatments of Psychiatric Disorders, 2nd Edition, Vol 2. Gabbard GO, Editor-in-Chief, Washington, DC, American Psychiatric Press, 1995

Peterson CB, Mitchell JE: Treatment of binge eating disorder in group cognitive-behavioral therapy, in Treating Eating Disorders. Edited by Werne J. San Francisco, CA, Jossey-Bass, 1996, pp 143–186

Pillay M, Crisp AH: The impact of social skills training within an established inpatient treatment program for anorexia nervosa. Br J Psychiatry 139:533–539, 1981

Pomeroy C, Mitchell JE: Medical complications and management of eating disorders. Psychiatric Annals 19:488–493, 1989

Rodin J, Silberstein LR, Striegel-Moore RH: Women and weight: a normative discontent. Nebr Symp Motiv 32:267–307, 1985

Rounsaville BJ, Chevron ES, Prusoff BA, et al: The relation between specific and general dimensions of the psychology process in interpersonal psychotherapy for depression. J Consult Clin Psychol 55:379–384, 1987

Russell G: Bulimia nervosa: an ominous variant of anorexia nervosa. Psychol Med 9:429–448, 1979

Schroeder HE, Black MJ: Unassertiveness, in Handbook of Clinical Behavior Therapy With Adults. Edited by Hersen H, Bellack AS. New York, Plenum, 1985, pp 509–530

Steel ZP, Farag PA, Blaszczynski AP: Interrupting the binge-purge cycle in bulimia: the use of planned binges. Int J Eat Disord 18:199–208, 1995

Striegel-Moore RH, Silberstein LR, Rodin J: Toward an understanding of risk factors for bulimia: the use of planned binges. Int J Eat Disord 41:246–263, 1986

Telch CF, Agras WS, Rossiter EM, et al: Group cognitive-behavioral treatment for the nonpurging bulimic: an initial evaluation. J Consult Clin Psychol 58:629–635, 1990

Thackwray DE, Smith MC, Bodfish JW, et al: A comparison of behavioral and cognitive-behavioral interventions for bulimia nervosa. J Consult Clin Psychol 61:639–645, 1993

Vitousek K, Hollon SD: The investigation of schematic content and processing in eating disorders. Cognitive Therapy and Research 14:191–214, 1988

Wilfley DE, Agras WS, Telch CF, et al: Group cognitive-behavioral therapy for the nonpurging bulimia individual: a controlled comparison. J Consult Clin Psychol 61:296–305, 1993

Wilson GT, Fairburn CG: Cognitive treatments for eating disorders. J Consult Clin Psychol 61:261–269, 1993

Wilson GT, Rossiter E, Kleifeld EI, et al: Cognitive-behavioral treatment of bulimia nervosa: a controlled evaluation. Behav Res Ther 24:277–288, 1986

Wolchik SE, Weiss L, Katzman MA: An empirically validated short-term psychoeducational group treatment program for bulimia. Int J Eat Disord 5:21–34, 1986

Wolf N: The Beauty Myth: How Images of Beauty Are Used Against Women. New York, William Morrow, 1991

Woolfolk RL, Lehrer PM: Stress and generalized anxiety, in Handbook of Clinical Behavior Therapy With Adults. Edited by Hersen H, Bellack AS. New York, Plenum, 1985, pp 89–107

Yates AJ, Sambrailo F: Bulimia nervosa: a descriptive and therapeutic study. Behav Res Ther 22:503–517, 1984

Chapter 5

Cognitive Therapy for Chronic and Severe Mental Disorders

Jan Scott, M.D., F.R.C.Psych., and
Jesse H. Wright, M.D., Ph.D.

The utility of *stress-diathesis models* of severe mental disorders has led to the acceptance of the role of systematic psychological interventions in the treatment of individuals with severe and chronic psychiatric disorders (Scott 1995c). Practitioners have recognized that structured, operationalized approaches such as cognitive-behavioral therapy (CBT) can be used to facilitate adjustment to the disorder, increase the acceptability of and adherence to prescribed medications, and reduce morbidity. In this chapter we give an overview of clinical and research activity in this field. We begin the chapter with a brief discussion of the applicability of CBT in the treatment of patients with chronic and severe disorders. We then detail a cognitive-behavioral approach for three conditions: chronic and severe depression, bipolar disorder, and schizophrenia. Examples are given of interventions that may help individuals with these disorders identify and control symptoms, reduce the risk of relapse, and improve how they cope with the disorder. We highlight available outcome data and the need for research in each of these three areas.

Applicability of Cognitive-Behavioral Therapy

Beck's model of CBT (Beck et al. 1979) is the most widely tested short-term psychotherapy for any psychological problem and offers a robust, empirically based approach (Scott 1995c). In addition to its well-known use for patients with affective disorders, CBT is also applicable for patients with substance dependence problems, personality disorders, and psychotic disorders (Beck 1993; Beck et al. 1990b; Kingdon and Turkington 1994). It may be used in a wide variety of formats such as alone or in combination with medication; in individual, couples, or family therapy; or for outpatients or inpatients (Scott 1995c, 1996; Thase 1993). This flexibility is important because patients with chronic and severe psychiatric disorders have heterogeneous and complex problems. Beck's approach (Beck et al. 1979) allows a consistent model to be applied to a broad spectrum of difficulties presented by such individu-

---

als, thus reducing the risk of confused messages about the treatment rationale.

Cognitive-behavioral therapy also has specific characteristics that may benefit patients with severe mental disorders. Its collaborative, educational style and its use of a step-by-step approach and of guided discovery make it acceptable to individuals who wish to take an equal and active role in their therapy (Beck et al. 1979; Scott 1995a). Many individuals with severe disorders resist and challenge a didactic approach to treatment (Miklowitz et al. 1988). If the structured approach to each session is maintained, patients may retain their focus on specific agenda items even when mildly elated or distractible (Scott 1995a) or when exhibiting psychotic symptoms (Kingdon and Turkington 1994). CBT also can encourage skill development and an increased sense of self-efficacy and control. These features of CBT may be particularly helpful to individuals who perceive a loss of identity because they are viewed as a person with a severe or chronic mental disorder (Fowler et al. 1995).

Chronic and Severe Depression

Rationale for Cognitive-Behavioral Therapy

Studies of treatment outcome have found that significant proportions of patients do not respond well to standard therapeutic interventions. For example, only 64% of the subjects in the National Institute of Mental Health (NIMH) collaborative psychobiological study were judged to be recovered after 2 years (Keller et al. 1982). A somewhat better remission rate was observed by Sargeant and co-workers (1990), who noted that 19.1% of patients in the naturalistic follow-up of the Epidemiologic Catchment Area (ECA) investigation still had major depression after 1 year. Scott (1988) has suggested that the percentage of depressed patients who have a chronic course is 15%–20%. Although different rates of treatment resistance have been described, there appears to be no question that therapy is not fully effective in a significant minority of cases of depression.

Reviews of factors associated with chronicity (Paykel 1994; Scott 1988) concluded that chronicity could be predicted by the following: old age, longer duration of illness before treatment, psychotic symptoms, positive family history of depression, high neuroticism scores, and a preponderance of negative life events occurring after the onset of the index depressive episode. Thase (1994) has identified several additional contributors to a poor therapeutic response, including high scores on measures of dysfunctional attitudes, lack of social support, personality pathology, and severity of the index episode of illness.

A variety of biological treatments are available for patients with chronic or severe depression. For example, a combination of antidepressant and antipsychotic medication or electroconvulsive therapy (ECT) has been shown to be especially effective for individuals who suffer from depression with psychotic features (Guscott and Grof 1991). Lithium or thyroid hormone augmentation may be helpful for patients with treatment-resistant depression (Kennedy and Joffe 1989; Thase and Rush 1995). Also, monoamine oxidase inhibitors are useful in some individuals who do not improve after treatment with other antidepressants (Thase and Rush 1995). Nevertheless, a significant number of patients do not respond, or only partially respond, to such interventions.

Several other factors in addition to biological treatment resistance suggest the need for a psychotherapeutic approach to chronic and severe depression. As noted by Scott (1988) and Thase (1994), variables such as neuroticism, stressful life events, dysfunctional attitudes, and interpersonal difficulties are associated with chronicity. These types of problems may be addressed directly in CBT. Also, patients with extreme or lasting symptoms often have high levels of hopelessness (Beck et al. 1985, 1990a); actual behavioral deficits, such as impaired work performance or reduced social skills (Scott 1992); and significant reductions in self-esteem (Ludgate et al. 1993). Noncompliance with pharmacotherapy is another problem that can be approached with cognitive and behavioral procedures (Basco and Rush 1996; Cochran 1986; Rush 1988). Potential targets for CBT of chronic or severe depression are summarized in Table 5–1.

Table 5–1.   Potential cognitive-behavioral therapy (CBT) targets in chronic and severe depression

Agitation

Behavioral and social skills deficits

Comorbid disorders

Dysfunctional attitudes (schemas)

Hopelessness and suicidality

Interpersonal problems

Lack of pleasurable activities

Low self-esteem

Psychomotor retardation

Psychotic features

Sleep disturbance

Stressful life events

Treatment noncompliance

Overview of Therapy Procedures

The treatment procedures described in this section have been developed by clinicians who have worked extensively with hospitalized depressed patients (Bowers 1989, 1990; Cooper 1994; Ludgate et al. 1993; Scott 1992; Thase and Wright 1991; Wright et al. 1993), individuals with chronic depression (Scott 1992; Thase et al. 1994), and patients with psychotic features (Ludgate et al. 1993). CBT for these individuals uses many of the procedures described by Beck and co-workers (Beck and Rush 1995; Beck et al. 1979; Wright and Beck 1983, 1994) for less severe conditions. However, significant modifications are made in order to work more productively with people who have more pronounced or enduring symptoms.

A collaborative-empirical therapeutic relationship is at the core of the CBT treatment approach. Patients are socialized into the cognitive model and are then taught how to use cognitive restructuring and behavioral techniques to reduce symptoms. The therapy is structured and problem oriented. Usually, an agenda is set for each session. The therapist is quite active, but the patient is encouraged to take considerable responsibility for self-help exercises.

For patients with severe depression, treatment techniques may be adjusted to help deal with high levels of agitation, psychomotor retardation, difficulties with concentration, psychotic features, or profound hopelessness (Ludgate et al. 1993). For example, sessions may be reduced in length but held more frequently. Thase and Wright (1991) have recommended a behavioral emphasis early in treatment with inpatients. Techniques such as activity scheduling and graded task assignments may help activate the patient and reduce high levels of anxiety and agitation. More challenging cognitive interventions may be delayed until the patient is better able to concentrate on psychological issues. It should be emphasized, however, that severely depressed patients can often do at least some cognitive restructuring early in treatment (Ludgate et al. 1993; Shaw 1987; Thase and Wright 1991). One of the most important features of CBT for severe depression is the focus on hopelessness and suicidality. Interventions to curb hopelessness are often needed at the outset of treatment. Techniques for reducing hopelessness are described in more detail in the "examples" section of this chapter.

Cognitive-behavioral therapy procedures for depressed inpatients may also include the use of a "cognitive milieu" (Wright et al. 1993). Staff members are trained in CBT techniques so that the patient can be exposed to multiple opportunities to learn cognitive and behavioral procedures. Highly developed inpatient cognitive therapy programs usually include psychoeducation, individual therapy, and group CBT. Staff members may be assigned to assist with homework assignments, behavioral interventions, or other components of treatment. Before discharge, patients often participate in relapse-prevention exercises such as cognitive-behavioral rehearsal (Thase 1993). Most of these programs adopt a cognitive-biological model in which CBT and psychopharmacology are the predominate therapies. In a series of studies of severe, chronic depression, Scott (1992) noted that the introduction of a milieu approach to CBT improved treatment outcome.

Although CBT has been described as a procedurally specified or "manualized" approach, most cognitive therapists use considerable flexibility in developing a customized case conceptualization and treatment plan for each patient. With severely ill patients, the therapist may focus on specific targets (see Table 5–1) at different phases of the therapy. For a patient with severe depression, for example, the emphasis in the early portion of treatment may be on hopelessness and suicidal ideation, sleep disturbance, and managing agitation. In contrast, an individual with chronic depression may benefit most from intensive work on restructuring underlying dysfunctional attitudes. In general, CBT addresses the need for rapid symptom relief in the beginning of treatment and then shifts to issues such as schema modification, improved interpersonal functioning, and enhancement of social skills later in the therapeutic process.

Both cognitive and behavioral techniques are used for acute symptom relief. A patient with marked sleep problems that are not fully responsive to pharmacotherapy might be taught relaxation and imagery procedures in addition to methods of reducing intrusive negative thoughts. An agitated individual could be helped with distraction exercises, relaxation, and activity scheduling (Thase and Wright 1991). However, a person who has come to a catastrophic conclusion about the significance of a stressful life event may benefit most from cognitive-restructuring procedures such as recognition of "cognitive errors" or thought recording (Wright and Beck 1994). Many severely depressed patients have very low self-esteem, a reduced ability to participate in pleasurable activities, and a variety of self-defeating behavioral patterns. CBT addresses low self-esteem in a number of ways, including revision of distorted cognitive errors and automatic thoughts and use of behavioral exercises to increase self-efficacy. Pleasant-event scheduling and graded task assignments can help reverse inertia, boredom, and social isolation.

Patients with chronic depression present a challenge for clinicians, regardless of the form of therapy used. Cognitive therapy for individuals with treatment-resistant disorders may vary depending on the case formulation. The overall strategy is to look for possible roadblocks to recovery and to design interventions to help the patient revise long-standing negative self-constructs or self-defeating patterns of behavior. Individuals with chronic affective disorders often have stressed or dysfunctional relationships with significant others. Thus, attention to interpersonal issues in individual therapy (Safran and Segal 1990) and/or the use of conjoint or family CBT (Epstein 1982; Epstein et al. 1988) are frequently indicated.

A central theme of CBT for persons with chronic conditions is the attempt to uncover and modify underlying schemas or dysfunctional attitudes. Maladaptive schemas are thought to predispose individuals to recurrent depression and to be predominate features of personality disturbances (Beck et al. 1979, 1990b). A variety of procedures are used to identify and revise schemas, including *examining the evidence, listing advantages and disadvantages, generating alternatives,* and *keeping a positive data log* of evidence to support more adaptive beliefs (Greenberger and Padesky 1995; Wright and Beck 1994). Schema modification is usually considered an advanced cognitive-therapy technique. This process often requires more time and effort than other frequently used CBT interventions such as thought recording or activity scheduling.

Persons with chronic disorders may have comorbid disorders that add to the difficulty in obtaining a satisfactory treatment response. Individuals with substance abuse, personality disorders, panic attacks, or other conditions require a multifaceted treatment plan that addresses each problem. CBT methods have been developed for most Axis I and Axis II disorders (Beck et al. 1979, 1990b). If a patient has a significantly severe comorbid condition, treatment is directed at all of the forms of pathology. For example, it is likely that a chronically depressed person who also abuses alcohol and has panic attacks would be approached with a combination of CBT interventions specifically designed for each problem. (See Chapters 1 and 2, by Clark and Wells and by Thase, in this volume for description of CBT for panic disorders and substance abuse, respectively.)

An additional treatment method has recently become available for patients with chronic and severe depression. A multimedia form of computer-assisted cognitive therapy (CCT) developed by Wright and colleagues (1995) was designed to be used by a wide range of patients, including those with severe levels of symptoms. No previous computer or keyboard experience is required. The intent of this interactive program is to facilitate the work of the clinician by teaching the basic concepts and procedures of CBT. Patients participate in a variety of exercises that can help them learn methods of modifying dysfunctional cognitions and behavior. A study of CCT in combination with treatment-as-usual for severely depressed inpatients demonstrated high levels of patient acceptance and substantial reduction in symptoms (Wright et al. 1996). It is possible that computer-assisted therapy could improve the efficiency of treatment for patients with chronic or severe depression. Also, CCT could help engage individuals who have difficulty with more traditional therapy approaches. However, controlled research has not yet been performed on the multimedia form of CCT.

Cognitive-Behavioral Therapy for Chronic or Severe Depression

In this subsection, we illustrate specific procedures for three of the more important targets for CBT of chronic and severe depression: hopelessness, psychotic features, and behavioral deficits.

Hopelessness.   Hopelessness has been found to be a strong predictor of suicide risk (Beck et al. 1975, 1985, 1990a) and also is associated with self-defeating behaviors such as helplessness, withdrawal, isolation, and substance abuse. Thus, reduction in hopelessness is a major goal of CBT. The basic structure of CBT is designed to counter hopelessness by involving the patient in action-oriented exercises that can break patterns of inertia. An agenda is set collaboratively for each session, and patient and therapist work together as a team to reverse cognitive distortions and develop more effective behaviors. A problem-focused approach helps patients become more hopeful as they develop more effective coping strategies for their difficulties.

The use of cognitive therapy procedures for hopelessness is illustrated by the case of Mr. N. a 54-year-old man who had lost his job as a banker after a corporate takeover by a national banking system. Within 6 weeks after losing his job, Mr. N. became severely depressed and attempted suicide by carbon monoxide poisoning. His wife found him by accident when she came home early from choir practice. After being admitted to the hospital, Mr. N. reported that he was sorry his wife had found him. During the initial interview, the cognitive therapist elicited a number of cognitions associated with hopelessness, including "My life is over," "Nobody would want to have anything to do with me," "I wasted my life," and "I've let everybody down." It was also noted that Mr. N. had been acting in a counterproductive manner since hearing that his job would be eliminated. Instead of accepting the bank's offer of outplacement services, he stayed alone at home and refused to consider any suggestions for going ahead with his life.

Cognitive-behavioral therapy for Mr. N. included a series of interventions designed to help him identify and modify negatively distorted thoughts. One of the therapist's first initiatives was to ask Mr. N. to work on a list of reasons to live. This commonly used CBT procedure can rapidly break through intense hopelessness. Although Mr. N. had a preponderance of pessimistic cognitions, he was able to write down several items on this list, including 1) "My wife," 2) "My family," 3) "I could possibly still make something of my life," 4) "I might be able to enjoy hobbies and sports," and 5) "I have something to give to others." The clinician used *Socratic questioning,* a standard CBT technique (Beck et al. 1979), to help the patient step away from his intensely negative cognitions and focus on more adaptive cognitions. The list of "reasons to live," developed on the first day of hospitalization, served as a template for Mr. N.'s subsequent reinvestment in overcoming the severe episode of depression.

A specific behavioral assignment was made to follow up on the material of the first session. Mr. N. agreed to take two actions to commit to his "reasons to live." He planned 1) to call his wife to tell her that he was feeling better and that he had started to turn his situation around and 2) to ask her to bring books on some of his previous interests. In later sessions, Mr. N. learned to identify and revise automatic thoughts and negative schemas that were related to hopelessness and depression. For example, the thought "I've let everybody down" was recognized as an inaccurate and dysfunctional cognition. Mr. N. was encouraged to "examine the evidence" (Wright and Beck 1994) for this automatic thought and to develop a more balanced and rational way of viewing his job loss. After a brief hospitalization, he was able to return home and initiate the process of looking for another job. Although still faced with the situation of finding new employment, Mr. N. was considerably more hopeful and was able to view his assets and liabilities in a balanced manner.

Psychotic features.   Major depression with psychotic features is usually treated vigorously with pharmacotherapy (antidepressant plus antipsychotic medication) or ECT. Nevertheless, psychotherapeutic interventions can also be useful. Individuals with psychotic depression may be guarded and suspicious, delusional, and/or behaviorally regressed, and/or may have pronounced guilt, hopelessness, and suicidality. The techniques described elsewhere in this chapter for these types of problems can be applied to depressed patients with psychotic features. However, adjustments must be made in the therapeutic relationship and in the timing and implementation of techniques.

In the early phase of treating psychotic depression, the cognitive therapist usually focuses on establishing a good therapeutic relationship and choosing targets for intervention that do not directly challenge delusional thinking. Cognitive therapy procedures for delusions are delayed until progress has been made with more approachable problems. For example, the treatment plan for a patient with significant agitation might utilize behavioral techniques such as relaxation training, distraction, or activity scheduling. After symptoms are reduced with CBT procedures and/or biological therapies, the therapist can begin to work on delusions. Formation of a collaborative therapeutic relationship is a prerequisite for cognitive therapy of delusions.

Procedures used to modify delusional thoughts include using Socratic questioning, implementing thought recording, identifying cognitive errors, examining the evidence, and listing alternatives. An example of a cognitive-restructuring exercise is presented in Table 5–2.

This procedure of examining the evidence was used to help a 70-year-old patient who had delusions of financial ruin. Although this patient was being treated with a combined pharmacotherapy regimen of an antidepressant and antipsychotic, he still had delusional fears of losing his home. By systematically examining the evidence for and against this frightening occurrence, he was able to gain a better degree of reality testing.

Many of the methods used for treating positive symptoms in schizophrenia discussed later in this chapter can also be applied to psychotic depression. However, the therapist usually directs a major portion of the treatment effort at the features of depression (e.g., low self-esteem, psychomotor retardation or agitation, hopelessness, loss of interest). The overall strategy is to diminish the significance of the delusional material by focusing on areas of positive change.

Behavioral deficits. Persons with chronic or severe depression often have significant behavioral deficits such as social isolation, lack of

---

Table 5–2. "Examining the evidence" in cognitive-behavioral therapy for psychotic depression: an example

---

Thought: I've made some kind of horrible mistake with managing our finances—we'll lose our home and everything we have worked for our whole lives.

"Evidence for"	"Evidence against"
1. I haven't paid the bills for 2 months.	1. My wife says that there is no problem.
2. An overdue notice came from the bank.	2. My accountant tells me that we are financially secure.
3. I've always feared losing everything.	3. The company pension is solid.
4. I should still be working.	4. Social security is probably reliable.
	5. I planned carefully for retirement
	6. We have reduced our expenses and can live modestly.

Alternative thoughts

1. Being depressed has made me have extremely negative thoughts.
2. Treatment for depression should help.
3. I haven't stayed on top of our finances, but there is no real evidence that we will lose everything.
4. I can get my wife to help me straighten things out.
5. I don't really need to go back to work, but a part-time job might be good for me.

---

assertiveness, and reduced self-efficacy. In addition to having a negatively distorted self-image, they may have actual impairment in their functional capacity. For example, depressed subjects have been shown to have difficulty in sustaining effort in challenging tasks (Cohen et al. 1982). CBT includes a variety of procedures that can be used to stimulate more adaptive behavior or improved social skills (Beck et al. 1979; Scott 1988; Thase and Beck 1993).

Behavioral interventions in chronic depression are illustrated in the case of Ms. T., a 37-year-old woman who had failed to respond fully to appropriate courses of pharmacotherapy, including both lithium and thyroid hormone augmentation of antidepressants. After several full courses of antidepressant therapy, she continued to have moderately severe depression. Ms. T. was referred for CBT because she was reporting increased difficulty in functioning at work and home. Ms. T. had became increasingly overwhelmed by her life situation and had developed pessimistic attitudes and more passive patterns of behavior. A portion of the CBT for this patient included specific interventions to help reverse such behavioral pathology.

In the first session with the cognitive therapist, Ms. T. reported that she could not "enjoy anything anymore." After returning from work, she was "totally exhausted" and "collapsed without being able to do anything for the children or myself." Ms. T. functioned better in her job as an office supervisor than at home, but had allowed several projects to pile up. She had stopped virtually all her previous enjoyable activities such as exercise classes, hobbies, and social engagements with friends. Ms. T. was a single mother who had excellent relationships with her two children. However, she felt guilty because her participation in family activities had also reached a very low level.

The behavioral component of treatment with Ms. T. included activity scheduling, graded task assignments, and cognitive-behavioral rehearsal. The first stage was to obtain a baseline assessment of her actual level of functioning. She was asked to complete a Weekly Activity Schedule (Beck et al. 1979; Thase 1993) and to rate each activity on a 0–10 scale for mastery and pleasure. As is often the case, Ms. T.'s assessment of a pervasive inability to experience pleasure was found to be inaccurate. Although she was clearly experiencing decreased energy and interest, there were still a number of activities (e.g., reading to daughter, taking a short walk, looking at garden catalogs, taking a coffee break with a friend) that were associated with a modest increase in pleasurable feelings. The Weekly Activity Schedule was used to help Ms. T. make gains in several areas: 1) to recognize distorted negative thinking about her capacities, 2) to plan activities to increase her experiences of mastery and pleasure, 3) to reduce the frequency of dysfunctional activities, 4) to organize time more effectively, and 5) to select targets for graded task assignments and/or CBT rehearsal.

Graded task assignments can help patients tackle problems that at first may seem to be overwhelming or exceptionally challenging (Wright and Beck 1994). For example, Ms. T. noted that she had allowed the family finances to "get totally out of control." Over the last 4 months she had been letting mail accumulate without opening it, had not balanced her checkbook, and had paid bills in a sporadic and inconsistent fashion. Now she viewed the situation as "impossible." The cognitive therapist worked with Ms. T. on a behavioral plan to tackle this difficult situation in a stepwise fashion.

Cognitive-behavioral rehearsal can be used to improve coping strategies or social skills (Thase and Beck 1993). This technique helped Ms. T. manage a difficult situation at work. She had avoided a meeting with employees whom she supervised because of fears of questions they might raise about the backlog of work. The therapist encouraged her to visualize the scene in advance, identify potential questions, and rehearse possible responses. Coaching and role playing were used in the therapy session to prepare Ms. T. for the staff meeting. After participating in these cognitive-behavioral exercises, Ms. T. was able to effectively bring the work group together to help resolve the problem.

Outcome Research

There is a great deal of evidence that CBT is an effective treatment for depression (for reviews of outcome research, see Dobson 1989; Hollon et al. 1991; Scott 1996; Wright and Beck 1994). However, most studies have been conducted on mild to moderately symptomatic outpatient samples of patients who meet research criteria for the diagnosis of nonpsychotic major depressive disorder. Investigators that have examined the effect of severity of illness have found mixed results. Blackburn and co-workers (1981), Kovacs and colleagues (1981), and Teasdale and associates (1984) observed that severity of illness (or endogenous subtype) did not influence treatment outcome with CBT. However, Elkin and co-workers (1989) noted that CBT was somewhat less effective for severe depression than for milder forms of this disorder. Thase and co-workers (1991b) found that patients with severe depression were less likely than other subjects to have a full remission after a course of CBT. Nevertheless, both patient groups improved substantially, and there were only small differences in endpoint depression scores.

Thase and colleagues (1994) have also reported on the differential response of acutely and chronically depressed patients to CBT. Subjects who had either major depression superimposed on dysthymia ("double depression") or chronic major depression were less likely than patients with acute depression to reach full remission. However, the group with chronic depression had significant reductions in Hamilton Rating

Scale for Depression (Ham-D) and Beck Depression Inventory (BDI) scores. Other investigators have observed that chronic or double depression can be associated with a reduced response to CBT (Fennell and Teasdale 1982; Harpin et al. 1982; Mercier et al. 1992; Scott 1992). Findings that chronicity or comorbidity with dysthymia can complicate treatment with CBT are not surprising because these conditions are also more difficult to treat with biological therapies (Thase and Howland 1994). CBT for psychotic depression has not been investigated systematically, but it would be expected that patients with this type of depression would also be less responsive to treatment than would patients with uncomplicated major depression. As such, treatment of psychotic depression with CBT alone is not recommended unless pharmacotherapy and ECT are refused and involuntary treatment is not feasible.

Scott (1992) found that CBT for a sample of inpatients with chronic, treatment-resistant depression was somewhat more effective if given as a total treatment package (cognitively oriented hospital milieu) than in a standard individual therapy format. Other studies of depressed inpatients have shown that this treatment approach can be useful for individuals with marked levels of symptomatic distress. For example, Bowers (1990) found that inpatients who received either CBT plus nortriptyline or a behavioral intervention plus nortriptyline had lower BDI scores and were more likely to be recovered at the end of treatment than inpatients who received drug alone. Patients who were treated with CBT had a significantly higher recovery rate as judged by Ham-D score criteria than either of the other two groups.

Another study of depressed inpatients, reported by Miller and co-workers (1989), found that subjects treated with CBT plus antidepressants improved significantly. However, at the end of hospitalization, there were no significant differences between "treatment as usual," social skills training, and CBT. (All groups received concomitant antidepressants.) Six and 12 months posthospitalization, there was a trend for subjects who received standard treatment to have a higher rate of relapse. Also, the pooled group of psychotherapy patients had a significantly higher rate of recovery (68%) than did the standard treatment group (33%). Subsequent analyses of these data documented a preferable response to the combined regimen in patients with high levels of dysfunctional attitudes (Miller et al. 1990) and a significant advantage over the standard condition on measure of dysfunctional cognitions (Whisman et al. 1991).

Several groups of investigators have explored the effects of CBT without medication for depressed inpatients. The first open trial of CBT in this context was conducted by Shaw (1987), who observed a substantial decrease in BDI scores after 8 weeks of treatment. In a later trial, Thase and co-workers (1991a) observed a decrease of mean BDI scores, from 32.4 to 6.9, over 3 to 4 weeks of CBT in hospitalized patients with endogenous depression. An expanded study by this same research group found a response rate of 70% for inpatient CBT (Thase 1994).

The only controlled study of CBT without medication for depressed inpatients was carried out by DeJong and co-workers (1986). This study had significant limitations, including a small number of patients in each treatment condition and the use of an outpatient control group. Treatment response was higher in hospitalized patients who received a complete package of CBT compared with those who received either inpatient cognitive restructuring or outpatient supportive therapy.

The overall results of research on CBT for patients with chronic and severe depression indicate that these individuals may have a somewhat more difficult treatment course than those with acute or less extreme symptoms. However, the predominance of evidence supports the effectiveness of CBT for both chronic and severe depression. Studies of inpatients have found that CBT can work without antidepressants and that cognitive-behavioral approaches are at least as effective as standard treatments. Some investigators have found an additive effect for inpatient CBT. Severe and treatment-resistant cases of depression are a challenge for any therapy method. It is expected that there will be further development of CBT procedures for patients with this demanding condition.

Bipolar Disorder

Rationale for Cognitive-Behavioral Therapy

The prevalence of bipolar disorder in the general adult population is estimated to be 0.4%–1.6%. There is an equal gender distribution, and the median age at onset of first episode is about 21 years (Regier et al. 1988). About 80% of persons with bipolar disorder experience at least one recurrence following an index affective episode (Prien and Potter 1990). The advent of lithium, carbamazepine, and divalproex sodium has undoubtedly improved the quality of life of many individuals. However, lithium prophylaxis protects only 25%–50% of individuals with bipolar disorder against further episodes (Dickson and Kendall 1986), and the use of newer medications has not eliminated the problem of relapse (Scott 1995c). The use of adjunctive psychological interventions has been advocated as a method of providing improved coping skills to deal with bipolar symptoms and enhanced treatment adherence (Basco and Rush 1996; Jamison et al. 1979; Prien and Potter 1990).

Several reviews have reported on individual or interpersonal difficulties that arise as a consequence of bipolar disorder or that increase an individual's vulnerability to future relapse (Goodwin and Jamison

1990; Prien and Potter 1990; Scott 1995c). Most of these problems are amenable to a cognitive-behavioral approach. For example, CBT may be used for Axis II, substance abuse, or relationship problems. In adulthood, 50% of individuals with bipolar disorder meet the criteria for a personality disorder (Peselow et al. 1995). The prevalence of comorbid substance abuse disorders and bipolar disorder is about 35% (Goodwin and Jamison 1990). Relationships may also be severely strained as a result of unacceptable behaviors during a manic episode. Moreover, about 60% of patients with bipolar disorder eventually divorce or separate from their partners (Goodwin and Jamison 1990).

Reported noncompliance rates for mood-stabilizing drugs vary between 20% and 50% (Jamison and Akiskal 1983; Scott 1995c). One in five individuals discontinue medication despite a good response (Bech et al. 1976). Noncompliance rates are particularly high during the first year of prophylaxis and in those individuals who complain of missing "highs." Practical problems that can reduce adherence include unacceptable side effects and complicated treatment regimens.

There is a 50% risk of a further affective episode in the year immediately after an episode of bipolar disorder in patients who do not take prophylactic medication (American Psychiatric Association 1994; Prien and Potter 1990). Hammen and colleagues (Hammen et al. 1992; Swendsen et al. 1995) identified prospectively that interpersonal life events led to bipolar disorder symptom exacerbation in patients with high levels of "sociotropy" (i.e., those who attach a high value to relationships), even when they were complying regularly with medication. Miklowitz and co-workers (1988) found that relapse of bipolar disorder occurred if there was a high level of expressed emotion or a negative affective style within the family, regardless of other variables such as medication compliance or baseline symptoms.

There are a number of reasons to consider the adjunctive use of CBT for bipolar disorder, including lack of full response to pharmacotherapy, nonadherence to treatment recommendations, presence of cognitive and behavioral symptoms, reactivity to stressors, and a high propensity for relapse (Basco and Rush 1996). The CBT approach outlined in the following subsection is directed at augmenting and complementing biological treatments of bipolar disorder.

Overview of Therapy Procedures

There are general and specific reasons for the use of CBT that the therapist will wish to discuss with a patient with bipolar disorder. The general aims for using this approach are to facilitate adjustment to the condition, to increase or enhance coping skills, to help the individual recognize and manage psychosocial stressors, and to teach CBT strategies for dealing with cognitive and behavioral problems.

At a more specific level, a conceptualization based on Padesky and Mooney's (1990) "five areas" model may be used to help understand bipolar disorder and its impact on the individual. This formulation stresses the links between four aspects of the individual (cognitions, behavior, mood, and biology), as well as the interaction between these diatheses and the environment (past and present events or experiences). To use this approach for bipolar disorder, the therapist should first ask the patient to describe his or her own views about the causes of the disorder and the problems. The patient's etiologic theory is then incorporated within the framework of the model. Links between all five areas are repeatedly stressed. The therapist explains that changes in one of these five areas may lead to changes in another area (Padesky and Mooney 1990). This rationale is used to engage the patient in CBT through monitoring and linking changes in thoughts, behaviors, feelings, and the symptoms of bipolar disorder. Many individuals will have been given a "biological" explanation of bipolar disorder before coming to CBT sessions. When the connections between the biological and other aspects of his or her experience are illustrated, the patient is usually able to understand the rationale for the use of CBT without having to reject other causal models.

Specific difficulties and consequences of the disorder will usually form key aspects of the patient's problem list. It is often helpful to define problems under three broad headings: intrapersonal (e.g., low self-esteem), interpersonal (e.g., lack of social support, difficulties in relationships with family members), and basic problems (e.g., symptom frequency; severity or course; early warning signs for relapse; difficulties coping with work; housing problems).

The therapy often starts with developing coping strategies to deal with particular symptoms. For example, mood lability may be tackled by teaching affect regulation techniques, exploring automatic thoughts and behavioral accompaniments of mood change, and monitoring medication adherence and changes in mood. If symptoms are brought under better control, the patient and therapist may then move on to deal with problems such as low self-esteem. In later sessions, interventions focus specifically on relapse prevention. Prodromal symptoms of relapse are explored, and self-management skills are developed. It also is important to explore patients' underlying dysfunctional attitudes and beliefs about themselves, their world, and their future that may act as barriers to full recovery.

The CBT approach to bipolar disorder is similar in many respects to methods used for individuals with other severe or chronic conditions. Between episodes, however, many individuals with bipolar disorder function at a higher level than do individuals with schizophrenia or chronic depression. Because shifts in the level of functioning can occur quite rapidly, the cognitive therapist has to be prepared for significant variations in what can or cannot be tackled during a session. Ground-work must be done to reduce the risk of the patient's opting for premature termination of therapy on the basis of overly optimistic subjective assessments of improvement. Miklowitz and Goldstein (1990) observed that patients with bipolar disorder may interact in a more fast-paced, affective, and spontaneous manner than those with other severe mental health problems. Clinicians need to avoid the temptation to "join the rush." They should take responsibility for establishing a clear structure and realistic pace for sessions. Because CBT attempts to deal with relapse prevention in addition to acute symptoms, the course of CBT may require up to 20–30 sessions over a period of a year or more (Scott 1995b). Psychiatrists who perform maintenance therapy may use CBT procedures combined with medication for bipolar patients over a period of many years.

Examples of Cognitive-Behavioral Therapy for Bipolar Disorder

The following section briefly outlines some of the CBT interventions that may be used with patients with bipolar disorder. Many of these techniques draw on personal experience or have been learned by the authors from others working in this or related areas (Basco and Rush 1996; Ludgate 1994; Newman and Beck 1992; Palmer et al. 1995; Rush 1988; Wright and Thase 1992).

Education about bipolar disorder. Individuals with bipolar illness deserve a frank description of the disorder, the known facts about prognosis, and information about alternative treatment approaches. A number of leaflets, books, and videos have been produced (Bohn and Jefferson 1992; Manic Depression Fellowship 1995; McKeon 1992; Peet and Harvey 1991). These resources provide valuable material for early homework assignments and also may stimulate the patient to ask questions at later CBT sessions. Because attitudes of significant others may influence a patient's prognosis, educating family members or supplementing individual CBT with family sessions may be desirable (Scott 1992).

Ms. D. was a 28-year-old single woman, currently residing with her parents. She was referred for outpatient CBT, 6 weeks after hospitalization for her first episode of acute mania. During the first interview, Ms. D. had a sad mood but did not have full symptoms of major depressive disorder. She was distressed at receiving the diagnosis of bipolar disorder. However, when asked to outline her own knowledge of the disorder, it was clear she had limited facts at her disposal. Ms. D. believed that "all forms of breakdown are a consequence of personal inadequacy." Further exploration revealed that a number of people, particularly her father, had influenced her thinking about mental disorders. Her mother had a history of unipolar depression. However, her father had responded with dismissive comments and an obvious lack of support.

Over a period of 3 weeks, Ms. D. was encouraged to test out her beliefs about bipolar disorder. During these sessions, Ms. D. and her therapist examined the validity of her ideas. She collected additional information from local libraries and support groups and also wrote to a national organization for people with bipolar disorder. Ms. D. was encouraged to take the lead in gathering information and to come back to the therapist with a list of additional questions at each session. Her views of bipolar disorder were then reexamined in light of the new data. As a result, Ms. D.'s self-ratings of the accuracy of the belief that the disorder was a consequence of personal inadequacy fell from 85% to 25%.

Next, the patient was encouraged to develop alternative hypotheses about the etiology of bipolar disorder. Evidence was developed to support the view that "bipolar disorder is a mental disorder with significant genetic and biological contributions." Ms. D. was not convinced that biological models offered a full explanation of her own problems, but eventually she was able to conclude that bipolar disorder has a multifactorial etiology and can not be explained purely on the basis of personal inadequacy.

The final phase of the process of education involved Ms. D.'s talking with her family to help them understand the disorder. Because Ms. D.'s father was known to be skeptical about multifactorial models, Ms. D. and the therapist undertook role-plays in the therapy session. Although the role-play appeared to help considerably, Ms. D. was still worried about her ability to deal with any negative views expressed by her father. Her negative automatic thoughts, such as "I won't do this very well—I'll make a fool of myself," were only partly discounted by exploration in the CBT session. Therefore, it was agreed that the patient would practice presenting the information she wanted to get across by talking to her brother. For a homework assignment, Ms. D. visited her brother, explained the disorder to him, and then answered his questions. This exercise helped undermine the basis of Ms. D.'s negative automatic thoughts, and subsequently she was able to undertake the same exercise with her parents. She handled her father's questions well, and he became sufficiently interested to read booklets and watch an educational video about bipolar disorder. Ms. D.'s strong sense of mastery from this exercise and the subsequent reduction in negative comments from her father contributed to an improvement in her self-esteem.

Enhancing medication compliance.   Recurring cognitive themes among those who have adherence problems are that the use of psychotropic medications indicates personal weakness, loss of control, and/or heightened vulnerability (Scott 1995a; Wright and Schrodt 1992). Misunderstandings regarding the nature of the disorder, fears about medication side effects, and concern about the reactions of others may also be relevant (Beck et al. 1979; Cochran and Gitlin 1988; Wright and Schrodt 1992). These dysfunctional cognitions can be approached with commonly used CBT procedures such as thought recording and examining the evidence. Also, because complex treatment regimens may increase the risk of noncompliance, simple medication schedules should be negotiated whenever possible (Goodwin and Jamison 1990).

Mr. R. was a 43-year-old businessman who presented with a history of two episodes of hypomania and one episode of mania over the past 2 years. At the initial interview, Mr. R. openly acknowledged that his adherence to prescribed medication was erratic. However, he found it hard to explain why he frequently missed taking his tablets. At first, he and the therapist identified that Mr. R.'s busy lifestyle played a part. Before going to work in the mornings, Mr. R. took responsibility for a number of household tasks and also was responsible for taking his two children to school. A weekly diary demonstrated that Mr. R. often omitted the morning dose of lithium. Two behavioral strategies were used (Rush 1988; Wright and Thase 1992): 1) a behavioral prompt (a note attached to a bathroom mirror) was used to remind Mr. R. that he should take a morning dose of lithium, and 2) the ingestion of medication was "paired" with a routine morning activity—making a pot of coffee for the family breakfast. Mr. R.'s adherence to the morning dose of lithium improved from 35% to 80% after implementing these simple behavioral strategies. Subsequently, Mr. R. suggested that his wife might ask him a question as he left home in the morning as a final reminder.

Mr. R. took a second dose of lithium in the early evening. The nature of his employment meant that he was often still at work or was away from home in a hotel. Although Mr. R. rarely failed to take his medication supply with him, on average he took the early-evening treatment only on two out of five occasions. A detailed analysis was undertaken of times when Mr. R. did and did not take this dose of medication. It was noted that high-risk situations for nonadherence were the weekly meeting with his business partners and out-of-state conferences. A dysfunctional thought record revealed that a number of situation-specific negative automatic thoughts (e.g., "If I take lithium before the weekly meeting, I'll look like a zombie"; "If I'm not on the ball at this contract meeting, I'll make a fool of myself and lose this business") were acting as barriers to adherence. Disconfirmatory evidence was gathered within CBT sessions, but homework exercises most helped to undermine these thoughts. Before specific meetings, Mr. R. took his medication, monitored and challenged his own negative thoughts, and then observed his "performance." Mr. R. also discussed his behavior at the meetings by seeking feedback from a trusted colleague. His colleague confirmed that he had behaved in an alert and highly professional manner throughout the meetings. Mr. R. then was able to support an alternative view that "taking lithium, even before important meetings, does not impair my performance."

For individuals who demonstrate greater ambivalence toward medication, additional CBT approaches are available. First, a cost-benefit analysis, with a format like the one shown in Table 5–3, can be conducted to assess reactions to the use of medication. Advantages and disadvantages for taking or not taking medication are identified. Patients often identify more reasons for adherence than for stopping medication. However, some individuals remain unconvinced. A treatment trial followed by a "drug holiday" with continuous monitoring of symptoms throughout and increased frequency of CBT sessions may be the only compromise. If the patient and therapist are not in total agreement about the meaning of the data collected in this experiment, the option of seeking a "third-party opinion" from someone else whom the patient trusts may also be useful (Newman and Beck 1992). This approach may help the patient retain trust in the therapist and may prevent medication compliance from becoming a battleground.

Self-monitoring and self-regulation.   Self-monitoring with procedures such as a daily activity schedule is a well-known component of CBT for depression (Beck et al. 1979). Recording activities, rating them for mastery and pleasure, and scheduling adaptive activities can help break patterns of inertia and hopelessness. Self-monitoring can also be a useful component of CBT for hypomania or mania. The goals for hypomania or mania may be to reduce levels of activity, find adaptive outlets for excessive energy, or recognize and avoid potentially dangerous behaviors.

When individuals are hypomanic or manic, considerable negotiation may be required between therapist and patient to reduce the risk for extreme levels of activity. For example, Mr. S. had a pattern of excessive engagement, for many hours a day, in a wide variety of sports activities when he became hypomanic. This overinvolvement had caused job and family problems. It was found that 1 hour of swimming satisfied his need to be active and also made him feel he had used up a good deal of his extra energy. Mr. S. also noted that a short walk in the early evening helped him with sleep. However, the therapist needed to work intensively with Mr. S. for him to see the benefit of performing a reasonable amount of daily exercise. A careful analysis of the advantages and disadvantages of such behavioral changes can be a useful method of assisting bipolar patients to reduce dysfunctional patterns of activity.

Table 5 3. Cost-benefit analysis of taking lithium

Advantages of taking lithium	Advantages of not taking lithium
1. Treatment keeps me out of the hospital.	1. I have fewer things to carry around and fewer things to remember.
2. My family is less worried when I'm on lithium.	2. I'm in control of me, not the tablets.
3. I know I'm doing everything I can to keep my illness under control.	
Disadvantages of taking lithium	**Disadvantages of not taking lithium**
1. I hate blood tests.	1. There is a greater risk I'll have a relapse.
2. I've gained weight as a side effect.	2. I might have to go back into the hospital, and that might jeopardize my career.
3. Lithium can be toxic, and you can get irreversible kidney damage.	3. If my wife finds out, she'll be upset.
	4. The doctor has expressed concern for my well-being if I don't use medication.
	5. Once, when depressed, I thought of killing myself—it was a frightening experience that I'd rather not have happen again.

It has been reported that bipolar patients benefit from maintaining regular patterns of sleep, physical activity, and eating (American Psychiatric Association 1994). Thus, regularity of habits should be encouraged. Self-regulation appears to increase stability in an individual's mental state and enhances his or her sense of self-efficacy (Scott 1995a). Mr. S. benefited from using self-regulation procedures such as self-talk to slow down movements and speech. One example of this type of intervention is Mr. S.'s repetition of the statement "Take your time" on five occasions before embarking on any new activity. Mr. S. made himself take 5 seconds to say the statement and repeated it at 10-minute intervals during the activity.

Daily mood graphs were used to identify fluctuations in the quality and severity of Mr. S.'s mood shifts. Additional instructions were agreed on and noted on the mood charts. For example, if Mr. S.'s elated mood rating was greater than 40%, he would increase his self-monitoring and mood-regulating self-talk. Additional self-talk statements used by Mr. S. included "Always sit down before getting into animated discussions" (which reduced the frequency and magnitude of accessory body movements). If Mr. S.'s elation ratings exceeded 60%, he would contact his therapist for additional help.

Relapse prevention.   Identifying personal factors that may make an individual more vulnerable to episodes of bipolar disorder (e.g., underlying sociotropic beliefs) or high-risk situations for relapse (e.g., work stress or increased alcohol consumption) can be of value to the patient. Many life events, particularly those related to loss, signal a period of increased risk for relapse.

Ms. B. was a single parent with two children aged 16 and 19 years. A relapse of her bipolar disorder 18 months previously had coincided with her older child's leaving home to go to college. When Ms. B. entered CBT, she was preoccupied with the imminent move of her younger child, who was also going to college in a few months. Ms. B. and her therapist explored the specific meaning of these life events and discovered that she felt insecure about her relationship with her children and feared that they would abandon her once they moved away from home. When her first child left, underlying beliefs about being unlovable were reactivated. Ms. B.'s father had left home when she was a child, and Ms. B. believed her mother blamed her for this. Ms. B. reported that when her own child left home, she had become so distressed that she could not get through the day or sleep at night without consuming half a bottle of gin. Ms. B. also became easily distracted and often failed to take her mood-stabilizing medication.

Ms. B. and her therapist worked on the underlying negative beliefs about abandonment and unlovability with CBT techniques such as keeping a "positive data log." The patient kept a daily record of any evidence (no matter how small) compatible with her belief that "I am lovable." Then, strategies were developed to cope with the forthcoming separation of Ms. B. from her second child. Adaptive coping methods were rehearsed in detail (Scott 1995a). Also, high-risk behaviors for relapse, such as excess use of stimulants (alcohol or caffeine intake) or noncompliance, were discussed, and alternative safer activities (e.g., phoning a trusted friend when distressed) were also developed.

Virtually all bipolar patients are able to learn to recognize the signs and symptoms of relapse and identify positive actions they can take. Retrospective examination of prodromal symptoms in previous episodes suggests that 85% of individuals with bipolar disorder can identify at least two prodromal symptoms specific to depressive swings and 75% can identify two symptoms specific to hypomanic swings (Smith and Tarrier 1992). These prodromal symptoms may be viewed as a "relapse signature." For example, Mr. F. identified that in the early stages of hypomania, his mood became elated, he did not need much sleep, and his spending became excessive. Only two of these features, poor sleep and excessive spending, were used as Mr. F.'s relapse signature.

My relapse signature is —
          lack of sleep.
          excessive spending.

When I start to go high, it helps if I —
          target my sleep pattern.
          cut out stimulants.
          actively calm myself.
          avoid major decisions.
          limit my spending.

My specific technique is —   48-hour delay rule.
The following individual may contact my doctor on my behalf —   John Dobson [telephone no., including area code, put here]

Figure 5–1. Flash card for relapse prevention.

Elated mood is a less reliable discriminator, because most patients in the early stages of relapse may misattribute feeling high to well-being rather than sickness (Smith and Tarrier 1992). Physical prodromal symptoms such as sleep disturbance (Wehr et al. 1987) or other features related to activation level are thus better symptoms to monitor than affective state (Bauer et al. 1991).

After identifying Mr. F.'s relapse signature, these symptoms were recorded on a flash card (Figure 5–1) so that the patient (and his relatives) could monitor early warning symptoms. In addition, a written hierarchy of coping responses was developed during the CBT sessions. The hierarchy started with strategies such as giving increased attention to self-regulation of activities, canceling meetings in which important (or irreversible) decisions might be made, and setting an agreed-on spending limit. Mr. F.'s special technique was "the 48-hour delay" rule, which discouraged him from acting impulsively on a "good" idea immediately. Instead, he practiced examining pros and cons and then reviewing the idea 2–3 days later with his therapist or a "third party" (Newman and Beck 1992). The flash card also included the name of a trusted individual whom Mr. F. would allow to contact mental health service professionals in situations where the patient was exhibiting poor judgment or denial of symptoms. Mr. F. and his family believed that this approach to relapse prevention proved extremely helpful.

Outcome Research

There are encouraging anecdotal and single-case reports on the use of CBT in patients with bipolar disorder (Chor et al. 1988; Jacob and

Cochran 1982; Scott 1995a; Wright and Schrodt 1992). Cognitive-behavioral approaches to enhancing medication compliance in patients with affective disorders also appear to be beneficial (Goodwin and Jamison 1990; Rush 1988; Wright and Thase 1992). Only two studies offer any outcome data on the use of CBT in bipolar disorder (Cochran 1984; Palmer et al. 1995); both were small-scale projects that used Beck's form of CBT (Beck et al. 1979).

Palmer and co-workers (1995) used a one-sample repeated-measure design to assess the benefits of using a 17-week group CBT program in combination with mood-stabilizing drugs and outpatient psychiatric clinic follow-up in a sample of six adults. The Internal State Scale (ISS; Bauer et al. 1991) was used to measure changes in manic and depressive symptoms. Social functioning was also assessed, but medication adherence was not measured. Two patients dropped out of the group after 1 week, but four individuals were followed up both during and after the conclusion of the CBT group. Outcome data suggested significant improvements on the well-being scale of the ISS for two patients, and for a third, a similar trend was reported. During the treatment phase, these three individuals had more ISS subscale scores in the remission category and more stable symptoms. Similar improvements occurred in social adjustment. During the 12-month follow-up phase, some of the social and symptomatic improvements had diminished.

Cochran (1984) studied the impact of six sessions of individual CBT on lithium compliance and clinical outcome in outpatients with bipolar disorder. Twenty-eight subjects with bipolar disorder who were newly referred to a lithium clinic were randomly assigned to CBT or to a control group (treatment as usual). Subjective and observer ratings (including serum lithium levels) indicated that compliance was significantly better at the 6-week and 6-month follow-up in the treatment-as-usual group. Only three CBT group subjects (21%), compared with eight (57%) control subjects, discontinued lithium against medical advice, and hospitalization rates were significantly lower in the CBT group.

Schizophrenia

Rationale for Cognitive-Behavioral Therapy

Lifetime prevalence rates for schizophrenia are between 0.5% and 1.0%. Full symptomatic remission probably occurs in fewer than 60% of individuals with this disorder (Shepherd et al. 1989), and despite appropriate antipsychotic medication, about 50% of patients experience a relapse within 5 years of an index schizophrenic episode (Remington and Adams 1994). Because few patients achieve a full restitution of function (i.e., freedom from positive symptoms, negative symptoms, and other emotional difficulties, such as depression or hopelessness) with pharmacotherapy alone, there are a number of potential targets for cognitive and behavioral interventions.

In many individuals with schizophrenia, positive symptoms (e.g., hallucinations and delusions) diminish in response to antipsychotic medication, but negative symptoms (e.g., affective flattening, poverty of thought, a decrease in goal-directed behaviors) may persist even after the acute episode has begun to remit. A significant minority of individuals may also exhibit "challenging behaviors." These are aberrant or inappropriate actions that isolate the individual from his or her social network and community. Behavioral procedures have been advocated for negative symptoms and challenging behaviors for a number of years, but cognitive interventions are increasingly being incorporated into treatment programs (Hogg and Hall 1992).

Although pharmacological advances have significantly reduced suffering, about 25% of persons with schizophrenia have a "treatment-resistant" disorder, and between 20% and 60% stop taking medication at some time (Curry 1985). In addition to treatment-refractory symptoms, factors such as premorbid personality, attitudes toward the use of medication, family and interpersonal problems, occurrence of life events, substance abuse problems, and negative reactions to the diagnosis of schizophrenia can adversely influence outcome. Also, psychosocial stressors may exacerbate symptoms or increase the risk for relapse. Each of these problems or issues can be a reason for using adjunctive psychological interventions.

Overview of Therapy Procedures

Therapy for persons with schizophrenia begins by trying to help the individual come to terms with his or her current situation. Discussing events that the patient often finds perplexing is a useful way in which to begin to develop the therapeutic relationship (Scott et al. 1993). If patients believe that the cognitive therapist is genuinely trying to understand their perspective, they are far more likely to engage in therapy in the long term. The CBT assessment process includes identifying any antecedents of the psychotic breakdown, establishing the patient's knowledge of the etiology of schizophrenia, and defining the effects of the disorder on the patient and his or her family (Beck 1952). A conceptualization is developed that encompasses cognitive (thoughts, images, and beliefs), behavioral, affective, biological, and environmental aspects of the individual's life. The approach described previously for bipolar disorder (Padesky and Mooney 1990), with its clear acknowledgment of biological factors, is particularly useful in working with individuals with severe mental disorders. It allows the therapist to emphasize a stress-diathesis model that includes biochemical factors as precipitants of symptoms.

A collaborative relationship is essential for CBT to proceed. A strong therapeutic alliance is associated with a reduction in symptoms and distress in its own right (Scott et al. 1993). In addition, as the individual with schizophrenia begins to trust the therapist, it is possible to start to jointly explore negative automatic thoughts about the disorder and its treatment. This process may allow hypotheses to be developed regarding idiosyncratic underlying beliefs. Identifying these beliefs may help to make sense of the specific content of delusions and hallucinations (Scott et al. 1993). However, it is important not to proceed too rapidly with reality testing of these symptoms. It is usually best initially to deal with anxiety, panic, or depressive symptoms and then to move gradually toward interventions targeting positive symptoms. The pace of CBT is usually dictated by the patient's ability to tolerate the process of guided discovery. If the therapist tries to hurry the process, the patient may find the sessions too difficult. Stress in response to application of overzealous therapy may actually exacerbate the symptoms of the disorder (Kingdon and Turkington 1993). Unless the patient can place substantial trust in the therapist, any attempts at collaborative exploration of delusional beliefs may be misconstrued as a challenge or confrontation. If therapist and patient have a good working relationship, it is usually possible to negotiate a withdrawal from the exploration of positive symptoms and to recommence this later, when this process is less threatening. A course of CBT may last considerably longer in the treatment of schizophrenia than in the treatment of nonpsychotic disorders (Fowler et al. 1995).

Hogg and Hall (1992) have observed that for many years, the interventions used to reduce challenging or aberrant behaviors were rather unsophisticated. This may have been a consequence of the fact that such behaviors were simply attributed to "the disorder," without any attempt to determine the underlying cognitive structures (core beliefs) or processes (logical errors) that might drive the individual's actions. If a cognitive framework is used, many challenging behaviors may be understood as a consequence of a "chain reaction" in which certain events activate an individual's underlying beliefs, which in turn lead to negative automatic thoughts, feelings of frustration or anger, and maladaptive behavior. Careful analysis of this sequence can identify triggering events (e.g., environmental factors, use of drugs or alcohol), idiosyncratic beliefs, and misinterpretations and can set the stage for the use of CBT interventions.

For some individuals, CBT sessions should be of short duration but held at frequent intervals to account for concentration difficulties and potential negative effects of overstimulation. Three 20-minute sessions per week may be more beneficial than one 1-hour session. Enhancing concentration through using graded task assignments, identifying and exploring fears about activities that have been avoided (such as new social ventures), or looking into general fears about the future may help overcome psychological factors that maintain negative symptoms (Kingdon and Turkington 1994).

Examples of Cognitive-Behavioral Therapy for Schizophrenia

Cognitive-behavioral interventions may be helpful for aspects of treatment such as providing individual and family education about schizophrenia, exploring attitudes toward the disorder and its treatment, facilitating adjustment, treating comorbid emotional disorders and hopelessness, developing self-management, and enhancing medication compliance. However, this section will concentrate on the use of CBT in dealing with positive and negative symptoms, because this work offers a new approach to the treatment of individuals with schizophrenia. A number of excellent manuals have recently been published that give detailed descriptions of the interventions outlined here (Birchwood and Shepherd 1992; Birchwood and Tarrier 1992; Fowler et al. 1995; Haddock and Slade 1996; Kingdon and Turkington 1994; Scott et al. 1993).

Delusions. To make appropriate interventions to modify positive symptoms, the therapist must first undertake a detailed collaborative assessment. For delusions, four dimensions are evaluated: conviction, accommodation (i.e., degree to which the delusion can be modified), persuasiveness, and level of encapsulation (Hole et al. 1979). Research suggests that individuals who experience delusions "jump to conclusions" when drawing inferences, underutilize disconfirming data, and tend to attribute negative events to external causes (Huq et al. 1988). Thus, delusions share many of the characteristics of distorted cognitions observed with affective disorders and theoretically should be amenable to structured reasoning and behavioral approaches (Scott et al. 1993; Turkington and Kingdon 1996).

Mr. H., a 43-year-old man with a 10-year history of schizophrenia, believed he was being followed by a leading member of the Mafia and that his life was in great danger. Initially, Mr. H. and the therapist investigated the approximate time of onset of the delusions and why his past or present experiences may have led him to attach significance to a specific event. Mr. H. had held this belief for about 8 years. He had been attacked in the street by a man with dark hair and brown eyes who Mr. H. said "looked Italian." The next day he had seen some graffiti on a garage wall in a local street stating "Newcastle United Mafia Rules OK." Since that time, Mr. H. was constantly on his guard. He believed that a man in a raincoat followed him persistently.

The therapist gently used Socratic questioning to help identify inconsistencies in the data being presented by Mr. H. Every piece of evidence identified as supporting his delusional belief was placed in rank order. First, the therapist asked Mr. H. to describe the person he thought was following him in great detail. Next, the graffiti on the wall was recorded on the list. Additional evidence offered by Mr. H. included "being jostled on the bus when I traveled to town, people talking in the street, and car doors being slammed at night." This supporting evidence was then examined in inverse order (starting with the least convincing data, "car doors slamming") with a reality-testing approach (Birchwood and Shepherd 1992).

Inconsistencies were initially explored through homework assignments, and alternative explanations were established that were more plausible. For example, Mr. H. established that car doors were not being slammed on his street every night and that not everyone shutting car doors at night slammed them. Mr. H. was also able to recognize that Newcastle United was the name of a local soccer team and that a group of the team's supporters had named themselves the "local Mafia." Mr. H. was thus able to generate an alternative explanation for the graffiti he had observed.

Lastly, Mr. H. kept a detailed diary regarding his view that he was being followed. He compiled a detailed document that demonstrated that there was no evidence that a man in a raincoat who "looked Italian" was following him. Mr. H. noted that a number of people regularly traveled on the same buses but that none of them looked Italian nor fit his original description. Mr. H.'s conviction in this delusion was significantly reduced, but he occasionally became worried when it rained and lots of people wore raincoats. To try to maintain his improvement, Mr. H. and the therapist developed a flash card for him to refer to whenever he began to think that "someone from the Mafia is following me" (Figure 5–2).

Hallucinations. The assessment of hallucinations in CBT is directed at the content, degree of variability, presence of antecedents or triggers, and any exacerbating or maintaining factors (Fowler et al. 1995).

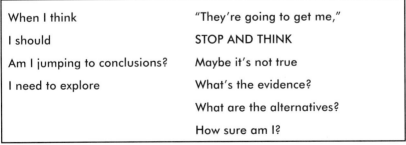

When I think	"They're going to get me,"
I should	STOP AND THINK
Am I jumping to conclusions?	Maybe it's not true
I need to explore	What's the evidence?
	What are the alternatives?
	How sure am I?

Figure 5–2. Flash card for coping with delusions.

Guided discovery is used to generate hypotheses regarding the origin of the hallucinations.

Ms. J., a 28-year-old university graduate, was employed as a senior clerk with a national bank. Ms. J. reported hearing voices telling her that "unless you follow our instructions, the economy will collapse." The therapist and Ms. J. first explored when she heard the voices. These usually occurred when she was alone in her apartment in the evenings, but there were some less-frequent occurrences in the staff restaurant at lunch time. Socratic questioning was used to get Ms. J. to evaluate possible explanations for the occurrence of the voices. Two hypotheses were generated: first, that the voices were "messages relayed by the government" and, second, that the voices were "symptoms of my illness and come from inside my head." Ms. J.'s belief that the voices were from the government was partly undermined when she was unable to explain how messages were relayed to her without others in the canteen hearing them. Ms. J. also kept a diary that revealed that the voices occurred more frequently when she was under stress (e.g., at the end of the financial year). After evaluating the evidence for the alternatives, Ms. J. began to believe that the most likely explanation of the voices was that they were internally generated symptoms of her illness.

Successful CBT interventions for hallucinations often involve the use of distraction techniques and stress management. Ms. J. found that the most effective distractions from the hallucinations were reading aloud or engaging in mental activities such as doing crossword puzzles or solving mathematical puzzles (Haddock and Slade 1996). "Personal stereo therapy" was also beneficial. Ms. J. was encouraged to play tapes of her choice whenever auditory hallucinations were particularly prominent. An additional strategy that may be helpful is to ask the individual to record rational responses to the comments made by the "voices" and to play this tape during symptom exacerbation (Turkington and Kingdon 1996).

Anxiety that was associated with Ms. J.'s auditory hallucinations was initially reduced with relaxation and breathing exercises. In addition, Ms. J. decided to follow the therapist's recommendation to lower her use of caffeine. She found these approaches helpful, but still expressed anxiety when experiencing "breakthrough" auditory hallucinations. Her fear that the national economy might suffer if she did not respond to the voices again became prominent. Experiments were developed to monitor what happened if Ms. J. did not obey the voices. The therapist and Ms. J. agreed that if stock prices did not fall by 10% and there were no news reports of a sudden downturn in the economy within 24 hours of each occasion that Ms. J. "disobeyed orders," they would be able to conclude that she did not have to respond to the demands of the voices. Monitoring over a period of 3 months demonstrated that on only 2 occasions out of 15 did Ms. J.'s refusal to comply with the demands of the voices coincide with the national press's reporting new difficulties in the economy, and on no occasion did the share prices fall by 10%. On the basis of this evidence, Ms. J. was able to conclude that she was not responsible for the nation's economic performance, and her emotional investment in the hallucinations was significantly reduced.

Negative symptoms. Hogg and Hall (1992) have given a comprehensive account of the techniques that may be used for negative symptoms. They emphasize that even if negative symptoms may arise as a consequence of neuropathology, this does not mitigate against the use of cognitive-behavioral approaches that have previously helped patients with other neurological disorders such as multiple sclerosis and individuals with learning difficulties. In designing CBT interventions for negative symptoms, it is important to distinguish between long-standing skills deficits and a more recent failure to use skills because of reduced motivation or cognitive distortion. The former may require the individual to engage in life skills and social skills training.

Helping individuals with schizophrenia to perform tasks or to enhance their ability to take on new tasks may be achieved through the use of a number of standard CBT interventions. For example, Mr. M., a 19-year-old male with a 4-year history of schizophrenia, presented following a number of arguments at home about his inactivity. Family education sessions were held to improve the family's understanding of Mr. M.'s problems, and individual CBT sessions were scheduled. In the early sessions, activity schedules and mastery and pleasure ratings were used to identify variability in Mr. M.'s activity levels and to develop a profile of tasks that he enjoyed doing. The therapist was very active in sessions, and positive reinforcement was offered for any task performed. Mr. M.'s mother also provided support and worked as a "cotherapist" to help the patient maintain his higher activity level between CBT sessions.

Next, the therapist and patient tried to identify any physical or psychological barriers to engaging in specific behaviors. Through collaborative exploration, Mr. M. and the therapist concluded that there was limited evidence for any physical illness or disability preventing Mr. M. from engaging in certain day-to-day activities. However, Mr. M. had a stream of negative automatic thoughts that interfered with task completion (e.g., "What's the point—my life is a waste of time—I'll only do this half as well as I used to"). Mr. M. and the therapist used daily thought records to challenge these thoughts. Although this technique was generally successful during therapy sessions, considerable practice and reinforcement were required before Mr. M. could effectively apply this technique in his everyday life. The cognitive-behavioral therapist usually must be patient and persistent to achieve significant levels of improvement in negative symptoms.

Outcome Research

Until the past few years, Beck's (1952) case study of the use of CBT for an individual with chronic schizophrenia was one of the only published papers on this topic. A number of single-case examples and uncontrolled treatment studies have now appeared (e.g., Bentall et al. 1994; Kingdon and Turkington 1991; Perris and Skagerlind 1994; Tarrier 1991). The encouraging results obtained from these studies have led to an expansion of research activity. Although to date only three controlled trials have been published, a large multicenter randomized control trial of CBT compared with "befriending" as an adjunct to medication for individuals with treatment-resistant schizophrenia is nearing completion ("The Newcastle–Charing Cross Study of Individuals With Treatment-Resistant Schizophrenia"; J. Scott, personal communication, 1996).

A small controlled trial was undertaken by Garety and colleagues (1994), who recruited 20 patients with "treatment-resistant" psychosis to an experimental group ($n = 13$) and a waiting-list control group ($n = 7$). The experimental group received approximately 16 sessions of CBT over 6 months. The treatment was aimed at educating the patient about schizophrenia, reducing hopelessness, modifying delusional beliefs, and developing coping strategies. Compared with the control group, the CBT group demonstrated significant reductions in preoccupation, conviction, and distress caused by delusions. Other measures of functioning showed a nonsignificant trend for the CBT group to do better.

A study of 58 subjects with acute, nonaffective psychotic disorders (mainly schizophrenia) was undertaken in a hospital inpatient unit by Drury and colleagues. Twenty randomly selected individuals were offered CBT comprising individual therapy that utilized techniques to modify delusional beliefs and activity programming, family and individual education and support sessions, and group CBT to develop coping skills. The other 38 subjects formed two "treatment as usual" control groups.

A preliminary data analysis (V. Drury, M. Birchwood, F. Macmillan, et al., "Promotion of Recovery From Acute Episodes of Psychosis," unpublished manuscript, 1996) suggested that although there were no significant differences between groups in medication received, the CBT group met the remission criteria significantly earlier than did either control group. The mean time to remission in the CBT group was 65 days, compared with 118–122 days for the two treatment-as-usual groups. In addition, mean length of inpatient stay was significantly shorter in the CBT group (less than half the duration of either control group).

The only published study that randomly allocated subjects to alternate CBT interventions was reported by Tarrier and co-workers (1993). One group of patients was offered a form of CBT directed toward problem solving; the other group was offered CBT targeted at relapse prevention. Twenty-seven individuals with schizophrenia who were experiencing chronic psychotic symptoms were offered 10 sessions of either problem-solving therapy (PST) or coping strategy enhancement (CSE). The former treatment was based on an approach similar to that adopted in family therapy and was aimed at enhancing problem-solving skills. The CSE therapy was designed to identify triggers of symptom exacerbation, to help the individual recognize and control these cues, and to develop techniques to reduce the impact of psychotic symptoms.

Compared with pretreatment baseline levels, both treatment groups showed significant reductions in delusional thinking and anxiety and depression ratings. Hallucinations and negative symptoms did not change significantly. Gains were for the most part maintained over 6 months of follow-up, and there was a trend for CSE to be more effective than PST.

Conclusions

The aims of therapy for psychiatric disorders are to alleviate acute symptoms, restore psychosocial functioning, and prevent relapse and recurrence. The recognition that individual vulnerability, in association with internal or external stressors, plays a critical role in the onset, maintenance, and relapse or recurrence of mental disorders has increased the acceptance of combined pharmacotherapy and CBT approaches. Systematic studies have been published that have examined treatment outcomes for individuals with treatment-resistant schizophrenia and severe and chronic depressive disorders (e.g., Scott 1992; Tarrier et al. 1993; Thase et al. 1991a, 1991b). Research on bipolar disorder has been relatively limited, but there is anecdotal evidence that CBT may also be beneficial (Chor et al. 1988; Cochran 1984; Palmer et al. 1995; Scott 1995a).

This chapter illustrates that CBT may be an effective approach but that there are gaps in our knowledge. More research on common underlying beliefs in individuals at risk of different syndromes and on attitudes toward the disorder and views about its treatment could aid our understanding of adjustment difficulties and psychological barriers to compliance and lead to better outcome.

Randomized controlled trials of individual and group CBT are required to establish what benefits accrue in both the short and long term and whether any reported gains exceed those of "treatment as usual." It also will be important to differentiate between specific and nonspecific benefits of such interventions and the mechanisms by which change is achieved. Ultimately, we will wish to know not only if the use of CBT is indicated for the patient with severe mental disorder but also whether, if indicated, it is effective because it enhances medication compliance, leads to the development of compensatory skills, or reduces vulnerability to relapse through change in core schemas. We will also wish to establish whether similar outcomes are obtained through the use of other manualized approaches such as interpersonal psychotherapy and behavioral family therapy.

In this chapter, we have explored the role of CBT in severe and chronic mental disorders. The material presented comments on the applicability of CBT and highlights how CBT may be used to address some of the problems encountered by individuals with these disorders. Our overall conclusion is that clinicians should be optimistic about the potential benefits of CBT for some of the most disabled and distressed patients seen by mental health service providers.

References

American Psychiatric Association: Practice guideline for the treatment of patients with bipolar disorder. Am J Psychiatry 151(suppl):1–36, 1994

Basco M, Rush AJ: Cognitive-Behavioral Therapy for Bipolar Disorder. New York, Guilford, 1996

Bech P, Vendesborg P, Rafaelson O: Lithium maintenance of manic-melancholic patients: its role in the daily routine. Acta Psychiatr Scand 53:70–81, 1976

Beck AT: Successful outpatient psychotherapy of a chronic schizophrenic with a delusion based on borrowed guilt. Psychiatry 15:305–312, 1952

Beck AT: Cognitive therapy: past, present, and future. J Consult Clin Psychol 61:194–198, 1993

Beck AT, Rush AJ: Cognitive therapy, in Comprehensive Textbook of Psychiatry/VI, 6th Edition. Edited by Kaplan HI, Sadock BJ. Baltimore, MD, Williams & Wilkins, 1995, pp 1847–1857

Beck AT, Kovacs M, Weissman A: Hopelessness and suicidal behavior: an overview. JAMA 234:1146–1149, 1975

Beck AT, Rush AJ, Shaw B, et al: Cognitive Therapy of Depression. New York, Wiley, 1979

Beck AT, Steer RA, Kovacs M, et al: Hopelessness and eventual suicide: a 10-year prospective study of patients hospitalized with suicidal ideation. Am J Psychiatry 142:559–563, 1985

Beck AT, Brown G, Berchick RJ, et al: Relationship between hopelessness and ultimate suicide: a replication with psychiatric outpatients. Am J Psychiatry 147:190–195, 1990a

Beck AT, Freeman A, and Associates: Cognitive Therapy of Personality Disorders. New York, Guilford, 1990b

Bentall R, Haddock G, Slade P: Cognitive behavior therapy for persistent auditory hallucinations: from theory to therapy. Behavior Therapy 25:51–66, 1994

Birchwood M, Shepherd G: Controversies and growing points in cognitive-behavioral interventions for people with schizophrenia. Behavioural Psychotherapy 20:305–342, 1992

Birchwood M, Tarrier N: Innovations in the Psychological Management of Schizophrenia. New York, Wiley, 1992

Blackburn IM, Bishop S, Glen AIM, et al: The efficacy of cognitive therapy in depression: a treatment trial using cognitive therapy and pharmacotherapy, each alone and in combination. Br J Psychiatry 139:181–189, 1981

Bohn J, Jefferson JW: Lithium and Manic Depression: A Guide. Madison, WI, Lithium Information Center, 1992

Bowers WA: Cognitive therapy with inpatients, in Handbook of Cognitive Therapy. Edited by Freeman A, Simon KM, Arkowitz H, et al. New York, Plenum, 1989, pp 583–596

Bowers WA: Treatment of depressed inpatients: cognitive therapy plus medication, relaxation plus medication, and medication alone. Br J Psychiatry 156:73–78, 1990

Chor P, Mercier M, Halper I: Use of cognitive therapy for treatment of a patient suffering from a bipolar affective disorder. Journal of Cognitive Psychotherapy 2:51–58, 1988

Cochran S: Preventing medical noncompliance in the outpatient treatment of bipolar affective disorder. J Consult Clin Psychol 52:873–878, 1984

Cochran SD: Compliance with lithium regimens in the outpatient treatment of bipolar disorder. Journal of Comprehensive Health Care 1:151–169, 1986

Cochran S, Gitlin M: Attitudinal correlates of lithium compliance in bipolar affective disorders. J Nerv Ment Dis 176:457–464, 1988

Cohen RM, Weingartner H, Smallberg SA, et al: Effort and cognition in depression. Arch Gen Psychiatry 39:593–597, 1982

Cooper M: Cognitive behaviour therapy in an in-patient with chronic difficulties: a case report. Behavioural and Cognitive Psychotherapy 22:171–176, 1994

Curry S: Commentary on the strategy and value of neuroleptic medication monitoring. J Clin Psychopharmacol 5:263–267, 1985

DeJong R, Treiber R, Henrich G: Effectiveness of two psychological treatments for inpatients with severe and chronic depression. Cognitive Therapy and Research 10:645–663, 1986

Dickson,W, Kendall R: Does maintenance lithium therapy prevent recurrence of mania under ordinary clinical conditions? Psychol Med 16:521–530, 1986

Dobson KS: A meta-analysis of the efficacy of cognitive therapy for depression. J Consult Clin Psychol 57:414–419, 1989

Elkin I, Shea MT, Watkins JT, et al: National Institute of Mental Health Treatment of Depression Collaborative Research Program: general effectiveness of treatments. Arch Gen Psychiatry 46:971–982, 1989

Epstein N: Cognitive therapy with couples. American Journal of Family Therapy 10:5–16, 1982

Epstein N, Schlesinger SE, Dryden W: Cognitive-Behavioral Therapy With Families. New York, Brunner/Mazel, 1988

Fennell MJV, Teasdale JD: Cognitive therapy with chronic, drug-refractory depressed outpatients: a note of caution. Cognitive Therapy and Research 6:455–460, 1982

Fowler D, Garety P, Kuipers E: Cognitive Behavior Therapy for Psychosis. New York, Wiley, 1995

Garety P, Kuipers L, Fowler D, et al: Cognitive behavioral therapy for drug-resistant psychosis. Br J Psychiatry 67:259–271, 1994

Goodwin FK, Jamison K: Manic-Depressive Illness. Oxford, UK, Oxford University Press, 1990

Greenberger D, Padesky CA: Mind Over Mood: A Cognitive Therapy Treatment Manual for Clients. New York, Guilford, 1995

Guscott R, Grof P: The clinical meaning of refractory depression: a review for the clinician. Am J Psychiatry 148:695–704, 1991

Haddock G, Slade P: Cognitive-Behavioral Interventions With Psychotic Disorders. London, Routledge, 1996

Hammen C, Ellicott A, Gitlin M: Stressors and sociotropy/autonomy: a longitudinal study of their relationship to course of bipolar disorder. Cognitive Therapy and Research 16:409–418, 1992

Harpin RE, Liberman RP, Marks I, et al: Cognitive-behavioral therapy for chronically depressed patients: a controlled pilot study. J Nerv Ment Dis 170:295–301, 1982

Hogg L, Hall J: Management of long-term impairments and challenging behaviors, in Innovations in the Psychological Management of Schizophrenia. Edited by Birchwood M, Tarrier N. New York, Wiley, 1992, pp 220–235

Hole R, Rush A, Beck AT: A cognitive investigation of schizophrenic delusions. Psychiatry 42:312–319, 1979

Hollon SD, Shelton RC, Loosen PT: Cognitive therapy and pharmacotherapy for depresion. J Consult Clin Psychol 59:88–99, 1991

Huq S, Garety P, Helmsley D: Probabilistic judgements in deluded and non-deluded subjects. Q J Exp Psychol 40:801–812, 1988

Jacob MK, Cochran SD: The effects of cognitive restructuring on assertive behavior. Cognitive Therapy and Research 6:63–76, 1982

Jamison K, Akiskal H: Medication compliance in patients with bipolar disorders. Psychiatr Clin North Am 6:175–192, 1983

Jamison K, Gerner R, Goodwin F: Patient and physician attitudes towards lithium: relationship to compliance. Arch Gen Psychiatry 36:866–869, 1979

Keller MB, Shapiro RW, Lavori PW, et al: Recovery in major depressive disorder: analysis with the life table and regression models. Arch Gen Psychiatry 39:905–910, 1982

Kennedy SH, Joffe RT: Pharmacologic management of refractory depression. Can J Psychiatry 34:451–456, 1989

Kingdon D, Turkington D: The use of cognitive behavioral therapy with a normalizing rationale in schizophrenia. J Nerv Ment Dis 179:207–211, 1991

Kingdon D, Turkington D: Cognitive Behavior Therapy for Schizophrenia. New York, Guilford, 1994

Kovacs M, Rush AJ, Beck AT, et al: Depressed outpatients treated with cognitive therapy or pharmacotherapy: a one-year follow-up. Arch Gen Psychiatry 38:33–39, 1981

Ludgate JW: Cognitive behavior therapy and depressive relapse: justified optimism or unwarranted complacency? Behavioural and Cognitive Psychotherapy 22:1–12, 1994

Ludgate JW, Wright JH, Bowers WA: Individual cognitive therapy with inpatients, in Cognitive Therapy With Inpatients: Developing a Cognitive Milieu. Edited by Wright JH, Thase ME, Beck AT, et al. New York, Guilford, 1993, pp 91–120

Manic Depression Fellowship: Inside Out. Surrey, UK, Manic Depression Fellowship, 1995

McKeon P: Coping With Depression and Elation. London, Sheldon Press, 1992

Mercier MA, Stewart JW, Quitkin FM: A pilot sequential study of cognitive therapy and pharmacotherapy of atypical depression. J Clin Psychiatry 53:166–170, 1992

Miklowitz D, Goldstein M: Behavioral family treatment for patients with bipolar affective disorder. Behav Modif 14:457–489, 1990

Miklowitz D, Goldstein M, Nuechterlein K, et al: Family factors and the course of bipolar affective disorder. Arch Gen Psychiatry 45:225–231, 1988

Miller IW, Norman WH, Keitner GI: Cognitive-behavioral treatment of depressed inpatients. Behavior Therapy 20:25–47, 1989

Miller IW, Norman WH, Keitner GI: Treatment response of high cognitive dysfunction depressed inpatients. Compr Psychiatry 30:62–71, 1990

Newman C, Beck A: Cognitive Therapy of Rapid Cycling Bipolar Affective Disorder: A Treatment Manual. Philadelphia, PA, Center for Cognitive Therapy, 1992

Padesky C, Mooney K: Clinical tip in presenting the cognitive model to clients. International Cognitive Therapy Newsletter, No 6, 1990, pp 13–14

Palmer A, Williams H, Adams M: Cognitive behavior therapy in a group format for bipolar affective disorder. Behavioural and Cognitive Psychotherapy 23:153–168, 1995

Paykel ES: Epidemiology of refractory depression, in Refractory Depression: Current Strategies and Future Directions. Edited by Nolen WA, Zohar J, Roose SP, et al. New York, Wiley, 1994

Peet M, Harvey N: Lithium maintenance, 1: a standard education program for patients. Br J Psychiatry 158:197–200, 1991

Perris C, Skagerlind L: Cognitive therapy with schizophrenic patients. Acta Psychiatr Scand 382:65–70, 1994

Peselow E, Sanfilipo M, Fieve R: Relationship between hypomania and personality disorders before and after successful treatment. Am J Psychiatry 152:232–238, 1995

Prien R, Potter W: NIMH workshop report on treatment of bipolar disorder. Psychopharmacol Bull 26:409–427, 1990

Regier D, Boyd J, Burke J: One-month prevalence of mental disorders in the United States. Arch Gen Psychiatry 45:977–982, 1988

Remington G, Adams M: Depot neuroleptics, in Schizophrenia: Exploring the Spectrum of Psychosis. Edited by Ancill R, Holliday S, Higenbotham J. New York, Wiley, 1994, pp 51–71

Rush A: Cognitive approaches to adherence, in American Psychiatric Press Review of Psychiatry, Vol 7. Edited by Frances AJ, Hales RE. Washington, DC, American Psychiatric Press, 1988, pp 627–642

Safran JD, Segal ZV: Interpersonal Process in Cognitive Therapy. New York, Basic Books, 1990

Sargeant JK, Bruce ML, Florio LP, et al: Factors associated with 1-year outcome of major depression in the community. Arch Gen Psychiatry 47:519–526, 1990

Scott J: Cognitive therapy with depressed inpatients, in Developments in Cognitive Psychotherapy. Edited by Dryden W, Trower P. London, British Journal of Psychiatry, 1988

Scott J: Chronic depression: can cognitive therapy succeed when other treatments fail? Behavioural Psychotherapy 20:25–34, 1992

Scott J: Cognitive therapy for clients with bipolar disorder: a case example. Cognitive and Behavioral Practice 3:1–23, 1995a

Scott J: Psychological treatments of depression: an update (editorial). Br J Psychiatry 167:289–292, 1995b

Scott J: Psychotherapy for bipolar disorder: an unmet need? Br J Psychiatry 167:581–588, 1995c

Scott J: Cognitive therapy of affective disorders: a review. J Affect Disord 37:1–11, 1996

Scott J, Byers S, Turkington D: The chronic patient, in Cognitive Therapy With Inpatients: Developing a Cognitive Milieu. Edited by Wright JH, Thase ME, Beck AT, et al. New York, Guilford, 1993, pp 357–390

Shaw BF: Cognitive therapy with an inpatient population, in Cognitive Therapy: Applications in Medical and Psychiatric Settings. Edited by Freeman A, Greenwood VB. New York, Human Sciences Press, 1987, pp 74–88

Shepherd M, Watt D, Falloon I, et al: The Natural History of Schizophrenia: A Five-Year Follow-up of Outcome and Prediction in a Representative Sample of Schizophrenics (Psychol Med Monogr 16). Cambridge, UK, Cambridge University Press, 1989

Smith J, Tarrier N: Prodromal symptoms in manic depressive psychosis. Soc Psychiatry Psychiatr Epidemiol 27:245–248, 1992

Swendsen J, Hammen C, Heller T, et al: Correlates of stress reactivity in patients with bipolar disorder. Am J Psychiatry 152:795–797, 1995

Tarrier N: Some aspects of family intervention programs in schizophrenia, I: adherence to intervention programs. Br J Psychiatry 159:475–480, 1991

Tarrier N, Beckett R, Harwood S, et al: A trial of two cognitive-behavioral methods of treating drug-resistant residual psychotic symptoms in schizophrenic patients. Br J Psychiatry 162:524–532, 1993

Teasdale JD, Fennell MJV, Hibbert GA, et al: Cognitive therapy for major depressive disorder in primary care. Br J Psychiatry 144:400–406, 1984

Thase ME: Transition and aftercare, in Cognitive Therapy With Inpatients: Developing a Cognitive Milieu. Edited by Wright JH, Thase ME, Beck AT, et al. New York, Guilford, 1993, pp 414–435

Thase ME: The roles of psychosocial factors and psychotherapy in refractory depression: missing pieces in the puzzle of treatment resistance? in Refractory Depression: Current Strategies and Future Directions. Edited by Nolen WA, Zohar J, Roose SP, et al. New York, Wiley, 1994, pp 83–95

Thase ME: Cognitive-behavioral therapy of severe unipolar depression, in Severe Depressive Disorders. Edited by Grunhaus L, Greden JF. Washington, DC, American Psychiatric Press, 1994, pp 269–296

Thase ME, Beck AT: An overview of cognitive therapy, in Cognitive Therapy With Inpatients: Developing a Cognitive Milieu. Edited by Wright JH, Thase ME, Beck AT, et al. New York, Guilford, 1993, pp 3–34

Thase ME, Howland R: Refractory depression: relevance of psychosocial factors and therapies. Psychiatric Annals 24:232–240, 1994

Thase ME, Rush AJ: Treatment-resistant depression, in Psychopharmacology: The Fourth Generation of Progress. Edited by Bloom FE, Kupfer DJ. New York, Raven, 1995, pp 1081–1097

Thase ME, Wright JH: Cognitive-behavior therapy manual for depressed inpatients: a treatment protocol outline. Behavior Therapy 22:579–595, 1991

Thase ME, Bowler K, Harden T: Cognitive behavior therapy of endogenous depression, Part 2: preliminary findings in 16 unmedicated inpatients. Behavior Therapy 22:469–477, 1991a

Thase ME, Simons AD, Cahalane J, et al: Severity of depression and response to cognitive behavior therapy. Am J Psychiatry 148:784–789, 1991b

Thase ME, Reynolds CF III, Frank E, et al: Response to cognitive behavior therapy in chronic depression. Journal of Psychotherapy Practice and Research 3:204–214, 1994

Turkington D, Kingdon D: Using a normalizing rationale in the treatment of schizophrenic patients, in Cognitive-Behavioral Interventions With Psychotic Disorders. Edited by Haddock G, Slade P. London, Routledge, 1996

Wehr T, Sack D, Rosenthal N: Sleep reduction as a final common pathway in the genesis of mania. Am J Psychiatry 144:201–203, 1987

Whisman MA, Miller IW, Norman WH, et al: Cognitive therapy with depressed inpatients: side effects on dysfunctional cognitions. J Consult Clin Psychol 59:282–288, 1991

Wright JH, Beck AT: Cognitive therapy of depression: theory and practice. Hosp Community Psychiatry 34:1119–1127, 1983

Wright JH, Beck AT: Cognitive therapy, in The American Psychiatric Press Textbook of Psychiatry. Edited by Hales RE, Yudofsky SC, Talbott JA. Washington, DC, American Psychiatric Press, 1994, pp 1083–1114

Wright JH, Schrodt R: Combined cognitive therapy and pharmacotherapy, in Handbook of Cognitive Therapy. Edited by Freeman A, Simon K, Beutler L, et al. New York, Plenum, 1992, pp 267–282

Wright JH, Thase M: Cognitive and biological therapies: a synthesis. Psychiatric Annals 22:451–458, 1992

Wright JH, Thase ME, Beck AT, et al (eds): Cognitive Therapy With Inpatients: Developing a Cognitive Milieu. New York, Guilford, 1993

Wright JH, Salmon P, Wright AS, et al: Cognitive Therapy: A Multimedia Learning Program. Louisville, KY, Mindstreet, 1995

Wright JH, Wright A, Zickel MB, et al: Tracking in computer-assisted cognitive therapy. Presented at the 148th annual meeting of the American Psychiatric Association, New York City, May 1996

Afterword to Section I

Jesse H. Wright, M.D., Ph.D., and
Michael E. Thase, M.D., Section Editors

The cognitive-behavioral therapies are the product of at least three convergent forces of the 1960s and 1970s: 1) the aim (as typified by the work of Aaron T. Beck) to develop more specific psychotherapies for depression that are more explicit and active (and, it is hoped, more rapidly effective) than traditional insight-oriented psychotherapy; 2) the broader need to make the target symptoms and outcomes of psychotherapies more objective so that efficacy (i.e., accountability) could be tested and demonstrated empirically; and 3) the tidal wave–like ascendence of the behavior therapy movement within academic clinical psychology. Today, slightly more than 20 years after the publication of Beck's initial (1976) landmark work, we can take stock in what has been accomplished and what work still needs to be done.

The chapters of this section illustrate the growth of the cognitive-behavioral therapies over the past decade and the breadth of psychiatric disorders to which this therapy is applicable. From its roots linking cognition with the affective and behavioral disturbances of depressive disorders, models of cognitive-behavioral therapy (CBT) have now been adapted for treatment of panic disorder and other anxiety disorders, substance abuse disorders, personality disorders, eating disorders, and several psychotic mental disorders, including bipolar affective disorder and schizophrenia. In the case of major depressive disorder and panic disorder, CBT has been established as an effective, first-line treatment option for ambulatory patients (Jacobson and Hollon 1996; Persons et al. 1996; Wolfe and Maser 1994). As discussed in the chapter by Scott and Wright (Chapter 5), CBT offers a viable approach to complement pharmacotherapy for treatment of the seriously and persistently mentally ill. Moreover, CBT is among the most promising of all nonpharmacological strategies available for substance abuse disorders and eating disorders. As suggested in Thase's chapter (Chapter 2), CBT may be a particularly useful approach for addictive disorders if a treatment package can be "welded" together that includes motivational enhancement, self-help activities, contingency management, and relapse-prevention skills.

Schools of therapy rise and fall, and it is sometimes difficult to separate a "real thing" from a fad or passing fancy. However, two characteristics of the cognitive-behavioral therapies will help to ensure a more enduring impact on the field: 1) a grounding in empirical studies (concerning both the role of cognition and affective regulation in psychopathology and the effectiveness of therapy for specific mental disorders), and 2) the operationalization of the methods and techniques of the therapy. The value of developing and refining therapies that are theory driven, generate testable hypotheses, have empirically validated outcomes, and are appropriate for assessments of adherence and quality cannot be underestimated.

For example, empiricism requires that the assumptions of the cognitive and behavioral models of symptom maintenance and etiology be tested, and necessitates that both the absolute and relative efficacy of CBT be demonstrated. These qualities help to differentiate a "school" based on clinical observation and experience from one with a more rigorous scientific basis. Empiricism also sometimes yields unexpected results that shape further revisions of theory and refinements of methodology. We consider such an empirical grounding to be essential in the cost-conscious 1990s, when "unproven" may ultimately translate into "not covered by your policy." Importantly, society should not be expected to support health care reimbursement for indefinite courses of therapy that achieve uncertain benefit. As practitioners of an applied clinical science, it is our obligation to provide cost-effective treatments whenever they are available. Further, for conditions such as the personality disorders, for which no such standard treatments have been empirically established, we see the model of treatment described in the chapter by Judith Beck (Chapter 3) to be an excellent place to start.

The operationalized nature of the cognitive-behavioral therapies both facilitates training and, eventually, offers an objective means of quality assurance. Results linking treatment outcomes with aspects of the fidelity or quality of the interventions also provide a clear indication that the therapy offers something more than the core qualities of empathy, genuineness, and restoration of morale. Although training in CBT is now commonplace among graduate schools approved by the American Psychological Association, most psychiatric residency programs lag far behind in the incorporation of such training. This is unfortunate, not only because of the relatively strong empirical basis of CBT but also because it is important that psychiatrists be knowledgeable about all of the major forms of therapy so that they can supervise and collaborate effectively with nonmedical mental health professionals.

Do we consider CBT to be the psychotherapy of first choice for most specific DSM-IV (American Psychiatric Association 1994) disorders? No—certainly this has not been established across the board. But a strong case can be made for this ranking for treatment of several of the anxiety disorders and, on the basis of controlled studies, for at least a coequal status with interpersonal psychotherapy (IPT) for outpatient treatment of major depressive disorder. By contrast, however, the empirical basis for CBT in the area of the more severe and persistent mental disorders lags far behind that for the major classes of pharmacotherapy. It is hoped that further research will help to better identify those patients who respond more favorably to CBT, IPT, pharmacotherapy, or combinations of the three.

What other areas of research are vital during the coming decade? First, it has been suggested that the additive effects of combined CBT and pharmacotherapy for anxiety, depressive, and eating disorders are not well defined (e.g., Persons et al. 1996). It remains to be seen if it is more efficient to conduct treatments in sequence or to judiciously limit the combined therapies for use with patients with more severe, complicated, or chronic disorders.

Second, the cost-effectiveness of CBT, both as a primary treatment of mild-to-moderate anxiety, eating, and depressive disorders and in combination with pharmacotherapy for treatment of bipolar disorder and schizophrenia, still needs to be established. What does CBT offer over and above nonspecific support that will justify its higher cost? In this regard, the suggested relapse-prevention value of CBT may yield a late-emerging benefit that helps to offset costs during acute-phase therapy. Of course, additional clinical research is still required to evaluate the efficacy of CBT for substance abuse and personality disorders.

Third, the "exportability" of models of CBT for use by nonacademic mental health professionals requires further attention. Specifically, the somewhat disappointing showing of CBT in the National Institute of Mental Health (NIMH) Treatment of Depression Collaborative Research Program (TDCRP) (e.g., Elkin et al. 1989) may point to a greater need for training and supervision of therapists than previously appreciated, particularly when compared with IPT and pharmacotherapy (Thase 1994).

Finally, is it possible to streamline CBT to enhance its efficiency for treatment of milder mood, anxiety, and eating disorders? Again, the results of the NIMH TDCRP study are informative in that patients with milder acute depressions responded equally well to CBT, IPT, and clinical management plus either placebo or active imipramine (Elkin et al. 1989). Unfortunately, clinical management plus placebo administered by board-certified psychiatrists is not a particularly relevant treatment strategy for practicing clinicians, and most controlled clinical trials have documented that waiting-list control conditions or "treatment as usual" by family practitioners does not achieve results comparable to those observed in the TDCRP. Thus, practical, efficient, and lower-cost initial treatments still need to be developed. The promise of more streamlined therapies is illustrated by Jacobson et al.'s (1996) recent outpatient study, in which a simpler treatment focus on "behavioral activation" yielded outcomes similar to those obtained with the full CBT package.

Options to reduce the labor intensity of individual CBT could include use of group sessions, self-help manuals to facilitate homework, and interactive CD-ROM video programs.

In summary, much has been accomplished over the past 20 years to broaden the scope and impact of CBT. Nevertheless, much work still needs to be done to better define the indications for, and limitations of, this model of therapy.

References

American Psychiatric Association: Diagnostic and Statistical Manual of Mental Disorders, 4th Edition. Washington, DC, American Psychiatric Association, 1994

Beck AT: Cognitive Therapy and the Emotional Disorders. New York, International Universities Press, 1976

Elkin I, Shea MT, Watkins JT, et al: National Institute of Mental Health Treatment of Depression Collaborative Research Program: general effectiveness of treatments. Arch Gen Psychiatry 46:971–982, 1989

Jacobson NS, Hollon SD: Cognitive-behavior therapy vs pharmacotherapy: now that the jury's returned its verdict, it's time to present the rest of the evidence. J Consult Clin Psychol 64:74–80, 1996

Persons JB, Thase ME, Crits-Christoph P: The role of psychotherapy in the treatment of depression. Arch Gen Psychiatry 53:283–290, 1996

Thase ME: After the fall: cognitive behavior therapy of depression in the "post-collaborative" era. The Behavior Therapist 17:48–52, 1994

Wolfe BE, Maser JD (eds): Treatment of Panic Disorder: A Consensus Development Conference. Washington, DC, American Psychiatric Press, 1994

II

Repressed Memories

II
Repressed Memories

Section II

Repressed Memories

Foreword

David Spiegel, M.D., Section Editor

Can those subjected to traumatic stressors forget to remember? Is traumatic memory too malleable to be trusted or too accurate to be avoided? The discussion and exploration of memory in psychotherapy has become a traumatic topic in itself in recent years. Prominent court cases involving recovered memories of sexual abuse and even murder have brought the phenomenon to national attention. Some doubt the veracity of any repressed memory, and others insist that the very absence of memory proves that a traumatic event occurred. These issues are at the heart of psychotherapy, the daily currency of which is the mining and working through of memories, be they of childhood experience, trauma, recent stressors, relationship problems, or existential dread. Memory is a complex but remarkable aspect of mental function, allowing us to organize a huge amount of information. Affect helps us do this, labeling certain memories as critically important and others as forgettable. However, the evidence reviewed below suggests that emotion may have other effects on memory and that the very association between mood and memory may make the regulation of conscious retrieval of memories a means of managing uncomfortable emotion. The authors examine both the research and clinical literature, providing evidence that memory of trauma is less than perfect but more than fantasy. Those who have experienced trauma and those who treat these people must come to grips with the vagaries and accuracies of memory.

In Chapter 6 (Butler and Spiegel), we examine the relationship between laboratory research on memory in cognitive psychology and clinical investigation of traumatic amnesia and other memory impairments. Mr. Justice Frankfurter once warned against the "cross-sterilization of disciplines." We caution that certain questionable assumptions underlie the facile application of laboratory findings to clinical problems: 1) the continuum fallacy: that childhood sexual abuse is simply more stressful than watching an upsetting movie; 2) the population generalizability problem: that college undergraduates provide findings salient to clinical populations; and 3) the difference between what is reported and what is remembered. Furthermore, we argue that a false dichotomy has been constructed in the literature using laboratory studies of suggested misinformation to argue that memory is unreliable and therefore, in particular, that repressed memories are suggested memories. After reviewing literature documenting repression of traumatic memories, we point out that suggested intrusion of false memory is the other side of the coin of suggested repression of real memory. Indeed, recent misinformation research has provided laboratory models of repression of real, if minor, traumatic memory. We argue that the nature of traumatic dissociative amnesia is such that it is not subject to the same rules of ordinary forgetting: it is more, rather than less, common after repeated episodes; involves strong affect; and is resistant to retrieval through salient cues. Laboratory research shows that stressful affect generally enhances memory for central information at the expense of peripheral details. In contrast to this general rule, dissociative amnesia involves central and peripheral information. We find that laboratory investigators are moving in the direction of assessing clinical problems, and clinicians are seeking systematic information with independent verification of memories. Both are salutary directions and should move the field toward the resolution of apparent contradictions.

In Chapter 7, Dr. McConkey points out that the laboratory and the clinic are complementary rather than competing venues. He notes that repressed memories can be distorted in the same way that non-repressed memories can. The fact that repressed memories are not completely accurate does not render them completely inaccurate. He notes that trauma affects cognitive function when it occurs and may affect brain systems afterward, as research showing reduced size of the hippocampus in veterans with posttraumatic stress disorder indicates. Thus, distortion of one cognitive function—memory—in the aftermath of trauma is not surprising. He reviews literature documenting memory distortion or amnesia for traumatic events. His own work has demonstrated that suggestive effects of memory retrieval facilitators such as hypnosis may affect confidence in memory more than content, producing "confident errors." He recommends that therapists be cautious about either accepting or rejecting memories of trauma and that more research be devoted to the usefulness of memory retrieval in the psychotherapy of posttraumatic stress syndromes.

In Chapter 8, by Koutstaal and Schacter, we are treated to a thorough and thoughtful examination of an aspect of memory processing and trauma that is often overlooked. The debate often involves two relatively discontinuous analyses of the response to trauma: such memories either are not likely to be forgotten, or, if they are not remembered, they did not happen. In this chapter, the authors explore the middle ground. It is not at all uncommon, as the authors note, for people to use various strategies to avoid thinking about trauma. They make dramatic moves—staying with a friend, changing apartments, or even leaving town—as a way of removing themselves from clues that will trigger memories of a rape. Koutstaal and Schacter remind us that such strategies work with varying degrees of success. Under certain circumstances, people can reduce the frequency with which they recall information by simply instructing themselves to forget. However, in some circumstances, particularly with neutral information, there tends to be a rebound—a return of the suppressed—and they remember it more later on. This may come from cue contamination, when people distract themselves from the memory to be avoided but wind up creating associations to the distracters. The authors note that a particularly unsuccessful strategy is often used by depressed individuals, who find themselves avoiding one depressive contact by focusing on another one, which produces an affective link that may stimulate cued recall. However, the experimental literature suggests that neutral stimuli are more likely to rebound than emotional stimuli. Of course, the kind of emotional triggers that one can mobilize in the laboratory are far different in intensity and even valence from those that one sees clinically in the aftermath of trauma.

The instincts of a psychotherapist are quite consistent with their observation at the end of Chapter 8 that the most effective suppression of thought may well come with its initial expression. This finding provides experimental support for the idea of critical incident debriefing after trauma and for more traditional psychotherapy. This chapter is an important contribution to the developing literature on effects of traumatic stress on memory and provides a useful bridge between conscious strategies enacted to control traumatic memories and the traditional literature on defense mechanisms.

In Chapter 9, Williams and Banyard review research on traumatic amnesia, noting the logical necessity that patients have both true and false memories of the presence and absence of abuse. That is, if it is possible to construct a false memory that abuse happened when it did not, it also must be possible to construct a false memory that abuse did not happen when in fact it did. Williams's own important research provided evidence that a substantial minority of women with documented histories of abuse requiring an emergency room visit did not recall the episode some 17 years later. They have thus shown that amnesia for real episodes occurs. This amnesia is not always continuous, and many women did recall the episode (although not necessarily continuously from the time it happened). In their chapter, the theme of the previous one is amplified, noting that forgetting of trauma may well be more than the aftermath of a conscious strategy of suppression, although it may derive from that as well.

In Chapter 10, Coons and colleagues provide a useful and important review of the clinical literature on traumatic amnesia. They point out that memory gaps are not uncommon in the aftermath of traumatic stressors, ranging from incest to the Holocaust. They provide data showing that histories of sexual and physical abuse in childhood are far more common among patients with dissociative disorders than in those with affective disorders. Traumatic amnesia occurred in both groups but was far more common among patients with dissociative disorder. The authors make a series of sensible and practical recommendations regarding memory in the psychotherapy of patients with recovered memories of trauma. These recommendations are very much in keeping with the American Psychiatric Association's Statement on Memories of Sexual Abuse, referred to in Chapter 7. This statement is well thought out, sensible, and practical. Much support for it can be found in the chapters in this section, and, for this reason, I include it below:

Statement on Memories of Sexual Abuse[1]

This *Statement* is in response to the growing concern regarding memories of sexual abuse. The rise in reports of documented cases of child sexual abuse has been accompanied by a rise in reports of sexual abuse that cannot be documented. Members of the public, as well as members of mental health and other professions, have debated the validity of some memories of sexual abuse, as well as some of the therapeutic techniques which have been used. The American Psychiatric Association has been concerned that the passionate debates about these issues have obscured the recognition of a body of scientific evidence that underlies widespread agreement among psychiatrists regarding psychiatric treatment in this area. We are especially concerned that the public confusion and dismay over this issue and the possibility of false accusations not discredit the reports of patients who have indeed been traumatized by actual previous abuse. While much more needs to be known, this *Statement* summarizes information about this topic that is important for psychiatrists in their work with patients for whom sexual abuse is an issue.

Sexual abuse of children and adolescents leads to severe negative consequences. Child sexual abuse is a risk factor for many classes of psychiatric disorders, including anxiety disorders, affective disorders, dissociative disorders and personality disorders.

Children and adolescents may be abused by family members, including parents and siblings, and by individuals outside of their families, including adults in trusted positions (e.g., teachers, clergy, camp counselors). Abusers come from all walks of life. There is no uniform "profile" or other method to accurately distinguish those who have sexually abused children from those who have not.

---

[1] APA Board of Trustees' Statement on Memories of Sexual Abuse. Copyright by the American Psychiatric Association, 1993. Reprinted with permission.

Children and adolescents who have been abused cope with trauma by using a variety of psychological mechanisms. In some instances, these coping mechanisms result in a lack of conscious awareness of the abuse for varying periods of time. Conscious thoughts and feelings stemming from the abuse may emerge at a later date.

It is not known how to distinguish, with complete accuracy, memories based on true events from those derived from other sources. The following observations have been made:

- Human memory is a complex process about which there is a substantial base of scientific knowledge. Memory can be divided into four stages: input (encoding), storage, retrieval, and recounting. All of these processes can be influenced by a variety of factors, including developmental stage, expectations and knowledge base prior to an event; stress and bodily sensations experienced during an event; post-event questioning; and the experience and context of the recounting of the event. In addition, the retrieval and recounting of a memory can modify the form of the memory, which may influence the content and the conviction about the veracity of the memory in the future. Scientific knowledge is not yet precise enough to predict how a certain experience or factor will influence a memory in a given person.

- Implicit and explicit memory are two different forms of memory that have been identified. *Explicit memory* (also termed declarative memory) refers to the ability to consciously recall facts or events. *Implicit memory* (also termed procedural memory) refers to behavioral knowledge of an experience without conscious recall. A child who demonstrates knowledge of a skill (e.g., bicycle riding) without recalling how he/she learned it, or an adult who has an affective reaction (e.g., a combat veteran who panics when he hears the sound of a helicopter, but cannot remember that he was in a helicopter crash which killed his best friend) are demonstrating implicit memories in the absence of explicit recall. This distinction between explicit and implicit memory is fundamental because they have been shown to be supported by different brain systems, and because their differentiation and identification may have important clinical implications.

- Some individuals who have experienced documented traumatic events may nevertheless include some false or inconsistent elements in their reports. In addition, hesitancy in making a report, and recanting following the report can occur in victims of documented abuse. Therefore, these seemingly contradictory findings do not exclude the possibility that the report is based on a true event.

- Memories can be significantly influenced by questioning, especially in young children. Memories also can be significantly influenced by a trusted person (e.g., therapist, parent involved in a custody dispute) who suggests symptoms/problems, despite initial lack of memory of such abuse. It has also been shown that repeated questioning may lead individuals to report "memories" of events that never occurred.

It is not known what proportion of adults who report memories of sexual abuse were actually abused. Many individuals who recover memories of sexual abuse have been able to find corroborating information about their memories. However, no such information can be found, or is possible to obtain, in some situations. While aspects of the alleged abuse situation, as well as the context in which the memories emerge, can contribute to the assessment, there is no completely accurate way of determining the validity of reports in the absence of corroborating information.

Psychiatrists are often consulted in situation in which memories of sexual abuse are critical issues. Psychiatrists may be involved in a variety of capacities, including as the treating clinician for the alleged victim, for the alleged abuser, or for other family member(s); as a school consultant; or in a forensic capacity.

Basic clinical and ethical principles should guide the psychiatrist's work in this difficult area. These include the need for role clarity. It is essential that the psychiatrist and the other involved parties understand and agree on the psychiatrist's role.

Psychiatrists should maintain an empathic, nonjudgmental, neutral stance towards reported memories of sexual abuse. As in the treatment of all patients, care must be taken to avoid prejudging the cause of the patient's difficulties, or the veracity of the patient's reports. A strong prior belief by the psychiatrist that sexual abuse, or other factors, are or are not the cause of the patient's problems is likely to interfere with appropriate assessment and treatment. Many individuals who have experienced sexual abuse have a history of not being believed by their parents, or other in whom they have put their trust. Expression of disbelief is likely to cause the patient further pain and decrease his/her willingness to seek needed psychiatric treatment. Similarly, clinicians should not exert pressure on patients to believe in events that may not have occurred, or to prematurely disrupt important relationships or make other important decisions based on these speculations. Clinicians who have not had the training necessary to evaluate and treat patients with a broad range of psychiatric disorders are at risk of causing harm by providing inadequate care for the patient's problems and by increasing the patient's resistance to obtaining and responding to appropriate treatment in the future. In addition, special knowledge and experience are necessary to properly evaluate and/or treat patients who report the emergence of memories during the use of specialized techniques (e.g., the use of hypnosis or amytal), or during the course of litigation.

The treatment plan should be based on a complete psychiatric assessment, and should address the full range of the patient's clinical needs. In addition to specific treatments for any primary psychiatric condition, the patient may need help recognizing and integrating data that informs and defines the issue related to the memories of abuse. As in the treatment of patients with any psychiatric disorder, it may be important to caution the patient against making major life decisions during the acute phase of treatment. During the acute and later phases of treatment, the issues of breaking off relationships with important attachment figures, of pursuing legal actions, and of making public disclosures may need to be addressed. The psychiatrist should help the patient assess the likely impact (including emotional) of such decisions, given the patient's overall clinical and social situation. Some patients will be left with unclear memories of abuse and no corroborating information. Psychiatric treatment may help these patients adapt to the uncertainty regarding such emotionally important issues.

The intensity of public interest and debate about these topics should not influence psychiatrists to abandon their commitment to basic principles of ethical practice, delineated in *The Principles of Medical Ethics With Annotations Especially Applicable to Psychiatry*. The following concerns are of particular relevance:

- Psychiatrists should refrain from making public statements about the veracity or other features of individual reports of sexual abuse.
- Psychiatrists should vigilantly assess the impact of the conduct on the boundaries of the doctor/patient relationship. This is especially critical when treating patients who are seeking care for conditions that are associated with boundary violations in their past.

The APA will continue to monitor developments in this area in an effort to help psychiatrists provide the best possible care for their patients.

This statement was approved by the Board of Trustees of the American Psychiatric Association on December 12, 1993.

Chapter 6

Trauma and Memory

Lisa D. Butler, Ph.D., and David Spiegel, M.D.

We forget because we must
And not because we will.

Matthew Arnold, "Switzerland,"
Empedocles on Etna, and Other Poems (1852)

The debate over memories of traumatic experience has itself become a traumatic experience for clinicians, patients, family members, and researchers. Increasingly, it has come to pit therapists, trauma survivors, and researchers on child abuse against families, sociologists, and researchers on memory. As is often the case in such situations, each side has come to take a rather one-dimensional view of the other. The "recovered memory" movement sees criticism as a shield behind which child abusers hide, whereas the "false memory" movement accuses psychotherapists of using their professional credentials as a hunting license, with family reputations being fair game.

This issue is too important to be left to the domain of accusation. The very concept of psychotherapy is built on the reexamination of memories. Classic psychoanalytic and modern psychodynamic psychotherapy—not just so-called recovered memory therapy—assume that current problems may reflect memories of life experiences, such as traumatic events (incest, assault, accidents), family stresses, or warded-off fears and wishes, which may be only partially accessible to consciousness at a given time. In some cases, people simply may not connect an available memory with a symptom; in other cases, they may not consciously remember the event. Consequently, many of the essential elements of psychotherapy—transference, working through, and re-

The authors wish to thank Elizabeth Bowman, M.D., Robert Garlan, A.B., and Cheryl Koopman, Ph.D., for their extremely helpful suggestions on earlier versions of this manuscript. The authors also express their great appreciation to Gordon Bower, Ph.D., for his critical reading of the manuscript and his extensive and invaluable recommendations for its improvement.

Supported by a National Institute of Mental Health National Research Service Award MH-19908 (L. D. B.) and a grant from the John D. and Catherine T. MacArthur Foundation (D. S.).

structuring—involve working with memories. The need for psychotherapy, in turn, is greater when individuals have had traumatic experiences. Psychotherapy remains the primary treatment for trauma victims, with pharmacological agents playing only a secondary role (Krystal et al., in press; Maldonado and Spiegel 1994). Understanding the effects of trauma on memory is critical to the therapeutic use of memory to affect the aftermath of trauma. Thus, this issue is of great practical and theoretical importance.

Fortunately, both experimental and clinical research offer considerable bodies of knowledge to inform our understanding of the effects of trauma on memory. However, they represent two distinct research traditions, and much of the debate that has arisen between them may be seen, at least in part, as a function of their differing perspectives. Experimental cognitive psychology and clinical psychology and psychiatry differ in so many fundamental respects that they often seem to inhabit different countries and speak different languages. Indeed, they actually study different populations, operate at different levels of analysis, use different tools, and proceed from quite different assumptions. These differences and their consequences must be considered in any analysis of the applicability of the findings of experimental research to clinical phenomena.

In this chapter, we focus on two broad areas: the effects of traumatic experience on memory and the status of laboratory findings of memory alteration and implantation as a model to explain recovered memories. We begin by briefly discussing problems in generalizing experimental research to clinical issues. As an example, we note that although cognitive research with nonclinical subjects has found that negative emotion tends to enhance memory for central details, there is evidence of significant memory disturbance in populations of trauma survivors. We also examine several of the explanations for traumatic amnesia offered by cognitive psychologists, emphasizing critical features that are not accounted for. Next, we describe the cognitive laboratory demonstrations of memory alteration and implantation in nonclinical subjects (known as misinformation effects) and outline some of the limitations of these effects relative to claims made about them. Then, we briefly discuss what the recent memory implantation findings may tell us about recovered memories. We propose that these findings are not inconsistent with a mechanism of dissociation to explain traumatic amnesia and recovered memories, and we argue that they may even be viewed as evidence in support of it. The following is necessarily a selective examination of these topics—we highlight issues that we believe are particularly important, especially to the currently polarized debate about repressed memories.

A few words about terminology are in order. We use the term *traumatic event* to refer to events that would be expected to evoke feelings of fear, helplessness, or horror and involve actual or threatened injury or threat to the physical integrity of self or others (see American Psychiatric Association 1994, pp. 427–428). Our use of the term *traumatic amnesia* implies many of the characteristics of the diagnostic term *dissociative amnesia* (American Psychiatric Association 1994). That is, it refers to a potentially reversible memory impairment characterized by an inability to recall important personal information of a traumatic or stressful nature and that seems too extensive to be explained by normal forgetfulness. Because diagnostic criteria have not been formally applied in most reported cases, we have chosen to use the general descriptive term rather than the specific diagnostic one. Use of the term *traumatic memories* is somewhat more complicated. In general, we use it to refer to memories of traumatic events. However, in some of the clinical literature, the term denotes specific types of posttraumatic memory disturbances such as intrusive memories (e.g., van der Kolk and van der Hart 1991). We have tried to point out when this change in usage occurs. Unfortunately, often there is little general agreement on terminology within disciplines and even less between them. Consequently, much of the clinical and experimental research described in this chapter employs different terms or similar terms with different meanings. Rather than trying to impose our definitions on these reports, we have elected in many cases to retain original terms.

Traumatic Memory and Amnesia

Before proceeding to a specific discussion of the effects of negative emotion on memory, we briefly review a number of the properties of memory that are relevant to an understanding of the effects of trauma on memory (for a more comprehensive review, see L. D. Butler, R. W. Garlan, D. Spiegel, "Some things experimental cognitive psychology can and cannot tell us about trauma and memory," unpublished manuscript, November 1996; Siegel 1995). First, the distinction between explicit and implicit memory (Schacter 1992; Squire 1992) suggests that experiences of abuse may be recorded—and then recalled and expressed—by different means (i.e., conscious/narrative vs. nonconscious/behavioral; Siegel 1995). Moreover, explicit adult autobiographical memory tends not to extend to events experienced during preverbal childhood (Nelson 1993), so caution should be used in considering narrative reports of memory from that period. Behavioral (implicit) memories, on the other hand, do not appear to be subject to infantile amnesia (Schacter and Moscovitch 1984) and therefore may be more reliable indicators of early childhood abuse (Terr 1988).

In addition, the processing of experience into memory is affected by a number of factors, including the degree to which it is elaborated, organized, and rehearsed (Kihlstrom 1994). In the case of sexual abuse, cognitive avoidance strategies (Bower 1990; see also Koutstaal and Schacter, Chapter 8, in this volume) or environmental prohibitions against verbalizing and sharing such information (Freyd 1993) may therefore undermine encoding, storage, and/or retrieval of these memories. Explicit memory, whether it be of generic event schemata or specific autobiographical episodes, may also be unwittingly influenced by vicariously learned information (e.g., Pynoos and Nader 1989). Consequently, one may have relatively elaborate cognitive structures for events that have not been personally experienced. Recovery of memories of childhood abuse is often precipitated by some environmental cue or trigger (Elliot and Fox 1994; Feldman-Summers and Pope 1994), and, in general, this appears consistent with the central role of cues in normal recall (Bower 1990; Kihlstrom 1994). Normal memory is undeniably reconstructive and imperfect (Bartlett 1932), with the clinical implication that findings of errors or inconsistencies in the recall of abuse experiences need not cast doubt on the central truth of the memory, any more than would be the case for nonabuse memories. However, confidence in a memory should not be taken as a reliable reflection of the truth of the memory (for a discussion, see Lindsay and Read 1994). With this background, we can begin our discussion of the cognitive literature on affect and recall.

Effects of Negative Affect on Recall: Cognitive Psychological Data

The literature describing the effects of emotion on memory is extensive, encompassing a number of research approaches that examine personal memories of negative or traumatic events, personal memories of significant public events ("flashbulb memories"), and memories of simulated negative events (shown on slides, videotapes, or staged) in laboratory settings. In the recent literature on memories of negative events, the general consensus is that such events seem to be better remembered than neutral events, and within negative events, central details or themes are better remembered than peripheral and contextual information (for an extensive review of memory for negative emotional events, see Christianson 1992).

Emotion and recall of details. In studies of the characteristics of naturally occurring memories of negative emotional ("traumatic") events in college populations (Christianson and Loftus 1990; Wessel and Merckelbach 1994), subjects report remembering more central than peripheral details, and the degree of emotion at the time of the event tends to be positively correlated with the amount of central, but not always peripheral, detail information that is remembered.

These findings are similar to the "weapon focus" effect (Loftus et al. 1987) reported by victims of and witnesses to crimes. Their descriptions suggest that one's attention during a crime is so focused on the weapon that little else is attended to; thus, poor recall of other details of the environment or event may be expected. The highly stressful nature of the situation presumably results in a narrowing of the range of the perceptual field, enhancing memory for the limited information attended to at the expense of information outside the range of this focus (Burke et al. 1992; Easterbrook 1959; for a discussion, see Christianson 1992). In the clinical literature, this phenomenon is also described in altered states of consciousness, such as during formal hypnosis or dissociative states (see Butler et al. 1996; D. Spiegel and Cardeña 1990). Termed *absorption*, it represents a state of highly focused attention (D. Spiegel 1992; Tellegen 1981; Tellegen and Atkinson 1974), which results in the exclusion of other experience or perceptual data that normally may be present in conscious awareness. This constriction of focus relegates other perceptual inputs to the periphery of consciousness, where they receive considerably less, if any, conscious cognitive processing and, therefore, are not committed to memory or may be more difficult to retrieve.

Emotion and accuracy. In addition to determining the primacy of recall for central versus peripheral details, when the facts about an event are known, memories may also be assessed for accuracy. In a study of actual witnesses to robberies, Christianson and Hubinette (1993) found relatively accurate memories for details associated with the robbery itself (action, weapon, clothing of the robber) but lower accuracy for other details (such as time, date, eye color of robber). In addition, higher accuracy rates were found for victims when compared with bystanders, although, surprisingly, different levels of emotion were not associated with differences in recollection.

The accuracy of personal memories for potentially upsetting public events has also been studied. *Flashbulb memory* (R. Brown and Kulik 1977; Pillemer 1984) is a term used to describe a vivid memory of a significant newsworthy event (e.g., learning of the Challenger explosion or the assassination of John F. Kennedy) and the circumstances surrounding learning of it (such as who told you, where you were, what you were doing, what time of day it was). Although the implication of the label is that a near-perfect "photographic" memory for the experience is retained, this has not been supported by all investigations (McCloskey et al. 1988; Neisser 1982). Nonetheless, Christianson (1992, p. 288) observed that "the loss of clarity and detail over time seems to be far less for these emotional memories than can be seen from the forgetting curve typically found in basic memory research (Murdock 1974)."

Laboratory studies of memory for emotional events have also produced mixed findings; however, Christianson (1992) concluded in his review of this literature that these findings are consistent overall with findings regarding memory for emotional events in real life. In one series of laboratory studies, Christianson and Loftus (1987) asked subjects to view slides/video of a traumatic event (e.g., witnessing someone being hit by a car or being shot during a bank robbery) or a neutral version of the same event. In the slide studies, subjects were instructed to pay close attention and rehearse the central detail of each slide (they wrote down a descriptive word). Subjects' memories were then tested after short (20 minutes) or longer (2 weeks) retention intervals. The results suggested that subjects who viewed the traumatic event were better able to remember the central details than those who viewed the neutral event. However, the traumatic group was less able to recognize the specific slides they had seen (they were varied by camera angle), indicating that memory was impaired in this group for some of the specific details, especially peripheral details (see also Burke et al. 1992). When tested again at 6 months, subjects who had initially viewed the traumatic event were more likely to recall the essence or theme of the event than subjects who had initially viewed the neutral event (see also Burke et al. 1992).

Because laboratory studies are controlled, they offer opportunities to study additional factors. For example, such studies have found that shocking events may impair memory for details present before the emotion-arousing event (Loftus and Burns 1982). In addition, some high-arousal events may be equally or less well remembered than low-arousal events at short retention intervals (which adds to some of the mixed findings in laboratory studies), but memory performance tends to be superior for high-arousal events compared with low-arousal events when testing intervals are delayed (Christianson 1992).

In summary, the cognitive literature on negative mood and memory, which includes studies of personal memories of negative or traumatic events, personal memories of significant public events (flashbulb memories), and memories of simulated negative events in laboratory settings, suggests that "highly negative events are relatively well retained, both with respect to the emotional event itself and with respect to the central critical information of the emotion-eliciting event—the information that elicits the emotional reaction" (Christianson 1992, p. 303). It is appropriate, then, to consider the degree to which these findings apply to clinical phenomena.

Application of Laboratory Research to the Clinical World

Bannister (1966, p. 24) noted that "in order to behave like scientists we must construct situations in which our subjects . . . can behave as little like human beings as possible and we do this in order to allow ourselves to make statements about the nature of their humanity." Just as dissection requires sacrifice of the living nature of the creature in favor of isolating and describing its physical components, so the controlled experimental study of human behavior often requires that it be plucked from its natural context and stripped of its rich, dynamic character to reveal basic processes and mechanisms.

This observation may have implications for the conclusions we may reasonably draw from experimental research. Campbell and Stanley introduced the concept of external validity three decades ago as one among many criteria that scientists should consider when choosing experimental designs. "*External validity* asks the question of *generalizability:* To what populations, settings, treatment variables, and measurement variables can this effect be generalized?" (Campbell and Stanley 1967, p. 5, quoted in Mook 1983, p. 379). In a lively discussion of the issue of external validity, Mook (1983) challenged the assumption that external validity is actually necessary in the case of much experimental psychological research, noting that "the distinction between generality of findings and generality of theoretical conclusions underscores what seems to me the most important source of confusion in all this, which is the assumption that the purpose of collecting data in the laboratory is to *predict real-life behavior in the real world. . . .* When it is, then the problem of [external validity] confronts us, full force" (p. 381). Mook suggests that the central distinction lies in the difference between claiming "what *can* happen, rather than what typically *does*" (p. 384). In other words, the conclusions of experimental research (that need not meet the standards of external validity) should be about a theory and not about a population. This is not to say that laboratory results cannot be generalized to the real world. Rather, we must ask how well the finding describes the phenomenon.

Artificial versus real events.   The issue of generalizability is critical when the findings of experimental laboratory studies of memory are extended to provide explanations of or predictions about clinical phenomena. In such cases, questions of the generalizability of manipulations, settings, measures, and subjects require attention. Many clinical and some experimental researchers have voiced substantial reservations about the application of findings from the experimental study of the effects of negative mood/arousal on memory to explicating real-world phenomena, such as eyewitness testimony in the forensic domain (Yuille and Cutshall 1986) or posttraumatic memory in the clinical domain (Olio and Cornell 1994; Tromp et al. 1995; van der Kolk and Fisler 1995). They note that laboratory studies use artificial events (e.g., slide, video, or staged incidents), and subjects know this. Consequently, experimental settings and manipulations may lack many of

the natural elements of an emotion-evoking experience such as immediacy, surprise, and personal consequence. In addition, the success of
the manipulation in evoking a degree of negative emotion or arousal
comparable to real-world situations is questionable. This may be unavoidable because it would be as unethical for cognitive researchers to
expose subjects to truly traumatizing manipulations as it would be for
clinical researchers to randomly assign children to abusive parents.
Nevertheless, the generalizability of research findings is predicated on
the assumption that the manipulation models the real-world event.

Laboratory events are also not personally relevant autobiographical
events in which subjects are active participants. Consequently, generalizing findings based on laboratory events requires the assumption
that the same basic processing characteristics apply across differing
situations. Moreover, laboratory studies of memory typically involve
recall and recognition assessment hours to days later, whereas forensic
settings may require that memory be assessed days to years after the
event in question occurred and clinical situations may include a time
frame of decades. These issues are central to the determination of
whether experimental findings may be appropriately generalized to
explain and predict phenomena beyond the confines of the laboratory.

Using nonclinical subjects.   Another condition of external validity—
the generalizability of the findings from one's sample to the population
of interest—is particularly nettlesome in discussions of trauma and
memory. A large number, perhaps the majority, of experimental cognitive psychology studies use college students as subjects. Yuille and Cutshall (1986) reported that, from 1974 to 1982, 92% of research articles
pertaining to eyewitness testimony used college students exclusively.
Therefore, legitimate questions of generalizability center on whether
findings with respect to this young, accomplished, and well-educated
sample can be assumed to apply to the general population. Presumably,
the assumption of experimental psychologists, as evidenced by their
faithful commitment to this pool of subjects, is that they can. Taking a
cue from Mook (1983), it would seem that this confidence rests on the
fact that experimentalists seek to describe and understand basic processes, to understand "what can happen."

Obviously, the issue of generalizability of experimental findings derived from studies of college students to clinical populations is more
complicated still. The generalization here is from a select group of nonclinical subjects to a select group of subjects with psychiatric disturbances that are the target of the generalization (e.g., depression,
posttraumatic reactions, dissociation) and that may be associated with
other characteristics that could vary between clinical and nonclinical
populations (e.g., level of functioning, motivation). To support such a
generalization, one must assume that the variable under study lies on

a psychological continuum that spans these populations. In other words, the processes in pathological conditions are fundamentally the same as those in nonpathological conditions—the difference is quantitative rather than qualitative. This critical assumption has not gone entirely unnoticed or unquestioned in the experimental mood and memory research that seeks generalization to clinical depression. Commentators have cautioned about generalizing from laboratory-induced depressed mood or naturally occurring nonpathological dysphoric affect to clinical depression (e.g., Ingram 1989).

This issue comes into particularly sharp focus, we believe, in discussions of the findings of experimental study of memories for events associated with negative affect/high arousal. If we adhere to the experimental findings and Christianson's (1992) conclusions from his extensive review of this literature, then we would conclude that high-stress events seem to be better remembered than low-stress events, especially in memory of the central details. However, a survey of 63 experts in eyewitness psychology found a different opinion (Kassin et al. 1989). Specifically, almost 80% of these experts agreed with a statement that the available evidence suggested that very high levels of stress impair the accuracy of eyewitness testimony, and most of them believed that nonviolent acts were better remembered than violent ones. Christianson (1992) suggested that this apparent expert consensus may be due to experts' selective attention to several widely cited eyewitness studies (those considered most relevant to forensic concerns) that failed to disambiguate reporting of central and peripheral details or found impairment only in recall of peripheral material. On the other hand, expert opinion is not inconsistent with clinical descriptions of those who have endured profound traumatic experiences and subsequently developed posttraumatic symptomatology—a different population from the one typically used in cognitive research.

Stress versus traumatic stress.   One of the major limitations to the applicability of the experimental literature to the clinical issue of traumatic memories has been the failure to consistently examine the memory characteristics of populations that have been *significantly* traumatized rather than just emotionally perturbed or upset. In the studies described earlier in this chapter, "traumatic events" are variously defined to include anything from watching a stranger being injured in a series of slides, to hearing about a presidential assassination, to actually being the victim of a violent assault. Obviously, for virtually everyone, the first two events are not equivalent to the third in their personal relevance or significance, immediacy, perceptual experience, emotion-evoking potential, or personal consequences. It seems reasonable, therefore, to consider that they may not be equivalent in their memorability or perhaps even in the kind of processing they evoke.

Even to generalize findings regarding personal memories of events that college students and others label as traumatic to those of individuals who have experienced events that would fulfill Criterion A of the DSM-IV (American Psychiatric Association 1994) diagnosis of posttraumatic stress disorder (PTSD)[1] assumes a dose-response relationship between negative emotional experience and memory that begs the question.[2] This is particularly problematic because about one-quarter of this latter group are estimated to go on to develop PTSD symptomatology (Green 1994), which may include significant and diagnostic *disturbances* in memory, such as flashbacks and/or amnesia for some or all of the traumatic event.

This unexamined factor—the differing prevalences of PTSD symptoms in the populations in different studies—may account for some of the discrepant findings in the eyewitness literature. Some studies have reported that witnesses to a murder, even those reporting the highest amount of stress, were highly accurate in their reports (the memories were "detailed, accurate and persistent") when interviewed soon after the event and when reinterviewed 4–5 months later (Yuille and Cutshall 1986, p. 181) and that victims of a post office robbery (i.e., the teller facing the gun) were significantly more accurate than bystanders who witnessed the event (Christianson and Hubinette 1993). However, other studies have found decrements in memory for traumatic experiences. For example, in a recent report examining characteristics of intensely pleasant, intensely unpleasant (nonrape), and rape memories, Tromp and her colleagues (1995) found that although memories of rape were more affectively negative than the other reported unpleasant memories, they were actually less clear and vivid, were less well remembered, had less meaningful order, and were less thought and talked about. Similarly, in a study of victims of violent crimes, Kuehn (1974) found that victims of more serious crimes (e.g., rape or assault) provided less rich descriptions of the crime to the police than victims of less serious crimes (e.g., robberies), and injured victims provided less information than uninjured victims regardless of the type of crime.

To reconcile these disparate findings, it seems reasonable to speculate that victims of more serious or injurious crimes would be more likely

---

[1] Criterion A in the DSM-IV diagnosis of PTSD requires that "the person has been exposed to a traumatic event in which both of the following were present: (1) the person experienced, witnessed, or was confronted with an event or events that involved actual or threatened death or serious injury, or a threat to the physical integrity of self or others," and "(2) the person's response involved intense fear, helplessness, or horror" (American Psychiatric Association 1994, pp. 427–428).

[2] Interestingly, a dose-response relationship has been established between physical proximity to a traumatic event and the development and severity of PTSD symptoms (Mueser and Butler 1987; Pynoos et al. 1987).

to have posttraumatic symptoms than victims of less serious or injurious crimes or than witnesses to crimes.[3] In other words, emotional arousal may enhance memory but only up to a point; after that point, negative emotion or high arousal (or their combination) may have a qualitatively different, disorganizing effect on memory function, and posttraumatic symptomatology may represent its residue. This is a view that the descriptive clinical literature has long and widely recorded (e.g., Brett and Ostroff 1985; Harvey and Herman 1994; Horowitz 1986; Janet 1889, 1909b, cited in van der Kolk and van der Hart 1991; Janet 1907; D. Spiegel and Cardeña 1991; van der Kolk and Fisler 1995; van der Kolk and van der Hart 1989, 1991).

Two central aspects of memory disturbance in posttraumatic conditions are not reflected in the empirical cognitive literature descriptions of memory for emotional events. These aspects reflect the clinical observation that, with respect to trauma, patients seem to remember either too much (intrusion symptoms) or too little (avoidance symptoms, specifically amnesia) (Horowitz 1986; van der Kolk and van der Hart 1991). We briefly examine these aspects in turn.

Effects of Negative Affect on Recall: Clinical Data

Memory disturbance in posttraumatic conditions: intrusion symptoms. The questions posed above about the applicability of laboratory findings regarding normal memory function to clinically significant traumatic memories are underscored when the features of posttraumatic memory are described. van der Kolk and van der Hart (1989, 1991; Janet 1889, 1919/1925, cited in van der Kolk and van der Hart 1991; Janet 1907; van der Kolk and Fisler 1995) proposed that the "traumatic memories" described in clinical populations as intrusion symptoms are qualitatively different from normal narrative memory and include sensory, affective, and motoric reliving experiences, flashbacks, nightmares, and behavioral reenactments. They appear to represent a distinct departure from normal memory processing.

The unbidden, vivid, and absorbing experience of a flashback or reliving of the traumatic event is one of the most profoundly disturbing intrusion symptoms in posttraumatic reactions. During these episodes, which may last from a few seconds to several hours, the traumatic event is not just remembered but reexperienced in the moment. This event presumably reflects a state of absorption into the content or fragment of a memory or belief and its attendant affect that is so profound that

---

[3] An alternative explanation of these particular findings could be that victims may be focusing their attention on their pain or injuries and consequently not encoding other characteristics of the event (G. Bower, personal communication, April 1996).

the current environment is largely ignored and the individual temporarily does not distinguish memory from present experience (Butler et al. 1996; Maldonado and Spiegel 1994). Such flashbacks, or relivings of the event, may be triggered by environmental stimuli reminiscent of the trauma and may occur even decades after the original event (Brockway 1988). Traumatic memories also may be experienced as distressing nightmares, either identical in experience to waking flashbacks or as more regular dreams intermixing traumatic and other material (van der Kolk and Fisler 1995). Sometimes such dreams can only be inferred from the patient's reports of having disturbing dreams for which he or she remembers few specifics or from accounts of his or her bed partner who witnessed the patient's utterances, screams, and movements (Maldonado and Spiegel 1994). Studies of posttraumatic nightmares indicate that the traumatic scenes may be repeated without modification, even for extended periods (e.g., 15 years) (van der Kolk et al. 1984).

Freud (1914/1958) observed that for some traumatized patients the memory of the event is experienced in the form of a motoric behavioral reenactment of the actions originally taken in the face of trauma. This reenactment "reproduces [the experience] not as a memory but as an action: he repeats it, without knowing, of course, that he is repeating," and in the end, we understand that this is his way of remembering" (quoted in van der Kolk and van der Hart 1991, p. 436). Terr (1988) described a related phenomenon, which she termed *behavioral memories,* in 18 of 20 children she studied who had experienced psychic trauma before age 5 years. She noted that for more than three-quarters of the children, their play, fears, or personality changes "strikingly mirrored" (p. 98) what had been documented about their histories.[4] Terr also observed that these behavioral memories were quite accurate and true to the events that stimulated them regardless of whether the trauma had occurred before or after language acquisition.

Differences in encoding, storage, and retrieval of traumatic memories. To explain these distressing and bizarre posttraumatic symptoms, investigators have proposed that some experiences may be so overwhelming that they cannot be integrated into existing normal mental frameworks and consequently are encoded differently (D. Spiegel 1984, 1986; van der Hart and Spiegel 1993; van der Kolk and Fisler 1995; van der Kolk and van der Hart 1991). Siegel (1995) enumerated the following factors that may be present in traumatic experiences and may influence the differential memory processing of these events:

---

[4]Note, however, that the rater was not blind in this study, thus a confirmation bias may have increased the likelihood of her noting a correspondence between the children's behaviors and the documentation of their traumatic experiences.

- The overwhelming emotions and extreme stress or physical pain during the event may impede processing of perceptual inputs.
- If the event is novel in the individual's experience, it may also overwhelm perceptual attention processes and/or deviate from preestablished schemata or mental models, thereby limiting possible encoding.
- Cognitive adaptations (such as perceptual avoidance, divided attention, escape fantasy, somatic numbing), the meaning of the event (loss, betrayal, abandonment), and the social context in which it occurs may all disrupt the processing necessary for consolidation of normal long-term memory.

Clearly, most of these features are absent (for ethical reasons) in laboratory studies of emotion and memory.

Janet (1889, 1907, 1919/1925, described in van der Kolk and van der Hart 1989, 1991) first proposed that traumatic memories represent the intrusive return of unassimilated material in fragmentary sensory, affective, and motoric form. van der Kolk and van der Hart (1991), in summarizing Janet's views, noted

> that the ease with which current experience is integrated into existing mental structures depends on the subjective assessment of what is happening; familiar and expectable experiences are automatically assimilated without much conscious awareness of details of the particulars, while frightening or novel experiences may not easily fit into existing cognitive schemes and be remembered with particular vividness, or totally resist integration. Under extreme conditions, existing meaning schemes may be entirely unable to accommodate frightening experiences, which causes the "memory" of these experiences to be stored differently, and not be available for retrieval under ordinary conditions: it becomes dissociated from conscious awareness and voluntary control. . . . When that occurs, fragments of these unintegrated experiences may later manifest recollections or behavioral reenactments. (p. 427)

van der Kolk (1987) also observed that people who are exposed to significant trauma experience a "speechless terror," and organization of the experience, at least initially, is without semantic representation. "The experience cannot be organized on a linguistic level and this failure to arrange the memory into words and symbols leaves it to be organized on a somatosensory or iconic level: as somatic sensations, behavioral reenactments, nightmares, and flashbacks" (van der Kolk and van der Hart 1991, p. 443). Schacter (1987; see also Siegel 1995) has suggested that traumatic memories, such as those that Janet described, may represent implicit memories of the trauma.

To remedy the intrusion of "the unassimilated scraps of overwhelming experiences" (p. 447) that present as traumatic memories, van der

Kolk and van der Hart (1991) suggested that these experiences need to be integrated with existing mental structures and transformed into narrative language. van der Kolk and Ducey (1989, p. 271) concluded that "a sudden and passively endured trauma is relived repeatedly, until a person learns to remember simultaneously the affect and cognition associated with the trauma through access to language."

Based on Janet's observations and their own, van der Kolk and colleagues (van der Kolk and Fisler 1995, see Table 2, p. 521; van der Kolk and van der Hart 1991) have enumerated four features that distinguish traumatic (intrusive) memories and normal narrative memories:

1. Traumatic memories are composed of images, sensations, and affective and behavioral states, whereas narrative memory is semantic and symbolic and may be conveyed verbally.
2. Traumatic memories are inflexible and invariant over time, whereas narrative memories serve social and adaptive functions.
3. Traumatic memories cannot be evoked at will but are automatically elicited under specific circumstances reminiscent of the original event; once one element of the memory is stimulated, the retrieval floodgates open, and the other elements are recalled (reexperienced). In contrast, narrative memories are generally accessible without triggers, and they do not bring with them an irrepressible constellation of associated affective, somatic, and motoric experiences.
4. Traumatic memories, which effectively reconstitute some or all of the trauma through behavioral reenactment or intrapsychic replay, take time to "remember," whereas narrative memories are verbal distillations that may be condensed or expanded on social demands.

A fascinating recent exploratory study further examined the differences between intrusive memories for traumatic events and nontraumatic memories. In this study, van der Kolk and Fisler (1995) recruited and assessed 46 nonclinical adults "who were haunted by memories of terrible life experiences" (p. 514). All subjects' symptoms met DSM-III-R (American Psychiatric Association 1987) criteria for PTSD. The subjects were interviewed to assess a variety of characteristics of their traumatic memories and then were asked the same questions about an intense, nontraumatic experience of their choice (e.g., birthdays, graduations, weddings, births of children). Of the subjects whose traumatic memories were of childhood events (more than 75% of the sample), 42% had endured significant or total amnesia for the experience at some time in their lives. More than 75% of the entire sample reported nightmares, some of which were identical to their flashbacks and others that were dreams incorporating non-trauma-related material or illogical combinations of material. *All* subjects claimed that they initially "remembered" the traumatic event as somatosensory flashback experiences, presenting in a variety of somatosensory modalities and emotions, rather than in coherent narrative form. These traumatic memories were reported to develop over time, involving more and more modalities, and ultimately were constructed into a narrative by the subject (although 11% of the sample were still unable to convey a coherent narrative of the event—all of these subjects had endured childhood traumas). The authors concluded that "traumatic 'memories,' per se, consist of emotional and sensory states, with little verbal representation" (p. 520). Interestingly, none of the significant *nontraumatic* memories were experienced as dreams, flashbacks, or somatosensory relivings; none were associated with amnesic periods; none had a photographic quality; none were reexperienced as vivid memories after environmental triggers; and in no case did subjects attempt to suppress them. van der Kolk and Fisler (1995, p. 520; see also Siegel 1995; van der Kolk and Ducey 1989) concluded that "traumatic experiences in people with PTSD are initially imprinted as sensations or feeling states that are not immediately transcribed into personal narratives. This failure to process information on a symbolic level following trauma is at the very core of the pathology of PTSD."

In the preceding section, we describe the intrusive traumatic memory symptoms of flashbacks, nightmares, and behavioral reenactments that characterize some posttraumatic conditions. These clinically significant traumatic memories represent what appears to involve a breakdown or qualitative shift in processing that occurs in the face of extreme affect rather than a quantitative enhancement of memory such as the experimental literature would suggest. These traumatic memories are unique in that they are represented in nonverbal modalities, they are accompanied by intense affect, and their retrieval is outside of conscious control. In the next section, we discuss the most severe posttraumatic memory disturbance—another memory presentation that is not accounted for in the experimental literature—amnesia.

Memory disturbance in posttraumatic conditions: traumatic amnesia. Although amnesia for childhood sexual abuse is currently an issue of much debate (e.g., Loftus 1993; Loftus and Ketcham 1994; Ofshe and Singer 1994; Ofshe and Watters 1994), cases of amnesia after traumatic or highly emotional events have been widely reported in relation to many different traumatic experiences, such as natural disasters and accidents (e.g., van der Kolk and Kadish 1987; Wilkinson 1983), and seem to be especially common after physical or psychological assaults, such as combat (e.g., Grinker and Spiegel 1945; Kardiner 1941; Kardiner and Spiegel 1947), concentration camp experiences (Jaffe 1968), and torture (Goldfield et al. 1988).

In the last two decades, the documentation of child sexual abuse has increased greatly (e.g., Finkelhor et al. 1990; Russell 1983; Wyatt 1985); along with this, a number of studies of adult survivors who claim periods of not remembering some or all of their abuse history at some time in their lives have been published. Among these are reports of partial to complete traumatic amnesia among 59%–64% of help-seeking childhood sexual abuse survivors (Albach 1993, 1995, reported in Bowman, in press a; Briere and Conte 1993; Herman and Schatzow 1987), 34%–40% of therapists with childhood sexual abuse histories (Feldman-Summers and Pope 1994; Polusny and Follette 1996), and 31%–44% of samples of adult survivors who were not therapists or seeking treatment for sexual abuse (Elliot and Briere 1995, community sample; Elliot and Fox 1994, college students; Loftus et al. 1994b, substance abuse patients; van der Kolk and Fisler 1995, subjects recruited because of traumatic memories).

The most compelling evidence to date of traumatic amnesia for childhood sexual abuse has been presented by Williams (1994a, 1995; see also Williams and Banyard, Chapter 9, in this volume). In this study, Williams (1994a) contacted women with established histories of childhood sexual abuse documented in emergency room records of a major city hospital during the early 1970s. Subjects were asked detailed questions about their childhood and life experiences, including childhood experiences with sex. The results of these interviews were striking: 38% of these women did not report the abuse that had been recorded 17 years earlier nor did they report any sexual abuse by the same perpetrator (this includes 12% of the entire sample who reported no abuse at all) (Williams 1994a). If the analysis was conservatively restricted to only those subjects with recorded medical evidence of genital trauma and whose accounts were rated as most credible (in the 1970s), 52% did not remember the sexual abuse. Of the women who did remember the abuse, 16% (10% of the entire sample) reported that there was a time when they did not remember the abuse (Williams 1995).

The Williams study (1994a) also has implications for the levels of reporting in the other studies described above. In each of those, the subjects had to remember the abuse to be able to report that they had at some point forgotten it. The findings of the Williams study suggest that some women who do not remember childhood sexual abuse may well have endured it and currently have traumatic amnesia for the experience. This group, however small or large it might be, is not represented in the rates of amnesia reported in most studies, suggesting that, as startling as prevalences reported above may be, they are likely to be underestimates of the true prevalence of traumatic amnesia among childhood sexual abuse survivors. Because no comparison groups were used in these studies, it is impossible to determine the extent to which the findings deviate from normal forgetting of non-abuse-related childhood events.

There is also evidence for more generalized memory impairment in some traumatized individuals. In an unpublished study (Vardi, cited in D. Brown 1995), memory performance was compared among women who had a history of incest, women who were raped as adults, and women who had no history of sexual molestation. The results indicated that both molested groups had acute PTSD symptoms, but only the incest survivors had chronic PTSD symptoms and significant impairments in personal autobiographical memory nonspecific to the abuse, such as remembering names of teachers, schools attended, and significant public events. These impairments occurred especially for the period of life associated with the incest—a finding reminiscent of the central versus peripheral detail recall evidence. Additionally, Bremner et al. (1993) found that patients with combat-related PTSD had deficits in short-term memory; these deficits may be related to the lower hippocampal volume also found in this population (Bremner et al. 1995b).

In summary, the experimental psychological literature on emotion/stress and memory seems to be correct up to a point: In general, memory for the central details and overall theme of a traumatic event may be enhanced by the increased negative affect associated with an event, whereas memory for peripheral or contextual information may be diminished. Christianson (1992) rejected the notion of a Yerkes-Dodson (1908) inverted U relationship between increasing stress and memory function, because the conclusions of his review did not support it (i.e., he did not find the descending arm of the association). It appears, however, that his literature survey was generally limited to nonclinical samples, and consequently, his conclusions describe a rather truncated portion of the possible sample of traumatizing experiences and traumatized individuals.

The clinical literature, on the other hand, suggests that with respect to individuals with posttraumatic conditions, the quantitative association (of increasing stress and improved retention/recall) may be replaced by a qualitatively different one in which intense fear, helplessness, or horror overwhelms the individual and exerts a destabilizing effect on the process of memory consolidation and/or accessibility (Horowitz 1986; van der Kolk and van der Hart 1991). Individuals who have experienced significant trauma, especially those with PTSD symptomatology, seem to represent a different population, exhibiting a contrasting response, in what are likely incomparable conditions, when compared with subjects in experimental studies of emotional arousal and memory. We concur with Harvey and Herman's (1994) somewhat understated conclusion that "future research into the nature of traumatic memory should be informed by clinical observation" (p. 295).

Some cognitive psychologists have argued that memory failure in survivors of childhood sexual abuse can be explained by theories of normal forgetting and that no special process need be inferred. We consider these arguments next.

Explanations for Traumatic Amnesia

Some cognitive psychologists (Bower 1990; Loftus 1993; Loftus et al. 1994a) have suggested that the concepts of repression or dissociation do not need to be invoked to explain the findings of memory inaccessibility among trauma victims. Rather, they suggest that ordinary forgetting (Loftus 1993; Loftus et al. 1994a), motivated forgetting (Bower 1990), or inadequate retrieval cues (Bower 1990) may account for the phenomenon.

Ordinary forgetting and motivated forgetting. Put simply, the "ordinary forgetting" explanation suggests that a survivor may just forget that she or he was repeatedly and violently molested over the course of years by her or his father. In support of this view, Loftus (1993) noted that people routinely forget important events, such as car accidents and hospitalizations. Bower (1990; see also Koutstaal and Schacter, Chapter 8, in this volume) adds the element of motivation to his analysis, thereby accommodating the aversive nature of the experience. He suggests that motivated nonlearning (through lack of attention, nonrehearsal, or automatized avoidance of unpleasant cognitions) or motivated overwriting of memories (learning new associations) may interfere with encoding or storage and thus make some memories difficult to retrieve. As Koutstaal and Schacter (Chapter 8 in this volume) point out, a motivated forgetting explanation of traumatic amnesia is consistent with the anecdotal descriptions of attempting to "block out" memories reported by some of the childhood sexual abuse survivors in the Williams study (1995). However, this hypothesis has no direct experimental support. Findings to date suggest that the more traumatizing the event (e.g., presence of PTSD in those who experienced it), the less successful attempts may be not to remember or think of it (for a discussion, see Koutstaal and Schacter, Chapter 8, in this volume). In addition, as Bower (1990) concedes, this model does not specify the conditions under which these types of mechanisms would come into operation and consequently does not explain why some unpleasant memories are (too) well recalled, whereas others are seemingly unretrievable. (It can be said that the repression and dissociation models of traumatic amnesia also fail to specify the conditions that would predict when these defense mechanisms would operate.)

Retrieval cue insufficiency. Bower (1990) suggested that inadequate retrieval cues probably contribute most to forgetting. Memory retrieval depends largely on the amount and appropriateness of the information contained in the cue (Bower 1990, 1991; Kihlstrom 1994). The adequacy of a cue also depends on the characteristics of the encoding (Tulving and Thompson 1973) and storage of that memory—if it has few or weakened associations, as might be the case with events that elicit motivated nonlearning or overwriting, then more will be required of the cue for successful retrieval. In simple terms, the cue insufficiency argument (Bower 1990) implies then that asking a woman if she had ever been molested may not be an adequate retrieval cue to elicit the memory that her father sexually molested her when she was a child. In addition, Bower (1990) suggested that there may be a motivated avoidance of certain lines of self-cues that might elicit unpleasant memories, thereby reducing the likelihood of an individual's simply coming upon such memories through a natural stream of consciousness.

Normal memory failure versus amnesia. Some of these investigators' resistance to considering or describing such memory inaccessibility as evidence of amnesia may be due to a misunderstanding of the characteristics of dissociative amnesia. For example, in a discussion of the Williams study (1994a), Loftus et al. (1994a) reject the notion of amnesia to describe the findings, stating:

> One could, of course, say that the women whom Williams studied constitute cases of complete amnesia. . . . This would mean, however, that when we forget anything, it is an example of complete amnesia for that thing. It dilutes the meaning of the term "amnesia," which has often been reserved for discussing a pathological sort of forgetting. It is rather similar to using the word "assassination" to describe the squashing of a bug. Given the new broad-ranging definition of amnesia, how would we describe what happens to the person who goes into the supermarket specifically to get aspirin and leaves 10 minutes later with a Snickers bar, a magazine, a box of Pop-Tarts, and no aspirin? Is this amnesia, or is it simply a case of forgetting? (p. 1178)

We find this logic difficult to follow and the analogies rather perverse. Moreover, the argument ignores the characteristics that define "pathological forgetting" (i.e., dissociative amnesia) outlined below, and it belittles the significance of the event and of the forgetting (see also Williams 1994b). Five central features of dissociative amnesia (as an isolated condition or as part of another dissociative disorder) should be considered (American Psychiatric Association 1994; Butler et al. 1996):

1. It involves the inability to recall important personal information.
2. The memory loss is "too extensive to be explained by normal forgetfulness" (American Psychiatric Association 1994, p. 481).
3. The unretrievable content is "usually of a traumatic or stressful nature" (American Psychiatric Association 1994, p. 481).

4. The amnesia is functional rather than organic and, therefore, potentially reversible (i.e., the information is inaccessible rather than lost, as would be the case if it had never been encoded or was somehow erased).
5. The information may still exert an influence on cognitive function, even though it is inaccessible to consciousness—it is out of sight but not out of mind (as is suggested by the heightened reactivity and other posttraumatic symptoms that bring some amnesic survivors of childhood sexual abuse into treatment).

All of these features may be identified in many adults who are amnesic for their histories of childhood sexual abuse. Consequently, although in this chapter we have used the term *traumatic amnesia* to describe extensive forgetting of childhood sexual abuse, it may be that many of these individuals would have symptoms that meet criteria for a formal DSM-IV diagnosis of dissociative amnesia.

Also, note that traumatic amnesia among adult survivors of childhood sexual abuse is not randomly distributed, as might be consistent with an ordinary forgetting or cue insufficiency explanation. Instead, in most studies in which amnesia has been examined, it is associated with factors that would presumably make the event more memorable, such as more violent or more chronic abuse (Briere and Conte 1993; Herman and Schatzow 1987), or factors that would conceivably have a greater effect on the child's developing identity and life experience, such as being younger at the time of the abuse and being molested by someone he or she knew, especially a family member (Briere and Conte 1993; Feldman-Summers and Pope 1994; Herman and Schatzow 1987; Williams 1994a, 1995). In other words, the greater the predictable psychological or developmental effect, the more likely the life experience will be forgotten by these individuals—clearly, this is contrary to what might be predicted from normal processes of memory failure, and it is inconsistent with the extensive cognitive literature on increased memorability of emotional events in nonclinical subjects (Christianson 1992).

Of course, the preceding observation assumes that sexual molestation in childhood is a significant, often life-altering, experience for most people. And that certainly seems to be what many adult survivors report—both those who continuously remember their abuse histories and those who recover memories as adults—particularly those who seek treatment for its ongoing effects on their lives. Childhood sexual abuse is associated with higher rates of many adult psychopathological sequelae, including depression, sexual dysfunction, substance abuse, interpersonal difficulties, revictimization, and PTSD (reviewed in Beitchman et al. 1992; Polusny and Follette 1995; Rowan and Foy 1993; Rowan et al. 1994) in both clinical and nonclinical samples. Some investigators debate, however, whether a distinct post–sexual abuse syndrome exists (Beitchman et al. 1992; cf. Finkelhor 1988), and others even question the basic claim of child sexual abuse as an etiological factor in adult psychiatric disorders, because studies reporting such associations are inadequately controlled (Pope and Hudson 1995).

Repetition and memory.   The association between chronic abuse and amnesia for the event also raises another issue that we believe challenges even the motivated forgetting explanation—that is, one of rehearsal. Bower's (1990) description of motivated forgetting would seem most applicable in cases of memories for isolated events, because it depends on the limitation or relative weakening of associations. It would seem to be hard pressed, however, to accommodate the memory effects of repeated abuse experiences, which may be viewed as rehearsals of the event in experience and memory (P. Jasiukaitis, personal communication, April 1996).

To reiterate the general point, it would seem that "single blow" traumas (Terr 1991) should be the events most likely to be forgotten because they are single events and presumably, therefore, less existentially meaningful and less likely to prompt the development of a memory category or cognitive schema for such an episode, they would not fit into preexisting schemata, and their rehearsal could be avoided or minimized. Repeated traumatic events (such as chronic childhood sexual abuse occurring for years), on the other hand, would represent unavoidable rehearsals of the experience and associated memories. They would accumulate as a store of autobiographical memories with elaborate associations, and consequently, they would be more likely to result in changes in general knowledge about the self and the world, in self-concept, and in schemata for the perpetrator (if he or she is known to the victim) and others perceived as being involved (e.g., denying family members) or for particular events (e.g., going to bed at night). However, the opposite often appears to be the case—the more chronic is the abuse (as well as other factors described previously), the more likely is the development of memory disturbances such as traumatic amnesia (Briere and Conte 1993; Herman and Schatzow 1987; Terr 1991).

Based on these considerations, the ordinary forgetting, motivated forgetting, or cue insufficiency arguments do not seem to offer reasonable alternative explanations for not remembering that one was sexually molested as a child or adolescent. It does seem reasonable, however, to suggest that events that might be expected to change one's life or that would change it if one knew of them would not *ordinarily* be forgotten or very difficult to retrieve and that if such information is inaccessible, then some cognitive processes are not, in fact, functioning normally.

Recovered Memory

In the preceding sections, we discussed the conflicting experimental and clinical views regarding the effects of strong negative affect on memory and some of the possible reasons for the inaccessibility of memories of childhood sexual abuse. An even more contentious debate has been prompted by cognitive research into memory alteration and implantation. In the following section, we review some of this literature and then discuss what we believe are its limitations, urging caution in generalizing from it to account for the clinical phenomenon of recovered memories.

Suggestion Effects: The Alteration of Memory With Postevent Information

A considerable body of empirical literature documents that memories for events may be altered in a variety of ways in experimental settings; this family of effects is commonly described as the *misinformation effect* (Garry et al. 1994). The misinformation effect generally refers to the finding that subjects who are misled about witnessed events may incorporate inaccurate postevent information into their accounts of those events (Garry and Loftus 1994). Another, more recent, misinformation effect is one in which wholly new memories may be implanted through suggestion. We briefly discuss several ways in which extant memories may be altered and new memories introduced (adapted, in part, from Garry and Loftus 1994; Garry et al. 1994).

The influence of leading questions on subject responses.   Loftus and Palmer (1974) found that when subjects were shown films of car accidents, the wording of the postviewing questioning could influence subjects' answers about the event. For example, subjects were more likely to report greater speeds for the moving cars they had seen if they were asked how fast the cars were going when they *smashed* into each other than if they were asked how fast the cars were going when they *hit* each other. Subjects in the former condition were also more likely to report seeing broken glass at the scene (32% for "smashed" subjects vs. 14% for "hit" subjects—a difference of 18%), even though none was shown, suggesting an alteration of the memory representation of the event.

Interestingly, in a study of accounts of real witnesses to a murder (Yuille and Cutshall 1986), the vast majority (83%) of witnesses resisted misleading information incorporated into interviews conducted 4–5 months later. In this study, subjects were asked whether they saw "*a* broken headlight" or "*the* broken headlight" on the perpetrator's car (when there was no broken headlight) or whether they saw "*a* yellow quarterpanel" or "*the* yellow quarterpanel" (when the off-color quarterpanel was blue)—virtually all of them correctly reported that there was no broken headlight or yellow quarterpanel or that they had not noticed the detail.

The insertion by suggestion of items or objects into a previously observed scene. Misleading but plausible information embedded in questions about a viewed scene may also influence the content of subsequent recall. For example, Loftus (1975) found that when subjects were asked, "How fast was the white sports car going when it passed the barn while traveling along the country road?" (when no barn had been in the scene that was viewed), they were more likely than control subjects to report remembering seeing a barn when queried about it later (17% for misled subjects vs. 3% for control subjects—a difference of 14%).

The manipulation of details about an item or object that appeared in a previously observed scene. Loftus et al. (1978) showed subjects slides of an automobile-pedestrian accident scene in which a red car stopped at either a stop sign or a yield sign and then struck a pedestrian at a crosswalk. After viewing the slides, half of the subjects were asked a question in which the nature of the sign was altered (e.g., the stop sign was now a yield sign, and vice versa). When subjects were asked to identify the slide they had seen (given a forced choice), those subjects who had received the misleading information were less likely to choose the actual slide they had seen than subjects who had not received misleading information (41% vs. 75% were correct, respectively—a difference of 34%).

In a related line of misinformation research, Ceci and Bruck and their colleagues have presented a variety of evidence indicating that children are quite suggestible (i.e., susceptible to misinformation), and more so than adults (see Ceci and Bruck 1993, for a review). In a recent study, Bruck et al. (1995) examined the influence of postevent suggestions on children's reports of stressful events involving their own bodies—in this case, a visit to a pediatrician for an inoculation. These children were recontacted an average of 11 months after the inoculations and visited on four separate occasions over 2 weeks. During each of the first three visits, the children were given pain-denying or neutral feedback about their original experience of the inoculation and were also given misleading information or no information about the actions of the pediatrician and of a research assistant who had been present at the time of the inoculation (e.g., who had given them the shot and who had showed them a poster). On the fourth visit, they were asked to state everything they could remember about the time they got their shot, to report everything that the research assistant and the pediatrician had done, and to rate how much the shot had hurt and how much they had cried at the time.

The results indicated that suggestion after a year's delay significantly influenced children's reports. Children receiving the pain-denying feedback reported less pain and crying than those receiving neutral feedback. Those who were misinformed were also more likely to make mistakes about who had done what during the original event. The authors suggest that although it is difficult to disambiguate whether these effects reflect a *change in how children report* their experiences (a social influence effect) or a *change in actual memory* for the events (a cognitive effect), some evidence suggested that reasoning-based inferential processes may have been at work. The addition of new information or of particular inaccuracies in the children's stories suggested they were trying to construct congruent mental scripts based on the misinformation and their own expectations about what must have happened. Note, however, that this last point does not necessarily indicate a change in what they remember, but rather it involves a construction of an explanation (i.e., what they believe) in the present that may or may not overwrite or alter the original memory.

Interestingly, this study also shows that suggestion effects on memory or its report may be bidirectional; that is, suggestion may deflate as well as inflate claims—in this case, pain-denying feedback resulted in retrospective reports of less pain. This is more analogous to a clinical situation in which a victim of abuse denies that an event happened than it is to one in which a psychotherapy patient falsely accuses a parent of abuse. The subjects in Bruck et al.'s study downplayed real, if mild, trauma.

Suggestion Effects: The Implantation of Memories

Clearly, the most relevant and controversial area of experimental research related to the clinical issue of recovered memories is whether individuals can be falsely convinced that something happened to them and come to "remember" experiencing that event. Although some anecdotal reports of false memories have been published (e.g., Piaget 1962; Pynoos and Nader 1989), Loftus and her colleagues (Loftus and Coan, unpublished data, reported in Loftus 1993; Loftus and Pickrell 1995; Loftus et al., in press) were the first to succeed in implanting memories in laboratory subjects without hypnosis. The implantation of memories is the only misinformation effect that involves the creation of new "memories" rather than the manipulation of existing ones.

The suggestion of entire episodes purportedly from the subject's past. In what has become the paradigmatic memory implantation protocol, confederate graduate students attempt to lead an offspring or sibling

---

to believe that he or she was lost in a shopping mall when he or she was 5 years old by telling the subject that they themselves remembered the event and asking the subject to try to recall and describe the event on repeated occasions. Loftus and Pickrell (1995) reported that 25% of their subjects claimed to remember the false event of being lost in a shopping mall at age 5, either fully or partially, and generated additional details about the event (see also Loftus and Coan, described in Loftus 1993; Loftus and Ketcham 1994; Loftus et al., in press). Hyman and colleagues (Hyman et al. 1995; Hyman and Billings, unpublished manuscript, reported in Loftus et al., in press) also reported implanting false childhood memories in 20%–27% of college students. In their study, the memories included having a birthday party at age 5 at which a clown visited and pizza was served; staying overnight at the hospital for a high fever and earache; attending a wedding and accidentally spilling a punch bowl; and evacuating a grocery store because a sprinkler had been activated—events chosen because they were presumably more unusual than the common experience of being lost or fearing being lost in a mall as a child.

In a study of source misattribution in children, Ceci et al. (1994) were also able to implant and study false memories. In this experiment, children were instructed to identify the events they actually remembered among four actual (parent-supplied) and four fictional (experimenter-contrived) events (one positive, negative, neutral-participant, neutral-nonparticipant for each type) described to them by the investigator. For each event, the children were told that their mothers had said it had occurred, were asked to try to visualize it, and were instructed to try to recall it on 12 separate occasions approximately 1 week apart. The results indicated that children almost always remembered the actual events, and more than 40% of them reported remembering at least one fictional event by the final session. The children were *least* susceptible to assenting to negative fictional events (e.g., falling off a tricycle and getting stitches) than to any other type of fictional event. Ceci et al. (1994, p. 315) noted that this finding is consistent "with claims that abusive or threatening events may be more resistant to false suggestions than neutral ones."

Pezdek (1995) proposed that the probability of suggestively implanting a memory may depend on the extent to which the event is familiar because of experience or knowledge and whether one has script knowledge already accessible. To test this hypothesis, she modified the Loftus et al. paradigm by having confederates suggest to their siblings or relatives three memories—one true event, one false yet familiar event (being lost at the mall), and one false and unfamiliar event (receiving a rectal enema). The results confirmed the prediction: three subjects "remembered" being lost at the mall (15%) and recalled additional details of this event, but *not a single subject remembered receiving an enema*. Because prior testing with different subjects had revealed differences in expected frequency and in the amount of information contained in the average mental script for each event, the author concluded that false memories involving familiar events are more easily planted than false memories of unfamiliar events. As Pezdek observed, "because the findings of Loftus and Coan . . . are frequently applied to cases involving adults' memory for childhood sexual abuse (Loftus 1993), it is especially important to evaluate the appropriateness of this generalization. The results of the present study suggest that it should be far more difficult to plant false memories of childhood sexual abuse than false memories of being lost in a mall as a child" (pp. 19–20).

Pezdek also noted another implication of her findings: "It should be easier to implant false memories of childhood sexual abuse with people for whom childhood sexual contact with an adult was more familiar than with people for whom childhood sexual contact with an adult was less familiar" (p. 20). It is worth reiterating, however, that familiarity with a particular type of event may be acquired by means other than personal experience (e.g., through vicarious learning of the experiences of others or reading or viewing material about such an event).

In summary, several recent studies have reported that false memories for some childhood events may be implanted in up to 27% of adult subjects (Hyman and Billings, unpublished manuscript, reported in Loftus et al., in press; Hyman et al. 1995; Loftus and Pickrell 1995; Pezdek 1995); however, some preliminary evidence indicates that the memory creation may depend on the individual's familiarity with the event.

The alteration and implantation of memories with hypnosis. The alteration and implantation of memories have also been achieved during hypnotic trance states, and this fact is of particular significance to therapists who use hypnosis as a tool for memory recovery. Hypnosis is a state of highly focused attention, usually coupled with physical relaxation. It is also characterized by a tendency to dissociate information (keep it out of conscious awareness) that would ordinarily be conscious and by a heightened responsiveness to social cues or suggestibility (H. Spiegel and Spiegel 1987). The ability to experience this state, termed *hypnotizability*, is a stable and measurable trait (Hilgard 1965; H. Spiegel and Spiegel 1987). Hypnotizability is as consistent over a 25-year interval in adulthood as is intelligence, with test-retest correlations in the range of .7 (Piccione et al. 1989). Hypnotizability is highest in late childhood and declines gradually throughout adulthood (Morgan and Hilgard 1973). This age difference is important, because it means that children are likely to be more vulnerable to suggestive influence.

Hypnotic phenomena may occur without a formal induction (H. Spiegel and Spiegel 1987); consequently, children and others could respond suggestively either to traumatic events or to suggestive influence about them (e.g., "it did not happen, it wasn't so bad"). Because the focus of attention is narrowed in hypnosis (Tellegen 1981; Tellegen and Atkinson 1974), hypnotized individuals are more likely than others to incorporate a central idea or image rather than judge it. They would thus seem to be at elevated risk for incorporating a deliberate or unwitting suggestion into their memory reports. Indeed, Laurence et al. (1986) noted that Janet used hypnosis explicitly to alter some of a patient's memories so that the events contained in them were no longer as traumatic (see also van der Kolk and van der Hart 1989; for descriptions, see Ellenberger 1970, pp. 361–364).

Laurence and Perry (1983) experimentally demonstrated that memories for fictitious events may be created with hypnosis. In this study, 27 hypnotized subjects were age regressed to a night during the previous week in which they reported sleeping soundly. The investigators then subtly suggested, through questioning, that these now "sleeping" subjects had heard a noise. While hypnotized, almost two-thirds of subjects reported that they had indeed heard a noise. After termination of the trance state, almost half of all subjects still believed that they had heard the noise that night. Even after being told that the noise had been suggested by the hypnotist and was not in fact real, more than one-fifth of subjects retained their belief. It should be noted that the investigators' efficacy in implanting the memory was likely enhanced by the fact that it was suggested to have occurred when the subjects were asleep; that is, there was no competition from a real memory, which might have made the implanted one less plausible.

In a recent replication of this study, Lynn et al. (1994) compared responses of highly hypnotizable subjects with simulating low hypnotizable subjects. The authors concluded that because "the simulating subjects were able to role-play the responses of the hypnotized subjects successfully . . . this raises the possibility that the memory reports of hypnotic subjects may reflect their response to situational demands or reporting biases rather than actual memory changes" (p. 124).

Spanos and his colleagues (reviewed in Spanos et al. 1994) have examined the ways in which some subjects construct elaborate and complex fantasies of past-life experiences, UFO alien contact/abduction, and childhood ritual satanic abuse that they believe to be memories. Their investigations have focused on these (usually hypnotically created) pseudomemories as a means to study the processes involved in the development of what Spanos believes is an analogous condition— dissociative identity disorder (formerly known as multiple personality disorder; see also Ganaway 1989). Spanos contends that all these conditions are learned and socially constructed. Evidence for this comes from findings that characteristics of these "memories" are influenced by expectations transmitted by the experimenter. For example, in one study of "past-life regression" (Spanos et al. 1991), half of the subjects wcrc told, before the regression, that children in earlier historical periods had frequently been abused. During the regression, these subjects reported significantly higher rates of abuse in their past-life identities than subjects not receiving this information. On termination of the hypnotic regression procedure, some subjects still reported believing that their experiences were actual memories of reincarnations.

The above studies notwithstanding, in reviewing the literature on pseudomemories and hypnotic suggestibility, D. Brown (1995, p. 6) concluded that "it is quite clear that hypnotizability, not a formal hypnotic induction, contributes significantly to PM [pseudomemory] production; PM rates are about the same in high-hypnotizable subjects, whether or not formal hypnotic procedures or waking instructions are used." D. Brown proposed that pseudomemory production in hypnosis is best understood as an interaction of hypnotizability and social influence and that therapists should carefully assess the risk factors for pseudomemory production in their patients, especially if they have posttraumatic stress symptoms without an identifiable stressor and with limited memories (see also Bowman, in press b).

It is important to recognize that hypnotic phenomena, including memory distortion, can occur even in the absence of a formal induction, especially among highly hypnotizable individuals (D. Spiegel 1995). Indeed, the structure of the hypnotic state, with its narrowing of focal attention, dissociation, and heightened responsiveness to social cues, shares many features with the acute dissociative state seen during and immediately after trauma (Bremner et al. 1995a; Koopman et al. 1994; Marmar et al. 1994; D. Spiegel and Cardeña 1991; for a review, see Butler et al. 1996). Therefore, it is logical that hypnotizable individuals may have spontaneously entered hypnotic-like states during traumatic experiences and, thus, be more prone to remembering them in a subsequent state of formal hypnosis. By the same token, the structure of the experience of entering a hypnotic state may elicit traumatic schemata independent of any specific content. Thus, vulnerability to the implantation of pseudomemories is higher among highly hypnotizable individuals, especially during hypnosis, because the mental state is similar in traumatic and hypnotic situations. Similarly, receptivity to the retrieval of veridical memories may also be increased because of the similarity of mental states. Consequently, hypnotized individuals may be more likely to report both suggested and veridical traumatic memories.

In short, there is mounting evidence that suggestion may cause some individuals to report false memories of past events with and without the use of hypnosis. The relative contributions of actual cognitive changes versus social conformity effects in these events have yet to be fully elucidated and may well differ depending on the nature of the reported memory alteration and the characteristics of the individual. Nevertheless, these findings have fueled much of the current public debate about recovered memories, so we turn now to a discussion of their limitations.

Some Limitations to the Misinformation Effect

To support their claims, critics of the veracity of recovered memories have relied heavily on the misinformation effects found by cognitive psychologists. But, we question the direct application of these experimental findings to clinical phenomena both because of the generalizability issues we raised earlier in this chapter (incomparable settings, measures, manipulations, and subjects) and because we believe that there are important limitations to these effects. Referring again to Mook (1983) and his suggestion that what laboratory research does best is illuminate "what can happen, rather than what typically does happen," the following section outlines some of the limitations of the misinformation effects and challenges some of the claims made about them.

In cognitive psychology, the focus is on understanding mental processes such as memory—processes common to all of us. The emphasis is on identifying and understanding the operation of fundamental mechanisms, for example, the conditions that enhance or undermine the encoding, storage, or retrieval of memories. Researchers are seeking universal effects (i.e., what is generally true across individuals). To the degree that they identify such general processes and basic mechanisms, they can make general claims.

This experimental focus on basic processes and mechanisms is typified in the following—not completely facetious—statement of Loftus and Hoffman (1989):

> We believe that the misinformation effect is sufficiently pervasive and eventually may be so highly controllable that we are tempted to propose a Watsonian future for the misinformation effect (see Watson 1939, p. 104, cited in Loftus and Hoffman 1989): Give us a dozen healthy memories, well-formed, and our own specified world to handle them in. And we'll guarantee to take any one at random and train it to become any type of memory that we might select—hammer, screwdriver, wrench, stop sign, yield sign, Indian chief—regardless of its origin or the brain that holds it. (p. 103)

In other words, the authors have found their evidence compelling enough to make an expansive claim and prediction about its generalizability.

More recently, the misinformation findings (now including the memory implantation results) have led Garry and Loftus (1994) to conclude that "it is not hard at all to make people truly believe they have seen or experienced something they have not" (pp. 365–366). This broad claim, we believe, lays the foundation for many of the attacks on memory recovery. However, does it really summarize or do justice to the empirical evidence? Let us examine it. (We undertake this exercise not for the sake of quarrelsomeness, but because this particular statement summarizes so many of the issues that we believe deserve further discussion.)

"It is not hard at all ... " How difficult is it? First, note that the misinformation findings are consistently rather small, implicating only a minority of subjects (0%–34%; typically fewer than one-quarter of adult subjects tested show them). (In all fairness, this clause may instead have been intended to convey the reliability of the findings rather than their generalizability—although we doubt this, given the previous "Watsonian" claim.) In contrast, consider an analogy in the clinical domain. It is unlikely that researchers would claim that "it is not hard at all" to treat disorder X, if only one-quarter of patients responded to the treatment. This contrast in what is considered an appropriate claim is, we believe, grounded in a fundamental difference in the two research traditions.

The experimental focus on identifying basic processes or mechanisms embraces statistical significance as the measure of the meaningfulness of a finding, sometimes irrespective of its real-world implications. In clinical research, *statistically significant* and *clinically significant* are distinct terms—the latter is a more stringent and appropriate criterion for clinical issues. In other words, as William James observed, the difference has to make a difference to be a difference. For example, in treatment outcomes, a drug is judged not only by whether it ameliorates symptoms to a statistically significant degree but also by whether treated patients show a reliable change from dysfunction to functionality (i.e., ideally, after treatment, patients should fall within the normal range; e.g., Ogles et al. 1995). These two contrasting research agendas serve their respective goals and need not conflict. They will conflict, however, if their limits are not specified. For the reasons described above, extreme caution must be used in generalizing from limited findings derived under such artificial circumstances to discussions of false memory creation in therapy.

" ... to make people ... " Who is susceptible? Obviously, based on the preceding, we believe it would be more prudent to say "to make *some* people"; however, another issue is involved. The experimental focus on identifying basic processes or mechanisms also tends to ignore the possible role of specific characteristics of the individual in mediating the effect (i.e., "which people?"). The question of which people are vulnerable to misinformation effects seems a reasonable one to pose, given that only a limited proportion of subjects succumb to the effect. In other words, why them and why only them?

Experimentalists might argue that the numbers merely reflect the limits of their present knowledge and technique in instilling misleading information (as the "Watsonian" quote above would suggest) or the limitations inherent in single trial designs (G. Bower, personal communication, April 1996). However, alternative explanations are also possible. For example, if the misinformation effects actually represent reporting differences caused by factors such as compliance, suggestibility (D. Spiegel 1995), demand characteristics, or "misinformation acceptance" (subjects trusting the experimenters' information over their own memories) rather than actual memory alterations (for discussions, see Ceci and Bruck 1993; Loftus and Hoffman 1989; Zaragoza and Koshmider 1989), then individual differences in traits related to these factors could illuminate who would be susceptible to the effect—that is, what is it about those subjects?

Two recent findings lend credence to the reasonableness of this query and indicate that some experimentalists have begun to ask such questions. In a replication of Hyman et al.'s (1995) study, Hyman and Billings (unpublished, reported in Loftus et al., in press) found that hypnotizability/vividness of mental imagery and the tendency to have dissociative experiences were strongly correlated with the experimental implantation of false childhood memories. As we mentioned earlier in this chapter, hypnotizability is a known risk factor for the creation of pseudomemories (for discussions, see D. Brown 1995; D. Spiegel 1995). Consider also the Pezdek (1995) finding in which the implantation of false memories seemed to depend on the subject's degree of experience or knowledge about the nature of the event being implanted. In the case of a rectal enema, for which most subjects had a limited prior knowledge base, none of the attempted implantations was successful. The findings of Hyman and Billings and of Pezdek suggest that trait or knowledge differences may well play a role in the development of false memories. By asking and answering the question "What is it about those subjects?" with experimental and clinical research, we may begin to be able to predict with greater precision who is at risk for implantation of false memories. This development would bring a level of specificity to this literature that has been sorely lacking.

" . . . truly believe . . . "   How truly are false beliefs held? There is little question that this issue is still the crux of significant debate. In a replication of the classic misinformation paradigm (Loftus et al. 1978), Zaragoza and Koshmider (1989) examined whether subjects exposed to misleading postevent information actually come to believe that they remember seeing that information at the time of the original event (i.e., that the memory is actually altered). They found that misled subjects were no more likely than subjects who were not misled to actually believe that they remembered seeing the misinformation as part of the original event. In addition, postevent exposure to misleading information did not reduce subjects' ability to accurately identify the original source of the information (i.e., they were no more likely to make source confusion errors). Zaragoza and Koshmider concluded that reporting misinformation does not necessarily indicate that subjects remember seeing it or have come to believe it to be true, and they note several possible alternative explanations for the misinformation effect (see also Loftus and Hoffman 1989). When a subject *does not* remember the original detail (e.g., that it was a stop sign), he or she may come to believe that the yield sign, introduced in the postevent information, was part of the original event either because it was introduced by a source that presumably has accurate information (the experimenter) or because the information simply fills a gap (and therefore does not conflict with anything) in his or her memory. Subjects who *do* remember the original detail may also report the misinformation either because it was offered by the experimenter, and they trust that source more than their own memory (*misinformation acceptance*; Loftus and Hoffman 1989), or because of social desirability or experimental demand characteristics (e.g., being cooperative, perceptions of how to do well on the test).

Likewise, in the study of implanting memories of fictional events in children, Ceci and his colleagues (1994) concede that it is impossible to determine from their data the degree to which any or all of the following factors contributed to the children's false reports: repeatedly being asked to think about the fictional event, being told that one's mother said that the event occurred, or repeatedly being asked to create images of the event. (In a footnote, they report that few children assent to fictional events if they are not given either of the latter two instructions.) The authors stated that "notwithstanding this inability to provide explanation, we do believe that not all false assenting reflected children's actual beliefs in the false events, because some children recanted these false assents after being told they were wrong in the final session" (Ceci et al. 1994, p. 317). In other words, the misinformation findings may well represent influences other than the alteration of true beliefs.

" . . . they have seen or experienced something they have not." How false is the false belief? Again, we refer to the studies previously described and note that the Pezdek study (1995) offers preliminary but suggestive evidence that a specific knowledge base may indeed be necessary before subjects can be convinced that have experienced something they have not (i.e., they must have some kind of experience of it already).

In the interests of clarity and circumspection then, we suggest that the statement, "It is not hard at all to make people truly believe they have seen or experienced something they have not," might be better rephrased as "It is possible to make some people mistakenly report that they have seen or experienced some things under certain (experimental) circumstances."

A Reconsideration of the Misinformation Effect

What do the misinformation and suggestibility effects reported by Loftus, Bruck, Ceci, and their colleagues in the experimental studies described above suggest? If we agree, as we do, that some memories could be altered or inserted in some people, what does it really tell us with respect to our considerations of recovered memory? For one thing, these findings underscore the necessity for significant caution in using suggestive "memory recovery" techniques in therapeutic situations, particularly with patients who have no memory of the abuse (for an extensive review, see Lindsay and Read 1994). These findings also offer some possible ways in which false or distorted memories "recovered" in therapy may be created (although, as we have emphasized, what a "false memory" actually represents—be it actual memory alteration, demand characteristics affecting reporting, or a belief in the new information rather than an actual memory of the implanted event—is far from established).

However, do these findings really challenge the credibility of recovered memories per se? Are they applicable to individuals who recover memories of childhood sexual abuse outside of a "recovered memory" therapy context? The factors that argue for the generalizability of experimental findings to therapy offices (such as suggestion of past events, perceived authority of the source, repetition of suggestions, perceived plausibility of suggestions, mental rehearsal, guided imagery, use of hypnosis; Lindsay and Read 1994) are less apparent in other settings where therapy is not involved (e.g., Stanton 1995), and therefore the generalizability argument seems uncomfortably stretched in these instances. Some experimentalists acknowledge this; for example, Lindsay and Read (1994) caution, in the beginning of their review, that their comments "are directed only to recollections of abuse that are the products of extensive use of memory recovery techniques and ancillary practices. People who have always remembered being sexually abused as children, or who spontaneously come to remember previously forgotten abuse, are on those bases different from clients who require months of guidance and memory recovery techniques prior to their first recollection" (p. 282). The possibility that some recovered memories may be created does not imply that all recovered memories are, in fact, created. Indeed, the experimental findings seem to be a rather clear example of experimental research showing what can happen rather than what typically does happen.

D. Spiegel (1995) offered an alternative conceptualization of what the misinformation studies may be revealing about memory. The fact that memory is malleable and subject to internal needs for comprehensibility and consistency and/or external suggestions and pressures is in no way inconsistent with the notion that traumatic memories may be dissociated or repressed. Contrary to the common assumption that these memory alteration findings are sufficient grounds for attacking the veracity of recovered memories, these studies may provide additional converging evidence in support of the possibility of dissociated memories, such as those seen in traumatic amnesia.

As a matter of pure logic, it should be equally easy to insert false information or to suppress true information (D. Spiegel 1995). Indeed, the former often requires the latter. The misinformation effect studies (reviewed in Garry and Loftus 1994) and the suggestion study of Bruck and associates (1995) offer cases in point. It may be argued that "to falsely remember a stop sign in an automobile accident, it is necessary to suppress veridical recollection of the yield sign that was there" (D. Spiegel 1995, p. 139). Similarly, for the misled children in the Bruck study to report remembering less crying at the time of the inoculation or to misidentify who gave them their shot suggests that the misinformation may be supplanting what they really remembered. This argument, however, requires that a true memory did exist and would have been reported if the postevent suggestions had not been inserted. Otherwise, it could be argued that the new information suggested by the questioner simply filled a memory gap, as in the Laurence and Perry (1983) "noises in the night" study (see also McCloskey and Zaragoza 1985), and would not be evidence of prior memories being displaced.

On this point, Loftus et al. (1978, p. 27) reported that, for at least half of their subjects, the initial information "got into memory in the first place" (i.e., they encoded the street sign). In the Bruck et al. (1995) study of children's memories for inoculations, reports of the amount of crying at 1 week and 1 year were highly stable for those children who were not given pain-denying feedback, and children who had not been misled about the actions of the pediatrician or research assistant were highly accurate about events for which they had memories. In other words, their memories for the event were intact—and could have been reported had they not been influenced—which suggests that those memories were suppressed at some level so that the suggested misinformation could be reported instead. This latter experiment is a particularly cogent example of the fact that misinformation is a two-edged sword: it may suppress veridical memories of traumatic experiences or create pseudomemories of traumatic experiences under certain circumstances. Additionally, the dissociation argument requires not only that a memory be supplanted but also that it remain retrievable. Zaragoza and Koshmider's (1989) finding, that subjects fed misleading information are not impaired in their ability to identify the original information, is consistent with this (i.e., the memory remains somewhere).

Conclusion

We discussed two large empirical literatures describing the effects of negative emotion and misinformation on memory. The issues we have examined urge use of caution in making inferences from experimental research to the clinical situation. Laboratory studies and surveys with nonclinical subjects indicate that negative affect tends to enhance memory, particularly for central details of an event. We considered several issues concerning the applicability of these research findings to clinical populations. In particular, we described some ways in which laboratory manipulations of emotion and memory appear to lack the "necessary nearness to life" (Stern 1910, p. 270, quoted in Yuille and Cutshall 1986, p. 291) that would allow the findings to be extrapolated to clinical populations with significant traumatic memories. This is important because the experimental findings seem to be at odds with the well-established clinical literature describing significant disturbances in memory associated with trauma. We also described several normal memory failure explanations that have been offered to account for traumatic amnesia and memory recovery—clinical phenomena that are often attributed to psychopathological processes of dissociation or repression. In this discussion, we concluded that these explanations are contradicted by the predictions that might be reasonably made about the memorability of events such as childhood sexual abuse. Furthermore, these explanations appear inadequate when measured up to the significance and extensiveness of the traumatic amnesia that they seek to explain.

The misinformation literature suggests that some memories (or reports of them) may be altered by postevent information or may even be implanted anew, both with and without hypnosis. We noted that the implications of misinformation effects for recovered memories are far from clear. These misinformation effects, real and important ones, may apply to only a minority of the population that has to date been little characterized—although recent studies indicate that suggestibility and proneness to dissociation may be predisposing factors. The literature also suggests that distortion of memory is most likely to occur when schemata similar to the imposed information preexist. Thus, those who are most likely to create false memories of trauma are those who also have real memories of it or elaborate (perhaps vicariously learned) schemata for it. The actual mechanisms and, therefore, meaning of the effects—whether the memory or the report is altered—have also not been established. To the extent that current social influence over memory retrieval distorts memory, such effects may occur in nature, as when an abusing parent denies to the child that the abuse occurred or threatens the child if she or he talks about it. Moreover, because both cognitive and social influences may be considerable in the therapist's office, clinicians should note the general cautions implied by these findings. We proposed that the misinformation phenomenon may be seen as consistent with the mechanisms of dissociation or repression, in that it requires the supplanting of one memory with another, particularly in cases in which the original information may still be reported. Misinformation pressure may as easily suppress as create traumatic memory. Misinformation may, then, be the other side of the coin of dissociation and repression.

Loftus and colleagues stated that "cognitive psychologists who question the idea of repressed and recovered memories naturally want some empirical evidence" (Garry et al. 1994, p. 449). We agree with the sentiment; however, given the ethical limitations on experimentally manipulating dissociation, memory implantation, or memory recovery of truly traumatic events, we need to find the reasonable balance between what laboratory analog studies offer as explanations of what may be happening and what clinical research and observation offer as descriptions of what is happening. In addition, the development of programmatic research dedicated to investigating these topics by, for example, using closer approximations of the clinical phenomena in the laboratory and by investigating some of the classic experimental findings with clinical subjects could yield findings that span the present information gap between these two disciplines.

References

American Psychiatric Association: Diagnostic and Statistical Manual of Mental Disorders, 3rd Edition, Revised. Washington, DC, American Psychiatric Association, 1987

American Psychiatric Association: Diagnostic and Statistical Manual of Mental Disorders, 4th Edition. Washington, DC, American Psychiatric Association, 1994

Bannister D: Psychology as an exercise in paradox. Bulletin of the British Psychological Society 19:21–26, 1966

Bartlett FC: Remembering: A Study in Experimental and Social Psychology. Cambridge, MA, Cambridge University Press, 1932

Beitchman JH, Zucker KJ, DaCosta GA, et al: A review of the long-term effects of child sexual abuse. Child Abuse Negl 16:101–118, 1992

Bower GH: Awareness, the unconscious, and repression: an experimental psychologist's perspective, in Repression and Dissociation—Implications for Personality Theory, Psychopathology, and Health. Edited by Singer JL. Chicago, IL, The University of Chicago Press, 1990, pp 209–231

Bower GH: Mood congruity of social judgments, in Emotion and Social Judgments. Edited by Forgas JP. Oxford, UK, Pergamon, 1991, pp 31–53

Bowman ES: Delayed memories of child abuse, part I: an overview of research findings on forgetting, remembering, and corroborating trauma. Dissociation (in press a)

Bowman ES: Delayed memories of child abuse, part II: an overview of research findings relevant to understanding their reliability and suggestibility. Dissociation (in press b)

Bremner JD, Scott TM, Delaney RC, et al: Deficits in short-term memory in posttraumatic stress disorder. Am J Psychiatry 150:1015–1019, 1993

Bremner JD, Bennett A, Southwick AM, et al: Toward a cognitive neuroscience of dissociation and altered memory functions in post-traumatic stress disorder, in Neurobiological and Clinical Consequences of Stress: From Normal Adaptation to Post Traumatic Stress Disorder. Edited by Freidman MJ, Charney DS, Deutch AY. Philadelphia, PA, JB Lippincott, 1995a, pp 239–271

Bremner JD, Randall P, Scott TM, et al: MRI-based measurement of hippocampal volume in patients with combat-related posttraumatic stress disorder. Am J Psychiatry 152:973–981, 1995b

Brett EA, Ostroff R: Imagery and posttraumatic stress disorder: an overview. Am J Psychiatry 142:417–424, 1985

Briere J, Conte J: Self-reported amnesia for abuse in adults molested as children. J Trauma Stress 6:21–31, 1993

Brockway S: Case report: flashback as a post-traumatic stress disorder (PTSD) symptom in a World War II veteran. Mil Med 153:372–373, 1988

Brown D: Pseudomemories: the standard of science and the standard of care in trauma treatment. Am J Clin Hypn 37:1–24, 1995

Brown R, Kulik J: Flashbulb memories. Cognition 5:73–99, 1977

Bruck M, Ceci SJ, Francoeur E, et al: "I hardly cried when I got my shot!" Influencing children's reports about a visit to their pediatrician. Child Dev 66:193–208, 1995

Burke A, Heuer F, Reisberg D: Remembering emotional events. Memory and Cognition 20:277–290, 1992

Butler LD, Duran REF, Jasiukaitis P, et al: Hypnotizability and traumatic experience: a diathesis-stress model of dissociative symptomatology. Am J Psychiatry 153 (suppl):42–63, 1996

Ceci SJ, Bruck M: Suggestibility of the child witness: a historical review and synthesis. Psychol Bull 113:403–439, 1993

Ceci SJ, Loftus EL, Leichtman MD, et al: The possible role of source misattributions in the creation of false beliefs among preschoolers. Int J Clin Exp Hypn 42:304–320, 1994

Christianson S-A: Emotional stress and eyewitness memory: a critical review. Psychol Bull 112:284–309, 1992

Christianson S, Hubinette B: Hands up! A study of witnesses' emotional reactions and memories associated with bank robberies. Applied Cognitive Psychology 7:365–379, 1993

Christianson S-A, Loftus EF: Memory for traumatic events. Applied Cognitive Psychology 1:225–239, 1987

Christianson S-A, Loftus EF: Some characteristics of people's traumatic memories. Bulletin of the Psychonomic Society 28:195–198, 1990

Easterbrook JA: The effect of emotion on cue utilization and the organization of behavior. Psychol Rev 66:183–201, 1959

Ellenberger HF: The Discovery of the Unconscious: The History and Evolution of Dynamic Psychiatry. New York, Basic Books, 1970

Elliot DM, Briere J: Posttraumatic stress associated with delayed recall of sexual abuse: a general population study. J Trauma Stress 8:629–647, 1995

Elliot DM, Fox B: Child abuse and amnesia: prevalence and triggers to memory recovery. Poster presented at the annual meeting of the International Society of Traumatic Stress Studies, Chicago, IL, November 1994, pp 1–8

Feldman-Summers S, Pope KS: The experience of "forgetting" childhood abuse: a national survey of psychologists. J Consult Clin Psychol 62:636–639, 1994

Finkelhor D: The trauma of child sexual abuse: two models. Journal of Interpersonal Violence 2:348–366, 1988

Finkelhor D, Hotaling G, Lewis IA, et al: Sexual abuse in a national survey of adult men and women: prevalence, characteristics, and risk factors. Child Abuse Negl 14:19–28, 1990

Freud S: Remembering, repeating and working-through (further recommendations on the technique of psycho-analysis II) (1914), in The Standard Edition of the Complete Psychological Works of Sigmund Freud, Vol 12. Translated and edited by Strachey J. London, Hogarth Press, 1958, pp 145–156

Freyd JJ: Theoretical and personal perspectives on the delayed memory debate. Paper presented at The Center for Mental Health at Foote Hospital's Continuing Education Conference: Controversies Around Recovered Memories of Incest and Ritualistic Abuse, Ann Arbor, MI, August 1993, pp 1–40

Ganaway GK: Historical versus narrative truth: clarifying the role of exogenous trauma in the etiology of MPD and its variants. Dissociation 2:205–220, 1989

Garry M, Loftus EF: Pseudomemories without hypnosis. Int J Clin Exp Hypn 42:363–378, 1994

Garry M, Loftus EF, Brown SW: Memory: a river runs through it. Consciousness and Cognition 3:438–451, 1994

Goldfield AE, Mollica RF, Pesavento BH, et al: The physical and psychological sequelae of torture: symptomatology and diagnosis. JAMA 259:2725–2729, 1988

Green BL: Psychosocial research in traumatic stress: an update. J Trauma Stress 7:341–362, 1994

Grinker RR, Spiegel JP: Men Under Stress. Philadelphia, PA, Blakiston, 1945

Harvey MR, Herman JL: Amnesia, partial amnesia, and delayed recall among adult survivors of childhood trauma. Consciousness and Cognition 3:295–306, 1994

Herman JL, Schatzow E: Recovery and verification of memories of childhood sexual trauma. Psychoanalytic Psychology 4:1–14, 1987

Hilgard ER: Hypnotic Susceptibility. New York, Harcourt Brace Jovanovich, 1965

Horowitz MJ: Stress Response Syndromes. New York, Jason Aronson, 1986

Hyman IE, Husband TH, Billings FJ: False memories of childhood experiences. Applied Cognitive Psychology 9:181–197, 1995

Ingram RE: External validity issues in mood and memory research. Journal of Social Behavior and Personality 4:57–62, 1989

Jaffe R: Dissociative phenomena in former concentration camp inmates. Int J Psychoanal 49:310–312, 1968

Janet P: The Major Symptoms of Hysteria. London, MacMillan, 1907

Kardiner A: The Traumatic Neuroses of War. New York, Basic Books, 1941

Kardiner A, Spiegel H: War Stress and Neurotic Illness. New York, Paul Hoeber, 1947

Kassin SM, Ellsworth PC, Smith VL: The "general acceptance" of psychological research on eyewitness testimony: a survey of the experts. Am Psychol 44:1089–1098, 1989

Kihlstrom JF: Hypnosis, delayed recall, and the principles of memory. Int J Clin Exp Hypn 42:337–345, 1994

Koopman C, Classen C, Spiegel D: Predictors of posttraumatic stress symptoms among survivors of the Oakland/Berkeley, Calif., firestorm. Am J Psychiatry 151:888–894, 1994

Krystal JH, Bremner JD, Southwick SM, et al: The emerging neurobiology of dissociation: implications for the treatment of PTSD, in Trauma, Memory and Dissociation. Edited by Bremner JD, Marmar C. Washington, DC, American Psychiatric Press (in press)

Kuehn LL: Looking down a gun barrel: person perception and violent crime. Percept Mot Skills 39:1159–1164, 1974

Laurence JR, Perry C: Hypnotically created memory among highly hypnotizable subjects. Science 222:523–524, 1983

Laurence JR, Nadon R, Nogrady H, et al: Duality, dissociation, and memory creation in highly hypnotizable subjects. Int J Clin Exp Hypn 34:295–310, 1986

Lindsay DS, Read JD: Psychotherapy and memories of childhood sexual abuse: a cognitive perspective. Applied Cognitive Psychology 8:281–338, 1994

Loftus EF: Leading questions and the eyewitness report. Cognitive Psychology 7:560–572, 1975

Loftus EF: The reality of repressed memories. Am Psychol 48:518–537, 1993

Loftus EF, Burns T: Mental shock can produce retrograde amnesia. Memory and Cognition 10:318–323, 1982

Loftus EF, Hoffman HG: Misinformation and memory: the creation of new memories. J Exp Psychol Gen 118:100–104, 1989

Loftus EF, Ketcham K: The Myth of Repressed Memories. New York, St Martin's Press, 1994

Loftus EF, Palmer JC: Reconstruction of automobile destruction: an example of the interaction between language and memory. Journal of Verbal Learning and Verbal Behavior 13:585–589, 1974

Loftus EF, Pickrell JE: The formation of false memories. Psychiatric Annals 25:720–725, 1995

Loftus EF, Miller DG, Burns HJ: Semantic integration of verbal information into a visual memory. J Exp Psychol Hum Learn 4:19–31, 1978

Loftus EF, Loftus GR, Messo J: Some facts about "weapon focus." Law and Human Behavior 11:55–62, 1987

Loftus EF, Garry M, Feldman J: Forgetting sexual trauma: what does it mean when 38% forget? J Consult Clin Psychol 62:1177–1181, 1994a

Loftus EF, Polonsky S, Fullilove MT: Memories of childhood sexual abuse: remembering and repressing. Psychology of Women Quarterly 18:67–84, 1994b

Loftus EF, Coan JA, Pickrell JE: Manufacturing false memories using bits of reality, in Implicit Memory and Metacognition. Edited by Reder L. Hillsdale, NJ, Lawrence Erlbaum (in press)

Lynn SJ, Rhue JW, Myers BP, et al: Pseudomemory in hypnotized and simulating subjects. Int J Clin Exp Hypn 42:118–129, 1994

Maldonado JR, Spiegel D: The treatment of post-traumatic stress disorder, in Dissociation: Clinical and Theoretical Perspectives. Edited by Lynn SJ, Rhue JW. New York, Guilford, 1994, pp 215–241

Marmar CR, Weiss DS, Schlenger WE, et al: Peritraumatic dissociation and posttraumatic stress in male Vietnam theater veterans. Am J Psychiatry 151:902–907, 1994

McCloskey M, Zaragoza M: Misleading postevent information and memory for events: arguments and evidence against memory impairment hypotheses. J Exp Psychol Gen 114:1–16, 1985

McCloskey M, Wible CG, Cohen NJ: Is there a special flashbulb-memory mechanism? J Exp Psychol Gen 117:171–181, 1988

Mook DG: In defense of external validity. Am Psychol 38:379–387, 1983

Morgan AH, Hilgard ER: Age differences in susceptibility to hypnosis. Int J Clin Exp Hypn 21:78–85, 1973

Mueser KT, Butler RW: Auditory hallucinations in combat-related chronic posttraumatic stress disorder. Am J Psychiatry 144:299–302, 1987

Murdock BB: Human Memory: Theory and Data. Potomac, MD, Lawrence Erlbaum, 1974

Neisser U: Snapshots or benchmarks?, in Memory Observed. Edited by Neisser U. San Francisco, CA, WH Freeman, 1982, pp 43–48

Nelson K: The psychological and social origins of autobiographical memory. Psychological Science 4:7–14, 1993

Ofshe RJ, Singer MT: Recovered-memory therapy and robust repression: influence and pseudomemories. Int J Clin Exp Hypn 42:391–410, 1994

Ofshe RJ, Watters E: Making Monsters: False Memory, Psychotherapy, and Sexual Hysteria. New York, Scribners, 1994

Ogles BM, Lambert MJ, Sawyer JD: Clinical significance of the National Institute of Mental Health Treatment of Depression Collaborative Research Program data. J Consult Clin Psychol 63:321–326, 1995

Olio KA, Cornell WF: Making meaning not monsters: reflections on the delayed memory controversy. Journal of Child Sexual Abuse 3:77–94, 1994

Pezdek K: What types of false childhood memories are not likely to be suggestively implanted? Paper presented at the meeting of the Psychonomic Society, Los Angeles, CA, November 1–23, 1995

Piaget J: Paleys, Dreams and Imitation in Childhood. New York, WW Norton, 1962

Piccione C, Hilgard ER, Zimbardo PG: On the degree of stability of measured hypnotizability over a 25-year period. J Pers Soc Psychol 56:289–295, 1989

Pillemer DB: Flashbulb memories of the assassination attempt on President Reagan. Cognition 16:63–84, 1984

Polusny MA, Follette VM: Long term correlates of child sexual abuse: theory and review of the empirical literature. Applied and Preventative Psychology 4:143–166, 1995

Polusny MA, Follette VM: Remembering childhood sexual abuse: a national survey of psychologists' clinical practices, beliefs, and personal experiences. Professional Psychology: Research and Practice 27:41–52, 1996

Pope HG, Hudson JI: Does childhood sexual abuse cause adult psychiatric disorder? Essentials of methodology. Journal of Psychiatry and Law 23:363–381, 1995

Pynoos RS, Nader K: Children's memory and proximity of violence. J Am Acad Child Adolesc Psychiatry 28:236–241, 1989

Pynoos RS, Frederick C, Nader K, et al: Life threat and posttraumatic stress in school-age children. Arch Gen Psychiatry 44:1057–1063, 1987

Rowan AB, Foy DW: Post-traumatic stress disorder in child sexual abuse survivors: a literature review. J Trauma Stress 6:3–19, 1993

Rowan AB, Foy DW, Rodriguez N, et al: Posttraumatic stress disorder in a clinical sample of adults sexually abused as children. Child Abuse Negl 18:51–61, 1994

Russell DEH: The incidence and prevalence of intrafamilial and extrafamilial sexual abuse of female children. Child Abuse Negl 7:133–146, 1983

Schacter DL: Implicit memory: history and current status. J Exp Psychol Learn Mem Cogn 13:510–518, 1987

Schacter D: Understanding implicit memory: a cognitive neuroscience approach. Am Psychol 47:559–569, 1992

Schacter D, Moscovitch M: Infants, amnesia, and dissociable memory systems, in Infant Memory. Edited by Moscovitch M. New York, Plenum, 1984, pp 173–216

Siegel DJ: Memory, trauma, and psychotherapy. Journal of Psychotherapy Practice and Research 4:93–122, 1995

Spanos NP, Menary E, Gabora NJ, et al: Secondary identity enactments during hypnotic past-life regression: a sociocognitive perspective. J Pers Soc Psychol 61:308–320, 1991

Spanos NP, Burgess CA, Burgess MF: Past-life identities, UFO abductions, and satanic ritual abuse: the social construction of memories. Int J Clin Exp Hypn 42:433–446, 1994

Spiegel D: Multiple personality as a post-traumatic stress disorder. Psychiatr Clin North Am 7:101–110, 1984

Spiegel D: Dissociating damage. Am J Clin Hypn 29:123–131, 1986

Spiegel D: The use of hypnosis in the treatment of PTSD. Psychiatr Med 10:21–30, 1992

Spiegel D: Hypnosis and suggestion, in Memory Distortion—How Minds, Brains, and Societies Reconstruct the Past. Edited by Schacter DL. Cambridge, MA, Harvard University Press, 1995, pp 129–149

Spiegel D, Cardeña E: Dissociative mechanisms in posttraumatic stress disorder, in Posttraumatic Stress Disorder: Etiology, Phenomenology, and Treatment. Edited by Wolf ME, Mosnaim AD. Washington, DC, American Psychiatric Press, 1990, pp 22–34

Spiegel D, Cardeña E: Disintegrated experience: the dissociative disorders revisited. J Abnorm Psychol 100:366–378, 1991

Spiegel H, Spiegel D: Trance and Treatment: Clinical Uses of Hypnosis. Washington, DC, American Psychiatric Press, 1987

Squire LR: Memory and the hippocampus: a synthesis from findings with rats, monkeys, and humans. Psychol Rev 99:195–231, 1992

Stanton M: Bearing witness: a man's recovery of his sexual abuse as a child. Providence Journal-Bulletin, May 7–9, 1995, pp 1A and following

Tellegen A: Practicing the two disciplines for relaxation and enlightenment: comment on "Role of the feedback signal in electromyograph biofeedback: the relevance of attention" by Qualls and Sheehan. J Exp Psychol Gen 110:217–226, 1981

Tellegen A, Atkinson G: Openness to absorbing and self-altering experiences ("absorption"), a trait related to hypnotic susceptibility. J Abnorm Psychol 83:268–277, 1974

Terr L: What happens to early memories of trauma? A study of twenty children under age five at the time of documented traumatic events. J Am Acad Child Adolesc Psychiatry 27:96–104, 1988

Terr L: Childhood traumas: an outline and overview. Am J Psychiatry 148:10–20, 1991

Tromp S, Koss MP, Figueredo AJ, et al: Are rape memories different? A comparison of rape, other unpleasant, and pleasant memories among employed women. J Trauma Stress 8:607–627, 1995

Tulving E, Thompson DM: Encoding specificity and retrieval processes in episodic memory. Psychol Rev 80:352–373, 1973

van der Hart O, Spiegel D: Hypnotic assessment and treatment of trauma-induced psychoses: the early psychotherapy of H. Breukink and modern views. Int J Clin Exp Hypn 41:191–209, 1993

van der Kolk BA: Psychological Trauma. Washington, DC, American Psychiatric Press, 1987

van der Kolk BA, Ducey CR: The psychological processing of traumatic experience: Rorschach patterns in PTSD. J Trauma Stress 2:259–274, 1989

van der Kolk BA, Fisler R: Dissociation and the fragmentary nature of traumatic memories: overview and exploratory study. J Trauma Stress 8:505–525, 1995

van der Kolk BA, Kadish W: Amnesia, dissociation, and the return of the repressed, in Psychological Trauma. Edited by van der Kolk BA. Washington, DC, American Psychiatric Press, 1987, pp 173–190

van der Kolk BA, van der Hart O: Pierre Janet and the breakdown of adaptation in psychological trauma. Am J Psychiatry 146:1530–1540, 1989

van der Kolk BA, van der Hart O: The intrusive past: the flexibility of memory and the engraving of trauma. American Imago 48:425–454, 1991

van der Kolk BA, Blitz R, Burr W, et al: Nightmares and trauma: a comparison of nightmares after combat with lifelong nightmares in veterans. Am J Psychiatry 141:187–190, 1984

Wessel I, Merckelbach H: Characteristics of traumatic memories in normal subjects. Behavioral and Cognitive Psychotherapy 22:315–324, 1994

Wilkinson CB: Aftermath of a disaster: the collapse of the Hyatt Regency Hotel skywalks. Am J Psychiatry 140:1134–1139, 1983

Williams LM: Recall of childhood trauma: a prospective study of women's memories of child sexual abuse. J Consult Clin Psychol 62:1167–1176, 1994a

Williams LM: What does it mean to forget child sexual abuse? A reply to Loftus, Garry, and Feldman (1994). J Consult Clin Psychol 62:1182–1186, 1994b

Williams LM: Recovered memories of abuse in women with documented child victimization histories. J Trauma Stress 8:649–673, 1995

Wyatt G: The sexual abuse of Afro-American and white American women in childhood. Child Abuse Negl 9:507–519, 1985

Yerkes RM, Dodson JD: The relation of strength of stimulus to rapidity of habit-formation. Journal of Comparative Neurology and Psychology 18:459–482, 1908

Yuille JC, Cutshall JL: A case study of eyewitness memory of a crime. J Appl Psychol 71:291–301, 1986

Zaragoza M, Koshmider JW III: Misled subjects may know more than their performance implies. J Exp Psychol Learn Mem Cogn 15:246–255, 1989

Chapter 7

Memory, Repression, and Abuse: Recovered Memory and Confident Reporting of the Personal Past

Kevin M. McConkey, Ph.D.

Memory provides us with an account of the past, helps us operate in the present, and helps us prepare for the future. Sometimes our memories are perfect; sometimes they are not. Sometimes we recover memories and remember things that we had forgotten; sometimes we create accounts of events that we had never experienced. Memory is a constructive and reconstructive process that serves us reasonably well in everyday life but sometimes misleads us and others. The biological, cognitive, and social influences that shape memory are intertwined in the debate about recovered memory and confident reporting of the personal past. The problems of memory, repression, and abuse are at the core of this debate, which in recent years has polarized the psychiatric and psychological communities, as well as patients and their family members. In the civil war that is being fought over this issue in homes, clinics, laboratories, and courts—and reported on and fueled by the media—the focus is the validity of recovered memories of childhood sexual abuse.

In this debate, the central issue is neither the occurrence of nor the possible harm done by childhood sexual abuse. There is no question that sexual abuse during childhood may be associated with major physical and mental health problems during adulthood (e.g., Kendall-Tackett et al. 1993; Levitt and Pinnell 1995; Nash et al. 1993; Roesler and McKenzie 1994; Romans et al. 1995; Schulte et al. 1995; Walker et al. 1995). Also, the central issue is not the reporting of always held, but previously unreported, memories of childhood sexual abuse. There is no question that some individuals do not report childhood sexual abuse even though they have memories of that abuse (e.g., Femina et al. 1990;

Preparation of this chapter was supported in part by a grant to the author from the Australian Research Council. The author is grateful to Amanda Barnier, Karen Bishop, Richard Bryant, Jacquelyn Cranney, Fiona Maccallum, and David Spiegel for comments and assistance during its preparation.

Freyd 1994; Kuyken and Brewin 1995; Loftus et al. 1994a). Rather, the central issue is the reporting of recovered memories of childhood sexual abuse by adults who had not previously indicated any memories of abuse. For some, this type of reporting involves the therapeutic recovery of repressed true memories. For others, this type of reporting involves the iatrogenic creation of false memories.

In recent years, a large and rapidly increasing number of publications on memory, repression, and suggestion have appeared in the context of this debate about recovered and false memory. These include professional and popular books (e.g., Bass and Davis 1994; Blume 1990; Dawes 1994; Fredrickson 1992; Goldstein 1992; Goldstein and Farmer 1993; Herman 1992; Kaminer 1993; Loftus and Ketcham 1994; Lynn and Rhue 1994; MacLean 1993; McConkey and Sheehan 1995; Ofshe and Watters 1994; Pendergrast 1994; Singer 1990; Spiegel 1994; Terr 1994; Wright 1994; Yapko 1994), special issues of journals (e.g., *American Journal of Clinical Hypnosis* 36(3), 1996; *Applied Cognitive Psychology* 8(4), 1994; *Consciousness and Cognition* 3(3–4), 1994; *International Journal of Clinical and Experimental Hypnosis* 42(4), 1994, and 43(2), 1995; *Journal of Traumatic Stress* 8(4), 1995; *The Counseling Psychologist* 23(2), 1995), and major journal articles (e.g., Bloom 1994; Bowers and Farvolden 1996; Freyd 1994; Loftus 1993; Lynn and Nash 1994; McConkey 1995; Pope and Hudson 1995). This publication trend will continue. It is hoped, however, that a shift will occur toward more reasoned and reasonable positions than some of those seen in the literature to date. That shift will require the motivation, time, and effort of all of us, and, in that sense, it will be similar to the processes of both therapy and science.

With an overall aim of contributing to that shift, this chapter has three objectives: 1) to provide an evaluative summary of core concepts and selected findings, 2) to comment on the relevance for clinical practice of current knowledge, and 3) to indicate the preferred directions for research to expand current knowledge. With those objectives in mind, in this chapter, I discuss 1) memory and repression, 2) traumatic memory and recovered memory, 3) recovered memory and well-being, and 4) guidelines for practice and directions for research. At the outset, it is important to recognize the difficulties that are involved in presenting a balanced position on the issues associated with recovered memories of childhood sexual abuse (e.g., Banks and Pezdek 1994; Enns et al. 1995; Green 1995; Grossman and Pressley 1994; Lindsay 1994, 1995; Lindsay and Read 1994). Across the literature, there is wide variation, for instance, in definitions of abuse, trauma, and repression. In addition, there is wide variation in what is considered acceptable evidence for the occurrence and validity of recovered memories of childhood sexual abuse. Given the imprecision and variation on these and other issues, we should not underestimate the difficulties involved in finding common ground, but we should continue to try.

Memory and Repression

Memory experts agree on many issues, including the fact that memory can be accurate, fallible, incomplete, malleable, and susceptible to external factors. Each of these points of agreement and the psychological principles that underscore them can be documented in a variety of ways (e.g., Bekerian and Goodrich 1995; Kihlstrom 1994; Kihlstrom and Barnhardt 1993; Neisser and Fivush 1994). By its nature, memory is a constructive process that is influenced by a wide range of cognitive and social events (e.g., Bartlett 1932; Cialdini 1993), including information that is provided during the encoding of the original event, during the storage of that memory, and during the retrieval of that memory (e.g., Garry et al. 1994; Johnson and Raye 1981; Johnson et al. 1993; Weingardt et al. 1995). Moreover, the use of techniques such as hypnosis to enhance retrieval can lead to major changes in individuals' reported recall and in their confidence in the accuracy of their memory (Krass et al. 1988; McConkey 1992, 1995; McConkey and Sheehan 1995). Put simply, individuals can believe strongly in the accuracy of their hypnotically enhanced memories, even though those memories are inaccurate (e.g., Barnier and McConkey 1992; Nogrady et al. 1985). In terms of the use of hypnosis to enhance memory, McConkey (1992) concluded that "it should be understood clearly that the experimental findings provide no guarantee that any benefits (e.g., increased accurate recall) will be obtained through its use, and that some costs (e.g., inaccurate recall, inappropriate confidence) may well be incurred through its use" (p. 426).

Although hypnosis causes problematic effects on memory, it is important to note that these effects have been recognized by and documented in research. The research that is desperately needed to determine the precise positive and negative effects on memory of other memory enhancement techniques, such as journal keeping and group discussion, has not been done. We should not assume that such techniques are problem-free in terms of their effects on memory, but we should acknowledge that we do not know what the problems are. In addition to the problems of particular techniques, particular types of patients may be especially vulnerable to memory confusions. For example, Bryant (1995) observed a relationship between fantasy proneness and reports of childhood sexual abuse; in particular, reports of abuse at a younger age were associated with a higher level of fantasy proneness. This finding, as well as others (e.g., Lynn and Rhue 1988), indicates that fantasy proneness may be a central process variable involved in the reconstruction of memories of childhood sexual abuse and underscores that patients who are prone to fantasy engagement may be especially vulnerable to factors that lead to the creation of memories.

Although substantial research has established that memories are malleable and should not be accepted as self-validating, this research is sometimes rejected as irrelevant to the debate about recovered memory because it has not involved memory for severely traumatic events (e.g., Herman 1992; Olio 1989; Terr 1994; van der Kolk 1994). This rejection, however, misses the point of the research. Recognizing that memory is malleable does not mean that recovered memories of childhood sexual abuse are necessarily false; rather, it means that they are not necessarily accurate. Moreover, there is no reason that memory for traumatic events should follow entirely different psychological principles from those followed by memory for nontraumatic events. Although a case for that possibility is made by some (e.g., Terr 1994; van der Kolk and Fisler 1995), evidence indicates that traumatic memories can be influenced by the same range of cognitive and social events that influence nontraumatic memories (e.g., Foa et al. 1995; Garry and Loftus 1994; Ofshe and Singer 1994). Recognition of this latter point is especially needed because it should make clinicians think more carefully about the techniques used in therapy and the inferences drawn from memories reported during therapy.

The focus by some on the distinctiveness of memory for traumatic events is linked to the central role of the concept of repression in the debate about recovered memories of childhood sexual abuse (e.g., Herman 1992; Olio 1989; Terr 1994). Repression, in a general sense, involves the motivated forgetting of information that is threatening to the self (e.g., Bowers and Farvolden 1996; Erdelyi 1993; Singer 1990). Note, however, that there are many variants in conceptualizing repression and related constructs such as dissociation and that variation is one of the problems of this debate (e.g., Lynn and Rhue 1994; Singer 1990; Spiegel 1994). Moreover, analyses of the original concept of repression in the writings of Freud have typically highlighted its internal inconsistencies and its limited value beyond a very general description of assumed processes (e.g., Bowers and Farvolden 1996; Brenneis 1994; Crews 1996; Ganaway 1994, 1995; Macmillan 1991). Overall, the relative impreciseness of the concept of repression, and the difficulty in testing it, has led some to argue that it is theoretically meaningless and without scientific support (e.g., Holmes 1974, 1990). In his review of relevant empirical research, Holmes (1990), for instance, concluded that "despite over sixty years of research . . . there is no controlled laboratory evidence supporting the concept of repression" (p. 96) and suggested, perhaps only a little facetiously, that those who choose to continue using the notion should precede it with a warning that "the concept of repression has not been validated with experimental research and its use may be hazardous to the accurate interpretation of clinical behavior" (p. 97).

The limitations of the concept of repression (and of dissociation) must be recognized, but it is impossible to ignore the substantial amount of clinical observation and personal anecdote that point to the ways in which individuals can set aside or avoid thoughts and memories that are unpleasant or threatening to them (e.g., Bower 1990; Davis 1990; Erdelyi 1993; Freyd 1994; Nemiah 1984; Weinberger 1990). Careful clinical observation plays a central role in conceptualizing many ideas in the domain of psychopathology, and systematic clinical observation of unreported, forgotten, and repressed memories of childhood sexual abuse is needed. Thoughts about and memories of important personal events can be set aside from normal awareness, and a concept such as repression or dissociation is needed to help understand that process. Accepting the value of such a concept, however, does not necessarily require an acceptance of the accuracy of reports of those thoughts and memories. As Bowers and Farvolden (1996) noted, "Endorsing the concept of repression does not commit theorists to the belief that recovered memories must be historically accurate in all particulars. A memory, by virtue of having been repressed, does not somehow escape the distortions and constructive features of memories in general" (p. 361).

Despite clinical anecdotes, the repression or dissociation of a memory of a traumatic childhood event may be relatively rare. Indeed, it seems that traumatic events are more likely to lead to recurrent and intrusive memories, in which biological, cognitive, and social processes may be involved (e.g., Bremner et al. 1995; Cotton 1994; Frankel 1994; LeDoux 1991; LeDoux et al. 1989; Nash 1994; Schachter et al. 1995; van der Kolk 1994; van der Kolk and Fisler 1995; van der Kolk and Saporta 1991). The fact that we sometimes remember events that we had forgotten does not mean that those events were traumatic, nor does it mean that those particular memories were repressed. Much of the non-reporting of such events may occur because of normal forgetting, embarrassment about reporting the events, the consequences of reporting the events, or other reasons that relate to factors other than repression (e.g., Freyd 1994; Loftus 1993). Currently, we cannot "distinguish between those [patients] who do not recall actual abuse and those who do not report on it, and among the former, between memory failures that reflect repression, dissociation, and other pathological processes, and those that are benign" (Kihlstrom 1995, p. 66). In other words, we should not assume that newly reported material indicates the lifting of repression that is linked to negative emotional experiences of childhood. As Nash (1994) concluded,

> when we are faced with patients who experience themselves as suddenly and agonizingly remembering a previously forgotten trauma . . . we should above all else recognize the enormous clinical importance of this material . . . [but recognize also that] memories do not literally return in pristine form, unsullied by contemporary factors like suggestion, transference, values, social context, and fantasies elaborated at the time of (and subsequent to) the event. (p. 357)

Traumatic Memory and Recovered Memory

The effects of trauma on memory apparently can range from individuals "being overwhelmed with unbidden memories of past events to [their] having no memory at all of the traumatic event or any aspect thereof" (Green 1995, p. 502). Recent research on traumatic memory has included an examination of the breakdown of cognitive functioning when trauma is occurring (e.g., Nachmani 1995), the neuroanatomical correlates of stress on memory (e.g., Bremner et al. 1995), the characteristics of traumatic memories (e.g., van der Kolk and Fisler 1995), the retention of personal experiences by children and the effects of repeated questions on their recall (e.g., Fivush and Schwarzmueller 1995; Ornstein 1995), the nature of memories of female sexual assault and the influence of therapy on those memories (e.g., Foa et al. 1995; Tromp et al. 1995), and the use of traumatic memories in the clinical setting when they are known to be accurate or inaccurate (e.g., Fowler 1994; Nash 1994). I illustrate recent research by summarizing selected studies and drawing out the relevance of the findings.

Howe et al. (1994) studied the nature and onset of early personal memories for traumatic events. In an analysis of children's recall of emergency room treatment, these authors concluded that children younger than 2 years retained very limited memories and that coherent memories did not develop until a sense of self was established after that age. Moreover, they reported that the pattern of recall for traumatic events was essentially similar to that for nontraumatic events; specifically, over time there was a loss of detail, but a retention of the gist, for both types of events. Goodman et al. (1994) interviewed young children after they had undergone a stressful procedure involving urethral catheterization. The strongest findings were related to the relevance of age differences. In particular, younger (3–4 years old) rather than older (7–10 years old) children recalled less about their experience, answered fewer questions, and made more errors in their answers. Also, factors such as the child's comprehension of the event, the mother's attention at the time, the communication between mother and child, and the child's emotional reaction at the time influenced the memory of this stressful event (Goodman et al. 1994).

Ceci et al. (1994a; see also Ceci et al. 1994b) reported that the difficulty in separating two or more sources of memory was a powerful mechanism underlying children's false beliefs about experiencing particular events; specifically, some children misattributed the source of their memory about a fictitious event. These authors interviewed children about real (parent-supplied) and fictitious (experimenter-contrived) events, and these interviews were conducted 7–10 times at intervals of 7–10 days for each child. The authors reported that all children were susceptible to source misattributions, but the younger children were particularly vulnerable when they were exposed to interview techniques that involved the creation of a mental image of the fictitious event. Such techniques increased the likelihood that younger children would believe that they had experienced those events, when, in fact, they had only imagined them in fantasy. This finding is consistent with other research on the way in which visual imagery about an event tends to lead to a belief in the existence of the event, independent of its actual occurrence (e.g., Dobson and Markham 1993; Markham and Hynes 1993).

To examine the effect of interviewing techniques, Fivush (1994) investigated how young children's recall of events may be changed through discussion with others. She interviewed children at ages 40, 46, 58, and 70 months about personal events and found that the children tended to incorporate relatively little of the information provided by the interview into their subsequent recall; however, they were generally inconsistent in the information that they recounted at the various interview times. Fivush (1994) acknowledged that her study raised more questions than it answered about the extent to which young children are susceptible to leading questions or the extent to which they retain accurate memories of personal events.

Hyman et al. (1995) conducted two experiments to investigate the creation of false memories of childhood experiences in response to misleading information and repeated interviews. Parents were asked to provide information about events that had occurred during the subjects' childhood, and subjects were interviewed about these events and about other events that were created and suggested by the experimenter. In the experiments, either 20% or 25% of the subjects created false memories; moreover, those individuals who had discussed background events relevant to the suggested false memories were more likely to subsequently incorporate those false memories into their own reporting. That is, a general discussion opened the way for the planting of a false memory in some, but not all, of the individuals.

In recognition of the potential influence on reported memory of interviewing techniques, Saywitz and Moan-Hardie (1994) tested a procedure to reduce children's distortion of their memories. In particular, they asked children to stop and think before answering questions and allowed them to indicate whether or not they remembered. The findings indicated that when this procedure was used, acquiescence was reduced and resistance was increased to misleading questions. Saywitz and Moan-Hardie (1994) noted the potential value of adopting such a procedure when dealing with the recall of childhood trauma by adults.

The necessity and potential value of developing and using appropriate interview procedures must be underscored. This is especially so because, although existing procedures have been greatly criticized (e.g., Lindsay and Read 1994; Schooler 1994), there is relatively little guidance on the interview techniques that should be used to minimize distortion in the reporting of memories of childhood sexual abuse (Pennebaker and Memon 1996; however, see Fisher and Geiselman 1992; McConkey and Sheehan 1995). It would be helpful to the debate about recovered memory as a whole to shift away from indicating what should not be done in therapy to indicating more forcefully and in more detail what should be done and why. In this respect, therapists should use techniques that help patients consider and progress in a direct way with their present problems and their hopes for the future and should limit the degree to which they create an imbalance in the lives of patients by inappropriately focusing on uncertain events of the past. Therapists and patients should collaborate on the deeds of the future rather than the assumed misdeeds of the past. Moreover, therapists should convey clearly to patients that they can work effectively with them without becoming involved in debates about the personal past. Hearing and working with what patients say about their beliefs is quite different from encouraging and seeking to validate the patients' reported memories.

In terms of the characteristics of the traumatic memories reported by adults, van der Kolk and Fisler (1995) used a structured interview to question adults about a traumatic and a nontraumatic memory. They found that people reported experiences of traumatic memories in different ways from how they reported experiences of nontraumatic memories. In particular, these investigators observed that sensory modalities were more likely to be associated with the reporting of traumatic memories. Given this finding, they argued that traumatic memories are invariable and do not change over time because of the nature of the sensory information associated with them; however, they also considered that "once . . . the sensations are transcribed into a personal narrative they presumably become subject to the laws that govern explicit memory: to become a socially communicable story that is subject to condensation, embellishment, and contamination" (van der Kolk and Fisler 1995, p. 521).

In other work on the characteristics of traumatic memories, Tromp et al. (1995) surveyed women's memories of rape, other unpleasant events, and pleasant events. They found that unpleasant and pleasant memories differed in terms of a range of feelings and consequences and that rape memories differed from other unpleasant memories by being less clear and vivid, less well remembered, and less thought and talked about and by having a less meaningful order. This study raised important questions about the reasons that rape memories had these characteristics and also raised issues about the way in which memories of different types of events should be dealt with clinically.

In this respect, Foa et al. (1995) examined female rape victims in terms of the changes in their narratives of rape during therapy. They found that the length of the victims' narratives increased across treatment, that the percentage of reported actions and dialogue decreased, and that the percentage of thoughts and feelings increased. In particular, the reported thoughts that attempted to organize and structure the memory of rape substantially increased. This finding indicated that rape victims' narratives of traumatic memories changed over time with the imaginal reliving of the trauma. In particular, the individuals sought to make sense of their memory of the rape and their feelings about that event by structuring their recall in a way that provided a sense of coherence. That sense of coherence may provide a strong feeling of narrative truth and may feel right for both the patient and the therapist, as it were, but it may not provide an unblemished indication of the historical truth of the event, especially given the changes that occur to memory over time (Sarbin 1995; Spence 1982, 1994). The fact that narrative and historical truth may not coincide is nonproblematic and manageable in the clinic by those therapists with relevant knowledge and skill but becomes problematic in nonclinical settings, such as the courtroom, in which the focus of activity and the demands of proof are quite different from those in the clinic (Schutte 1994; Spiegel and Scheflin 1994). As Spiegel and Scheflin (1994) commented, "it is just as possible to dissociate and then retrieve a real memory as it is to convince oneself of a false belief. In the absence of independent corroboration, especially in criminal cases, memory alone cannot fully be trusted" (p. 422).

A number of studies, which have examined whether memories of childhood sexual abuse can be repressed, have raised questions about the trust that can be placed in recovered memory and the utility of such memory in the clinic and in the courtroom (for reviews, see Lindsay and Read 1994; Pope and Hudson 1995). Lindsay and Read (1994) provided a comprehensive analysis of psychotherapy and memory of childhood abuse and argued, in particular, that therapies that involve the recovery of memory can lead to the creation of illusory memories. They focused their comments on memories of abuse that could be said to be the outcome of the use of particular therapeutic techniques, which Lindsay and Read (1994) referred to as "memory recovery therapies." In contrast, Pezdek (1994) argued that the type of memory recovery therapy that was criticized by Lindsay and Read (1994) was not used to a significant degree in psychotherapy and that no clear evidence existed for the creation of illusory memories of sexual abuse by therapists. Pezdek (1994) indicated that many individuals come to therapy with reasonably clear memories of childhood sexual abuse and that other individuals come to therapy after the spontaneous recovery of memory in the absence of any therapeutic intervention. Nevertheless, Banks and Pezdek (1994) considered that "recovered memories can be accurate . . . and compelling memories can be completely unfounded" (p. 267), and these memories may even coexist (Baars and McGovern

1995). Ceci and Loftus (1994) stated that the problem of the creation of illusory memories was pervasive and was not limited to particular individuals or approaches to therapy. They argued strongly that "clients can be led to co-construct vivid memories of events that never transpired; repeated suggestions, imagery instructions, journal writing, and trance inductions are potent psychological mechanisms that we are beginning to realise can lead to false memories" (Ceci and Loftus 1994, p. 362).

Pope and Hudson (1995) reported a detailed analysis of four studies (Briere and Conte 1993; Herman and Schatzow 1987; Loftus et al. 1994b; Williams 1994) and sought to determine whether confirmatory evidence of the abuse had been presented and whether amnesia for the abuse had been demonstrated in these four studies. Note that these were the only relevant studies that Pope and Hudson (1995) could locate, and they concluded that the four studies did not present confirmatory evidence of the abuse and did not demonstrate amnesia for the abuse. Therefore, Pope and Hudson (1995) argued that the "present evidence is insufficient to permit the conclusion that individuals can 'repress' memories of childhood sexual abuse" (p. 126). Notwithstanding this conclusion, it is useful to consider these and other relevant studies for the information that they convey. At the very least, these studies present the difficult conceptual, methodological, and inferential issues that are involved in conducting research on recovered memory of childhood sexual abuse.

In an early study, Herman and Schatzow (1987) reported on the recovered (or suspected) memories of childhood sexual abuse of women who were in group therapy. Because of the problems in understanding the nature of the sample of women, the nature of the memory deficits that they had experienced or were experiencing, the corroboration of abuse claimed by some subjects, and the fact that some cases that were presented by the authors were apparently composites of several cases, it is very difficult to draw meaningful inferences from this study.

More recently, Harvey and Herman (1994) reported on the memories of three adults with childhood trauma. The first case involved the continuous recall of sexual abuse, but with different interpretations and understandings of the events that were said to constitute the abuse; the second case involved a mixture of partial recall and shifts in the individual's understanding of childhood sexual abuse; and the third case involved substantial amnesia by the individual of childhood sexual abuse. Harvey and Herman (1994) highlighted the multiple pathways that can lead to the reporting of memories of childhood sexual abuse in the clinical setting and the different clinical approaches that should be used in these different types of cases. Moreover, they underscored that these different types of cases relate to issues concerning the forensic implications of different pathways to a memory, and they usefully argued that "a science of memory must be able to account for the aberrations of memory and consciousness [and that] effective treatment of these [aberrations] can and must be informed by basic research" (Harvey and Herman 1994, p. 305). Many would agree with this point, but it is difficult to keep it in focus in the politically charged nature of current culture (e.g., Dershowitz 1994; Herman 1995; Hughes 1993; Kaminer 1993; Loftus et al. 1995; Sykes 1992).

In this respect, Briere (1995; see also Brown 1995; Herman 1995) saw limitations with a scientific approach in resolving debate about recovered memory and argued that much of the debate revolved around political issues such as public education, improved professional training, and the marginalization of abuse survivors. Importantly, Briere (1995) highlighted the need for increased attention to standards of professional practice in the area of trauma-oriented psychotherapy, which is a point that needs to be underscored.

Briere and Conte (1993) reported findings from a sample of individuals who were in therapy and indicated that 59% of these patients had identified a period in their lives when they had no memory of the occurrence of childhood molestation. Moreover, the findings suggested that the more violent the abuse and the earlier the abuse occurred, the more likely it was that a period of amnesia had been experienced. Also, the findings indicated that patients who had experienced periods of amnesia had more current psychological symptoms than those who had not. Briere and Conte (1993) acknowledged that their research was limited in several ways, including problems with the selection of their sample (e.g., the individuals were in therapy, and the therapist chose whom to include in the sample) and with the accuracy of the individuals' reports of childhood molestation and periods of amnesia (e.g., they were asked whether there was ever a time when they could not remember an abuse experience). Moreover, it is clear that the corroboration of the patients' reports of childhood sexual abuse was problematic; of course, this is a major issue in this area of research in general (Briere and Conte 1993).

In a somewhat similar study, Loftus et al. (1994b) interviewed women with a history of abuse and asked them whether they had forgotten the abuse for a period of time. Although, and in contrast to Briere and Conte (1993), only 19% of these women indicated such a period, the meaning of this finding is not clear because of the same methodological problems that characterize the study by Briere and Conte (1993). In other research, Elliott and Briere (1995) examined the recall of childhood sexual abuse in a sample of the general population and found that 42% of the respondents with a history of sexual abuse had experienced less memory of the abuse at some time in their life than at other times. Moreover, delayed recall or the recovery of memory was associated with the reported use of threats at the time of the childhood sexual abuse. Finally, those respondents who had recently recovered memories of abuse were reported to have more clinical symptomatology than those who had not. In their focus on a nonclinical sample, Elliott and Briere (1995) importantly suggested the need for a closer examination of the recovery of memory away from the therapeutic setting.

Williams (1994; see also Williams 1995) interviewed women who had histories of sexual abuse in childhood that had been documented in hospital records. She found that 38% of the women did not recall the abuse that had been documented 17 years previously. In particular, those women who were younger at the time of the abuse and those who had been molested by someone they knew were more likely not to recall the previously documented abuse. Given these findings, Williams (1994) argued that the recovery of memories of childhood sexual abuse by some women should not be surprising and that the absence of a memory of abuse should not be seen as necessarily indicating that no abuse occurred during childhood. Loftus et al. (1994a) reviewed and highlighted many of the strengths and weaknesses of this important study. In particular, they indicated how the findings supported the claim that individuals can forget a sexually abusive experience but did not support any claim that childhood sexual abuse is typically set aside from awareness and reliably recovered during adulthood. As Loftus et al. (1994a) noted, some of the women were so young when they were abused that the information was probably not encoded adequately, and others who were abused when older may have simply forgotten the events, as they had forgotten many other events of childhood.

Williams's (1994) research emphasized that some individuals who were sexually abused in childhood may not report such abuse during a clinical examination because they have forgotten it. This study is important not only because it provided information of value and indicated some of the problems involved in conducting meaningful research, but also because the reception and discussion of the findings by both scientists and practitioners interested in this issue indicated how easy it is to mislead and to be misled in this debate (see Loftus et al. 1994a). That is, the complexity of the findings is occasionally masked by overly simplified statements about the inferences that can be drawn from them.

The findings of these various studies underscore that recovered memories of abuse should not be seen as self-validating. Their nature and accuracy must be determined independently rather than being simply assumed by the patient, the therapist, or others. Unfortunately, as Bowers and Farvolden (1996) have stated, "what complicates the situation is that many therapists accept such abuse memories at face value, in part because they feel they are rejecting the patient unless they confirm each and all of his or her ideas, memories, and beliefs" (p. 361). This tendency by some therapists is unfortunate, not only because it may provide the essential approval for the patient to assume the validity of memories that may not be accurate, but also because it conveys that the therapist knows the truth about the patient. For instance, Herman (1992) considered that the "therapist should make clear that the truth is a goal constantly to be striven for, and that while difficult to achieve at first, it will be attained more fully in the course of time" (p. 148). We should recognize, and be comfortable with, the fact that therapists do not know historical truth (Spence 1982, 1994), and to convey otherwise is professional arrogance of the worst kind. As Bowers and Farvolden (1996; see also Lynn and Nash 1994; Lynn et al. 1994) highlighted, "neither the therapist nor the patient has privileged access to the origins of a patient's distress. The therapist can have more or less plausible theories regarding why the patient is distressed, but such theories should not be mistaken for the Truth—however compelling the theory may seem" (p. 373).

Recovered Memory and Well-Being

For some, the recovery of memories of sexual abuse is an essential part of the therapeutic experience and central to the successful outcome of therapy (Courtois 1992, 1995; Olio 1989). For others, the assumption that memories of childhood sexual abuse need to be recovered encourages an attitude of victimization and is counterproductive to the successful outcome of therapy (Loftus et al. 1995; Nash 1994). For instance, Loftus et al. (1995) commented, "[T]herapy that focuses exclusively on the past and what might have been done to the client, still leaves the client wallowing in the victim role. We have only traded one cultural myth for another: that we are never responsible for our own problems or our own healing" (pp. 307–308).

Therapy that focuses on recovered memory may, in fact, have negative effects on well-being. For instance, McElroy and Keck (1995) provided case analyses of three women with eating or obsessive-compulsive disorders who were told that their symptoms were based on childhood sexual abuse and that the recovery of memories of this abuse would be important in treatment. Two of the women were unable to recover any such memories, and their conditions deteriorated; their conditions improved in response to traditional treatment. McElroy and Keck (1995) argued that pressuring patients to recover memories of abuse when they do not believe that they have been abused may have significant negative consequences for treatment. In other work, Byrne and Sheppard (1995) presented 11 case histories of individuals who either made allegations of childhood sexual abuse or had such allegations made against them; in each case, the allegations were either withdrawn or disproved. Based on their analysis of these cases, Byrne and Sheppard (1995) argued for the need for particular guidelines to be developed to identify the possible occurrence of false memory and to treat individuals who are experiencing false memories of childhood sexual abuse.

Brenneis (1994) highlighted how a psychoanalyst who strongly believes in the recovery of early traumatic experiences may make direct and indirect suggestions that will encourage patients to produce false beliefs about such experiences. He indicated that analysts should be aware of the potential risks and benefits of having a strong belief in the possibility of recovering traumatic memories and that the current evidence suggests that the risks to the patient's well-being are likely to be greater than the potential benefits (see also Haakrn 1995). Relatedly, Person and Klar (1994) argued that psychoanalytic notions have blurred distinctions between unconscious fantasies and repressed memories of sexual abuse, and they used a case analysis to discuss problems that psychoanalytically oriented therapists have in dealing with this distinction. Although Person and Klar (1994) argued that memory and fantasy can be disentangled, it must be noted that in the absence of corroboration, little evidence supports the reliability of any such method of differentiation.

In the relevant studies and case reports in the literature, a major issue is the difficulty in obtaining a clear understanding of the "presumed therapeutic benefits of various memory recovery techniques" (Grossman and Pressley 1994, p. 279). No convincing studies or individual cases appear to clearly demonstrate the nature of the benefits that would be derived from the recovery of memory. It may be that techniques do lead to benefit when used by appropriately trained individuals but not by those who are essentially incompetent. There may be value in the recovery of memory if it occurs in the context of genuinely therapeutic activities rather than as a therapeutic activity in its own right. Enns et al. (1995) stated that the experienced and knowledgeable therapist "does not imply that childhood sexual abuse is the only issue that contributes to the client's current psychological status or that this issue must receive greater attention than other issues that the client faces" (p. 229) and also that "major gaps in the client's memory for the past should be noted but the [therapist] should not assume that these gaps necessarily signify a troubled past" (p. 232).

At present, we simply have no convincing evidence that recovered memory leads to improvements in well-being. Thus, as Grossman and Pressley (1994) indicated, the crucial question of whether the potential benefits outweigh the potential costs of attempts to recover memories of childhood sexual abuse cannot be answered at this stage. Read and Lindsay (1994, p. 430) concluded that

> research evidence does not support the idea that a large percentage of clients who have no conscious recollections of childhood sexual abuse

were in fact abused; [that there is] no compelling evidence in support of the idea that therapeutic approaches designed to help clients recover suspected repressed memories are helpful; [and that] there is substantial evidence consistent with the idea that overzealous use of such techniques and ancillary practices may lead some clients who were not abused as children to come to believe that they were abused.

Similarly, and forcefully, Lindsay (1995) emphasized the need to determine whether the recovery of memory is actually associated with positive therapeutic outcomes and concluded that "there is not a single controlled study demonstrating any beneficial effect of therapeutic efforts to recover hidden memories of [child sexual abuse] in clients who report no abuse history, and there is no convincing evidence to support the claim that practitioners can discriminate between clients with no awareness of abuse histories and clients with no abuse histories" (p. 288).

Guidelines for Practice and Directions for Research

The extent to which guidelines for practice are needed depends in part on the degree to which the knowledge and activities of practitioners are at odds with the evidence that is available about recovered memories of childhood sexual abuse. Poole et al. (1995) conducted two surveys of the opinions and practices of therapists in the United States and the United Kingdom concerning psychotherapy and the recovery of memories of childhood sexual abuse. The findings overall raised concerns about the assumptions held and the suggestive approaches used by some therapists when dealing with recovered memory. For instance, the findings indicated that some practitioners believed that they could identify individuals who had been sexually abused, even when those individuals denied such abuse, and that some practitioners used a range of procedures to encourage patients to recover memories of childhood sexual abuse. Notably, some practitioners saw a very wide range of presenting complaints as being associated with childhood sexual abuse. Most respondents considered that it was important to remember abuse for therapy to be effective, but the vast majority also believed that it was possible to develop illusory memories. It is important to acknowledge that most of the respondents to Poole et al.'s (1995) survey indicated that childhood sexual abuse was relevant to only some of their patients, and there was general concern about the possibility of inadvertently leading patients to create false memories or illusory beliefs about childhood sexual abuse.

Because their members need information and because of their responsibility to patients and society more broadly, various organizations have made formal statements or offered formal guidelines about recovered memories of childhood sexual abuse (e.g., American Medical Association 1994; American Psychiatric Association 1993; American Psychological Association 1994; Australian Psychological Society 1994; British Psychological Society 1995; the "Statement on Memories of Sexual Abuse" by the American Psychiatric Association Board of Trustees [1993] appears in the Foreword to Section II in this volume.) After examination of these statements and guidelines, as well as those offered by individuals (e.g., Bloom 1994; Lindsay and Read 1994; Yapko 1994), the particular points of convergence can be summarized as follows:

- Childhood sexual abuse is an unfortunate reality that sometimes has devastating consequences.
- Memory is potentially unreliable, and people can have memories that are not consistent with historical fact.
- Repression should not be rejected as a possibility, but it cannot be accepted without question.
- The presence of particular problems in adulthood cannot be used as a reliable way of inferring that sexual abuse occurred in childhood.
- Therapists should make sure that in attempting to help their patients, they do not do more harm than good; therapists' responsibilities to their patients are best met through an approach of caution and care about the assumptions that they make and the techniques that they use.
- Recovered memories of childhood sexual abuse may or may not be accurate, and independent corroboration is the only way to determine this.
- Therapists should be mindful that different assumptions, procedures, and demands operate in the clinical and legal contexts; professional and ethical responsibilities are best met by avoiding the excessive encouragement or discouragement of reports of childhood sexual abuse.

Of course, knowing how to work effectively in a setting and climate of ambiguity, uncertainty, and demand from patients is one of the most difficult skills that a therapist has to learn, and a strong argument can be made that specific training is needed to help therapists develop and maintain these skills. Moreover, development of comprehensive manuals for the treatment of those who suspect or recover memories of childhood sexual abuse is necessary, and those treatment manuals must be evidence-based and specify best-practice standards (Beutler and Hill 1992; Lindsay and Read 1994). Consistent with this view, Enns et al. (1995) highlighted the need for competent ethical practice and underscored how competent practice must involve a knowledge of memory research; an understanding of trauma, dissociation, and memory loss; and the development of specific intervention skills and practices. Bowers and Farvolden (1996) offered two essential safeguards for therapy that should be heeded regardless of the problem being treated and the technique being used. First, "Do not define the possibility for healing in terms that require the therapist and the patient to understand the latter's problems in the same way" (p. 373). In other words, convey clearly to patients that although you may have a plausible hypothesis about the reasons for their problems, and the strategies for resolving those problems, the patients do not have to necessarily agree with your view. Equally, therapists should not need to accept the reasons given by patients in order to work in a therapeutically effective way with those patients. Second, "Entertain alternative hypotheses to account for the patient's problems, so as not to fixate on one of them" (Bowers and Farvolden 1996, p. 373). In other words, therapists should consider the various reasons that may account for the problems of patients and should ensure that each of these reasons is given appropriate consideration. Therapists should ensure that their reaction to the essential ambiguity of clinical work is not to adopt a position of ultimately indefensible certainty.

Although many researchers and practitioners are striving to understand the issues involved in memory, trauma, and repression, we have a substantial distance to travel before we can agree on what the relevant data are and how to understand the meaning of those data. When faced with finding our way through the maze surrounding the reporting of recovered memories of childhood sexual abuse, the best approach is one that involves a caring application of scientific knowledge. We need to fill the gaps in our knowledge about the processes involved in the reporting of accurate and inaccurate recovered memories, and particular research is needed to understand more about the encoding, storage, and retrieval of memory of trauma (Wolfe 1995). This research should be conducted in the laboratory and in naturalistic settings, and a balanced analysis of the biological, cognitive, and social processes that are involved in such memory is needed. There are also gaps in our knowledge about therapeutic practices that involve the recovery of memory, and particular research is needed to understand more about the ways in which practices may or may not shape the reported recovered memories of patients. Most basic of all, however, we need to move beyond ideology and belief and determine whether therapy that involves the recovery of memory of childhood sexual abuse is effective in improving the well-being of patients.

After reviewing their survey findings, Poole et al. (1995) derived three major issues that research needs to focus on:

1. Whether memory recovery is helpful for patients
2. Criteria to differentiate patients whose adult problems are based in childhood sexual abuse as opposed to other etiology

3. Particular features and influences of different clinical techniques intended to recover memories of childhood sexual abuse

In focusing more specifically on the hypothesis of repression, Pope and Hudson (1995) drew attention to the need for studies that 1) identify individuals whose sexual abuse had been well documented, 2) identify individuals who had experienced sexual abuse after age 5 years, 3) interview these individuals about any history of trauma, and 4) re-interview those individuals who did not comment on the sexual abuse, and ask them about that abuse. According to Pope and Hudson (1995), this type of rigorous methodology is needed to allow meaningful comment to be made about the existence of repression. The comments provided by many in the field about critical research suggest that we need

- Research that more carefully investigates the differences among the memory reports of patients who do not report, forget normally, and repress memories of particular events of childhood
- Systematic case studies of patients who recover memories of childhood sexual abuse where those memories have been independently determined to be accurate
- Systematic case studies of patients who recover memories of childhood sexual abuse where those memories have been independently determined to be inaccurate
- Research that more carefully investigates the differential effects of therapeutic practices that are used to recover memories of particular events of childhood

Primarily, however, research is needed to address the basic question of whether the recovery of memory of particular events of childhood is of genuine therapeutic benefit. To date, no appropriate large-scale research has investigated this issue. For this—and other—research to be conducted, people must work together rather than in opposition; that is, scientists, practitioners, those reporting recovered memories, and those affected by such reports all have to contribute so that we can gather the necessary data.

Conclusion

In some areas of activity, it is difficult to separate the perspectives of the personal and the professional, and that point has been recognized in this debate. Our personal and professional experiences sometimes shape the way in which we frame questions, interpret responses, and practice therapy. We need to recognize, nevertheless, that therapy with patients who report recovered memories of childhood sexual abuse should proceed with an open attitude, a commitment to evidence-based therapy, and a recognition of the experience of patients in a way that conveys the concern and care that is required when dealing with any reports of childhood sexual abuse.

References

American Medical Association: Report of the Council on Scientific Affairs: Memories of childhood abuse. Chicago, IL, American Medical Association, June 1994

American Psychiatric Association Board of Trustees: Statement on memories of sexual abuse. Washington, DC, American Psychiatric Association, December 1993

American Psychological Association: Interim report of the APA working group on investigation of memory of childhood abuse. Washington, DC, American Psychological Association Public Affairs Office, November 1994

Australian Psychological Society: Guidelines relating to the reporting of recovered memories. Melbourne, VIC, Australian Psychological Society, October 1994

Baars BJ, McGovern K: Steps toward healing: false memories and traumagenic amnesia may coexist in vulnerable populations. Consciousness and Cognition 4:68–74, 1995

Banks WP, Pezdek K: The recovered memory/false memory debate. Consciousness and Cognition 3:265–268, 1994

Barnier AJ, McConkey KM: Reports of real and false memories: the relevance of hypnosis, hypnotizability, and context of memory test. J Abnorm Psychol 101:521–527, 1992

Bartlett FC: Remembering: A Study in Experimental and Social Psychology. Cambridge, MA, Cambridge University Press, 1932

Bass E, Davis L: The Courage to Heal: A Guide for Women Survivors of Child Sexual Abuse, 3rd Edition. New York, HarperPerrenial, 1994

Bekerian DA, Goodrich SJ: Telling the truth in the recovered memory debate. Consciousness and Cognition 4:120–124, 1995

Beutler LE, Hill CE: Process and outcome research in the treatment of adult victims of childhood sexual abuse: methodological issues. J Consult Clin Psychol 60:204–212, 1992

Bloom PB: Clinical guidelines in using hypnosis in uncovering memories of sexual abuse: a master class commentary. Int J Clin Exp Hypn 42:173–178, 1994

Blume ES: Secret Survivors: Uncovering Incest and Its Aftereffects in Women. New York, Wiley, 1990

Bower GH: Awareness, the unconscious, and depression: an experimental psychologist's perspective, in Repression and Dissociation: Implications for Personality Theory, Psychopathology, and Health. Edited by Singer JL. Chicago, IL, University of Chicago Press, 1990, pp 209–231

Bowers KS, Farvolden P: Revisiting a century-old Freudian slip—from suggestion disavowed to the truth repressed. Psychol Bull 119:355–380, 1996

Bremner JD, Krystal JH, Southwick SM, et al: Functional neuroanatomical correlates of the effects of stress on memory. J Trauma Stress 8:527–553, 1995

Brenneis CB: Belief and suggestion in the recovery of memories of childhood sexual abuse. J Am Psychoanal Assoc 42:1027–1053, 1994

Briere J: Child abuse, memory, and recall: a commentary. Consciousness and Cognition 4:83–87, 1995

Briere J, Conte J: Self-reported amnesia for abuse in adults molested as children. J Trauma Stress 6:21–31, 1993

British Psychological Society: Recovered Memories. Leicester, UK, British Psychological Society, January 1995

Brown LS: Toward not forgetting: the science and politics of memory. The Counseling Psychologist 23:310–314, 1995

Bryant RA: Fantasy proneness, reported childhood abuse, and the relevance of reported abuse onset. Int J Clin Exp Hypn 43:184–193, 1995

Byrne P, Sheppard N: Allegations of child sexual abuse: delayed reporting and false memory. Irish Journal of Psychological Medicine 12:103–106, 1995

Ceci SJ, Loftus EF: "Memory work": a royal road to false memories? Applied Cognitive Psychology 8:351–364, 1994

Ceci SJ, Huffmann MLC, Smith E, et al: Repeatedly thinking about a non-event: source misattributions among preschoolers. Consciousness and Cognition 3:388–407, 1994a

Ceci SJ, Loftus EF, Leichtman MD, et al: The possible role of source misattributions in the creation of false beliefs among preschoolers. Int J Clin Exp Hypn 42:304–320, 1994b

Cialdini R: Influence: Science and Practice, 3rd Edition. Glenview, IL, HarperCollins, 1993

Cotton P: Biology enters repressed memory fray. JAMA 272:1725–1726, 1994

Courtois CA: The memory retrieval process in incest survivor therapy. Journal of Child Sexual Abuse 1:15–31, 1992

Courtois CA: Scientist-practitioners and the delayed memory controversy: scientific standards and the need for collaboration. The Counseling Psychologist 23:294–299, 1995

Crews F: The verdict on Freud. Psychological Science 7:63–68, 1996

Davis PJ: Repression and the inaccessibility of emotional memories, in Repression and Dissociation: Implications for Personality Theory, Psychopathology, and Health. Edited by Singer JL. Chicago, IL, University of Chicago Press, 1990, pp 387–403

Dawes RM: House of Cards: Psychology and Psychotherapy Built on Myth. New York, Free Press, 1994

Dershowitz AM: The Abuse Excuse. Boston, MA, Little, Brown, 1994

Dobson M, Markham R: Imagery ability and source monitoring: implications for eyewitness memory. Br J Psychol 32:111–118, 1993

Elliott DM, Briere J: Posttraumatic stress associated with delayed recall of sexual abuse: a general population study. J Trauma Stress 8:629–648, 1995

Enns CZ, McNeilly CL, Corkery JM, et al: The debate about delayed memories of child sexual abuse: a feminist perspective. The Counseling Psychologist 23:181–279, 1995

Erdelyi M: Repression: the mechanism and the defense, in Handbook of Mental Control. Edited by Wegner DM, Pennebaker JW. Englewood Cliffs, NJ, Prentice-Hall, 1993, pp 126–148

Femina DD, Yeager CA, Lewis DO: Child abuse: adolescent records vs adult recall. Child Abuse Negl 14:227–231, 1990

Fisher RP, Geiselman RE: Memory Enhancing Techniques for Investigative Interviewing: The Cognitive Interview. Springfield, IL, Charles C Thomas, 1992

Fivush R: Young children's event recall: are memories constructed through discourse? Consciousness and Cognition 3:356–373, 1994

Fivush R, Schwarzmueller A: Say it once again: effects of repeated questions on children's event recall. J Trauma Stress 8:555–580, 1995

Foa EB, Molnar C, Cashman L: Change in rape narratives during exposure therapy for posttraumatic stress disorder. J Trauma Stress 8:675–690, 1995

Fowler C: A pragmatic approach to early childhood memories: shifting the focus from truth to clinical utility. Psychotherapy 31:676–686, 1994

Frankel FH: The concept of flashbacks in historical perspective. Int J Clin Exp Hypn 42:321–336, 1994

Fredrickson R: Repressed Memories: A Journey to Recovery From Sexual Abuse. New York, Simon & Schuster, 1992

Freyd JJ: Betrayal trauma: traumatic amnesia as an adaptive response to childhood abuse. Ethics and Behavior 4:307–329, 1994

Ganaway GK: Transference and countertransference shaping influences on dissociative syndromes, in Dissociation: Clinical and Theoretical Implications. Edited by Lynn SJ, Rhue JW. New York, Guilford, 1994, pp 317–337

Ganaway GK: Hypnosis, childhood trauma, and dissociative identity disorder: toward an integrative theory. Int J Clin Exp Hypn 4:127–144, 1995

Garry M, Loftus EF: Pseudomemories without hypnosis. Int J Clin Exp Hypn 42:363–378, 1994

Garry M, Loftus EF, Brown SW: Memory: a river runs through it. Consciousness and Cognition 3:438–451, 1994

Goldstein E: Confabulations: Creating False Memories—Destroying Families. Boca Raton, FL, SIRS Books, 1992

Goldstein E, Farmer K: True Stories of False Memories. Boca Raton, FL, Upton Books, 1993

Goodman GS, Quas JA, Batterman Faunce JM, et al: Predictors of accurate and inaccurate memories of traumatic events experienced in childhood. Consciousness and Cognition 3:269–294, 1994

Green BL: Introduction to special issue on traumatic memory research. J Trauma Stress 8:501–504, 1995

Grossman LR, Pressley M: Introduction to the special issue on recovery of memories of childhood sexual abuse. Applied Cognitive Psychology 8:277–280, 1994

Haakrn J: The debate over recovered memory of sexual abuse: a feminist-psychoanalytic perspective. Psychiatry: Interpersonal and Biological Processes 58:189–198, 1995

Harvey MR, Herman JL: Amnesia, partial amnesia, and delayed recall among adult survivors of childhood trauma. Consciousness and Cognition 3:295–306, 1994

Herman J: Trauma and Recovery. New York, Basic Books, 1992

Herman JL: Crime and memory. Bull Am Acad Psychiatry Law 23:5–17, 1995

Herman J, Schatzow E: Recovery and verification of memories of childhood sexual trauma. Psychoanalytic Psychology 4:1–14, 1987

Holmes DS: Investigations of repression: differential recall of material experimentally or naturally associated with ego threat. Psychol Bull 81:632–653, 1974

Holmes D: The evidence for repression: an examination of sixty years of research, in Repression and Dissociation: Implications for Personality Theory, Psychopathology, and Health. Edited by Singer JL. Chicago, IL, University of Chicago Press, 1990, pp 85–102

Howe ML, Courage ML, Peterson C: How can I remember if "I" wasn't there: long-term retention of traumatic experiences and emergence of the cognitive self. Consciousness and Cognition 3:327–355, 1994

Hughes R: Culture of Complaint: The Fraying of America. New York, Oxford University Press, 1993

Hyman IE, Husband TH, Billings FJ: False memories of childhood experiences. Applied Cognitive Psychology 9:181–197, 1995

Johnson MK, Raye CL: Reality monitoring. Psychol Rev 88:67–85, 1981

Johnson MK, Hashtroudi S, Lindsay DS: Source monitoring. Psychol Bull 114:3–28, 1993

Kaminer W: I'm Dysfunctional, You're Dysfunctional: The Recovery Movement and Other Self-Help Fashions. New York, Vintage Books, 1993

Kendall-Tackett KA, Williams LM, Finkelhor D: Impact of sexual abuse on children: a review and synthesis of recent empirical studies. Psychol Bull 113:164–180, 1993

Kihlstrom JF: Hypnosis, delayed recall, and the principles of memory. Int J Clin Exp Hypn 42:337–345, 1994

Kihlstrom JF: The trauma-memory argument. Consciousness and Cognition 4:63–67, 1995

Kihlstrom JF, Barnhardt TM: The self-regulation of memory: for better and for worse, with and without hypnosis, in Handbook of Mental Control. Edited by Wegner DM, Pennebaker JW. Englewood Cliffs, NJ, Prentice-Hall, 1993, pp 88–125

Krass J, Kinoshita S, McConkey KM: Hypnotic memory and confident reporting. Applied Cognitive Psychology 2:35–51, 1988

Kuyken W, Brewin CR: Autobiographical memory functioning in depression and reports of early abuse. J Abnorm Psychol 104:585–591, 1995

LeDoux JE: Systems and synapses of emotional memory, in Memory: Organization and Locus of Change. Edited by Squire LR, Weinberger NM, Lynch G, et al. New York, Oxford University Press, 1991, pp 205–216

LeDoux JE, Romanski L, Zagoraris A: Indelibility of subcortical memories. J Cognitive Neuroscience 1:238–243, 1989

Levitt EE, Pinnell CM: Some additional light on the childhood sexual abuse–psychopathology axis. Int J Clin Exp Hypn 43:145–162, 1995

Lindsay DS: Contextualizing and clarifying criticisms of memory work in psychotherapy. Consciousness and Cognition 3:426–437, 1994

Lindsay DS: Beyond backlash: Comments on Enns, McNeilly, Corkery, and Gilbert. The Counseling Psychologist 23:280–289, 1995

Lindsay DS, Read JD: Psychotherapy and memories of childhood sexual abuse: a cognitive perspective. Applied Cognitive Psychology 8:281–338, 1994

Loftus EF: The reality of repressed memories. Am Psychol 48:518–537, 1993

Loftus EF, Ketcham K: The Myth of Repressed Memory: False Memories and Allegations of Sexual Abuse. New York, St Martin's Press, 1994

Loftus EF, Garry M, Feldman J: Forgetting sexual trauma: what does it mean when 38% forget? J Consult Clin Psychol 62:1177–1181, 1994a

Loftus EF, Polonsky S, Fullilove MT: Memories of childhood sexual abuse: remembering and repressing. Psychology of Women Quarterly 18:67–84, 1994b

Loftus EF, Milo EM, Paddock JR: The accidental executioner: why psychotherapy must be informed by science. The Counseling Psychologist 23:300–309, 1995

Lynn SJ, Nash MR: Truth in memory: ramifications for psychotherapy and hypnotherapy. Am J Clin Hypn 36:194–208, 1994

Lynn SJ, Rhue J: Fantasy-proneness: hypnosis, developmental antecedents, and psychopathology. Am Psychol 43:35–44, 1988

Lynn SJ, Rhue J (eds): Dissociation: Clinical and Theoretical Perspectives. New York, Guilford, 1994

Lynn SJ, Myers B, Sivec H: Psychotherapists beliefs, repressed memories of abuse, and hypnosis: what have we really learned? Am J Clin Hypn 36:182–184, 1994

MacLean HN: Once Upon a Time: A True Story of Memory, Murder, and the Law. New York, HarperCollins, 1993

Macmillan M: Freud Evaluated: The Completed Arc. Amsterdam, North-Holland, 1991

Markham R, Hynes L: The effect of vividness of imagery on reality monitoring. Journal of Mental Imagery 17:159–170, 1993

McConkey KM: The effects of hypnotic procedures on remembering: the experimental findings and their implications for forensic hypnosis, in Contemporary Hypnosis Research. Edited by Fromm E, Nash MR. New York, Guilford, 1992, pp 405–426

McConkey KM: Hypnosis, memory, and the ethics of uncertainty. Australian Psychologist 30:1–10, 1995

McConkey KM, Sheehan PW: Hypnosis, Memory, and Behavior in Criminal Investigation. New York, Guilford, 1995

McElroy SL, Keck PE: Misattribution of eating and obsessive-compulsive disorder symptoms to repressed memories of childhood sexual or physical abuse. Biol Psychiatry 37:48–51, 1995

Nachmani G: Trauma and ignorance. Contemporary Psychoanalysis 31:423–450, 1995

Nash MR: Memory distortion and sexual trauma: the problem of false negatives and false positives. Int J Clin Exp Hypn 42:346–362, 1994

Nash MR, Hulsey TL, Sexton MC, et al: Long-term sequelae of childhood sexual abuse: perceived family environment, psychopathology, and dissociation. J Consult Clin Psychol 61:276–283, 1993

Neisser U, Fivush R: The Remembering Self. Cambridge, MA, Cambridge University Press, 1994

Nemiah JC: The unconscious and psychopathology, in The Unconscious Reconsidered. Edited by Bowers KS, Meichenbaum D. New York, Wiley, 1984, pp 49–87

Nogrady H, McConkey KM, Perry C: Enhancing visual memory: trying hypnosis, trying imagination, and trying again. J Abnorm Psychol 94:195–204, 1985

Ofshe RJ, Singer MT: Recovered-memory therapy and robust repression: influence and pseudomemories. Int J Clin Exp Hypn 42:391–410, 1994

Ofshe RJ, Watters E: Making Monsters: False Memories, Psychotherapy, and Sexual Hysteria. New York, Charles Scribner's Sons, 1994

Olio KA: Memory retrieval in the treatment of adult survivors of sexual abuse. Transactional Analysis Journal 19:93–100, 1989

Ornstein PA: Children's long-term retention of salient personal experiences. J Trauma Stress 8:581–605, 1995

Pendergrast MH: Victims of Memory: Incest Accusations and Shattered Lives. Hinesburg, VT, Upper Access Books, 1994

Pennebaker JW, Memon A: Recovered memories in context: thoughts and elaborations on Bowers and Farvolden. Psychol Bull 119:381–385, 1996

Person ES, Klar H: Establishing trauma: the difficulty distinguishing between memories and fantasies. J Am Psychoanal Assoc 42:1055–1081, 1994

Pezdek K: The illusion of illusory memories. Applied Cognitive Psychology 8:339–350, 1994

Poole DA, Lindsay DS, Memon A, et al: Psychotherapy and the recovery of memories of childhood sexual abuse: U.S. and British practitioners' opinions, practices, and experiences. J Consult Clin Psychol 63:426–437, 1995

Pope HG, Hudson JI: Can memories of childhood sexual abuse be repressed? Psychol Med 25:121–126, 1995

Read JD, Lindsay DS: Moving toward a middle ground on the false memory debate: reply to commentaries on Lindsay and Read. Applied Cognitive Psychology 8:407–435, 1994

Roesler TA, McKenzie N: Effects of childhood trauma on psychological functioning in adults sexually abused as children. J Nerv Ment Dis 182:145–150, 1994

Romans SE, Martin JC, Anderson JC, et al: Factors that mediate between child sexual abuse and adult psychological outcome. Psychol Med 25:127–142, 1995

Sarbin TR: A narrative approach to "repressed memories." Journal of Narrative and Life History 5:51–66, 1995

Saywitz KJ, Moan-Hardie S: Reducing the potential for distortion of childhood memories. Consciousness and Cognition 3:408–425, 1994

Schachter DL, Kagan J, Leichtman MD: True and false memories in children and adults: a cognitive neuroscience perspective. Psychology, Public Policy, and Law 1:411–428, 1995

Schooler JW: Seeking the core: the issues and evidence surrounding recovered accounts of sexual trauma. Consciousness and Cognition 3:452–469, 1994

Schulte JG, Dinwiddie SH, Pribor EF, et al: Psychiatric diagnoses of adult male victims of childhood sexual abuse. J Nerv Ment Dis 183:111–113, 1995

Schutte JW: Repressed memory lawsuits: potential verdict predictors. Behavioral Sciences and the Law 12:409–416, 1994

Singer JL (ed): Repression and Dissociation: Implications for Personality Theory, Psychopathology, and Health. Chicago, IL, University of Chicago Press, 1990

Spence DP: Narrative Truth and Historical Truth. New York, WW Norton, 1982

Spence DP: Narrative truth and putative child abuse. Int J Clin Exp Hypn 42:289–303, 1994

Spiegel D (ed): Dissociation: Culture, Mind and Body. Washington, DC, American Psychiatric Press, 1994

Spiegel D, Scheflin AW: Dissociated or fabricated? Psychiatric aspects of repressed memory in criminal and civil cases. Int J Clin Exp Hypn 42:411–432, 1994

Sykes CJ: A Nation of Victims: The Decay of the American Character. New York, St Martin's Press, 1992

Terr L: Unchained Memories: True Stories of Traumatic Memories, Lost and Found. New York, Basic Books, 1994

Tromp S, Koss MP, Figueredo AJ, et al: Are rape memories different? A comparison of rape, other unpleasant, and pleasant memories among employed women. J Trauma Stress 8:607–627, 1995

van der Kolk BA: The body keeps the score: memory and the evolving psychobiology of posttraumatic stress. Harvard Review of Psychiatry 1:253–265, 1994

van der Kolk BA, Fisler R: Dissociation and the fragmentary nature of traumatic memories: overview and exploratory study. J Trauma Stress 8:505–525, 1995 van der Kolk BA, Saporta J: The biological response to psychic trauma: mechanisms and treatment of intrusion and numbing. Anxiety Research 4:199–212, 1991

Walker EA, Gelfand AN, Gelfand MD, et al: Medical and psychiatric symptoms in female gastroenterology clinic patients with histories of sexual victimization. Gen Hosp Psychiatry 17:85–92, 1995

Weinberger DA: The construct validity of the repressive coping style, in Repression and Dissociation: Implications for Personality Theory, Psychopathology, and Health. Edited by Singer JL. Chicago, IL, University of Chicago Press, 1990, pp 337–386

Weingardt KW, Loftus EF, Lindsay DS: Misinformation revisited. Memory and Cognition 23:72–82, 1995

Williams LM: Recall of childhood trauma: a prospective study of women's memories of child sexual abuse. J Consult Clin Psychol 62:1167–1176, 1994

Williams LM: Recovered memories of abuse in women with documented child sexual victimization histories. J Trauma Stress 8:649–674, 1995

Wolfe J: Trauma, traumatic memory, and research: where do we go from here? J Trauma Stress 8:717–725, 1995

Wright L: Remembering Satan. New York, Knopf, 1994

Yapko MD: Suggestions of Abuse: True and False Memories of Childhood Sexual Trauma. New York, Simon & Schuster, 1994

Chapter 8

Intentional Forgetting and Voluntary Thought Suppression: Two Potential Methods for Coping With Childhood Trauma

Wilma Koutstaal, Ph.D., and Daniel L. Schacter, Ph.D.

> My strongest asset through all my experiences was my ability to "block out" whatever I didn't want to remember. If I didn't talk about them, or even think about them, I was able to survive.
>
> *Anonymous incest victim (Silver et al. 1983, p. 97)*

Extreme trauma often evokes equally extreme responses. In the effort to cope, and faced with a life-threatening or world-view shattering traumatic event, an individual may find herself or himself vulnerable to radical alterations in cognitive, emotional, and neurophysiological responses. Posttraumatic stress disorder (PTSD) (e.g., Krystal et al. 1995), psychogenic amnesia (e.g., Schacter et al. 1982), fugue states (e.g., Eisen 1989), and dissociative identity disorder (e.g., Putnam 1993; Schacter et al. 1989) are among such responses. Yet not all individuals respond to trauma with such "extreme" coping mechanisms, nor are all sources of trauma immediately and consistently identified as such. Some forms of trauma, including childhood sexual abuse, may assume a more chronic, ambiguous, and intermittent course, interspersed with periods of comparative normality (see Conte et al. 1989; Trickett and Putnam 1993). What forms of coping might a child attempt to draw on in dealing with such abuse? If abuse is (for the moment) not occurring, and the individual is "expected" to continue with social, familial, and other roles and responsibilities as if nothing had happened, how might the individual attempt to manage thoughts and memory of the abuse?

In this chapter, we specifically focus on two less extreme responses—intentional forgetting and voluntary thought suppression—that represent more commonplace, but potentially important, possible responses to abuse. Although clear evidence supports the role of pro-

Preparation of this chapter was supported by National Institute on Aging Grant AG08441.

cesses similar to intentional forgetting and thought suppression in cases of both childhood sexual abuse and adult trauma (and we begin by reviewing some of this evidence), we also attempt to address a further question. What evidence is available from empirical laboratory research that would help us determine when such strategies might or might not prove successful?

We do not assume that intentional forgetting and thought suppression are the only, or even the most important, methods used in coping with sexual abuse or other forms of trauma (although this may be true for some individuals). Equally important, we do not assume that there is evidence for a form of massive and unconscious repression of trauma, in which individuals allegedly become entirely amnesic for repeated or prolonged periods of severe abuse. There is little evidence for such massive repression (see Holmes 1990; Loftus 1993; Ofshe and Singer 1994; Pope and Hudson 1995), and instances of broadly encompassing amnesia may be more likely to involve dissociative pathology than unconscious "repression" (for discussion, see Schacter 1996; Schacter et al., in press; Spiegel 1995). Rather, we are specifically concerned with deliberate and *conscious* efforts at curtailing one's thoughts and memories. We ask: 1) Is there evidence or reason to believe that intentional forgetting and thought suppression are sometimes used (either alone or as a supplement to other methods) in coping with sexual abuse or other forms of trauma? and 2) What does research from laboratory paradigms reveal about the probable effects of these methods on later thinking and memory?

This chapter has four major sections. We begin by briefly reviewing several sources of evidence suggesting that intentional and conscious efforts to suppress one's thoughts and memory of traumatic experiences are, indeed, sometimes used by individuals in attempting to cope with the trauma. In the main part of this chapter, we focus on the empirical literature regarding directed forgetting and thought suppression. In these sections, we assess evidence of the degree to which, and the conditions under which, intentional forgetting and voluntary thought suppression can produce their intended effects. We also provide an assessment of the processes believed to underlie successful intentional forgetting and thought suppression. In the final section, we attempt briefly to interrelate key findings from these two paradigms with clinical and other reports of trauma and suggest several questions that future research should examine.

Evidence Regarding Conscious Efforts to Suppress or to Forget Trauma

Evidence from several sources converges in suggesting that traumatic events—including childhood sexual abuse—may sometimes be followed by deliberate and conscious efforts to suppress thoughts and memories of the abuse. Three general sources of evidence supporting such efforts include

1. Retrospective self-reports obtained during interviews or from questionnaires asking how individuals responded to childhood abuse or other forms of trauma
2. Observations reported by others after a traumatic event, indicating that traumatized individuals sought to avoid reminders or thoughts of the incident or actively denied that it had occurred
3. General background information about the conditions often surrounding revelations of childhood abuse

Excerpts from follow-up interviews recently reported by L. M. Williams (1995) with women who had a documented history of sexual abuse during childhood clearly implicate deliberate and intentional efforts not to think about the abuse as a potential contributor to poor recall of some abuse episodes. In an earlier study, L. M. Williams (1994) found that of 129 women with a documented incident of abuse in childhood, 62% recalled the particular abuse episode that had occurred some 17 years earlier, which had resulted in their being brought to the attention of the investigators. However, additional questioning of these women revealed that not all of them had always remembered the abuse. Of the 75 women who recalled the abuse and who were also asked additional questions, 12 women (16%) reported that there was a time in their past when they had forgotten the abuse—in some cases, after a deliberate and purposeful effort to do so. One woman said, "I blocked it out right away, the first time it happened (age 12). . . . I didn't remember until it happened again—I was raped when I was 17" (p. 663). Two other women used the identical expression of "blocking it out" and further noted how, after a time, they specifically stopped thinking of the abuse: "I don't know how old I was, I used to think about it for the first two years, then I just blocked it out. I may not have completely forgot, I just didn't think about it" (p. 663); "Well I guess I may not have *completely* forgotten about it after my mother talked to me, but blocked it out most of the time, just stopped thinking about it" (p. 666).

These responses are remarkably similar to the efforts at suppression reported by adult rape victims (Burgess and Holmstrom 1979). Some adult victims reported that they attempted to dispel all memory of the rape from their minds through a deliberate and conscious effort. They did not like to be reminded of the rape ("Don't refresh my mind to it") and spoke of being able to "block the thoughts" from their minds (Burgess and Holmstrom 1979, p. 1280). These responses are also similar to that of one woman, anonymously questioned by Silver et al. (1983), about how she had coped with father-daughter incest that had occurred years earlier and who wrote: "My strongest asset through all my experiences was my ability to 'block out' whatever I didn't want to remember. If I didn't talk about them, or even think about them, I was able to survive" (p. 97).

There is also at least some evidence of denial of traumatic events during childhood, soon after those events occurred. For example, in their study of children's memory for an invasive and painful medical procedure (involving urinary tract catheterization), Goodman et al. (1994, p. 288) reported that "a few" of the children from a sample of 46 denied that they had ever undergone the procedure. Likewise, a recently reported and corroborated case of recovered memory for an incident of childhood sexual abuse (Nash 1994) indicated at least *behavioral* denial of the event directly after it occurred.

Children may also actively avoid reminders associated with other forms of trauma. For example, Nader et al. (1990) found that 14 months after a sniper attack on a school playground, of all the children—including those who were on the playground, in the school, or away from the school on that day—66% reported avoidance of reminders of the attack. Of those who were on the playground itself during the attack, nearly 90% still reported avoidance of reminders. In the entire group, avoidance of reminders was the most common symptom still present at 14 months, and the next two most frequently occurring symptoms were fear when thinking of the event (48% of the entire group) and becoming upset by thoughts of the event (47%).

The need or desire to keep abuse secret, either absolutely, so that no one is ever told of the abuse, or selectively, so that only a few trusted others learn of it, may also encourage deliberate efforts at thought suppression and avoidance of reminders that might prompt memories and thoughts of the abuse (see Lane and Wegner 1995). In a national survey of childhood sexual abuse in adult men and women, Finkelhor et al. (1990) found that fewer than 50% of the men and women reporting abuse also reported that they had told anyone about it within a year of its occurrence. Of 169 men who reported a childhood sexual abuse experience, 42% reported that they had never told anyone of the abuse; likewise, of 416 women reporting abuse, 33% indicated that they had never told anyone.

In some cases of childhood abuse, the perpetrator or others who learn of the abuse may actively encourage thought suppression or forgetting by urging secrecy, telling the child that the event never happened, or refusing to discuss the incident (e.g., Adams-Tucker 1982; Browne and Finkelhor 1986; Everson et al. 1989). For example, researchers who have sought to determine the degree of maternal support offered to sexually abused children in clinical samples have found that relatively few mothers are supportive, with the proportion of mothers deemed supportive ranging between 25% and 56% (e.g., Adams-

Tucker 1982; Everson et al. 1989). In a sample of 84 mothers of children with substantiated occurrences of intrafamilial sexual abuse, Everson et al. (1989) found that only 44% of the mothers provided consistent support during the period following disclosure of the abuse (e.g., made clear and public statements of belief in their child, or actively demonstrated disapproval of the perpetrator's abusive behavior). An additional 32% provided ambivalent or inconsistent support (e.g., wavered in believing the child, or remained passive, refusing to take sides), and 24% were unsupportive or rejecting of their children (e.g., were threatening or hostile, or totally denied that the abuse occurred).

Based on questionnaire results anonymously asking a large (non-clinical) sample of women how they had attempted to make sense of their earlier experiences of father-daughter incest, Silver et al. (1983, p. 97) concluded that "the ability to block or interrupt thoughts of a negative event may be crucial in living with events that have, in fact, no resolution." Based on her interviews with women with documented instances of abuse, L. M. Williams (1995, p. 668) concluded that "forgetting about the child sexual abuse is for some a motivated, volitional forgetting (in a conscious attempt to deal with the abuse by blocking it out)."

Deliberate and conscious efforts to minimize thinking about an abusive episode or to purposefully block it from awareness may—at least in some instances—provide an immediate means of coping with the abuse. Do such efforts also reduce the ease and likelihood that the abuse will be remembered?

Evidence accumulated across decades of experimental research on memory has shown that the more a stimulus or event is cognitively elaborated on and interassociated with other aspects of one's knowledge, the more likely it is that the stimulus or event will be remembered (e.g., Craik and Tulving 1975; Fivush and Schwarzmueller 1995; Tessler and Nelson 1994; for review, see Schacter 1996). Research on the degree to which individuals can forget when instructed or "directed" to do so points to a similar conclusion. However, research on directed forgetting has also emphasized other factors that may—sometimes quite substantially—alter the likelihood and ease with which events will be accessed. Prominent among these factors are aspects of the *retrieval environment* in which memory is probed, including both the degree to which item-specific cues are present (i.e., features or aspects similar to the to-be-remembered event or stimulus itself) and the degree to which the more general environmental and cognitive context of the individual corresponds to that present during the initial encounter with the material (for review and discussion, see Davies and Thomson 1988; Koutstaal and Schacter, in press). Intriguingly, the physical and mental circumstances present during an individual's efforts to suppress a particular thought have also emerged as prominent considerations in the experimental work on voluntary thought suppression, influencing the likelihood that suppression will be successful or will lead to the exact *opposite* of the hoped-for result: greater rather than diminished preoccupation with the unwanted thought.

We next review findings from these two laboratory paradigms. In each case, we first examine basic outcome data on the degree to which the intended outcome (forgetting or reduced frequency of the unwanted thought) can be achieved and then consider possible mechanisms underlying those effects. We examine experiments using both emotionally neutral and emotionally significant materials; in addition, in the case of directed forgetting, we also briefly consider studies that investigated whether children can intentionally forget.

Intentional Forgetting

Can Adults Intentionally Forget Emotionally Neutral Materials?

Clear and consistent experimental evidence indicates that instructing an individual to forget something can subsequently result in diminished memory for that material compared with memory for information that was never subjected to an intention to forget (for reviews, see Bjork 1989; H. M. Johnson 1994). However, whether intentional forgetting will be successful depends on a variety of factors relating both to the conditions present during the encoding of the to-be-forgotten information and to the conditions under which retrieval is attempted.

One factor that has emerged as particularly important in determining the extent to which memory for the to-be-forgotten items is, indeed, impaired relative to memory for items that were designated as to-be-remembered concerns the manner in which the instruction to forget is given. Two methods of providing the instruction to forget have been most frequently explored by cognitive researchers in recent years. In one method, individuals are first presented an entire set or block of items under intentional learning conditions. They are then unexpectedly told that this information should be forgotten—usually under the guise that the first block of items were "practice" items. In this method—hereafter referred to as the "block-cuing" directed forgetting procedure—the instruction to forget is given only after subjects have already encountered and actively attempted to remember many stimuli. In contrast, in a second method, individuals are told at the outset that the experiment is concerned with how well people can selectively remember some information while forgetting other information. In this method—hereafter referred to as the "item-cuing" directed forgetting procedure—each stimulus item is designated either as to-be-remembered or as to-be-forgotten soon after it is presented (usually within a few seconds).

The second of these methods, in which some of the stimulus items are cued as to-be-forgotten soon after they are encountered, generally results in more forgetting than in the first method, in which the instruction to forget is postponed until after a larger set of items has been presented. Table 8–1 presents a comparison of the amount of forgetting observed on free- or cued-recall tests with the item-cuing versus block-cuing procedure. Results are shown for eight experiments or experimental conditions in which both of these cuing procedures were used within the same experimental design (Basden et al. 1993a, 1994; Koutstaal 1996). As can be seen in Table 8–1, both procedures resulted in greater recall of the remember-cued than the forget-cued items. However, the differences were consistently larger in the item-cuing than in the block-cuing procedure, resulting in an average difference of 27% for the item-cuing (range, 14%–45%) compared with only 12% for the block-cuing method (range, 6%–21%).

With the item-cuing procedure, forgetting is also generally found during recognition testing (e.g., Bjork and Geiselman 1978; Golding et al. 1994). In contrast, the strong retrieval cues provided by the recognition test items usually eliminate the disadvantage for the forget-cued

Table 8–1. Magnitude of directed forgetting on recall tests under item cuing and block cuing

Experiment and type of test	Item cuing			Block cuing		
	Rem	For	Diff	Rem	For	Diff
Basden et al. (1993a)						
Expt. 1 cued recall	.35	.14	.21	.33	.24	.09
Expt. 2 cued recall	.82	.59	.23	.74	.65	.09
Expt. 3 free recall	.50	.05	.45	.41	.20	.21
Expt. 4 free recall, short list	.25	.11	.14	.33	.22	.11
Expt. 4 free recall, long list	.23	.08	.15	.19	.10	.09
Basden et al. (1994)						
Expt. 1 free recall	.53	.12	.41	.44	.24	.20
Koutstaal (1996)						
Expt. 4 free recall	.37	.12	.25	.35	.24	.11
Expt. 5 free recall	.42	.07	.35	.34	.28	.06
Average directed forgetting effect			.27			.12

Note. All results are for the first test administered only.
Rem = remember cued; For = forget cued; Diff = difference in remember-cued and forget-cued performance (Rem − For).

items under block cuing (e.g., Basden et al. 1993a, 1994; Geiselman et al. 1983; Koutstaal 1996, Experiments 3 and 4). Table 8–2 presents the outcome of 12 experiments that used the item-cuing method, in which subjects were tested by using recognition, and in which recognition was the first test administered. In these experiments, the average directed forgetting effect was 18% (range, 7%–35%). In contrast, a set of 8 experiments that used the block-cuing method yielded an average directed forgetting effect of only 2% (range, −2%–9%).

Do these differences in memory performance for the to-be-remembered versus the to-be-forgotten items arise from *impaired* memory for the *forget-cued* items? Or do they primarily reflect *enhanced* memory for the *remember-cued* items? As will be seen, comparisons of the data provided in Tables 8–1 and 8–2 as well as other sources of evidence suggest that the answer to this question depends on the method that is em-

Table 8–2. Magnitude of directed forgetting on recognition tests under item cuing and block cuing

Experiment and condition	Item cuing			Block cuing		
	Rem	For	Diff	Rem	For	Diff
Basden et al. (1993a)						
Expt. 1	.88	.77	.11	.92	.89	.03
Expt. 2	.92	.77	.15	.90	.89	.01
Expt. 4, short list	.81	.67	.14	.86	.88	−.02
Expt. 4, long list	.75	.59	.16	.76	.74	.02
Basden et al. (1994)						
Expt. 1	.86	.67	.19	.89	.83	.06
Koutstaal (1996)						
Expt. 1	.86	.67	.19	—	—	—
Expt. 2	.94	.87	.07	—	—	—
Expt. 3	—	—	—	.98	.97	.01
Expt. 4	.89	.70	.19	.85	.86	−.01
Expt. 5	.93	.58	.35	.87	.78	.09
Gardiner et al. (1994)						
Short cue delay	.68	.43	.25	—	—	—
Long cue delay	.67	.55	.12	—	—	—
MacLeod (1989)						
Expt. 1, immediate test	.76	.55	.21	—	—	—
Average directed forgetting effect			.18			.02

Note. All results are for the first test administered only. Dashes indicate that the relevant procedure (item cuing or block cuing) was not included in a particular experiment and condition.
Rem = remember cued; For = forget cued; Diff = difference in remember-cued and forget-cued performance (Rem − For).

ployed. Whereas the differences found in the item-cuing procedure may primarily result from preferentially thinking about and elaborating on the remember-cued items, this account does not seem to apply as well to the forgetting observed in the block-cuing procedure. With block cuing, the to-be-forgotten items may be less readily retrieved from memory *despite* having been initially processed and encoded to the same degree as the to-be-remembered items. However, further discussion of the possible processes underlying directed forgetting will be postponed until evidence regarding forgetting of emotionally significant materials and directed forgetting in children has been examined. At this point, however, we can draw five conclusions from the above discussion and from the data provided in Tables 8–1 and 8–2 concerning the forgetting of emotionally neutral material:

1. There is clear evidence that the intention to forget certain experimentally presented materials can lead to reduced memory performance for those items compared with stimuli that were not subjected to an intention to forget.

2. Under conditions of relatively little retrieval support (such as during free-recall or cued-recall testing), the decrease in memory for the forget-cued items has been observed both when individual items are cued as to-be-forgotten soon after their presentation (item cuing) and when the instruction to forget is given only after several stimuli have already been actively processed (block cuing).

3. Under conditions of greater retrieval support (such as recognition testing), the decrease in memory for the forget-cued items has most often been seen only under item cuing and not with block cuing.

4. Despite the presence of sometimes quite substantial differences in memory performance for the to-be-remembered and to-be-forgotten items, *some* of the to-be-forgotten items are still recalled and recognized. For example, the average level of recall for the forget-cued items in Table 8–1 was 16% under item cuing and 27% under block cuing; likewise, the average level of recognition for the forget-cued items in Table 8–2 was 65% under item cuing. Thus, directed forgetting seems to involve a relative rather than absolute phenomenon.

5. The directed forgetting effects obtained with item cuing tend to be greater than those found with block cuing and are also greater under free- or cued-recall test conditions than under recognition testing. The latter observation is important because it partially addresses the concern that directed forgetting effects are simply due to voluntary response withholding—that is, a failure to report information about the to-be-forgotten items even though that information is, in fact, remembered. If individuals were merely fail-

ing to report the to-be-forgotten items, it is not clear why they would more often fail to report that information during one testing situation (e.g., under recall testing) than another (e.g., recognition testing; see, for example, Brandt et al. 1985; Spanos et al. 1990; Williamsen et al. 1965; see also Schacter 1986).

Can Adults Intentionally Forget Emotional or Traumatic Stimuli?

The findings concerning intentional forgetting of emotional materials are somewhat mixed but, on the whole, indicate that forgetting can also occur for emotionally significant materials, at least under some circumstances. Two studies have specifically reported failures to forget emotionally negative materials or a failure to forget either emotionally negative or emotionally positive materials. In one study (Geiselman and Panting 1985, Experiment 2), undergraduate students were presented a list of words, one-half of which were judged to be positive in meaning (e.g., clown, butterfly, love) and one-half of which were judged to be negative in meaning (e.g., garbage, disease, dirt). The item-cuing method was used, with the positive and negative words presented in intermixed fashion for 3 seconds each, and immediately followed by an instruction either to remember or to forget (also for 3 seconds). Analyses of subjects' free-recall responses revealed a significant interaction of cue type with word affect, indicating that for the remember-cued items, positive words were significantly more likely to be recalled (mean, 64%) than negative words (mean, 43%), but the reverse was true for the forget-cued items; when given an instruction to forget, negative words were significantly more likely to be recalled (mean, 31%) than were positive words (mean, 16%).

More recently, Ochsner and Schacter (unpublished observations, February 1996) used a modified block-cuing procedure to determine whether recollection of emotionally charged photographs could be affected by intentional forgetting. Subjects were instructed to either remember or forget six-item blocks of photographs that depicted scenes and objects with neutral emotional content (e.g., a rolling pin or an office scene), positive content (e.g., a happy family), or negative content (e.g., a mutilated limb). All items in a given block were of the same emotional valence. On a subsequent recognition test, when subjects indicated that an item was old (i.e., was previously presented in the experiment), they were asked to indicate whether they could also "recollect" particular details regarding the photograph's prior occurrence, such as its appearance or their reaction to it, or whether they simply "knew" that the item had been previously presented, without being able to recollect any specific episodic details about it. (For a general review of this procedure, known as the *remember/know* distinction but here referred to as *recollect/know* so as to avoid confusion with the instruction cue, which is also designated as *remember,* see Gardiner and Java 1993.) The key finding was that directed forgetting affected only memory for neutral items. In general, negative photographs produced the most, and neutral photographs the fewest, recollections, but when subjects were instructed to forget, recollections of negative and positive items were unchanged, whereas recollections of neutral items were reduced by 40%.

This study suggests that, under certain conditions, both positive and negative emotional information may be resistant to conscious attempts to forget. However, three other studies have yielded either more mixed conclusions or evidence of successful forgetting of emotionally significant materials. Using the block-cued directed forgetting procedure, Myers et al. (1992) found no effect of emotional valence on the recall of words. In this study, a manipulation of the valence of the words (positive, negative, or neutral) was combined with another individual differences factor. The subjects (female undergraduate students) were classified on the basis of their performance on the Marlowe-Crowne Social Desirability Scale (Crowne and Marlowe 1964) and the short version of the Taylor Manifest Anxiety Scale (Taylor 1953) into four groups: 1) repressors (high defensiveness and low anxiety, $n = 15$), 2) low anxious (low defensiveness and low anxiety, $n = 15$), 3) high anxious (low defensiveness and high anxiety, $n = 12$), and 4) defensive high anxious (high defensiveness and high anxiety, $n = 12$) (for the original development of this classification scheme, see Weinberger et al. 1979). Two blocks of items, each composed of six positive, six negative, and six neutral words, were presented. Subjects were required to rate each of the words for pleasantness and then were told, after the first block, that those items were for practice and could be forgotten. Averaging across the groups, there was significant directed forgetting (average recall of to-be-remembered items, 32%; average recall of to-be-forgotten items, 19%). However, there was no interaction of group with instruction cue, indicating that the magnitude of the directed forgetting effect was similar for all four subject groups. Also, although there were too few observations for the differently valenced words to be analyzed separately, examination of the mean number of to-be-forgotten words that were recalled showed no evidence that negative words were either more or less likely to be forgotten than positive or neutral words (average recall of to-be-forgotten negative, positive, and neutral words of 9%, 7%, and 3%, respectively; average recall of to-be-remembered negative, positive, and neutral words of 11%, 13%, and 8%, respectively).

Using a quite different procedure, in which individuals were administered shocks for retrieving to-be-forgotten items, Weiner (1968, Experiments 6, 7, and 8) found that individuals were modestly but significantly less likely to retrieve information when they knew they would be shocked for doing so (average recall across three experiments, 55%) than when no shock would follow on retrieval (average recall, 60%). Although the investigators attempted to ensure that these differences were not simply due to voluntary response withholding, this alternative cannot be definitively ruled out.

The most directly relevant study to address the issue of directed forgetting and trauma arising from childhood sexual abuse is that of McNally et al. (unpublished observations, February 1996). These investigators used the item-cuing procedure to examine the extent to which women who had been sexually abused as children could selectively remember or forget trauma-related words (e.g., molested, scream), positive words (e.g., healthy, secure), and neutral words (e.g., curtain, desk). Performance was examined separately for those women who had a current diagnosis of PTSD ($n = 14$) and those who did not currently have PTSD ($n = 12$). The words (10 from each category) were presented in intermixed fashion, with each word presented for 2 seconds, followed by the instruction cue to remember or to forget for 3 seconds. All subjects were tested first on free recall, then on cued recall (the recall cues consisted of the first three letters of each word), and finally on a yes/no recognition test (composed of the 30 studied items and 30 new nonstudied distractor items, with the distractor items also being drawn from the trauma-related, positive, and neutral categories).

In the PTSD participants, although memory for the trauma-related words was greater with an instruction to remember (38%) than with an instruction to forget (26%), the overall level of recall of the trauma-related words (32%) significantly exceeded that for the positive and neutral words (mean, 15%), which were entirely unaffected by the instruction cue (mean for remember cue, 15%; mean for forget cue, 15%). PTSD participants recalled significantly fewer positive to-be-remembered words (11%) and significantly fewer neutral to-be-remembered words (19%) than did control participants (29% and 45%, respectively). In contrast, the non-PTSD participants recalled a similar number of trauma-related and non-trauma-related words overall and had better memory for the to-be-remembered items than for the to-be-forgotten items, regardless of the valence of the words (to-be-remembered recall for trauma-related, positive, and neutral words of 33%, 29%, and 45%, respectively; to-be-forgotten recall for the same categories, respectively, of 23%, 15%, and 20%). A very similar pattern was found in cued recall. The PTSD participants tended to recall more of the trauma-related words (54% remember, 48% forget) than the neutral or positive words (average, 28%), and this trend was largely unaffected by the instruction, whereas the non-PTSD control subjects showed overall directed forgetting. On the recognition test, PTSD participants recognized significantly fewer of the to-be-remembered words than did the control subjects; also, whereas PTSD participants showed no overall directed forgetting in recognition, the non-PTSD control subjects again showed directed forgetting.

On the one hand, considering the participants with PTSD, this study indicates a *failure* of selective forgetting of trauma-related material: these participants tended to remember trauma-related words that they were supposed to forget and failed to remember non-trauma-related words that they were supposed to remember. On the other hand, considering the participants who did not have PTSD, this study also suggests that successful intentional forgetting of trauma-related material is possible. Despite having a history of childhood abuse, the non-PTSD participants *were* able to selectively remember and to forget, with that ability manifested for both the trauma-related items and non-trauma-related items.

Extrapolation of these findings to settings outside the laboratory must be done cautiously. The ability to selectively remember or forget the presentation of single word cues in an experimental setting—even words semantically associated with a form of trauma that an individual experienced—is clearly not equivalent to the ability to remember or forget the trauma itself or even the environmental and other cues actually associated with the trauma. Furthermore, in themselves, these results cannot explain why PTSD participants were less able to forget trauma-related words than were their non-PTSD counterparts who had also endured childhood abuse. For example, did PTSD participants have more extensive and more strongly activated general schemata for abuse, thus making it both more difficult to forget the trauma-related words and more difficult to remember the non-trauma-related words? Nonetheless, these results suggest that the effectiveness of intentional forgetting of abusive episodes might be moderated by factors relating to the psychological status of the individual at the time. Voluntary forgetting of trauma-related materials may not be possible for some individuals (e.g., those with PTSD) but may be possible for others (e.g., those without PTSD). Other factors, possibly correlated with the presence or absence of PTSD, such as the severity or nature of the abuse, may, of course, also be important.

Can Children Show Intentional Forgetting?

Is intentional forgetting possible for young children? Because many incidents of abuse occur during childhood, this question is clearly important.

Four studies have examined children's ability to forget neutral materials (Bray et al. 1983, 1985; Harnishfeger and Pope 1996; Howard and

Goldin 1979), and each demonstrated that children may—under certain conditions—be able to successfully attend to, and remember, relevant rather than irrelevant information. However, if the information is designated as to-be-forgotten only after the child has already encountered it, then younger children (kindergarten children; 7-year-olds; and, to a lesser degree, 9-year-olds) prove largely unable to selectively forget.

Three of these studies used a somewhat different directed forgetting procedure, in which each child was presented with several trials, but some trials included an instruction to forget some of the items. Howard and Goldin (1979) showed kindergarten children (mean age, 5.8 years) a female doll, named "Amy," who (they explained) had to wear special items of clothing to signal that she was a secret agent. The child's task was to help Amy remember which items were special on any one day (i.e., experimental trial). This task was challenging because the items were always drawn from a set of 16 items, including 1 of 4 different hats (e.g., the hat could be a pillbox, beret, ski cap, or sailor hat), 1 of 4 different belts, 4 colors of flowers, and 4 types of neckpieces. Both the number of items that were said to be part of the "special signal" and the number of items that were presented but were not (for that trial) part of the special signal were varied across trials.

The investigators found that children could very efficiently selectively encode relevant information if they were told what types of items (e.g., hat and belt) were relevant *before* the doll was presented. In this case, children showed little interference from the presentation of other (but currently irrelevant) items. However, if children were told what types of items were relevant only after encoding, then they showed interference from the irrelevant items that were also presented.

Using a design in which children were repeatedly presented with one or two sets of pictures, but were sometimes told to forget one of the sets, Bray et al. (1983) also found that the youngest children (age 7 years) had no enhancement in the ability to remember the to-be-remembered items because the other items were cued as to-be-forgotten. For these children, performance was the same as if the child had been presented with both sets of items and was asked to remember both sets. However, 9-year-old children showed some ability to benefit from the forget cue, yet not as much as 11-year-olds, who showed complete elimination of the interference from the forget-cued items. (The latter result was also obtained with 11-year-olds in a subsequent study by Bray et al. 1985 and is also found with adults.)

More recently, the block-cuing directed forgetting procedure typically used with adults has also been studied in children. Harnishfeger and Pope (1996, Experiment 1) presented children (first-, third-, and fifth-graders) with a list of 20 unrelated words, with directions to repeat each word out loud as it occurred and to try to remember it. The children were interrupted after the first 10 words and were told either that the words presented up to that point had been "for practice" and so should be forgotten or that they should continue to remember the words while the next half of the list was presented. On a subsequent free-recall test, the fifth-graders (mean age, 11.5 years) showed consistent and significant directed forgetting, third-graders (mean age, 9.5 years) showed directed forgetting on one measure but not another (forgetting in a within-subjects comparison but not in a between-subjects comparison), and first-graders (mean age, 7.2 years) showed no directed forgetting. An essentially similar pattern was obtained in a replication study (Harnishfeger and Pope 1996, Experiment 2) that included an additional manipulation check to ensure that the children understood the directions given to them at the midpoint of the study list.

What do these findings imply about the ability of children to selectively encode—or remember—information in situations outside the laboratory, particularly situations involving abuse? Any form of direct extrapolation of these findings to such situations is clearly impossible. Nonetheless, they suggest that although even relatively young children may have the capacity to channel their efforts at remembering—provided that they know, at the outset, what it is that they are to try to remember—younger children may be less able to selectively forget information that they have already encoded and processed. By early adolescence, however, children may also be able to selectively forget stimuli or events even after that information has been encoded, effectively exercising control over information already present in memory rather than only precluding entry of information into memory in the first place.

What Processes Underlie Successful Intentional Forgetting?

Three processes have been postulated to underlie the successful forgetting of to-be-forgotten information that has been observed in the laboratory:

1. *Selective search of the to-be-remembered items,* according to which individuals are thought to initially code or "tag" to-be-remembered stimuli differently from to-be-forgotten stimuli and, then, during attempted retrieval, to somehow limit their search for a given item only to the to-be-remembered items
2. *Preferential encoding and rehearsal of the to-be-remembered stimuli,* according to which individuals more extensively process the to-be-remembered items than the to-be-forgotten items
3. *Retrieval inhibition,* according to which the intention to forget initiates a form of suppression such that the to-be-forgotten items are rendered less accessible during retrieval than the to-be-remembered items (Other processes that might render retrieval more dif-

ficult but that do not necessarily involve "inhibition" in a strict sense are also possible.)

Evidence supportive of a possible role for each of these processes has been found.

The strongest evidence for a contribution of selective search to successful forgetting has been obtained using a multitrial short-term memory procedure (e.g., Epstein and Wilder 1972; Homa and Spieker 1974; Howard 1976) that differs in several ways from the item-cuing and block-cuing directed forgetting procedures described earlier in this chapter. Although selective search may also contribute to enhanced memory for the to-be-remembered items under the block-cuing procedure (particularly when only the to-be-remembered items are tested), it does not seem sufficient to account for the full pattern of results under either that procedure or the item-cuing procedure. For example, it is not clear why—provided that individuals *know* that the to-be-forgotten items are being probed—memory for the to-be-forgotten items should be impaired. Why can individuals not just broaden their memory search to include both the to-be-remembered and the to-be-forgotten items?

Recent work has thus focused on evaluating the likely contribution of the second and third processes: preferential encoding of the to-be-remembered items on the one hand and disrupted access to the forget-cued items during retrieval on the other. The preponderance of the evidence suggests that intentional forgetting under the item-cuing method derives from more elaborative and extensive encoding of the remember-cued items. In contrast, several sources of evidence suggest that a form of inhibition or disruption of retrieval access is most likely involved in the block-cuing procedure.

The differential pattern of forgetting on recall versus recognition testing is perhaps one of the more important sources of data supporting this distinction. A pattern of impaired access to information during recall testing combined with intact performance during recognition testing has long been thought to indicate that the information must have been *available* in memory (or how could it have been recognized?) but for some reason was *inaccessible* during attempted recall (Tulving and Pearlstone 1966). Conversely, impaired performance despite the presence of strong and specific retrieval cues, such as those provided by a recognition test, has been thought to point to the possibility that the nonrecognized items were not stored in the first place (i.e., were not only inaccessible but also unavailable) (e.g., Roediger and Crowder 1972). Important caveats apply to this general rule (e.g., under certain conditions, the content or structure of the recognition test itself may make it more difficult to access information that is available in memory); nonetheless, impaired memory for the to-be-forgotten items during recognition testing under the item-cuing method—but not under the block-cuing method—is highly consistent with the notion that the to-be-forgotten items may have an encoding disadvantage with the former but not the latter method.

A comparison of the task demands under the two methods also supports the plausibility of this interpretation. On the one hand, the close proximity of the instruction cues to the initial presentation of the stimulus items under the item-cuing procedure leaves ample room for subjects to adopt a "wait-and-see" approach in their efforts to comply with the task. That is, before making a full-scale effort to remember a given item, subjects involved in the item-cuing procedure might "wait and see" if the instruction cue indicates that the item is, indeed, supposed to be remembered, fully elaborating on and actively rehearsing only those items that are subsequently cued as to-be-remembered and minimally processing the forget-cued items. On the other hand, the postponement of the forget instruction under the block-cuing procedure until many items have been processed and subjects' initial unawareness that a forget instruction will be given at all both suggest that these items were initially adequately encoded and processed but subsequently rendered less accessible.

Two further findings are consistent with the interpretation that the forget-cued items are less extensively elaborated on under item cuing but not under block cuing: 1) subjects' recollection for the forget-cued items is strongly impaired in item cuing but either not impaired or only minimally impaired in block cuing, and 2) conceptual priming for the forget-cued items may be reduced in item cuing but not block cuing. Subjects' memory for the to-be-forgotten items when they are instructed to remember or to forget on an item-by-item basis is much less often accompanied by additional information about the internal or external circumstances under which they first encountered the items than is true for the to-be-remembered items. Asked to indicate not only whether they recognize previously presented stimuli but also whether they can recollect any specific episodic details about their earlier encounter with the stimulus (e.g., what the item led them to think about), subjects involved in the item-cuing procedure had a very poor recollection of the items they were instructed to forget (Basden et al. 1993b; Gardiner et al. 1994; Koutstaal 1996; for a general review and description of this remember/know procedure, see Gardiner and Java 1993). In contrast, when subjects were instructed to forget using the block-cuing procedure, recollection of the circumstances surrounding the forget-cued items either was not impaired (Basden et al. 1993b) or was only slightly diminished, with a significant effect apparent only in a meta-analysis combining results across experiments (Koutstaal 1996). Likewise, recent reports suggesting diminished performance for forget-cued compared with remember-cued items on conceptual implicit tests, including word association (Basden et al. 1993b) and general knowledge questions (Basden and Basden, in press), with the item-cuing procedure but not the block-cuing procedure suggest that in item cuing but not block cuing, the to-be-forgotten stimuli are less elaboratively encoded and processed than the to-be-remembered stimuli. (For discussion of the distinction between perceptual and conceptual implicit tests, see, for example, Roediger et al. 1989; Schacter 1994.)

Nonetheless, it is possible that not *all* of the effects observed with the item-cuing procedure arise from enhanced encoding of the remember-cued items. For example, evidence also indicates that instructing subjects to use a more active form of forgetting—by mentally repeating "STOP" whenever a forget-cued item is presented—enhances the degree of forgetting observed compared with that observed for other strategies, including trying to think of nothing (i.e., trying to make one's mind "go blank") or deliberately rehearsing the to-be-remembered items (Geiselman et al. 1985, Experiment 2). Intriguingly, this enhancement of forgetting as a result of the use of the more active forgetting strategy was apparent only during free-recall testing. Although, overall, both recall and recognition of the to-be-remembered items were greater than that for the to-be-forgotten items, the more pronounced directed forgetting effect due to the use of the "STOP" procedure was apparent only on the recall test. A further experiment indicated that mentally repeating a nonsense word ("DAX") whenever a to-be-forgotten item was presented was less effective in reducing recall than was repetition of the conceptually more meaningful word "STOP" (Geiselman et al. 1985, Experiment 3). These findings suggest that under some conditions, the directed forgetting effect observed with the item-cuing method may also derive, in part, from depressed availability of the forget-cued items (as well as, or in addition to, enhanced memory for the remember-cued items) and that more specific and focused voluntary efforts at suppressing the to-be-forgotten material may more strongly impair memory.

If the intentional forgetting observed under the block-cuing procedure primarily involves a form of suppression or disruption in retrieval access to the to-be-forgotten items, rather than poorer initial storage or encoding, how—more specifically—might such disruption or inhibition "work"? For example, can any other indications of disrupted access be obtained, apart from the diminished ability to recall the items themselves? Although the precise nature of the processes involved is unclear, several findings suggest that the inhibitory or disruptive effects may be somewhat diffuse, encompassing not only the information that was specifically subjected to an intention to forget but also other stimuli or attributes that were associated with the to-be-forgotten information.

Initial evidence suggesting that the instruction to forget might result

in diminished access to the entire episode to which the forget instruction was applied was reported by Geiselman et al. (1983). In a series of
experiments, they found that subjects who were instructed to forget
the first of two blocks of items not only were less likely to recall the
items that were designated as to-be-forgotten but also were less likely
to recall other incidentally learned items that had been interspersed
among the to-be-forgotten items but were never specifically mentioned
as a target for forgetting. This diffuse form of forgetting was also observed, at least under some conditions, by Barnhardt (1993) after controlling for a potential artifact in the Geiselman et al. (1983) study and
may be similar to a diffuse form of forgetting recently reported by Allen
et al. (1995) with hypnotic virtuosos. Allen et al. found that hypnotic
virtuosos had posthypnotic recognition amnesia not only for a studied
word list for which amnesia was explicitly suggested but also for a word
list that was learned during the same hypnotic session but was not
covered by any amnesia suggestion—again suggesting that intentional
forgetting may assume a more general or broadly encompassing form
than is strictly required by the instruction.

Geiselman et al. (1983) noted that subjects who were instructed
to forget the first block of items were especially inaccurate at determining when those items had occurred. The order in which subjects
recalled the forget-cued items (as well as the incidentally learned
items that had been interspersed with those items) also tended to be
only weakly correlated with the order in which the items had originally been presented. This was not true for the remember-cued items
or for the first block of items in a control group asked to remember
the first block. These findings of both relatively poor source memory
for the forget-cued items (indicated by difficulties in determining
when they had occurred) and impaired retrieval organization for
those items (indicated by the tendency to recall the to-be-forgotten
items in an order that had little relation to the order in which they
had originally been encountered) suggested that access to the forget-cued items might be impeded because of a disruption in the association between the items and representations of the context in
which they had been learned.

A recent experiment conducted in our laboratory (Koutstaal 1996)
also found evidence of disrupted access to a form of contextual information concerning the forget-cued items. This experiment involved a manipulation that heightened the distinctiveness of the
to-be-forgotten versus the to-be-remembered items by associating
all of the forget-cued items with one contextual factor (one group of
people read all of these items) and all of the remember-cued items
with another contextual factor (a different group of people read all
of these items). Subjects were significantly less accurate at identifying the group of people who had been associated with the forget-

cued items than they were at determining the group of people who had been associated with the remember-cued items. Furthermore, and unlike nearly all previous experiments using block cuing, in this experiment (Experiment 5 in Table 8–2), directed forgetting was also observed during recognition testing.

The observation of impaired memory for the to-be-forgotten items even when retrieval cues were provided suggests that the intentional forgetting of entire episodes of previously encountered information might be facilitated if the to-be-forgotten episode is accompanied by contextual features that differentiate it from other experiences. Differentiating contextual features may allow the to-be-forgotten information to be more efficiently isolated from other information in memory and thus allow more selective forgetting. Contextual change may reduce the frequency with which external reminders of the to-be-forgotten information are encountered. Changes in context may also lead to more internal and possibly largely automatic processes wherein other information, goals, and intentions accompanying the to-be-forgotten information are more effectively deactivated (see Beckmann 1994; Goschke and Kuhl 1993) after environmental and cognitive change than in their absence. Additional research in this direction involving the manipulation of other forms of contextual features (e.g., mood state and general environmental characteristics, such as the place where information is learned) would allow assessment of the possibility that stronger and less readily reversed forgetting of entire episodes may occur if the contexts for the to-be-remembered and to-be-forgotten episodes are sufficiently distinctive.

Nonetheless, although manipulations of context might facilitate forgetting, we reiterate that these effects of intentional forgetting—when observed—involve relative rather than absolute differences. Memory for the to-be-forgotten materials may be diminished relative to memory for the to-be-remembered materials, but a considerable proportion of the to-be-forgotten information is still remembered, with greater memory generally apparent with more adequate retrieval support. Furthermore, although findings concerning directed forgetting have begun to be extended to emotional materials and, in some circumstances, directed forgetting has been observed for emotionally significant materials, this has not been consistently found, and definite counterexamples, with both item-cuing and a modified block-cuing procedure, have also been reported. Thus, whereas, on the whole, the evidence reviewed about intentional forgetting does point to processes that permit restricted encoding and to some extent diminished accessibility of information, these findings provide no evidence supporting the possibility that individuals' conscious attempts to forget will result in massive and complete amnesia for severely traumatizing events.

Voluntary Thought Suppression

The question of whether individuals can intentionally forget information about stimuli or events that they have already encountered and processed is closely linked with another question: To what extent can individuals successfully avoid or suppress conscious thoughts about an unwanted topic (independently of the effects this may have on memory)? Although some investigators have noted the connections between directed forgetting and thought suppression (e.g., Barnhardt 1993; H. M. Johnson 1994; Wegner et al. 1987), several differences in the experimental procedures used to study intentional forgetting and thought suppression have also been identified. Perhaps most important, investigations of voluntary thought suppression have typically involved instructions to suppress thoughts about a single topic or episode, whereas investigations of directed forgetting have most often involved instructions to forget many items of information that are usually entirely unrelated to one another or that are derived from several different semantic categories. (Note that for the block-cuing directed forgetting method, even though an entire set of previously encountered items is designated as to-be-forgotten—and so in one sense a single temporal episode is targeted for forgetting—many different and usually semantically unrelated items are in the block. This differs from having only a single topic or theme to be suppressed.)

Several experiments have investigated the degree to which individuals could successfully suppress thoughts about essentially neutral or innocuous topics. Specifically introduced by the experimenter as a target for attempted thought suppression, these topics have included both relatively whimsical and novel subjects (e.g., thoughts about a white bear or a story about a green rabbit) and more familiar and mundane matters (e.g., thoughts about vehicles or the Statue of Liberty). Can individuals successfully suppress such thoughts? What might experimental investigations of the suppression of such thoughts reveal about the suppression of more emotionally significant and personally relevant topics?

On the one hand, the processes involved in the suppression of thoughts that have considerable emotional and personal significance may well differ in important ways from the processes that allow the eradication or reduced frequency of more neutral thoughts. Emotionally neutral and experimenter-provided thoughts may differ from personally relevant thoughts in how familiar, how complex, and how easily imagined they are and in how much experience individuals have in attempting to control them (Kelly and Kahn 1994). Also, as Salkovskis and Campbell (1994) observed, the emotional effects of the intrusive thoughts may modify the ways in which such thoughts are processed (emotion may affect the nature of the thought itself), and the individual's cognitive appraisal of the meaning and implications of the thoughts may affect the intensity or nature of the motivation to suppress (i.e., thoughts about the thought may influence further affect and motivation about the thought).

On the other hand, exploration of the relative success with which individuals can suppress emotionally neutral or experimentally suggested thoughts allows greater experimental control than is otherwise possible. Such exploration may permit the isolation and identification of factors that may also moderate the suppression of personally relevant thoughts but that—given the idiosyncratic and often complex set of conditions involved in their formation and maintenance—may be very difficult to disentangle. Confining experimental examination of thought suppression to only those thoughts that individuals find intrusive and personally distressing in their lives clearly has its own hazards, not the least of which is sampling bias. When only thoughts that have been identified as intrusive and as recurrent sources of distress are used as objects of experimental investigation, whether (or how often) other thoughts have been successfully suppressed and what conditions allowed such suppression cannot be determined. Ascertaining how, when, and to what extent individuals are able to suppress comparatively unfamiliar and externally introduced thoughts may provide a "window" on the very early processes that are involved in suppression, allowing determination of the conditions that may lead *either* to a future and chronic course of unsuccessful suppression or to successful suppression.

Fortunately, investigators do not need to choose between these two alternatives, and several recent experiments have been reported using targets for suppression that have greater emotional and personal significance to the individuals. We next review some of the central findings from these investigations, beginning with emotionally neutral materials.

Can Adults Voluntarily Suppress Emotionally Neutral Thoughts?

Most of the evidence from studies using emotionally neutral materials indicates at least some degree of *initial* success in suppressing a target thought—when success is measured on the order of several minutes. For example, in one of the earliest studies of thought suppression, Wegner et al. (1987, Experiment 1) compared two groups of subjects. Both groups of subjects first participated in a 5-minute practice session with a stream-of-consciousness technique in which they were asked to verbalize continually what they were presently thinking, without attempting to explain or justify their thoughts. Then, one group of subjects—the *initial suppression* condition—was instructed to continue to verbalize their thoughts in the same manner as before with one important exception: subjects were told, "This time, try not to think of a white bear. Every time you say 'white bear' or have 'white bear' come to mind, please ring the bell on the table before you." Another group of subjects—the *initial expression* condition—were given similar instructions but, instead, were told to "try to think of a white bear." The results showed that the suppression instruction clearly reduced the frequency with which the target thought occurred. After combining all three possible ways in which thoughts of white bears might be indicated (bell ring plus verbal mention of a bear, bell ring only, and verbal mention only), subjects in the initial expression condition had an average of 16.38 overtly indicated thoughts of bears during the 5-minute period. In contrast, subjects in the initial suppression condition had only 6.3 such thoughts. Furthermore, most of these thoughts occurred during the first 2 minutes of the suppression period, such that by the end of 5 minutes, subjects in the suppression condition were overtly indicating fewer than 1 "unwanted" thought per minute.

Most other investigations (e.g., Clark et al. 1991; Wegner et al. 1990, 1991; Wenzlaff et al. 1991) have also found that subjects initially instructed to try to suppress a neutral thought are relatively—albeit not absolutely—successful in doing so. (Note that although the suppression instructions decreased the frequency of the target thought in the study described above, a number of such thoughts still occurred.) Successful suppression has also been observed in comparison to what may be a more natural "think of anything" baseline condition, in which subjects are not asked to express the target thought but instead are instructed to think of anything they like, including the target (Clark et al. 1991, 1993). For example, Clark et al. (1993) compared how often subjects thought about a tape-recorded story about a green rabbit that they had just heard when instructed to suppress all thoughts of the story ("Keep from your mind thoughts of anything that you heard on tape. . . . It is absolutely essential that you try to suppress this material from your mind") with subjects who were instructed to think of anything they wished, including the story ("Think about absolutely anything, with no restrictions, including material you heard on the tape"). Although some 46% of the thoughts verbalized by subjects in the think of anything condition referred to the tape, only 19% of the thoughts verbalized by subjects in the suppression condition referred to the taped material. Individuals in the suppression condition also provided lower ratings than did individuals in the think of anything condition when asked to subjectively rate the amount of time they had spent thinking about the tape. (For two cases in which suppression was not evident in either the expression or the think of anything condition, see, respectively, Muris et al. 1992, 1993.)

However, most of these studies also indicate a further phenomenon that provides an important qualification. Individuals who are first asked to suppress a neutral thought often show a "rebound" in the frequency with which the target thoughts occur, such that during a subsequent postsuppression period, they more often think of the thought than if they had not been asked to suppress. Individuals who earlier tried to suppress a neutral thought and were later either asked to express the thought (e.g., Kelly and Kahn 1994; Wegner et al. 1987, 1991) or were encouraged to think about anything they liked (Clark et al. 1991, 1993) showed significantly more frequent occurrences of the thought than did persons who were never asked to suppress the thought (but were first asked either to express the thought or to think about anything).

Why does this rebound effect occur? Is a resurgence of the frequency of the "unwanted" thought inevitable, or might rebound somehow be prevented, so that voluntary thought suppression would prove to be a more enduring remedy for unwanted thoughts? Most important, does a similar effect occur with emotionally and personally significant materials?

Two primary accounts of the rebound effect have been proposed, each of which has received some support. However, we discuss these accounts—and what the evidence concerning them tells us about the conditions under which successful thought suppression may occur—after a review of studies involving the suppression of emotional materials. Surprisingly, the evidence for rebound effects with emotional materials is considerably less strong than for neutral materials.

Can Adults Voluntarily Suppress Emotionally Significant and Personally Relevant Thoughts?

The findings as to whether adults can voluntarily suppress thoughts that are more intimately associated with their emotional, motivational, and personal lives are decidedly mixed and complex. Both the somewhat equivocal nature of the findings and the complexity arise from three factors: 1) variability in how particular thoughts were selected as targets for suppression, 2) differences in how long (and in what contexts) suppression instructions were maintained, and 3) differences in the characteristics of the individuals chosen for inclusion in the studies.

Unsuccessful suppression, involving a failure to suppress negative or aversive materials, has been reported by several investigators. Two such reports involved instructions to suppress a target thought over a period of several days—including contexts outside the laboratory setting. Muris and Merckelbach (1991, cited in Muris et al. 1992) first read subjects a transcription of Freud's Ratman obsession and then instructed one-half of the subjects to suppress all thoughts of the transcription; the remaining subjects were given no instructions about suppression. One week later, subjects were interviewed as to the frequency with which they had thought of the transcription over the past week. Subjects who had been given suppression instructions reported more intrusions of the thought than did subjects who had not been encouraged to suppress.

Although suggestive, the reliance on individuals' subjective and retrospective reports to determine thought occurrences in this study is clearly highly problematic. A more convincing indication that individuals' longer-term efforts at deliberately suppressing negative thoughts may prove unsuccessful has recently been reported by Trinder and Salkovskis (1994). Subjects in this study (undergraduates) were preselected from a larger population on the basis of a questionnaire describing and assessing negative intrusive thoughts; to be selected into the study, subjects had to report having experienced such thoughts during the preceding month. Individuals who met this criterion were then interviewed on two occasions, separated by 4 days. During the first session, subjects were asked to identify, and then evaluate, a specific negative intrusive thought on various dimensions (e.g., amount of discomfort experienced during the thought). They were also given a habituation sequence for the thought, in which they were repeatedly asked to imagine the thought as clearly as possible and then (again) to evaluate various aspects of the thought. Thereafter, they were assigned to one of three groups: 1) a suppression group, instructed to try to suppress the thought as quickly as possible whenever it came to mind; 2) a control group, instructed simply to record any occurrences of the target thought ("record only" group); or 3) a third group, instructed to think about the target thought as much as possible whenever it occurred without modifying the thought ("think through" group). Subjects were also given postcards on which to write any occurrences of the thought, with separate sections for each of the 4 days, and were given a distinctive reminder cue to wear on their watches to help them remember to record any target thoughts.

Subjects who were asked to suppress experienced *more* of the target thoughts than did subjects in either the record only group or the think through group, which did not differ from each other. Nonetheless, subjects' self-ratings of the degree to which they had attempted to suppress thoughts were higher for the suppression group than for the other groups, suggesting that greater frequency of the target thought occurred despite greater efforts at suppression.

Do these findings indicate that emotional materials cannot be suppressed and that suppression may even lead to precisely the opposite effect—increased rather than decreased cognitive and emotional involvement with the unwanted thought? In answering this question with regard to this study and other studies that have explored thought suppression of emotional materials, it is critical to keep in mind a point raised earlier in this chapter: When only thoughts that have been identified as intrusive and as recurrent sources of distress are used as objects of experimental investigation, whether (or how often) other thoughts have been successfully suppressed and what conditions allowed such suppression cannot be determined. Two forms of "selection bias" may operate in such cases: bias in the *thoughts* within individuals that are selected for examination and bias in the particular *persons* who are selected for the study. For example, in the Trinder and Salkovskis (1994) study, only slightly more than one-half (56%) of the larger population of students that was originally sampled reported having negative intrusive thoughts during the preceding month, and all of the subjects included in the study were selected from this subset of students. What about the other 44% of the sample? Why had they not experienced (or at least not reported having experienced) such thoughts? How might these individuals respond differently to negative or aversive thoughts than the 56% included in the study?

The experimental evidence on thought suppression may be examined with different questions in mind. To investigate whether thought suppression provides a viable model for the occurrence of ruminative or obsessive thinking, selection on the basis of the presence of intrusive and recurrent negative thoughts may well increase ecological validity. But to examine whether individuals—in general—can voluntarily suppress negative or aversive thoughts, preselection of subjects may prove misleading.

It is important that several additional studies that have reported unsuccessful attempts at thought suppression also preselected subjects (e.g., Mathews and Milroy 1994; Salkovskis and Campbell 1994). In contrast, of five studies that either reported successful initial suppression of emotionally significant or negative thoughts (Kelly and Kahn 1994; Roemer and Borkovec 1994; Wegner and Gold 1995; Wegner et al. 1990) or were ambiguous (Muris et al. 1992), none preselected subjects specifically on the basis of intrusiveness or nonintrusiveness of thoughts. Although in two cases, subjects were selected or assigned to particular experimental groups on the basis of the nature and intensity of emotional responses they had to particular situations or persons (Roemer and Borkovec 1994; Wegner and Gold 1995), subjects were not included precisely on the basis of the intrusiveness of particular target thoughts in any of these studies.

Muris et al. (1992) asked subjects (undergraduates) to read a story that involved a highly negative event (subjects were asked to imagine themselves being late for an appointment, speeding through a yellow traffic light, and causing an accident in which a child is killed) or a very similar story in which the emotional words and phrases were replaced by neutral elements. Thereafter, subjects in the emotional and neutral story conditions were assigned either to a suppression condition or to a "think of anything" condition, in which they were free to think or not to think about the story they had read. This first phase, which lasted for 5 minutes, was followed by two 5-minute "think of anything" phases, with the first free expression phase occurring immediately after the initial suppression or expression phase and the second occurring after a 20-minute unrelated task. (Thus, for both the emotional story and the neutral story, one group of subjects received a suppression phase immediately followed by a think of anything phase, followed 20 minutes later by an additional think of anything phase; another group of subjects received a think of anything phase on all three occasions.) During each of the three critical phases, subjects were told to press the button of a hand-held event marker each time they happened to think of the story.

There was no indication that subjects given the suppression instructions—for either the emotional or the neutral story—were successful in less often thinking about the story. Both of these groups tended to think about the story as often as subjects in the emotional think of anything condition, and all of these groups thought of the story more often than subjects in the neutral think of anything condition. In the former three groups (suppress–neutral, suppress–emotional, think of anything–emotional), there was a slight trend for fewer thoughts to occur during the second (think of anything) phase than during the initial phase, and thoughts of the story had clearly decreased by the third (think of anything) phase. On the one hand, the equivalence of the two suppression groups to the think of anything–emotional group during the initial phase does point to a failure of initial suppression. On the other hand, the largely parallel *decrease* in thoughts of the story in all three groups across the later two periods appears to indicate a form of habituation to thoughts of the story over time. Such habituation is clearly inconsistent with the notion that rebound would occur after attempted suppression.

Four studies, using quite different emotional topics as targets for suppression, have provided evidence for successful initial suppression of emotional thoughts. Wegner et al. (1990) examined mentions of target thoughts under suppression compared with expression instructions for an exciting topic (e.g., thoughts about sex) and a relatively less exciting topic (e.g., thoughts about dancing). Although suppression did not entirely eliminate the target thought, mentions were clearly less frequent during suppression than during expression instructions. Evidence also indicated that the frequency of the target thoughts decreased with both suppression and expression instructions for shorter- (4-minute) and longer-term (30-minute) periods, suggesting that thoughts about exciting topics were not especially susceptible to rebound.

Initially successful suppression has also been reported for thoughts about an "old flame" (i.e., a "significant past romantic relationship") (Wegner and Gold 1995), individuals' own intrusive thoughts (Kelly and Kahn 1994), and personal situations specifically associated with depression or anxiety (Roemer and Borkovec 1994). For example, Roemer and Borkovec (1994) found that the proportion of direct statements related to a to-be-suppressed topic situation under initial suppression instructions was 19% for a depressing situation, 26% for an anxious situation, and 17% for a neutral situation; under initial expression instructions, the corresponding proportions were 89%, 67%, and 45%. Suppression was also successful when negative affect statements were the dependent measure, such that under expression conditions, depressed and anxious groups expressed more negative affect than the neutral group, and under suppression instructions, negative affect for the depressed and anxious groups did not differ from that for the neutral group. However, suppression was not observed for *indirect* statements about the situation (e.g., if the subject's depression involved the loss of a friend, but the subject referred to some other loss); such indirect thoughts were not affected by the suppression instruction.

Little evidence of a rebound effect was found in the study by Kelly and Kahn (1994) involving subjects' own intrusive thoughts. In the study by Wegner and Gold (1995), a rebound effect was observed only for participants who suppressed thoughts about an individual they no longer desired or often thought about (a "cold flame"). Whereas cold flame participants reported more thoughts about the past romantic relationship if they had just suppressed thoughts of that relationship than if they had just suppressed thoughts about a neutral topic (e.g., thoughts about the Statue of Liberty), "hot flame" participants, when invited to talk about their past romantic relationship, often spoke about their old flame regardless of whether they had just suppressed thoughts of the flame or had just suppressed thoughts about a neutral topic. Thus, although both hot and cold flame participants were able to initially suppress thoughts about their past romantic relationships, this suppression bore no special costs of increased thinking about the relationship for the hot flame participants, but it did for cold flame participants. (A possible account of this result is provided in the final section.)

In summary, most studies with neutral stimuli indicate some degree of success in *initially* suppressing the target thought. Similar results have been obtained in most studies with more emotionally significant materials—*provided* that subjects were not preselected on the basis of their inability to suppress particular thoughts. However, especially in the case of neutral thoughts, but less so for emotionally significant thoughts, initial suppression is often followed by a rebound. When later given the opportunity either to specifically express the target thought or to think of anything at all, individuals who had earlier suppressed a neutral thought are especially likely to think of that very thought. What might account for this effect, and, equally important, why might it less frequently occur with emotionally significant materials?

What Processes Underlie Successful—and Unsuccessful—Voluntary Thought Suppression?

Analysis of subjects' reported thoughts during their attempts to suppress an unwanted thought revealed that many individuals were using an unfocused form of self-distraction. In their effort not to think about the "forbidden" thought, subjects often focused their attention on various apparently harmless aspects of their immediate surroundings (e.g., the wall, the light switch, their shoes). However, because subjects often focused on these environmental details immediately after they had failed to suppress the unwanted thought, these "would-be distractors" may have become associatively linked with the to-be-suppressed thought—and so may later act as *reminders* of the to-be-avoided topic.

Indirect support for this "association" hypothesis (Wegner and Gold 1995; Wegner et al. 1987) has been obtained from two sources. First, individuals have been found to show more resistance to a rebound of the unwanted thought if they are instructed to use a specific distractor thought. Rather than engaging in an unfocused and haphazard search for satisfactory alternative thoughts in which sundry things may—unwittingly—become cues to the thought, individuals may be encouraged to consistently replace unwanted thoughts with another specific thought. Rebound has been reduced in the presence of focused distraction both with a neutral target (e.g., thoughts of a white bear) as the to-be-suppressed item (Wegner et al. 1987) and with naturally occurring intrusive thoughts. Providing subjects with a specific distractor task to perform during their attempts to suppress a naturally occurring intrusive thought (Salkovskis and Campbell 1994) diminished the frequency with which intrusions occurred, both compared with a condition in which only general (unfocused) distraction instructions were given and compared with the usual suppression instructions (in which no distraction strategies are specifically mentioned). (Interestingly, the clinical use of thought suppression may involve both thought-stopping and instruction in the use of a pleasant distractor thought. See, for example, Kumar and Wilkinson 1971; Turner et al. 1983.)

Although consistent with the association hypothesis, these findings have alternative interpretations. For example, to the extent that reliance on a specific distractor thought results in fewer occurrences of the unwanted thought, then the unwanted thought is itself less elaborated and richly encoded. Less elaborated and richly encoded thoughts may themselves be less readily recalled independent of whether particular cues were associated with the thoughts to prompt their return.

Possibly stronger support for the association hypothesis derives from comparisons of the degree to which individuals are successful in maintaining thought suppression when they are either in an environment that closely matches that in which they initially tried to suppress an unwanted thought or in a situation that differs in important ways. Several studies have found that intrusions of an unwanted thought are less common after the individual's environment is altered, both when external features of the environment are changed and when the individual's mood or "mental context" (Lockhart 1988; Smith 1995) is changed. For example, Wegner et al. (1991) manipulated the external context that was present during thought suppression by showing color slides drawn from different themes (e.g., landscapes or household appliances) during subjects' efforts to suppress thoughts about a white bear and then by showing slides from the same theme or a different theme during a subsequent expression period. The rebound effect was considerably stronger if the slides during initial suppression and later expression were the same than if they were different. There was also evidence that the slides themselves were mentioned more frequently during initial suppression than initial expression instructions (i.e., at the point at which distraction was first occurring), and, during subsequent expression, references to the slides were more often directly followed by references to the white bear for initial suppression than for initial expression subjects.

During unfocused attempts at distraction, individuals may turn their attention not only to various aspects of the external environment but also to their current concerns, intentions, memories, and so forth. To the extent that these internal sources of distraction are filtered by the individual's present mood (e.g., such that depressed people tend to choose negative thoughts as distractors more than do nondepressed people), then altering an individual's mood might act in a manner similar to altering the external environment. By reducing the likelihood that previous distractor *thoughts* return to mind, alterations in an individual's mood should also reduce the likelihood that the *associations* between these earlier thoughts and the unwanted thought will prompt return of the unwanted thought. Alterations in mood have, indeed, been found to act in this way. For example, Wenzlaff et al. (1991) used a mood induction procedure to encourage ("induce") subjects to feel either relatively more or less positive during an initial suppression period and either more or less positive during a later expression period. Although initial suppression subjects showed a rebound effect regardless of whether their mood was the same or different between the earlier and later periods, the rebound effect was stronger if the subjects' mood was congruent in both phases (negative-negative, positive-positive) than if it was incongruent (negative-positive, positive-negative).

This effect was found for suppression of a neutral thought (i.e., thoughts of a white bear). Heightened rebound effects under mood-congruent conditions have also been established with positive and negative autobiographical events, both when mood was experimentally manipulated via a mood induction procedure (Howell and Conway 1992, Experiment 1) and when subjects were assigned to positive and negative mood conditions on the basis of their scores on a self-report measure (Beck Depression Inventory; Howell and Conway 1992, Experiment 2). Wenzlaff et al. (1988) reported that depressed individuals had an especially pronounced rebound effect during the latter part of a 9-minute suppression period if they were asked to suppress thoughts about a highly negative life-event description. Additional analyses of the emotional valence of subjects' thoughts immediately preceding and following negative thought intrusions indicated that nondepressed subjects' thoughts were significantly more positive after the intrusion of a negative target thought than before the thought, but the valence of the thoughts of the depressed subjects did not change. Thus, the nondepressed subjects tended to distract themselves from the negative target thought by focusing on a positive thought, whereas the depressed subjects turned from the negative target thought toward other negative thoughts—ultimately, a less effective strategy.

All of these findings regarding the effects of altered external and internal context on the effectiveness of suppression and the likelihood of rebound are clearly consistent with the association hypothesis. Nonetheless, evidence also suggests that the association hypothesis cannot explain all of the effects (or countereffects!) of suppression. Although diminished in magnitude, rebound effects have also been observed when the context has been different from the original suppression context (Wegner et al. 1991) and with an indirect measure that did not require conscious recollection of the stimulus (Macrae et al. 1994).

Based on these and several additional findings, investigators have proposed an alternative explanation for suppression: the "accessibility" hypothesis. The accessibility hypothesis suggests that rebound occurs because of an "ironic" and automatic mental process (Wegner 1994; Wegner et al. 1993) that is established during the initial intention to suppress. According to the accessibility hypothesis, in addition to suppression per se, successful suppression requires remembering the thought to be suppressed. Whereas suppression involves voluntary or "controlled" cognitive processes in which the individual expends cognitive effort in searching for and maintaining suitable distractor thoughts, remembering what is to be suppressed is an automatic process—a process that operates largely outside of awareness, with little conscious guidance beyond that involved in initiating suppression (e.g., Hasher and Zacks 1979; see Uleman 1989). This involves a constant vigilant monitoring for any occurrences of the to-be-suppressed thought—or of thoughts even remotely or weakly associated with it—so as to quickly suppress the unwanted thought. However, paradoxically, this second automatic process, because it renders the individual unusually attuned to internal and external stimuli associated with the unwanted thought, increases the likelihood that the thought will recur—even with very little prompting or cuing.

If both a controlled process of suppression and an automatic process of detecting stimuli associated with the unwanted thought are occurring, then a manipulation that interferes with the ability to consciously suppress should "uncover" the automatic process. More specifically, if the intention to suppress engenders an automatic process of hypervigilance for items associated with the unwanted thought, then—provided one can effectively circumvent or undermine conscious efforts at suppression through distraction—it might be possible to observe *hyperaccessibility* of the to-be-suppressed thought. Individuals instructed to suppress a target thought might show that thought (and possibly thoughts associated with it) to be even more accessible to them than to individuals who are deliberately attempting to concentrate on that same thought (concentration presumably requiring vigilance but not necessarily hypervigilance).

Consistent with this expectation, Wegner and Erber (1992) found that subjects who were attempting to suppress a particular neutral target thought (e.g., house or mountain) when placed under high "cognitive load" showed hyperaccessibility of the thought. Asked to very rapidly produce associations to various words, subjects who were attempting to suppress a given target word were more likely to give that word as an association than were subjects who were trying to concentrate on the word. Asked to perform the same task but without any particular time pressure, the reverse occurred: subjects concentrating on the topic more often provided it as a response than did subjects suppressing the topic. Additional evidence supportive of altered accessibility of the target thought has also been reported with a modified version of the Stroop task (Wegner and Erber 1992, Experiment 2; see Lavy and van den Hout 1994).

Taken together, all of these findings suggest that both associative cuing and alterations in the accessibility of the target thought may influence the likelihood of successful suppression. As suggested by Macrae et al. (1994), the accessibility hypothesis possibly can be extended or modified to include associative cuing factors. To the extent that features of one's internal or external context become associated with the to-be-suppressed target thought, then the target may receive additional activation when the context is maintained or reinstated. A modified account such as this might also more readily accommodate the findings that reinstatement effects (e.g., Davies and Thomson 1988) and reduced proactive and retroactive interference due to altered contexts (e.g., Kanak and Stevens 1992) may be observed in other paradigms even when no particular conscious or deliberate attention has been directed toward aspects of the environment. We next discuss the possible relevance of these findings and previously reviewed findings on directed forgetting in regard to traumatic situations.

Integration and Relation to Abuse Literature

Our comments in this section focus on three factors: 1) the importance of external and internal context as a moderating factor in both intentional forgetting and thought suppression, 2) the interconnectedness of intentional forgetting and thought suppression with other factors (including other forms of coping) that may affect memory, and 3) future directions and questions.

The Importance of External and Internal Context

The critical role of the amount of retrieval support offered by the environment during attempts to probe memory has long been recognized (e.g., McGeoch 1932; Tulving 1983). However, a review of findings on both intentional forgetting and voluntary thought suppression suggests that retrieval cues may assume a more than usually potent role in prompting the return of to-be-forgotten or to-be-suppressed thoughts. Encountering all (Basden et al. 1993a, 1994; Geiselman et al. 1983; Koutstaal 1996) or even only a few (Bjork and Bjork 1991; Goernert and Larson 1994) of the to-be-forgotten items following an attempt to forget an entire set or block of items may largely eliminate the mnemonic disadvantage for the forget-cued items that would otherwise have been observed. Such "release from retrieval inhibition" (Basden et al. 1993a; Bjork 1989) on reexposure to the to-be-forgotten stimuli is similar to the effect produced by encountering aspects of the environment that were present during earlier attempts at thought suppression. Rebound of thoughts is especially strong in external and internal conditions that closely parallel those prevailing during initial attempts at suppression.

These findings suggest that retrieval cues may also be especially important in prompting the reemergence of thoughts or memories of traumatic incidents when people attempt to suppress or forget those incidents. Many investigators have specifically pointed to the role of retrieval cues in prompting recall of previously forgotten or suppressed incidents of abuse (e.g., Feldman-Summers and Pope 1994) or have reported individual cases consistent with such a view (McNally et al., unpublished data, February 1996; Schooler 1994; see also Christenson et al. 1981; McGee 1984). For example, some anonymous women who were self-reported survivors of father-daughter incest that had occurred an average of 20 years earlier still reported recurrent, intrusive, and disruptive memories, and most respondents reported that memories, thoughts, and images of the experience were likely to be triggered by salient cues in their everyday interactions (Silver et al. 1983).

As the time from an original episode of abuse increases, an individual's external context is likely to have changed, thus increasing the likelihood of successful forgetting. Individuals may also deliberately alter their living or work circumstances to facilitate forgetting. Interviews of adults who had been raped 4–6 years earlier (Burgess and Holmstrom 1979) revealed several strategies that the victims used to cope with the rape. In addition to thought suppression, many individuals changed their residence or traveled. Some victims moved into a new apartment within the same neighborhood, others moved to a completely different neighborhood, and still others (often those with less financial independence) temporarily stayed with relatives or friends. Some of these individuals directly remarked on the positive aspects of moving. For example, one victim said, "I think it was easier for me because I went to another city and wasn't reminded of it. I didn't have to see it every day. I could forget it" (Burgess and Holmstrom 1979, p. 1280).

Nonetheless, complete avoidance of all reminders is unlikely to be successful, particularly when reminders may also include an individual's internal cognitions and feelings at the time of attempted suppression. Kuyken and Brewin (1994) found that women with a history of childhood sexual or physical abuse who were currently depressed reported both high levels of intrusive memories of the abuse and avoidance of those memories. This preliminary study did not permit the directionality of these effects to be determined (did intrusive memories lead to depression, or did depression encourage higher levels of intrusive memories?) nor did it include an assessment of the extent to which high intrusiveness and avoidance were especially true for memories of abuse as opposed to negative and stressful life events more generally. However, both the increased availability of negative thoughts and the decreased capacity for cognitive effort caused by depression could act to undermine attempts at suppression (see, for example, Conway et al. 1991; see also Freeston et al. 1995) by enhancing similarity to the original context in which suppression had occurred and by diminishing the ability to find or devise effective distractor thoughts.

The Interconnectedness of Intentional Forgetting and Thought Suppression With Other Factors That May Affect Memory

A self-initiated effort to avoid thoughts or memories of abuse may interact with and supplement factors in the environment that encourage thought suppression and forgetting. The press toward secrecy or discomfort experienced when discussing an incident may decrease the extent to which thoughts about the incident are elaborated and conceptualized (see Goodman et al. 1994; see also Fivush and Schwarzmueller 1995). Both self-initiated and externally encouraged efforts to suppress thoughts may either diminish or increase the formation of interassociations between thoughts about the abuse and other aspects of the individual's internal and external environment (e.g., Nelson 1993; Tessler and Nelson 1994). Although the latter possibility—that attempts at suppression will *increase* associative ties between the thought and the environment—is highlighted by the association hypothesis, the degree to which such interassociations are formed is also clearly moderated by the presence or absence of focused distractor techniques. For example, one account of the findings from Wegner and Gold (1995) that were discussed earlier in this chapter, in which only participants who had suppressed thoughts about a "cold flame" showed a rebound effect, focuses on the importance of environmental cuing together with distractors. Kelly and Kahn (1994) proposed that individuals thinking about a "cold flame" may not have been recently suppressing thoughts about him or her, so they were not prepared with salient or focused distractors. They may, therefore, have been more likely to use cues in the external laboratory environment to provide distraction, thereby also increasing the likelihood of later rebound due to environmental cuing.

Evidence indicates that individuals who have been abused may have fewer specific memories from childhood and may more often produce "overgeneral" autobiographical memories in response to word cues (see Kuyken and Brewin 1995; Parks and Balon 1995). These autobiographical memory deficits may partially result from diminished encoding or later elaboration and thinking of the times when abuse occurred (see J. M. G. Williams 1992). It is at least possible that poor memory for entire periods may reflect earlier efforts not to think of specific episodes by *also* not thinking of events, people, or places associated with abuse.

Likewise, cognitive changes due to development are not neatly separable from thought suppression or intentional forgetting. Although cognitive developmental changes may directly result in diminished memory caused by infantile or childhood amnesia (e.g., Howe et al. 1994; but cf. Nelson 1993), developmental factors may also affect the likelihood that intentional efforts at controlling memory will be undertaken and the probable success of such attempts. Discussing the interview responses of women with documented incidents of childhood abuse, L. M. Williams (1995) noted that some women reported that they did not immediately begin intentionally blocking out memories of the abuse but began doing so only some time later. On the one hand, as L. M. Williams (1995, p. 668) observed, this may be because developmental factors precluded the use of such strategies: "[D]eliberate forgetting may be available as a strategy only for the child who has attained more formal cognitive operations and has at least some limited verbal skills." On the other hand, as L. M. Williams also noted, because these reports were based on participants' subjective reports, documenting whether such *delayed* attempts at voluntary forgetting do, in fact, occur requires longitudinal research. More generally, the issue of the frequency of delayed attempts to forget trauma is important, especially because such delays may be more likely to be accompanied by aid from the environment in the form of contextual change and thus are more likely to be successful.

Self-reports including phrases such as "I blocked it out" or "I didn't think about it" do not convey how this occurs. Although, as observed at the outset, there is little reason to believe that there is a form of massive unconscious repression of traumatic incidents, the exact manner in which individuals use conscious efforts to not think about traumatic events is unclear. Does "blocking it out" involve a simple effort not to think about the event or the use of specific distractor thoughts? If so, how is distraction related to dissociation or to related factors such as imaginative involvement or absorption (e.g., Kihlstrom et al. 1994; Spiegel and Cardeña 1991; Tellegen and Atkinson 1974; see also Trickett and Putnam 1993)? Evidence from both the directed forgetting and thought suppression literature clearly shows that the use of focused distractors results in a more effective limitation of memory and thoughts than does unfocused distraction. How, more precisely, did individuals such as those cited earlier from the L. M. Williams study "block out" memories or thoughts of the abuse?

Finally, there is also a complex interplay of denial or blocking of *cognitive* information and the repression of *emotion* (e.g., Davis 1990; Weinberger et al. 1979). What role might the denial of the emotional effect of traumatic or stressful events, the isolation of affect, or affective blunting play in thought suppression or intentional forgetting? For example, in a recent case reported by Mann and Delon (1995, p. 503), a woman who had been raped at age 14 by her sister's fiancé confided that: "in previous years, memories of the rape had occasionally invaded her thoughts, but were infrequent and were associated with little affect." To what extent did emotional numbing render recall less likely to begin with? And—even if memories did invade her thoughts—to what extent did the emotional numbing preclude or curtail any cognitive processing and elaboration of those memories, thereby also rendering future retrievals less likely? Although some evidence indicates that successful cognitive suppression may not necessarily be accompanied by successful emotional suppression (Wegner et al. 1990), it is also probable that cognitive suppression may at times "benefit" from emotional suppression (see, for example, Holtgraves and Hall 1995; Kuhl 1985; Tomarken and Davidson 1994).

Future Directions and Questions

Research on voluntary thought suppression has been limited in that it has primarily examined factors that influence the frequency of the to-be-suppressed target thought on a short-term basis and following a *counterinstruction* that explicitly encourages or implicitly permits the occurrence of the target thought. However, this research cannot inform us as to what would happen if individuals persisted unabated in a continued attempt to suppress the target thought. To be effective, perhaps suppression does not need to be absolutely or entirely successful directly from the beginning. Initial expression or thinking about an episode followed by thought suppression ultimately might be a more effective way to forget. Research exploring the consequences of a more sustained long-term effort to suppress, particularly after different degrees of initial elaboration and expression of the thought, is especially needed.

Likewise, as noted earlier in this chapter, further research on contextual factors in directed forgetting, particularly when larger episodes are involved (block cuing), is also needed. Research employing multidimensional and complex materials, especially emotionally significant materials, would be particularly valuable. In addition, it would be informative to begin to explore item cuing and block cuing within individuals rather than only across individuals. If the processes involved in the two procedures are, indeed, fundamentally different, are individuals especially adept at one form and not the other? Can individuals become more proficient at forgetting with appropriate instructions? The results of the study by Geiselman et al. (1985), discussed earlier, in which subjects who were instructed to use the mental "STOP" procedure rather than other less active and less focused strategies showed greater forgetting, suggest that more explicit strategy instructions may well enhance forgetting. However, comparable studies using the block-cuing procedure would also be informative. Also, many studies would benefit from a focus not only on the consequences of suppression or attempted forgetting on recall or recognition of the to-be-forgotten information but also on the degree to which memory for the target episodes corresponds to the earlier events—memory accuracy as well as accessibility (see Koriat and Goldsmith 1996). Explorations of the accessibility of contextual information under directed forgetting with the block-cuing procedure suggest that errors in monitoring the source of information (e.g., M. K. Johnson et al. 1993) might be especially pronounced for material that was earlier subjected to the intention to forget. What are the hazards for memory accuracy arising from attempts to consciously forget? Are the impairments in source memory documented thus far with the block-cuing method (Geiselman et al. 1983; Koutstaal 1996) due to the involvement of contextual representations in initiating forgetting in the first place? Or might more general decrements in accuracy be observed?

Horowitz (1986, cited in Greenberg 1995, p. 1283) has differentiated three types of adaptive control that a traumatized individual might exercise over intrusive cognitions: "(a) control over when, where, in what manner, and for how long the trauma is contemplated; (b) control over the self-concepts and world views that guide the review; and (c) control over what information about the trauma is considered and what is disregarded." Neither obsessive rumination nor complete failure to cognitively and emotionally work through trauma is likely to result in optimal adjustment. Nonetheless, a certain degree of intentional forgetting may in some—possibly many—cases ultimately prove to be a healthy response. An intrusive and too pervasive concern with abuse may undermine what one hopes to establish: present and future relationships that move beyond exploitation, toward increasing strength and autonomy. On the one hand, insufficient conscious awareness and emotional and conceptual understanding of the nature and ramifications of the abuse may leave individuals vulnerable to harmful consequences of abuse, including the possibility of repeated abuse. On the other hand, excessive intrusiveness of the abuse into consciousness and preoccupation with the abusive episodes also may leave individuals vulnerable and diminish functioning at all levels. Seeking greater understanding of when it is best to remember and when it is best to suppress or to forget is to some degree not only an open empirical question at the nomothetic level but also a deep empirical question—in the sense of rooted in experience—at the idiographic level. Nonetheless, experimental research can also provide guidance at this level and may ultimately provide understanding not only of the conditions that may allow survival but also of successful overcoming and healing.

References

Adams-Tucker C: Proximate effects of sexual abuse in children: a report on 28 children. Am J Psychiatry 139:1252–1256, 1982

Allen JJ, Iacono WG, Laravuso JJ, et al: An event-related potential investigation of posthypnotic recognition amnesia. J Abnorm Psychol 104:421–430, 1995

Barnhardt TM: Directed forgetting effects in explicit and implicit memory. Ph.D. Dissertation, University of Arizona, 1993

Basden BH, Basden DR: Directed forgetting: further comparisons of the item and list methods. Memory (in press)

Basden BH, Basden DR, Gargano GJ: Directed forgetting in implicit and explicit memory tests: a comparison of methods. J Exp Psychol Learn Mem Cogn 19:603–616, 1993a

Basden BH, Basden DR, Torzynski R: Directed forgetting in conceptual and perceptual implicit tests. Paper presented at the meeting of the Psychonomics Society, St. Louis, MO, November 1993b

Basden BH, Basden DR, Coe WC, et al: Retrieval inhibition in directed forgetting and posthypnotic amnesia. Int J Clin Exp Hypn 42:184–203, 1994

Beckmann J: Ruminative thought and the deactivation of an intention. Motivation and Emotion 18:317–334, 1994

Bjork RA: Retrieval inhibition as an adaptive mechanism in human memory, in Varieties of Memory and Consciousness: Essays in Honour of Endel Tulving. Edited by Roediger HL III, Craik FIM. Hillsdale, NJ, Lawrence Erlbaum, 1989, pp 309–330

Bjork RA, Bjork EL: Dissociations in the impact of to-be-forgotten information on memory. Paper presented at the annual meeting of the American Psychological Association, San Francisco, CA, August 1991

Bjork RA, Geiselman RE: Constituent processes in the differentiation of items in memory. J Exp Psychol Hum Learn Mem 4:347–361, 1978

Brandt J, Rubinsky E, Lassen G: Uncovering malingered amnesia. Ann N Y Acad Sci 444:502–503, 1985

Bray NW, Justice EM, Zahm DN: Two developmental transitions in selective remembering strategies. J Exp Child Psychol 36:43–55, 1983

Bray NW, Hersh RE, Turner LA: Selective remembering during adolescence. Developmental Psychology 21:290–294, 1985

Browne A, Finkelhor D: Impact of child sexual abuse: a review of the research. Psychol Bull 99:66–77, 1986

Burgess AW, Holmstrom LL: Adaptive strategies and recovery from rape. Am J Psychiatry 136:1278–1282, 1979

Christenson RM, Walker JM, Ross DR, et al: Reactivation of traumatic conflicts. Am J Psychiatry 138:984–985, 1981

Clark DM, Ball S, Pape D: An experimental investigation of thought suppression. Behav Res Ther 29:253–257, 1991

Clark DM, Winton E, Thynn L: A further experimental investigation of thought suppression. Behav Res Ther 31:207–210, 1993

Conte JR, Wolf S, Smith T: What sexual offenders tell us about prevention strategies. Child Abuse Negl 13:293–301, 1989

Conway M, Howell A, Giannopoulos C: Dysphoria and thought suppression. Cognitive Therapy and Research 15:153–166, 1991

Craik FIM, Tulving E: Depth of processing and the retention of words in episodic memory. J Exp Psychol Gen 104:268–294, 1975

Crowne DP, Marlowe D: The Approval Motive: Studies in Evaluative Dependence. New York, Wiley, 1964

Davies G, Thomson DM (eds): Memory in Context: Context in Memory. Chichester, Sussex, England, Wiley, 1988

Davis PJ: Repression and the inaccessibility of emotional memories, in Repression and Dissociation: Implications for Personality Theory, Psychopathology, and Health. Edited by Singer JL. Chicago, IL, University of Chicago Press, 1990, pp 387–403

Eisen MR: Return of the repressed: hypnoanalysis of a case of total amnesia. Int J Clin Exp Hypn 37:107–119, 1989

Epstein W, Wilder L: Searching for to-be-forgotten material in a directed forgetting task. J Exp Psychol 95:349–357, 1972

Everson MD, Hunter WM, Runyan DK, et al: Maternal support following disclosure of incest. Am J Orthopsychiatry 59:197–207, 1989

Feldman-Summers S, Pope KS: The experience of "forgetting" childhood abuse: a national survey of psychologists. J Consult Clin Psychol 62:636–639, 1994

Finkelhor D, Hotaling G, Lewis IA, et al: Sexual abuse in a national survey of adult men and women. Child Abuse Negl 14:19–28, 1990

Fivush R, Schwarzmueller A: Say it once again: effects of repeated questions on children's event recall. J Trauma Stress 8:555–580, 1995

Freeston MH, Ladouceur R, Provencher M, et al: Strategies used with intrusive thoughts: context, appraisal, mood, and efficacy. Journal of Anxiety Disorders 9:201–215, 1995

Gardiner JM, Java R: Recognition memory and awareness: an experiential approach. European Journal of Cognitive Psychology 5:337–346, 1993

Gardiner JM, Gawlik B, Richardson-Klavehn A: Maintenance rehearsal affects knowing not remembering; elaborative rehearsal affects remembering, not knowing. Psychonomic Bulletin and Review 1:107–110, 1994

Geiselman RE, Panting TM: Personality correlates of retrieval processes in intentional and unintentional forgetting. Personality and Individual Differences 6:685–691, 1985

Geiselman RE, Bjork RA, Fishman DL: Disrupted retrieval in directed forgetting: a link with posthypnotic amnesia. J Exp Psychol Gen 112:58–72, 1983

Geiselman RE, Rabow VE, Wachtel SL, et al: Strategy control in intentional forgetting. Human Learning 4:169–178, 1985

Goernert PN, Larson ME: The initiation and release of retrieval inhibition. J Gen Psychol 12:61–66, 1994

Golding JM, Long DL, MacLeod CM: You can't always forget what you want: directed forgetting of related words. Journal of Memory and Language 33:493–510, 1994

Goodman GS, Quas JA, Batterman-Faunce JM, et al: Predictors of accurate and inaccurate memories of traumatic events experienced in childhood. Consciousness and Cognition 3:269–294, 1994

Goschke T, Kuhl J: Representation of intentions: persisting activation in memory. J Exp Psychol Learn Mem Cogn 19:1211–1227, 1993

Greenberg MA: Cognitive processing of traumas: the role of intrusive thoughts and re-appraisals. Journal of Applied Social Psychology 25:1262–1296, 1995

Harnishfeger KK, Pope RS: Intending to forget: the development of cognitive inhibition in directed forgetting. J Exp Child Psychol 62:292–315, 1996

Hasher L, Zacks RT: Automatic and effortful processes in memory. J Exp Psychol Gen 108:356–388, 1979

Holmes DS: The evidence for repression: an examination of sixty years of research, in Repression and Dissociation: Implications for Personality Theory, Psychopathology, and Health. Edited by Singer JL. Chicago, IL, University of Chicago Press, 1990, pp 85–102

Holtgraves T, Hall R: Repressors: what do they repress and how do they repress it? Journal of Research in Personality 29:306–317, 1995

Homa D, Spieker S: Assessment of selective search as an explanation for intentional forgetting. J Exp Psychol 103:10–15, 1974

Horowitz MJ: Stress Response Syndromes, 2nd Edition. Northvale, NJ, Jason Aronson, 1986

Howard DV: Search and decision processes in intentional forgetting: a reaction time analysis. J Exp Psychol Hum Learn Mem 2:566–576, 1976

Howard DV, Goldin SE: Selective processing in encoding and memory: an analysis of resource allocation by kindergarten children. J Exp Child Psychol 27:87–95, 1979

Howe ML, Courage ML, Peterson C: How can I remember when "I" wasn't there: long-term retention of traumatic experiences and emergence of the cognitive self. Consciousness and Cognition 3:327–355, 1994

Howell A, Conway M: Mood and the suppression of positive and negative self-referent thoughts. Cognitive Therapy and Research 16:535–555, 1992

Johnson HM: Processes of successful intentional forgetting. Psychol Bull 116:274–292, 1994

Johnson MK, Hashtroudi S, Lindsay DS: Source monitoring. Psychol Bull 114:3–28, 1993

Kanak NJ, Stevens R: PI and RI in serial learning as a function of environmental context. Applied Cognitive Psychology 6:589–606, 1992

Kelly AE, Kahn JH: Effects of suppression of personal intrusive thoughts. J Pers Soc Psychol 66:998–1006, 1994

Kihlstrom JF, Glisky MI, Anguilo MJ: Dissociative tendencies and dissociative disorders. J Abnorm Psychol 103:117–124, 1994

Koriat A, Goldsmith M: Memory metaphors and the real-life/laboratory controversy: correspondence versus storehouse conceptions of memory. Behavioral Brain Science 19:167–228, 1996

Koutstaal W: Beyond content: The fate—or function?—of contextual information in directed forgetting. Ph.D. Dissertation, Harvard University, 1996

Koutstaal W, Schacter DL: Inaccuracy and inaccessibility in memory retrieval: contributions from cognitive psychology and neuropsychology, in Trauma and Memory: Clinical and Legal Controversies. Edited by Appelbaum PS, Uyehara LA, Elin MR. New York, Oxford University Press (in press)

Krystal JH, Bennet AL, Bremner JD, et al: Toward a cognitive neuroscience of dissociation and altered memory functions in post-traumatic stress disorder, in Neurobiological and Clinical Consequences of Stress: From Normal Adaptation to PTSD. Edited by Friedman MJ, Charney DS, Deutch AY. Philadelphia, PA, Lippincott-Raven, 1995, pp 239–269

Kuhl J: Volitional mediators of cognition-behavior consistency: self-regulatory processes and action versus state orientation, in Action Control: From Cognition to Behavior. Edited by Kuhl J, Beckmann J. New York, Springer-Verlag, 1985, pp 101–128

Kumar K, Wilkinson JCM: Thought stopping: a useful treatment in phobias of 'internal stimuli.' Br J Psychiatry 119:305–307, 1971

Kuyken W, Brewin CR: Intrusive memories of childhood abuse during depressive episodes. Behav Res Ther 32:525–528, 1994

Kuyken W, Brewin CR: Autobiographical memory functioning in depression and reports of early abuse. J Abnorm Psychol 104:585–591, 1995

Lane JD, Wegner DM: The cognitive consequences of secrecy. J Pers Soc Psychol 69:237–253, 1995

Lavy EH, van den Hout MA: Cognitive avoidance and attentional bias: causal relationships. Cognitive Therapy and Research 18:179–191, 1994

Lockhart RS: Conceptual specificity in thinking and remembering, in Memory in Context: Context in Memory. Edited by Davies GM, Thomson DM. Chichester, Sussex, England, Wiley, 1988, pp 319–331

Loftus E: The reality of repressed memories. Am Psychol 48:518–537, 1993

MacLeod C: Directed forgetting affects both direct and indirect tests of memory. J Exp Psychol Learn Mem Cogn 15:13–21, 1989

Macrae CN, Bodenhausen GV, Milne AB, et al: Out of mind but back in sight: stereotypes on the rebound. J Pers Soc Psychol 67:808–817, 1994

Mann SJ, Delon M: Improved hypertension control after disclosure of decades-old trauma. Psychosom Med 57:501–505, 1995

Mathews A, Milroy R: Effects of priming and suppression of worry. Behav Res Ther 32:843–850, 1994

McGee R: Flashbacks and memory phenomena: a comment on "flashback phenomena—clinical and diagnostic dilemmas." J Nerv Ment Dis 172:273–278, 1984

McGeoch JA: Forgetting and the law of disuse. Psychol Rev 39:352–370, 1932

Muris P, Merckelbach H, van den Hout M, et al: Suppression of emotional and neutral material. Behav Res Ther 30:639–642, 1992

Muris P, Merckelbach H, de Jong P: Verbalization and environmental cuing in thought suppression. Behav Res Ther 31:609–612, 1993

Myers LB, Brewin CR, Power MJ: Repression and autobiographical memory, in Theoretical Perspectives on Autobiographical Memory. Edited by Conway MA, Rubin DC, Spinnler H, et al. Dordrecht, The Netherlands, Kluwer Academic, 1992, pp 375–390

Nader K, Pynoos R, Fairbanks L, et al: Children's PTSD reactions one year after a sniper attack at their school. Am J Psychiatry 147:1526–1530, 1990

Nash MR: Memory distortion and sexual trauma: the problem of false negatives and false positives. Int J Clin Exp Hypn 42:346–362, 1994

Nelson K: The psychological and social origins of autobiographical memory. Psychological Science 4:1–8, 1993

Ofshe RJ, Singer MT: Recovered-memory therapy and robust repression: influence and pseudomemories. Int J Clin Exp Hypn 42:391–410, 1994

Parks ED, Balon R: Autobiographical memory for childhood events: patterns of recall in psychiatric patients with a history of alleged trauma. Psychiatry 58:199–208, 1995

Pope HG Jr, Hudson JI: Can memories of childhood sexual abuse be "repressed"? Psychol Med 25:121–126, 1995

Putnam FW: Dissociative disorders in children: behavioral profiles and problems. Child Abuse Negl 17:39–45, 1993

Roediger HL III, Crowder RC: Instructed forgetting: rehearsal control or retrieval inhibition (repression)? Cognitive Psychology 3:244–254, 1972

Roediger HL III, Weldon MS, Challis BH: Explaining dissociations between implicit and explicit measures of retention: a processing account, in Varieties of Memory and Consciousness: Essays in Honour of Endel Tulving. Edited by Roediger HL, Craik FIM. Hillsdale, NJ, Lawrence Erlbaum, 1989, pp 3–41

Roemer L, Borkovec TD: Effects of suppressing thoughts about emotional material. J Abnorm Psychol 103:467–474, 1994

Salkovskis PM, Campbell P: Thought suppression induces intrusion in naturally occurring negative intrusive thoughts. Behav Res Ther 32:1–8, 1994

Schacter DL: Feeling-of-knowing ratings distinguish between genuine and simulated forgetting. J Exp Psychol Learn Mem Cogn 12:30–41, 1986

Schacter DL: Priming and multiple memory systems: perceptual mechanisms of implicit memory, in Memory Systems 1994. Edited by Schacter DL, Tulving E. Cambridge, MA, MIT Press, 1994, pp 233–268

Schacter DL: Searching for Memory: The Brain, the Mind, and the Past. New York, Basic Books, 1996

Schacter DL, Wang PL, Tulving E, et al: Functional retrograde amnesia: a quantitative case study. Neuropsychologia 20:523–532, 1982

Schacter DL, Kihlstrom JF, Kihlstrom LC, et al: Autobiographical memory in a case of multiple personality disorder. J Abnorm Psychol 98:508–514, 1989

Schacter DL, Norman KA, Koutstaal W: The recovered memory debate: a cognitive neuroscience perspective, in False and Recovered Memories. Edited by Conway MA. New York, Oxford University Press (in press)

Schooler JW: Seeking the core: the issues and evidence surrounding recovered accounts of sexual trauma. Consciousness and Cognition 3:452–469, 1994

Silver RL, Boon C, Stones MH: Searching for meaning in misfortune: making sense of incest. Journal of Social Issues 39:81–102, 1983

Smith SM: Mood is a component of mental context: comment on Eich (1995). J Exp Psychol Gen 124:309–310, 1995

Spanos NP, James B, DeGroot HP: Detection of simulated hypnotic amnesia. J Abnorm Psychol 99:179–182, 1990

Spiegel D: Hypnosis and suggestion, in Memory Distortion: How Minds, Brains, and Societies Reconstruct the Past. Edited by Schacter DL, Coyle JT, Fischbach GD, et al. Cambridge, MA, Harvard University Press, 1995, pp 129–149

Spiegel D, Cardeña E: Disintegrated experience: the dissociative disorders revisited. J Abnorm Psychol 100:366–378, 1991

Taylor J: A personality scale of manifest anxiety. J Abnorm Soc Psychol 48:285–290, 1953

Tellegen A, Atkinson G: Openness to absorbing and self-altering experiences ("absorption"), a trait related to hypnotic susceptibility. J Abnorm Psychol 83:268–277, 1974

Tessler M, Nelson K: Making memories: the influence of joint encoding on later recall by young children. Consciousness and Cognition 3:307–326, 1994

Tomarken AJ, Davidson RJ: Frontal brain activation in repressors and nonrepressors. J Abnorm Psychol 103:339–349, 1994

Trickett PK, Putnam FW: Impact of child sexual abuse on females: toward a developmental, psychobiological integration. Psychological Science 4:81–87, 1993

Trinder H, Salkovskis PM: Personally relevant intrusions outside the laboratory: long-term suppression increases intrusion. Behav Res Ther 32:833–842, 1994

Tulving E: Elements of Episodic Memory. Oxford, UK, Clarendon Press, 1983

Tulving E, Pearlstone Z: Availability versus accessibility of information in memory for words. Journal of Verbal Learning and Verbal Behavior 5:381–391, 1966

Turner SM, Holzman A, Jacob RG: Treatment of compulsive looking by imaginal thought-stopping. Behav Modif 7:576–582, 1983

Uleman JS: A framework for thinking intentionally about unintended thoughts, in Unintended Thought. Edited by Uleman JS, Bargh JA. New York, Guilford, 1989, pp 425–449

Wegner DM: White Bears and Other Unwanted Thoughts. New York, Guilford, 1994

Wegner DM, Erber R: The hyperaccessibility of suppressed thoughts. J Pers Soc Psychol 63:903–912, 1992

Wegner DM, Gold DB: Fanning old flames: emotional and cognitive effects of suppressing thoughts of a past relationship. J Pers Soc Psychol 68:782–792, 1995

Wegner DM, Schneider DJ, Carter SR III, et al: Paradoxical effects of thought suppression. J Pers Soc Psychol 53:5–13, 1987

Wegner DM, Shortt JW, Blake AW, et al: The suppression of exciting thoughts. J Pers Soc Psychol 58:409–418, 1990

Wegner DM, Schneider DJ, Knutson B, et al: Polluting the stream of consciousness: the effect of thought suppression on the mind's environment. Cognitive Therapy and Research 15:141–152, 1991

Wegner DM, Erber R, Zanakos S: Ironic processes in the mental control of mood and mood-related thought. J Pers Soc Psychol 65:1093–1104, 1993

Weinberger DA, Schwartz GE, Davidson RJ: Low-anxious, high-anxious, and repressive coping styles: psychometric patterns and behavioral and physiological responses to stress. J Abnorm Psychol 88:369–380, 1979

Weiner B: Motivated forgetting and the study of repression. J Pers 36:213–234, 1968

Wenzlaff RM, Wegner DM, Roper DW: Depression and mental control: the resurgence of unwanted negative thoughts. J Pers Soc Psychol 55:882–892, 1988

Wenzlaff RM, Wegner DM, Klein SB: The role of thought suppression in the bonding of thought and mood. J Pers Soc Psychol 60:500–508, 1991

Williams JMG: Autobiographical memory and emotional disorders, in The Handbook of Emotion and Memory: Research and Theory. Edited by Christianson S-A. Hillsdale, NJ, Lawrence Erlbaum, 1992, pp 451–477

Williams LM: Recall of childhood trauma: a prospective study of women's memories of child sexual abuse. J Consult Clin Psychol 62:1167–1176, 1994

Williams LM: Recovered memories of abuse in women with documented child sexual victimization histories. J Trauma Stress 8:649–673, 1995

Williamsen JA, Johnson HJ, Eriksen CW: Some characteristics of posthypnotic amnesia. J Abnorm Psychol 70:123–131, 1965

Chapter 9

Perspectives on Adult Memories of Childhood Sexual Abuse: A Research Review

Linda M. Williams, Ph.D., and Victoria L. Banyard, Ph.D.

Adult memories and recollection of childhood sexual abuse are the focus of both increasing interest and continuing controversy for researchers, clinicians, and lawyers in the field of child maltreatment. News of cases of recovered memories for sexual abuse and opposing views about the veracity of such accounts have appeared in media ranging from the popular press to academic journals and conference symposia. No longer is the focus of media attention on the incidence and prevalence of child sexual abuse, drawing attention to the seriousness of a long hidden problem. Indeed, a recent review of the coverage of the issue of child sexual abuse in the popular news media found that 73% of the articles about child sexual abuse during 1992–1994 were focused on the issue of false accusations in general. In 1994, 65% of the articles on child sexual abuse dealt with the specific issue of false memories (Beckett 1996), portraying recovered memories of abuse as unreliable and emphasizing the damage false accusations do to families and wrongly accused individuals. Beckett suggests that this refocus of public attention on false allegations may be a consequence of increased attention to cases of abuse in which family members were the perpetrators. When abuse is seen as a threat to children by dangerous "outsiders," then the societal response is unified or solidaristic. However, when alleged perpetrators are insiders such as family members (Beckett 1996), or community leaders such as priests, judges, and other professionals, the social fabric is disrupted and a social denial is elicited.

Achieving a better understanding of memory for traumatic events is crucial for both researchers who study the effects of child maltreatment and clinicians who work with trauma survivors. Andrews et al. (1995) surveyed British psychotherapists and found that 51% of therapists who worked with sexually abused patients reported that they had seen patients who, during some period, did not have a clear memory for the sexual abuse. Proponents of different sides of this debate have

This research was supported by the U.S. Department of Health and Human Services, National Center on Child Abuse and Neglect, Grant 90-CA-1552.

cautioned practitioners against what they see as the widespread use of *memory recovery therapy,* the danger of creating false memories in the minds of those in treatment for emotional problems (Lindsay and Read 1994), and the negative consequences of being unsupportive of memory recovery (Herman 1992). Clearly, the questions about memory and child sexual abuse are important for anyone practicing in the field of child maltreatment. To understand this issue, however, it is necessary to look beyond the rhetoric and to examine what we really know about this phenomenon. Such is the aim of this chapter. We review and synthesize recent empirical findings on the impact of childhood sexual abuse on adult memory by drawing from a diverse empirical literature from the fields of cognitive, developmental, and clinical psychology; psychiatry; and child maltreatment.

We consider several basic questions in this chapter:

1. Are memories of childhood events different from memories of adulthood experiences because of developmental differences in the structure of memory systems of children and adults?
2. Is memory for trauma different, or does it operate in different ways, from everyday, declarative memory?
3. Do memories of childhood sexual abuse at any age differ qualitatively from memories of other events, even memories of other trauma?

We must ask not only how the experience of trauma may influence memory but also how the experience of sexual abuse may influence memory. In the second section of this chapter, we consider the empirical evidence that supports the likelihood that childhood sexual abuse can be forgotten, that memories of childhood sexual abuse can be implanted, and that memories of such abuse, once forgotten, can be recovered.

A Developmental Perspective on Memory

An extensive body of research on adult memory and memory for autobiographical events has raised a number of important issues. Research on memory processes more generally, for example, has shown that memory is imperfect (Rogers 1995), although investigators disagree about the degree to which memory is fallible and under what conditions (Brewin et al. 1993; Henry et al. 1994). Various studies suggest that all experiences or aspects of experiences are not encoded and stored and that more experience is in fact forgotten than is remembered (Lindsay and Read 1994; Squire 1989). Other work has focused on the conditions under which memory errors occur. Research has shown that the memory of both adults and children may be affected by the way that questions are asked, the presentation of new or misleading information, or prior knowledge (Belli and Loftus 1994; Ceci et al. 1981; Hyman and Pentland 1996; Loftus and Davies 1984; Loftus et al. 1992).

In addition to the general comment that memory is fallible, to understand memory function more fully requires taking a developmental perspective. This is particularly true if we wish to understand the process of memory as it pertains to sexual abuse experienced in childhood. Many different theories exist about the development of the memory system in childhood and about when memories are possible and how accurate they are (see Howe and Courage 1993 or Pillemer and White 1989 for extensive reviews of this literature).

Of particular interest to developmentalists and memory researchers has been the observation that adults do not seem to have any memories of events that occurred earlier than age 2–4 years. This phenomenon has been called "infantile" or "childhood amnesia" (Nelson 1988) and has been the subject of much theoretical discussion. Some researchers have posited that memory operates differently in childhood and in adulthood and that this explains the lack of adult memories for early childhood events. Nadel and Zola-Morgan (1984), for example, stated that structural, neurological differences between memory systems available to infants and those available to older children/adults create this absence of early memories. Others assert that the main differences are cognitive in nature (Usher and Neisser 1993), suggesting that childhood memories are encoded differently from adult memories or that lack of verbal skills in young children makes retrieval of information from that time impossible (Nelson and Ross 1980). Pillemer and White (1989) have even posited the existence of two independent memory systems—one that operates from birth and can process very general memories for various skills and routines and a second that develops later in early childhood that enables the individual to retain memories for more specific events and information. In a recent article, Schacter et al. (1995) review research that draws some limited parallels between memory errors made by children and those of patients with damage to the frontal lobe. Although Schacter and colleagues raised more questions than they answered, their review suggested a hypothesis that developmental differences in frontal-lobe maturity may partially account for age differences in memory errors, and they urge more research to be conducted in this area. What all these researchers have in common is the shared hypothesis that the memory systems of infants and young children have some type of structural differences that interfere with the long-term retention or accessibility of memories of events that occurred during this time.

In contrast, another group of researchers dispute the notion of a phenomenon such as infantile amnesia. They assert that no empirical evidence indicates differences in the memory systems of young children and adults. Memory, according to this view, does not become reorganized at some point in childhood but remains the same for children as it is for adults (Fivush and Hammond 1990; Howe and Courage 1993; Nelson 1988). They explain adults' lack of early memories by examining other aspects of cognitive and social development that affect the memory system. Fivush and Reese (1992), for example, discuss the fact that children seem to learn social rules for what is important to remember through conversations with parents. The lack of these rules early in childhood may lead to memories that are fragmented and difficult to retrieve and the appearance of infantile amnesia. Howe and Courage (1993) pay particular attention to the cognitive development of the child's sense of self. They assert that children have all the required memory systems at birth, but it is not until around age 2 years, when a coherent sense of self has developed, that true autobiographical memories about the self are possible. These theorists suggest that children's memory is not structurally any different from that of adults and that forgetting of childhood events may be related to other aspects of social and cognitive development more than to any developmental immaturity of the child's memory systems. Even these theories, however, raise questions about whether children can be expected to retain complex memories for events that occur before age 4 years.

Indeed, Goodman and colleagues' (1994) review of the literature on children's memories seems to show that regardless of whether memory structures are the same or different from that of adults, a variety of evidence indicates that some long-term retention of childhood events, particularly those that occur after age 4, as well as inaccessibility of these memories, is possible. Goodman et al. (1994) cited evidence that memories of young children, even after the period of disputed "infantile amnesia," may be more open to distortion by outside influences, and these young children may need more cues from others or the environment to recall certain events or information. Some aspects of memory develop over the course of childhood as children become more skilled at processes such as attaching meaning to memories. Such research suggests that, for developmental reasons, childhood events cannot always be expected to be clearly remembered. Goodman et al. (1994) also empirically examined children's memories of a traumatic and invasive medical procedure. Age predicted accurate recall of the event, and children age 5 years and older had more accurate memories that were less open to modification by outside information than did children ages 3 or 4. However, other, more individual, differences were also important—factors such as the emotional reaction of the child to the procedure (children who reported high levels of embarrassment had more memory errors), social support by a parent (children whose mothers were less supportive and talked with them less about the event had less accurate recall), and the child's prior knowledge of the medical procedure (children who had more knowledge had more accurate recall).

What are the implications of these studies of general memory processes for memories of traumatic events such as child sexual abuse? Again, this area of study is characterized by considerable controversy and disagreement. Some researchers suggest that memories for traumatic events are the same as for other events, suggesting that normal developmental differences in memories for childhood events may explain why some survivors of abuse have no or impaired recall of the trauma. Others provide evidence for a distinction, stating that trauma has unique effects on memory that may result in impaired recall. One avenue of investigation has examined the effect of emotion on memory based on the notion that the emotional salience of traumatic events may exert particular effects on memory.

The Impact of Emotion on Memory

Memory researchers have studied the impact of emotion on memory and have examined the question: "Are memories for highly emotionally salient events more clearly remembered?" Brown and Kulik (1977), for example, discussed their discovery of what they termed *flashbulb memories*. These are memories for highly salient and surprising events that seem to create permanent memories of even minute details of the situation, such as an imprint of the details of where one was at the time one learned of John F. Kennedy's assassination. Others, such as Rubin and Kozin (1984), have looked more broadly at "vivid memories," which seem to be associated with surprising and important events. Some have critiqued these theories and this research and asserted that memories such as "flashbulb memories" may not be accurate (Neisser, cited in Rubin and Kozin 1984). Although some research reports that high emotional arousal can lead to narrowing of one's attention and less accurate memories for details of the event or can decrease recall for other stimuli around or previous to the event (Burke et al. 1992; Kramer et al. 1991; Loftus and Burns 1982), in a review of this literature, Koss et al. (1995) found that "emotional memories have been characterized as 'detailed, accurate, and persistent' and ratings of intense emotional reaction are predictive of better, not worse, recall" (p. 124). In terms of sexual abuse, such theories would suggest that the central elements of traumatic events may be better remembered than those of nontraumatic events because of their emotional salience.

Memory for Traumatic Events Is the Same as That for Other Events

Overall, the evidence seems to indicate that central details of emotionally salient events are well remembered by individuals over time, but these memories are not immune to modifying influences (Howe et al. 1994; Loftus and Christianson 1989). However, are memories for traumatic events—situations in which emotional arousal is extremely high—different in some way from memories for more neutral events? A number of researchers do not believe so. Loftus and Christianson (1989), for example, did not find evidence that traumatic or highly emotional stimuli are more well remembered than other events and even suggested that they may be less well remembered than neutral stimuli and may be more susceptible to misinformation given after the memory has formed. Loftus (1993) asserted that evidence of forgetting incidents of childhood sexual abuse may be the result of the same process of forgetting that affects individuals' memories for any event and that no unique process is at work because the event is traumatic. Howe et al. (1994) conducted a study of children's memories of a traumatic injury that led to an emergency room visit. They concluded that these traumatic events were not remembered differently from other events. The degree of stress of the child was not related to how well the event was recalled. Furthermore, although central details of the event were reasonably well remembered even 6 months later, children's recollection of more peripheral details declined over time, as would be predicted by theories of normal forgetting. They stated:

> This finding is consistent with our proposal that traumatic and autobiographical events enjoy no special status in long-term memory. That is, unlike what some theorists would have us believe (e.g., Freud 1953), these memories are not held in some secret repository that is immune to the ravages of normal forgetting. Rather, like all memories, early autobiographical memories and memories for traumatic events are subject to the same laws that govern the retention of memories in general. (Howe et al. 1994, p. 347)

The points raised by such research are important to consider and highlight the ways in which memory systems may operate similarly across a variety of situations. There are some limitations, however. As Goodman et al. (1994) have discussed in relation to their own work on children's memories for hospitalizations, qualitative differences may persist between these emotionally difficult events and the types of trauma caused by child abuse or other life-threatening experiences such as rape and combat that may produce symptoms of posttraumatic stress disorder. These extreme forms of trauma may have a more direct and noticeable effect on memory systems.

Memory for Traumatic Events Is Different From That for Other Events

In contrast to the view that memories for traumatic events are the same as for any other experience, a number of researchers have discussed the ways in which traumatic memories may be different. These researchers tend to focus on the most extreme forms of traumatic events—child sexual abuse and wartime combat. Their research provides evidence that trauma does influence memory at the biological, psychological, and social levels. It creates the conditions for the formation of both indelible memories that continually reappear in consciousness through processes such as flashbacks and nightmares and pockets of amnesia for aspects of the traumatic experience.

van der Kolk has been one of the major proponents of this point of view (van der Kolk, in press; van der Kolk and Fisler 1995; van der Kolk and van der Hart 1991). van der Kolk has raised questions about whether the typical studies of trauma and memory that are conducted in the laboratory, where participants are shown a series of slides, some of which contain traumatic material such as watching a shooting, are really comparable to memory for real-life traumatic events. He and others assert that trauma can have profound physiological effects on brain structures such as the hippocampus that are key components of the memory system (see Bremner et al. 1995; Hartman and Burgess 1993; Siegel 1995; van der Kolk, in press, for a more extensive review of this literature). Prolonged stress responses that occur when an individual is traumatized may alter normal physiological stress and memory processes. This can lead to both "a strengthening of particular memory traces related to traumatic events, as well as gaps in memory, which are known as amnestic episodes" (Bremner et al. 1995, p. 531). This research is in its early stages but is further supported by studies such as that conducted by Cahill et al. (1994). They examined the hypothesis that better memory for emotionally salient events was related to activation of the β-adrenergic system. Human participants were divided into two groups—those who saw slides depicting a neutral story and those who saw a more emotional story about a boy in a life-threatening accident. Some participants were given a substance (propranolol) that blocks the β-adrenergic system, and others were given a placebo. The inhibitory substance had no effect on memory for the neutral stimulus but did decrease recall for details of the more emotionally salient event. This study demonstrates a link between the β-adrenergic system and memory and suggests ways in which physiological stress responses triggered by emotionally salient events can enhance memory for these events. These studies contribute to an understanding of how memories for traumatic events may be different and more indelible and well remembered.

In addition to differences in the physiology of traumatic events and memories of such events, recent research has also focused on psychological factors that may differentiate traumatic memories from others and thus explain why traumatic events may be less well remembered. van der Kolk and Fisler (1995), for example, presented some preliminary findings from a study of differences between traumatic and nontraumatic memories in patients with posttraumatic stress disorder. He found that the traumatic memories tended to be initially remembered "in the form of somatosensory or emotional flashback experiences" (p. 517). Traumatic memories seem to be experienced more in terms of bodily sensations, visual images, sounds, and so on rather than as a verbal narrative. van der Kolk used this finding as preliminary evidence to support his theory that memories of trauma may be initially sensorimotor in nature and may not be completely well organized. An individual may be, therefore, unable to verbalize the memory although she or he has some access to it. Enns et al. (1995) reviewed a variety of other research on cognitive theories of traumatic memory. They discussed the idea that trauma may affect cognitive information processing systems in several ways. It may lead to the use of dissociation or repression, mechanisms that limit information that is taken in or that can be retrieved from memory for the event. They also highlighted the ways in which trauma can disturb one's assumptions about oneself and one's world (Janoff-Bulman, cited in Enns et al. 1995). This threatening and inconsistent material may not easily fit into existing schemata about one's experience, and incomplete processing of this information may result (Enns et al. 1995).

Freyd (1994) also presented a theoretical argument for the effect of trauma on cognitive processing. She argued that amnesia may be an important survival strategy when an individual is confronted with traumatic stress, and sexual abuse in particular. As a coping strategy, "forgetting" one's abuse may allow one to maintain needed attachments to a perpetrator who may also be an important caregiver. She focused on the impact of traumatic betrayal as an important influence of trauma on memory. Although her discussion is purely theoretical, she concludes that "the degree to which a trauma involves a sense of having been fundamentally cheated or betrayed by another person may significantly influence the individual's cognitive encoding of the experience of trauma, the degree to which the event is easily accessible to awareness, and the psychological as well as behavioral responses" (p. 308).

Finally, the social context in which the trauma occurs and the ways in which social factors may affect the formation of traumatic memories have begun to be discussed. Fivush and Schwartzmuller (1995) reviewed research on how children recall events and the effect of questioning on children's reported memories. In this review, they suggested that a child's rehearsal of an event by talking to another person about it may aid the memory process. In situations in which the event is an incident of child abuse, however, this verbal rehearsing often may not occur because the event is kept secret. This may lead to impaired or less clear memories for such events. A study by Tromp et al. (1995) also speaks to the powerful role that silencing may play in the processing of traumatic memories for rape. They conducted a survey of 3,210 women, asking them to describe memories of a rape experience or other significant life event. They found that rape memories were different from other unpleasant memories in several important ways. Rape memories were rated as being more unpleasant and were also reported to be less well remembered and less talked and thought about. In their discussion of these results, the authors noted that victims of rape often remain silent about their experiences, and this silence may affect the memory process. Although research has not shown that events must be frequently talked or thought about in order to be remembered for any length of time, some investigators believe that sharing memories of events with others helps to change memories—to make them more connected to other memories and more integrated into one's experience. Tromp et al. (1995) hypothesized that when rape memories are not discussed, either because the victim cannot put her experiences into words or because she fears being blamed for the rape, these memories may not be erased but are simply kept outside of awareness and continue to influence her behavior or emotions because they have not been integrated into the larger scheme of her experience. van der Kolk and van der Hart (1991, p. 431) asserted that "in contrast to narrative memory, which is a social act, traumatic memory is inflexible and invariable. Traumatic memory has no social component; it is not addressed to anybody, the patient does not respond to anybody; it is a solitary activity."

Recall of Childhood Sexual Abuse

Thus far, the discussion of the research on memory has not permitted us to reach any definitive conclusions about memories of sexual abuse in childhood. Indeed, in many respects, more questions have been raised than answered. For example, Bremner and colleagues (1995) have found that child sexual abuse is associated with long-term deficits in verbal short-term memory. Their findings add to a growing literature that supports a relation between stress and alterations in memory. Neurobiological correlates of the effects of stress on memory may provide potential explanations for delayed recall of memories of childhood sexual abuse, but studies to date have provided only an incomplete picture of this phenomenon.

Much of the current controversy around this issue is fueled by contradictory research findings and a wide variety of difficulties encountered in conducting research on this topic (Carlson 1996). One of the difficulties in understanding the nature of adults' memories of childhood sexual abuse is that these are real, not laboratory-derived, events. The characteristics of the abuse and its timing cannot be controlled by researchers. It is also difficult to construct good analogue studies of memories of abuse, although some research with children has examined memories of interpersonal touching (Leippe et al. 1991) and medical procedures that involve the genitalia (Goodman et al. 1994; Saywitz et al. 1991). A complication of naturalistic studies of memory for sexual abuse is that child molestation usually occurs in private, and only rarely are other adults or even other children present. Thus, follow-up studies of memories of such abuse are plagued by incomplete data on what actually transpired during the abuse. Corroboration may simply be unavailable in most cases.

Research has documented the relevant characteristics of child sexual abuse (e.g., secrecy, threats of harm to child or others, grooming of the child to accept the sexual contact) that might dramatically affect memories of these events in ways that differ from memories of other types of traumatic childhood events (e.g., witnessing the death of a parent). Nevertheless, most of what is known about the dynamics and patterns of child sexual abuse comes from retrospective reports of adults molested during childhood (Finkelhor 1979; Herman 1992; Russell 1986) or perpetrators of the abuse (Conte et al. 1989; Williams and Finkelhor 1995) and is subject to possible distortion, confabulation, and other errors of memory.

Researchers have used a simple 2 × 2 table to examine the intersection of true abuse status (not abused/abused) and memory status (recalls/does not recall) (McHugh 1994; Spiegel 1993). Figure 9–1 is a

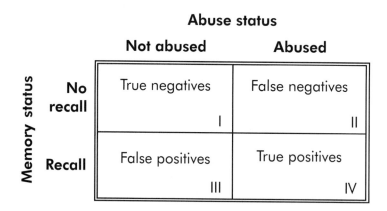

Figure 9–1. A 2 × 2 table of abuse and memory status.

diagram of this 2 × 2 table. Quadrant I represents those who were not abused and recall no abuse experiences (true negatives). Quadrant II includes those who were abused but do not recall the abuse (false negatives). Quadrant III represents those who were not abused but recall such experiences (false positives). Quadrant IV includes those who were abused and recall the abuse (true positives).

Consideration of the 2 × 2 table brings into focus a number of important issues in the debate about memories of childhood sexual abuse. The research and the theoretical focus of trauma researchers have centered on the right side of this table (false negatives and true positives), because these quadrants comprise all those who have been abused. The negative consequences of abuse and the symptomatology that brings many adult survivors of abuse in quadrant IV into contact with the medical and mental health systems have been well documented (Beitchman et al. 1992; Briere 1992; Browne and Finkelhor 1986). The work of trauma researchers has also focused on the problem of false negatives (quadrant II). At first, clinicians and researchers concentrated on false negatives attributable not to the victim's actual memory of the abuse but to the inadequacy of screening questions, for example, when a social and psychological history was taken on individuals presenting with psychiatric symptoms. It has been observed that asking behaviorally specific questions about abuse history or asking detailed questions about trauma history readily uncovers such histories in many patients (Briere and Zaidi 1989). Only relatively recently has attention been directed to the problems of truly forgotten abuse among clinical samples (Briere 1992; Courtois 1992; Herman 1992; L. Terr, "True memories of childhood trauma: quirks, absences, and returns," unpublished manuscript, Langley Porter Psychiatric Institute, University of California–San Francisco, 1994). Research in these areas has involved clinical, not laboratory, work.

On the other hand, researchers and practitioners concerned with the problem of false accusations have focused on the lower half of the 2 × 2 table, especially quadrant III (false positives). It is interesting that the label of "false memory" has come to be used to describe "false memories of abuse when such abuse did not really happen," but this label has not been used to refer to "false memories of no abuse when such abuse did indeed occur" (false negatives). In part, because the work of researchers in this area is driven by issues of criminal or civil defense (see Neimark 1996), significant attention has been given to examination of forensic issues, and laboratory research has attended to confabulation and errors of memory. Much of the work in this area has focused on suggestibility and problems of source attribution (i.e., the memory errors that arise when an individual recalls information that came from some source after the event and when that individual goes on to erroneously attribute the information to the original event).

Much of the debate about memory of childhood sexual abuse has focused on how cases are distributed among each of the quadrants in Figure 9–1 and on the explanations for how and why individuals come to falsely believe that they were not abused when, in fact, they were abused and to falsely believe that they were abused when, in fact, they were not. Some of the contentiousness (Berliner and Loftus 1992) in this false memory debate may have occurred because of communication errors, the differential attention paid to each quadrant by trauma researchers and memory researchers, different strategies for clinical and laboratory research, and the application of clinical research methods to quadrants II and IV and laboratory research designs to quadrant III. There has been little crossover in either direction to date. In the next several sections of this chapter, we review relevant research in the second, third, and fourth quadrants of the figure: false negatives, false positives, and true positives.

Forgetting Childhood Sexual Abuse—False Negatives

One critical research question at the root of the debate on "recovered" memory is, "How common is it to have no memory of sexual abuse that occurred in one's childhood?" People forget myriad ordinary experiences, but do people forget childhood sexual abuse, especially if the abuse was traumatic and occurred after the offset of infantile amnesia? This question has been raised repeatedly in the debate about memories of childhood sexual abuse. Loftus (1995) and others (Pope and Hudson 1995; Wakefield and Underwager 1991) have suggested that to have no recall of abuse is uncommon and argue that no evidence indicates that a child would forget a truly traumatic event unless the event occurred before age 3 years. However, other research documents the prevalence of this phenomenon.

Much of the research specifically focused on adults' experiences with forgetting childhood sexual abuse is based on naturalistic studies of clinical samples of women and men in treatment for the consequences of sexual abuse. This research reveals that many adults who recall sexual abuse in childhood report prior periods when they did not remember the abuse. Herman and Schatzow (1987) reported "severe memory deficits" for abuse in 28% of their clinical sample of women in group therapy for incest survivors. Approximately two-thirds of their sample (64%) reported some degree of "amnesia." Briere and Conte (1993) found that 59% of 450 women and men in treatment for sexual abuse reported that, at some time before age 18, they had forgotten the sexual abuse they endured during childhood. Loftus et al. (1994b) reported that a sizable minority (31%) of their sample of sexually abused women in treatment for substance abuse had at least partial forgetting or incomplete memory of their abuse, and 19% reported prior periods of total lack of recall of the abuse. Gold et al. (1994) reported that 30% of patients in outpatient psychotherapy for treatment of the traumatic effects of childhood sexual abuse claimed to have previously completely blocked out any recollection of the abuse for a year or more. These studies and many others now appearing in the published literature indicate that a significant minority of victims of child sexual abuse in treatment report prior periods of forgetting.

Even in nonclinical samples of adults, a high rate of prior periods of forgetting childhood sexual abuse is reported. Among a national sample of psychologists, Feldman-Summers and Pope (1994) found that of the 79 participants who experienced childhood sexual abuse, 40% reported that they could not remember some or all of their abuse during an earlier period. D. M. Elliott ("Traumatic Events: Prevalence and Delayed Recall in the General Population," unpublished manuscript, Harbor-UCLA Medical Center, 1995) conducted a study of a national, stratified, random sample of 505 women and men. Of the sample, 23% reported a history of childhood sexual abuse, and, of these, 20% reported a time when they had no memory of this event, and an additional 22% reported a time when they had less memory of this event than they did at the time of the interview.

It has been suggested that rather than providing evidence of false negatives, the fact that many respondents from clinical samples report prior periods of forgetting may simply be attributable to false positives. The argument is that these respondents' "memories" of abuse may have been recovered under the influence of therapists who believe that amnesia for sexual abuse is common. However, no evidence is found in the studies of clinical samples that most of the memories were recovered by therapy. It is perhaps more feasible that if prior periods of forgetting or recently recovered memories of childhood sexual abuse are associated with higher rates of symptomatology (Elliott and Briere 1995), then we would expect those individuals who were sexually abused in childhood and who are currently in treatment for such symptomatology to have a higher rate of prior forgetting than those who are not in treatment. Studies that rely on community samples overcome problems associated with sampling bias and the possibility of an elevated rate of prior forgetting in clinical samples. Both community studies and clinical samples, however, used a retrospective methodology to gather information about forgetting of childhood sexual abuse and, as a result, are subject to the problem that such abuse is usually uncorroborated. In addition, studies must rely on retrospective accounts of prior forgetting, yet the validity of these accounts is unknown.

Finally, retrospective designs are unable to examine instances in which sexual abuse experienced in childhood continues to be forgotten. Obviously, researchers cannot survey adults and ask whether they were abused in childhood but have now forgotten. For this reason, two prospective-cohorts-design studies of child sexual abuse, in which abused and neglected children were followed up prospectively into adulthood, have received much attention.

Williams (1994) followed up women and men (Williams and Banyard 1996) who, in the early 1970s, were seen in a hospital emergency room for child sexual abuse and found that (17 years post abuse) 38% of the women ($n = 129$) and 55% of the men ($n = 47$) did not recall the abuse. Williams also reported that of the 80 women who recalled the documented abuse, 16% stated that there was a time in the past when they did not remember that it had happened to them. In a similar study, C. S. Widom ("Accuracy of adult reports of child abuse," unpublished manuscript, State University of New York at Albany, 1996) found that 32% of women ($n = 70$) and 58% of men ($n = 19$) with court-substantiated reports of child sexual victimization did not report such abuse on re-interview some 20 years later.

Neither study design called for directly confronting participants who appeared to have forgotten the abuse with the evidence of abuse documented in their records from the 1970s (a decision based on concern for protection of human subjects). It is, of course, possible that some of the interviewed men and women in these studies simply did not wish to talk about the abuse or were too embarrassed or ashamed to do so. Femina et al. (1990) reported that adolescents, when confronted with a failure to report a history of childhood physical abuse, indicated they were too ashamed or embarrassed to talk about it to the interviewer. Those investigators (Lindsay and Read 1994; Pope and Hudson 1995) who cite Femina et al. as evidence of deliberate nondisclosure fail to note that the Femina study was a follow-up of not only individuals who denied their abuse histories but also those who reported but minimized their abuse. The critical subsample in this study was also very small. In fact, only 8 of the 18 subjects who denied or minimized the documented abuse were recontacted for the clarification interview to determine whether they were deliberately denying the event or had actually forgotten it.

Williams (1994) contends that it is unlikely that embarrassment was the reason that so many women did not report the abuse in her study. Of the women who did not recall the child sexual abuse that brought them into the study (the "index" abuse), 68% told the interviewer about other sexual assaults (clearly involving different perpetrators and circumstances) that they experienced in childhood. Of the women who did recall the "index" abuse, the same proportion (68%) reported other incidents of child sexual abuse, indicating that those who did not recall the index abuse were no less likely to reveal details of other personal, upsetting, or potentially embarrassing experiences. The two prospective studies (C. S. Widom, "Accuracy of adult reports of child abuse," unpublished manuscript, State University of New York at Albany, 1996;

Williams 1994) have remarkably similar findings and are also consistent with the data from clinical samples. Although we cannot conclusively report what proportion of abuse victims forget, these studies suggest that a significant proportion of those with documented histories of sexual abuse in childhood, when reinterviewed as young adults, do not recall the abuse.

Mechanisms for forgetting child sexual abuse. In earlier sections of this chapter, we reviewed some of the literature on memory and the mechanisms that may play a role in remembering or forgetting traumatic experiences. If many abuse survivors forget experiences of childhood sexual abuse or report periods of not remembering, what evidence do we have about the mechanisms for such forgetting? Various explanations are likely. Clinicians and researchers who have suggested that the findings from these studies provide evidence for certain theories about the actual mechanisms for the forgetting have been harshly criticized (Loftus and Ketcham 1994; Loftus et al. 1994a; Pope and Hudson 1995). These critics suggest that deliberate nondisclosure, allegations of amnesia for secondary gain (Pope and Hudson 1995), and normal forgetting (Loftus et al. 1994a) account for the "lack of recall" in these studies. They argue against any specific psychological mechanisms associated with abuse or other forms of traumatic stress. However, there is a growing body of scientific evidence on the psychological effects and memories of abuse (Briere and Conte 1993; Elliott and Briere 1995; Herman and Schatzow 1987) and clinical literature on survivors of child sexual abuse (see, for example, Briere 1992; Herman 1992; Terr 1988, 1990, 1991; van der Kolk and Fisler 1995) that provides support for trauma theory, which suggests that forgetting abuse reflects the use of psychological mechanisms such as cognitive avoidance, dissociation, and repression as coping strategies for the psychological distress associated with prior traumatic events.

In several studies, young age at the time of abuse has been associated with prior periods of forgetting (Briere and Conte 1993; Elliott, unpublished data, 1995; Herman and Schatzow 1987; Williams 1994). Although infantile amnesia and cognitive developmental processes could explain the forgetting by the youngest victims, several studies have documented such forgetting even among those who were older at the time of victimization (C. S. Widom, "Accuracy of Adult Reports of Child Abuse," unpublished manuscript, State University of New York at Albany, 1996; Williams 1994). Certainly, in some cases, the abuse may not be remembered because it was not very important, and a long time has passed. In cases of relatively less dramatic experiences, especially in people whose lives are full of other traumatic events, an episode or two of sexual touching by someone unimportant may simply be forgotten.

Clinical literature on adult survivors of child sexual abuse suggests that the aversiveness of the experience may lead some victims to engage in active strategies to avoid reminders of traumatic events and ultimately memories of the event. Over time, coping mechanisms may cause the experience to recede until it is accessible only with certain stimuli (Briere 1992). Both Briere and Conte (1993) and Herman and Schatzow (1987) found that, among their treatment-seeking respondents, having a prior period of no recall of the abuse was associated with *more violent episodes* of abuse and *younger age at the time of the abuse*. Herman and Schatzow suggested that massive repression was the main defensive resource available to their patients who were sexually and/or violently abused in early childhood. Briere and Conte suggested that the association they found between no recall and *trauma* (as measured by violence or injury) and the lack of association between no recall and *conflict* (as measured by guilt, shame, and enjoyment) fit better with the process of dissociation than with an active defensive process of repression. Similarly, Terr (1991) suggested that what she calls type II traumas (long-standing or repeated ordeals) may be more likely to result in denial and dissociation. Briere and Conte suggested that young age is associated with no recall for the abuse because younger children may be more likely to experience abuse as violent, thus motivating repression or dissociation, or may have fewer psychological defenses available to them other than forgetting. As evidence that the age–no recall association is not primarily attributable to cognitive developmental features of young children, Briere and Conte (1993) and Herman and Schatzow (1987) emphasized that many of their subjects who retrieved memories were very young at the time of abuse. Williams (1995) reported that those in her sample with recovered memories were on average 3 years younger at the time of abuse than those who reported continuous recollection of their abuse experiences.

In addition, memories of sexual abuse may be encoded, stored, and retrieved differently from other memories (van der Kolk and Fisler 1995), especially when the abuse occurs under circumstances of high arousal, terror, and extreme ambivalence; when escape is impossible; or when the meaning of the abuse, if confronted, could be devastating. The concepts of repression or dissociation as psychologically motivated defenses against knowing cannot be dismissed. Although the mechanisms that might explain such phenomena have not yet been confirmed in laboratory studies, this does not make them impossible.

In contrast to these findings, Williams (1994) reported that after controlling for age, no relationship was found between force used in the abuse and recall. On the other hand, the women in Williams's (1994) study who had been abused by someone with whom they had a closer relationship, a variable often associated with greater psychological distress, were more likely to have forgotten the abuse, even when abuse severity and age at time of abuse were controlled. Williams (1995) also found that women in her sample who recalled the abuse but reported prior periods of forgetting were more likely than women who reported continuous memories of the abuse to have had weak or no support from their mothers. These findings are consistent with Freyd's (1994) notion of betrayal trauma.

Even though none of the studies discussed in this section delineates the specific mechanisms for the forgetting, the findings do suggest that in some individuals, the lack of recall of the abuse is based on more than just ordinary forgetting associated with the passage of time, their young age when abused, or a lack of salience of the event. Indeed, there is some reason to believe that the process of forgetting childhood sexual abuse may differ from that of forgetting other traumatic events of childhood. After all, most child sexual abuse occurs in secret. The sexual contact may be associated with shame and guilt, and the responses of others who learn about the abuse often do little to ensure comfort and unconflicted memories of the event, because their responses often convey shock, disbelief, and denial (Berliner and Conte 1990; Browne and Finkelhor 1986). However, one important study (Elliott, unpublished data, 1995) suggested that such forgetting or delayed recall is not limited to sexual abuse. Elliott found that the phenomenon occurs across a variety of traumas and is most likely with particularly traumatic events. Because any examination of memories of traumatic events can only rely on observed behavior, we may never have conclusive proof that a specific mechanism is responsible for the observable forgetting. Nevertheless, the variables found to be associated with forgetting in the studies to date are consistent with the hypothesis that complex psychological processes affect memories of childhood sexual abuse.

False Reports, Beliefs, or Memory—False Positives

Investigators have suggested that estimates of the prevalence of child sexual abuse in community surveys are inflated by false reports (Grossman and Pressley 1994; Lindsay and Read 1995; Loftus et al. 1994b), but no empirical evidence has been accumulated to describe how frequently such false positives actually occur, and no information is available that would allow reasonable estimates of the magnitude of the problem. Research on fictitious reports of abuse by children or their parents suggests a fabrication rate of 4%–8% (for review, see Everson and Boat 1989), and 2% of the women in Williams's (1994) study reported that they or others had fabricated the report of child sexual abuse. However, there is no evidence that fabrication occurs at even this rate when adults are asked behaviorally specific questions about whether they were sexually abused in childhood. No scientific evidence shows that adults commonly make purely fabricated allegations of abuse in childhood when surveyed using standard victimization screening techniques. This frequently raised issue will remain only theoretical until specific research is done to assess its frequency.

The body of research on false positives has focused on the issue of suggestibility and recovered memories of abuse (Kihlstrom 1993; Lindsay and Read 1994; Loftus 1993) and therapists' use of techniques designed to recover such memories. Several books and articles have made claims that a majority of therapists will, on occasion, hunt for repressed memories and will use suggestive techniques to do so (Ofshe and Watters 1993; Poole et al. 1995; Yapko 1994). Poole et al. (1995) surveyed American and British psychologists and concluded that 25% of therapists believe that recovering memories of abuse is an important part of therapy, believe they can identify patients with hidden memories during the initial session, and toward this end use two or more techniques (such as age regression or dream interpretation) to help patients recover memories of child sexual abuse (Poole et al. 1995). The critique of these practices (Lindsay and Read 1994) has grown out of and is supported by a tradition of laboratory research by cognitive psychologists on the fallibility of memory.

A profusion of research on suggestibility and memory shows that memory is reconstructive and imperfect (Loftus and Loftus 1980; Spence 1984), that memory can be influenced and distorted (Dodson and Johnson 1993), that confabulation can occur to fill in memory gaps, and that subjects can be persuaded to believe they heard, saw, or experienced events that they have not (Johnson et al. 1988, 1993; Lindsay 1994). Inaccurate memories can be strongly believed and convincingly described (Winograd and Neisser 1992). Much of the laboratory research on suggestibility of memory has involved paradigms in which individuals view an item or event (e.g., the presence of a barn in a photograph or the speed of a vehicle before an accident), are later given incorrect information about the event, and, finally, are asked about what they saw. Individuals who are given incorrect information are likely to incorporate that information into later reports of their memories of the event. This process is termed the *misinformation effect*, and it is argued that this effect also applies to memories of childhood sexual abuse. Some researchers assert that similar processes may lead to a patient's false belief that he or she was sexually abused if such a history is suggested by a therapist (see Lindsay and Read 1994).

Criticisms of the application of laboratory research to investigations of memory of childhood sexual abuse have focused on the ecological validity of the studies—that is, its applicability to the real-world experience of child molestation and its aftermath (Berliner and Williams 1994). Just because an experimenter can make a person think that she or he saw a barn in a bucolic country scene when there was no barn, it does not necessarily mean that someone can be made to falsely believe that she or he was sexually abused when, in fact, the abuse did not occur. Changing or adding a feature to an event, as is the procedure in much of the laboratory research, is not the same as making someone believe that an entirely new event occurred (Olio 1994; Pezdek 1995). In addition, implanting memories for traumatic events and for self-referent events may be a very different matter. Self-involved memories may be less susceptible to the misinformation effect. Of course, research ethics preclude any experiment that would attempt to implant memories of something as serious as sexual abuse.

Recently, several studies have attempted to directly assess the implantation of memories for events that would be traumatic had they occurred, to examine types of events that are more likely to be implanted, and to investigate the factors associated with successful implantation of memories for events that did not occur. Several paradigms have been used, but all have in common an attempt to make younger family members of the researchers' collaborators "remember" events that did not occur. A "lost in a shopping mall" study (Loftus and Pickrell 1995) found that 25% of the adults ($n = 24$) could lead a child or other relative to believe that he or she had been lost in a shopping mall when he or she was 5 years old. Five of the six participants in this study who "remembered" the false event also generated additional details about the incident.

Hyman et al. (1995) attempted to address criticisms that the shopping mall study tests for a "memory" of a universally feared, high-base-rate childhood event (separation from a parent) by asking college students about their memories of false events that were more unusual, such as attending a wedding and knocking over a punch bowl or having to evacuate a grocery store when a sprinkler system was accidentally activated. None of the 51 subjects had false recalls during the first interview, but 25% (13) claimed to recall these events by the third interview (more information and increasing demands for recall were provided with each reinterview). In another study, Pezdek (1995) tested the hypothesis that it would be easier to implant memories for events for which one has a generic script. She used two false events that differed in the availability of scripts: 1) the familiar event—getting lost and 2) the unfamiliar event—receiving an enema. Pezdek found that 3 of the 20 participants remembered the familiar event, whereas none of the 20 participants remembered the unfamiliar event. Pezdek concluded that events will be suggestively implanted to the extent that the suggested event is familiar.

This research suggests that individuals can be made to believe that they had experiences that did not actually occur, but they are more resistant to the implantation of memories for events that are less familiar. I. E. Hyman and F. G. Billings ("Individual Differences and the Creation of False Childhood Memories," unpublished manuscript, Western Washington University, 1995) found that those who created false memories scored higher on measures of dissociation and creative imagination, suggesting that one's ability to engage in reality monitoring is related to acceptance of false events. Hyman and Pentland (1996) reported that individuals who were asked to form a mental image of an event and to describe it to an interviewer were more likely to create a false event. Interestingly, they were also more likely to recover memories of a previously unavailable true event.

It must be kept in mind that all of these studies involved fairly small samples and that most participants resisted implanted memory. It is unclear whether an actual memory is in fact recalled or whether it was created in response to the demand characteristics of the experiment (e.g., active confirmation of the truth of the experience by an older family member who claimed to have been present).

How generalizable these findings are to issues of false positives in cases of child sexual abuse is unclear. The demand characteristics of these experiments in which an older, more powerful adult directly asserts that the event took place, claims to have been present, and asks the individual to try hard to remember do not describe the demand characteristics of most therapy. If, however, such pressures were placed on a patient to remember childhood sexual abuse, subsequent recollections, although not necessarily untrue (Hyman and Pentland 1996), would be suspect. These findings have important implications for clinical practice, which are discussed below.

Remembering Childhood Sexual Abuse—True Positives

Taking the position that some women are amnesic for sexual abuse that happened in childhood does not mean that all or even most victims forget. Most individuals who were molested after the offset of infantile amnesia probably have continuous memories of the abuse (Terr 1988; Williams 1994). This does not mean that individuals remember every detail of the abuse experience nor that they remember it every waking hour, but they recall that it happened. Indeed, for some, the memories are all too vivid.

Williams (1994) found that 62% of the women and 45% of the men in her sample (Williams and Banyard 1996) recalled abuse that had been documented in their hospital records in childhood. Of the women who recalled the abuse, 84% reported that memories of the abuse had been continuous (Williams 1995). Williams was able to compare the accounts of adult women with the details of the abuse recorded in the 1970s and, therefore, was also able to examine an important subset of those who remembered their abuse—those who currently remembered their abuse but who had some prior period of forgetting. The experiences of these women can help us understand the variability of memory even among the true positive group and how complicated it is to distinguish between false positives and true positives.

Williams (1995) found that women with recovered memories were younger at the time of abuse than those who had continuous memories of the experience. Although the number of women in this sample with recovered memories of abuse was small ($n = 12$) and the findings must be treated as preliminary, this study suggests that women who report prior forgetting are able to recall the abuse. Although the women's reports of some details changed, their accounts of the abuse were surprisingly clear and true to the basic elements of the original incident. Interestingly, despite few gross inaccuracies, the women with recovered memories were often very unsure about their memories and made statements such as, "What I remember is mostly from a dream" or "I'm really not too sure about this." The woman's level of uncertainty about recovered memories was not associated with more inaccuracies in her account. In fact, the accounts of the women who reported their memories to be vague were no more inaccurate than those who reported their memories to be clear. This suggests that individuals who are recalling true events may be relatively unsure about these memories. Lack of clarity about abuse experiences, particularly those that occurred at a young age, should not be seen as evidence that the events did not occur. Of course, these findings cannot be used to assert the validity of *all* recovered memories of child abuse, but they do suggest that recovered memories of childhood sexual abuse reported by adults can be quite accurate.

Memory and Symptomatology

The previous sections provide some support for the notion that childhood sexual abuse can be forgotten, although the mechanisms that cause such memory lapses are much less clear. An important next question pertains to the mental health consequences of such forgetting. Theories that address this issue are closely linked to discussions of mechanisms that underlie the forgetting. For example, if we believe that survivors, such as those in Williams's study (1994) who did not report having been abused, either choose not to report their history or had forgotten the incident as a result of normal forgetting processes, then we might speculate that their mental health outcomes would not be significantly different from those of survivors who report continuous recall of their abuse. On the other hand, if we theorize that the forgetting is related to an avoidance coping style that may in some instances be adaptive (Tromp et al. 1995), then perhaps survivors with no reported memory for the abuse will actually have a better mental health outcome. Finally, if we follow theories that suggest that forgetting of trauma is a result of repression, dissociation, or physiological alterations in neurochemistry caused by extreme stress, then we would predict that individuals with memory problems would report higher levels of psychological symptomatology (Briere and Conte 1993; Herman 1992; Spiegel 1986; van der Kolk and Fisler 1995). Preliminary results from several studies raise more questions than they answer and suggest that some combination of these anticipated results may be expected.

Williams and Banyard (1995) have presented some preliminary exploratory analyses of the effects of remembering on mental health symptoms. Participants in the prospective study were divided into two groups: those who had continuous recall of their sexual abuse and those who either did not currently remember or reported some period in the past when they did not remember. The groups were further divided based on their age at the time of the index abuse. The investigators hypothesized that few differences would be found between subjects with and without memory problems who were young (9 years or younger) at the time of the abuse. A variety of mechanisms for forgetting might have been operating in this group, including the effects of childhood amnesia and other developmental interferences, making clear patterns of effects difficult to discern. On the other hand, the investigators hypothesized that those who were ages 10, 11, or 12 at the time of the abuse but did not remember it or had some prior period of forgetting would have more mental health symptoms if a mechanism such as repression or dissociation was at work. The study produced limited conclusions. Small sample sizes contributed to a lack of overall significance in the analyses. However, a descriptive examination of the magnitude of differences among the various groups showed a trend in the expected direction, with those participants who were older at the time of the abuse and had memory problems also reporting higher levels of sexual abuse trauma symptoms such as fear of men or sexual problems.

Studies by Briere and Conte (1993) and Elliott and Briere (1995) also address this issue. Briere and Conte studied a sample of 450 adults who had been sexually abused as children and were in treatment at the time of the study. They found that those individuals who did not have continuous recall of their abuse, but had some prior period of forgetting, also had higher scores on the General Symptom Index of the Symptom Checklist—90 (SCL-90). Elliott and Briere expanded this work and examined differences among sexual abuse survivors who had continuous recall of their abuse, those who had some prior period of forgetting but recovered the memory of their abuse very recently (less than 2 years before the interview), and those who had recovered memories more than 2 years before the research interview. Their results indicated that those individuals with more recent recall of their abuse reported the highest levels of symptomatology such as posttraumatic intrusion, avoidance, dissociation, and the highest scores on measures of posttraumatic stress. They discussed these findings as evidence that the process of recovering memories may produce a resurgence in posttraumatic symptoms, and individuals experiencing this phenomenon may require additional clinical support. They also highlighted the fact that such symptoms seem to abate over time, as evidenced by the lower rates of distress reported by the remote recall group. Elliott and Briere suggested that the increased symptoms associated with recall may be distressing, but they may also help to facilitate the healing process. This theory may support work by Pennebaker (1982, 1990), who discussed the curative effects of disclosing and discussing traumatic events rather than inhibiting their discussion or ruminating about them in silence. Such events can be discussed only if they are remembered.

This area of study requires much future research. Some data will come from studies that clarify the mechanisms that may produce amnesia for child sexual abuse in some individuals, whereas others have frequent intrusive flashbacks. Indeed, perhaps as we discover the variety of mechanisms that may lead to forgetting, we will have a better understanding of the full range of outcomes associated with this response. We may never be able to conclude that forgetting is either adaptive or problematic and may find that it can be either or both for any particular individual; also, it may vary in effect at different stages of the life course. Although Pennebaker (1982) emphasized the benefits of discussing traumatic experiences, he also cited evidence that in some cases, putting the experience behind one and finding the ability to not dwell on it may be very adaptive. We need to learn much more about the conditions under which forgetting sexual abuse may be adaptive and the conditions under which it may create difficulties.

Research Implications

Laboratory research indicates many reasons to be concerned about the accuracy of memories of childhood sexual abuse. These include the fallibility of memory and the passage of time. However, the concepts of source misattributions and misinformation effect could also be applied to studies designed to understand the false negatives and to explain the memory processes that could be involved in total amnesia for abuse or in false beliefs or false memories about an event (such as when a young woman misremembers actual sexual abuse only as an injury to her genitals caused by a fall from a bicycle or when a young man recalls his actual abuse as a consensual experience with an older woman). Problems of source monitoring, an influential interviewer, an interviewer seeking to confirm preconceived ideas, and repeated or persistent suggestion could result in false positives *or* false negatives.

Research studies designed to examine how the dynamics of sexual abuse, particularly abuse by a close, powerful family member, may contribute to the creation of false beliefs of nonabuse would be useful. Future research could examine what happens when subjects are encouraged or pressured to forget and the extent to which false memories of true events are influenced by fears and posttraumatic stress disorder; by feelings of guilt, shame, or betrayal; or by reframing an event to a more socially and personally acceptable scenario. Just as the social context can distort memory in the direction of falsely believing one was abused, it seems reasonable that it can distort memory in the direction of dissociation and forgetting.

Our review of the research suggests other interesting questions for future research: What accounts for forgetting some parts versus all of the abuse? What accounts for short periods versus long periods of forgetting? What accounts for complete lack of recall and never remembering the abuse? What is the association between such patterns of recall and social and psychological functioning in adulthood? These and other questions about the phenomenology and mechanism of forgetting about childhood sexual abuse and other childhood trauma require further study. Longitudinal research is needed to examine what happens to memory in childhood and throughout the life span.

The field of child abuse and neglect, in general, and child sexual abuse, in particular, would also benefit from well-designed treatment outcome studies (Finkelhor and Berliner 1995), including studies of the use and effect of techniques of memory recovery. Clinical research should also focus on not only the impact of memory on symptomatology but also the impact of false memories or beliefs of abuse on the individual and the family.

Treatment Implications

Although an assessment of the treatment issues in the area of memory for childhood sexual abuse is beyond the scope of this chapter, a number of important treatment implications emerge from this research review (for discussion of some treatment issues, see Bowman and Mertz 1996; Enns et al. 1995). Researchers who study the fallibility of memory and those advocates who are concerned with the problems of false positives have raised important questions for professionals who work with trauma survivors. Others have raised serious questions about the use of active memory recovery strategies that may lead to the development of false memories or false beliefs that one was abused when, in fact, no such abuse occurred. Surveys of clinical practitioners indicate that some clinicians need more information about normal memory processes and could benefit from specific guidance about potential problems of suggestibility and memories of childhood sexual abuse.

Although it is not easy to implant memories for events about which an individual is unfamiliar and it is not clear how generalizable the research is to memories of childhood sexual abuse, laboratory research indicates that false beliefs about childhood experiences can be generated by pressing for a memory, especially when the individual has a ready script available for that experience (Pezdek 1995) or when the individual is asked to form a mental image of an event and to describe it to an interviewer.

One interesting implication of Pezdek's findings is that those who were truly abused may also be more susceptible to false beliefs about abuse because these individuals have a ready script for child sexual abuse available. On the other hand, evidence from Hyman and Pentland (1996) indicates that techniques such as guided imagery may assist with recall of memories of previously forgotten true events. These paradoxical findings from laboratory research suggest that clinicians must proceed with caution in working with patients' memories of abuse and in drawing conclusions about abuse histories. However, the standards of proof or necessity for corroboration of any memory of a childhood event will vary for individual, therapeutic, and criminal justice or other legal system decision making (Bowman and Mertz 1996).

These cautions must be balanced by the research on the problem of false negatives, which has implied that it would be unwise and possibly harmful for therapists or others to dismiss patients' recollections of abuse simply because the memories are vague. Findings from Williams's (1995) study support the idea that when previously forgotten sexual abuse experiences are subsequently recalled, they contain many of the characteristics of remembering noted in clinical settings. The women's memories came not from therapy, but through environmentally triggered cues (see also Elliott, unpublished data, 1995). The women reported a gradual process of remembering, often initially characterized by vague and fragmentary images. Many said that these images were contained in dreams. Although the women who recovered memories were often not very confident about their memories, when their accounts of the abuse were compared with earlier documentation of abuse, they were accurate—as reliable as those of the women who had always remembered their abuse. Research on the experiences of those in the true positive group has verified that child sexual abuse has a wide range of negative consequences. Clinicians cannot afford to collude with families and society in silencing survivors' recollections of their abuse. Because knowledge of the effect of child sexual abuse on memory remains very limited, we must conduct more research to better understand this phenomenon and combine such research with an ongoing discussion of its implications for practitioners.

References

Andrews B, Morton J, Bekerian DA, et al: The recovery of memories in clinical practice: experiences and beliefs of British Psychological Society practitioners. The Psychologist, May 1995, pp 209–214

Beckett K: Culture and the politics of signification: the case of child sexual abuse. Social Problems 43(1):57–76, 1996

Beitchman JH, Zucker KJ, DaCosta GA, et al: A review of the long-term effects of child sexual abuse. Child Abuse Negl 16:101–118, 1992

Belli RF, Loftus EF: Recovered memories of childhood abuse: a source monitoring perspective, in Dissociation: Theory, Clinical, and Research Perspectives. Edited by Lynn SJ, Rhue JW. New York, Guilford, 1994, pp 415–433

Berliner L, Conte JR: The process of victimization: the victim's perspective. Child Abuse Negl 14:29–40, 1990

Berliner L, Loftus E: Sexual abuse accusations: desperately seeking reconciliation. Journal of Interpersonal Violence 7:570–578, 1992

Berliner L, Williams LM: Memories of child sexual abuse: response to Lindsay and Read. Journal of Applied Cognitive Psychology 8:379–387, 1994

Bowman CG, Mertz E: A dangerous direction: legal intervention in sexual abuse survivor therapy. Harvard Law Review 109:549–639, 1996

Bremner JD, Krystal JH, Southwick SM, et al: Functional neuroanatomical correlates of the effects of stress on memory. J Trauma Stress 8:527–554, 1995

Brewin CR, Andrews B, Gotlib IH: Psychopathology and early experience: a reappraisal of retrospective reports. Psychol Bull 113:82–98, 1993

Briere J: Child Abuse Trauma: Theory and Treatment of the Lasting Effects. Newbury Park, CA, Sage, 1992

Briere J, Conte J: Self-reported amnesia for abuse in adults molested as children. J Trauma Stress 6:21–31, 1993

Briere J, Zaidi LY: Sexual abuse histories and sequelae in female psychiatric emergency room patients. Am J Psychiatry 146:1602–1606, 1989

Brown R, Kulik J: Flashbulb memories. Cognition 5:73–99, 1977

Browne A, Finkelhor D: The impact of child sexual abuse: a review of the research. Psychol Bull 99:66–77, 1986

Burke A, Heuer F, Reisberg D: Remembering emotional events. Memory and Cognition 20:277–290, 1992

Cahill L, Brins B, Weber M, et al: β-Adrenergic activation and memory for emotional events. Nature 371:702–704, 1994

Carlson EB (ed): Trauma Research Methodology. Lutherville, MD, Sidran Press, 1996

Ceci SJ, Caves RD, Howe MJA: Children's long-term memory for information that is incongruous with their prior knowledge. Br J Psychol 72:443–450, 1981

Conte J, Wolfe S, Smith T: What sexual offenders tell us about prevention strategies. Child Abuse Negl 13:293–301, 1989

Courtois CA: The memory retrieval process in incest survivor therapy. Journal of Child Sexual Abuse 1:15–31, 1992

Dodson CS, Johnson MK: Rate of false source attributions depends on how questions are asked. Am J Psychol 106:451–557, 1993

Elliott DM, Briere J: Posttraumatic stress associated with delayed recall of sexual abuse: a general population study. J Trauma Stress 8:629–648, 1995

Enns CZ, McNeilly CL, Corkery JM, et al: The debate about delayed memories of child sexual abuse: a feminist perspective. The Counseling Psychologist 23:181–279, 1995

Everson M, Boat B: False allegations of sexual abuse by children and adolescents. J Am Acad Child Adolesc Psychiatry 28:230–235, 1989

Feldman-Summers S, Pope KS: The experience of "forgetting" childhood abuse: a national survey of psychologists. J Consult Clin Psychol 62:636–639, 1994

Femina DD, Yeager CA, Lewis DO: Child abuse: adolescent records vs. adult recall. Child Abuse Negl 14:227–231, 1990

Finkelhor D: Sexually Victimized Children. New York, Free Press, 1979

Finkelhor D, Berliner L: Research on the treatment of sexually abused children. J Am Acad Child Adolesc Psychiatry 34:1408–1423, 1995

Fivush R, Hammond NR: Autobiographical memory across the preschool years: toward reconceptualizing childhood amnesia, in Knowing and Remembering in Young Children. Edited by Fivush R, Hudson JA. New York, Cambridge University Press, 1990, pp 223–248

Fivush R, Reese E: The social construction of autobiographical memory, in Theoretical Perspectives on Autobiographical Memory. Edited by Conway MA, Rubin DC, Spinnler H, et al. Boston, MA, Kluwer Academic Press, 1992, pp 115–132

Fivush R, Schwartzmueller A: Say it once again: effects of repeated questions on children's event recall. J Trauma Stress 8:555–580, 1995

Freud S: The Standard Edition of the Complete Psychological Works of Sigmund Freud, Vol 7. Translated and edited by Strachey J. London, Hogarth Press, 1953

Freyd JJ: Betrayal trauma: traumatic amnesia as an adaptive response to childhood abuse. Ethics and Behavior 4:307–329, 1994

Gold SN, Hughes D, Hohnecker L: Degrees of repression of sexual abuse memories. Am Psychol 49:441–442, 1994

Goodman GS, Quas JA, Batterman-Faunce JM, et al: Predictors of accurate and inaccurate memories of traumatic events experienced in childhood. Consciousness and Cognition 3:269–294, 1994

Grossman LR, Pressley M: Introduction. Applied Cognitive Psychology 8:277–280, 1994

Hartman CR, Burgess AW: Information processing of trauma. Child Abuse Negl 17:47–58, 1993

Henry B, Moffitt TE, Caspi A, et al: On the "remembrance of things past": a longitudinal evaluation of the retrospective method. Psychological Assessment 6:92–101, 1994

Herman JL: Trauma and Recovery. New York, Basic Books, 1992

Herman JL, Schatzow E: Recovery and verification of memories of childhood sexual trauma. Psychoanalytic Psychology 4:1–14, 1987

Howe ML, Courage ML: On resolving the enigma of infantile amnesia. Psychol Bull 113:305–326, 1993

Howe ML, Courage ML, Peterson C: How can I remember when "I" wasn't there: long-term retention of traumatic experiences and emergence of the cognitive self. Consciousness and Cognition 3:327–355, 1994

Hyman IE, Pentland J: The role of mental imagery in the creation of false childhood memories. Journal of Memory and Language 35:101–117, 1996

Hyman IE, Husband TH, Billings FJ: False memories of childhood experiences. Applied Cognitive Psychology 9:181–197, 1995

Johnson MK, Foley MA, Suengas AG, et al: Phenomenal characteristics of memories for perceived and imagined autobiographical events. J Exp Psychol Gen 4:371–376, 1988

Johnson MK, Hashtroude S, Lindsay DS: Source monitoring. Psychol Bull 114:3–28, 1993

Kihlstrom JF: The recovery of memory in the laboratory and clinic. Paper presented at the joint convention of Rocky Mountain Psychological Association and Western Psychological Association, Phoenix, AZ, April 1993

Koss MP, Tromp S, Tharan M: Traumatic memories: empirical foundations, forensic and clinical implications. Clinical Psychology Scientific Practice 2(2):111–132, 1995

Kramer TH, Buckhout R, Fox P, et al: Effects of stress on recall. Applied Cognitive Psychology 5:483–488, 1991

Leippe M, Manion A, Romanczyk A: Eyewitness memory for a touching experience: accuracy differences between child and adult witnesses. Journal of Applied Cognitive Psychology 76:367–379, 1991

Lindsay DS: Memory source monitoring and eyewitness testimony, in Adult Eyewitness Testimony: Current Trends and Developments. Edited by Lindsay DC. New York, Cambridge University Press, 1994, pp 27–55

Lindsay DS, Read JD: Psychotherapy and memories of childhood sexual abuse: a cognitive perspective. Applied Cognitive Psychology 8:281–338, 1994

Lindsay DS, Read JD: "Memory work" and recovered memories of childhood sexual abuse: scientific evidence and public, professional, and personal issues. Psychology, Public Policy, and Law 1:846–908, 1995

Loftus EF: The reality of repressed memories. Am Psychol 48:518–537, 1993

Loftus EF: Remembering dangerously. Skeptical Inquirer. March/April, 1995, pp 20–29

Loftus EF, Burns TE: Mental shock can produce retrograde amnesia. Memory and Cognition 10:318–323, 1982

Loftus EF, Christianson S: Malleability of memory for emotional events, in Aversion, Avoidance, and Anxiety. Edited by Archer T, Nilsson L. Hillsdale, NJ, Lawrence Erlbaum, 1989, pp 311–322

Loftus EF, Davies GM: Distortions in the memory of children. Journal of Social Issues 40:51–67, 1984

Loftus EF, Ketcham K: The Myth of Repressed Memories. New York, St Martin's Press, 1994

Loftus EF, Loftus GR: On the permanence of stored information in the human brain. Am Psychol 35:409–420, 1980

Loftus EF, Pickrell JE: The formation of false memories. Psychiatric Annals 25:720–725, 1995

Loftus EF, Smith KD, Klinger MR, et al: Memory and mismemory for health events, in Questions About Questions: Inquiries Into the Cognitive Bases of Surveys. Edited by Tanur JM. New York, Russell Sage Foundation, 1992, pp 102–137

Loftus EF, Garry M, Feldman J: Forgetting sexual trauma: what does it mean when 38% forget? J Consult Clin Psychol 62:1177–1181, 1994a

Loftus EF, Polonsky S, Fullilove MT: Memories of childhood sexual abuse: remembering and repressing. Psychology of Women Quarterly 18:67–84, 1994b

McHugh PR: Reconciliation: scientific, clinical and legal issues of false memory syndrome. Conference Opening Remarks, Memory and Reality. Baltimore, MD, December 1994

Nadel L, Zola-Morgan S: Infantile amnesia: a neurological perspective, in Infant Memory: Its Relation to Normal and Pathological Memory in Humans and Other Animals. Edited by Moscovitch M. New York, Plenum, 1984, pp 145–172

Neimark J: The diva of disclosure: memory researcher Elizabeth Loftus. Psychology Today 29(1):48, 1996

Nelson K: The ontogeny of memory for real events, in Remembering Reconsidered: Ecological and Traditional Approaches to the Study of Memory. Edited by Neisser U, Winograd E. New York, Cambridge University Press, 1988, pp 244–276

Nelson K, Ross G: The generalities and specifics of long-term memory in infants and young children, in New Directions for Child Development: Children's Memory. Edited by Perlmutter M. San Francisco, CA, Jossey-Bass, 1980, pp 87–101

Ofshe RJ, Watters E: Making monsters. Society 3(3):4–16, 1993

Olio KA: Truth in memory. Am Psychol 49:442–443, 1994

Pennebaker JW: The Psychology of Physical Symptoms. New York, Springer Verlag, 1982

Pennebaker JW: Opening Up, the Healing Power of Confiding in Others. New York, William Morrow, 1990

Pezdek K: What types of false childhood memories are not likely to be suggestively planted? Paper presented at the meeting of the Psychonomic Society, Los Angeles, CA, November 1995

Pillemer DB, White SH: Childhood events recalled by children and adults. Adv Child Dev Behav 21:297–340, 1989

Poole DA, Lindsay DS, Memon A, et al: Psychotherapy and the recovery of memories of childhood sexual abuse: doctoral-level therapists' beliefs, practices, and experiences. J Consult Clin Psychol 63:426–437, 1995

Pope HG, Hudson JI: Can individuals "repress" memories of childhood sexual abuse? An examination of the evidence. Psychiatric Annals 25:715–719, 1995

Rogers ML: Factors influencing recall of childhood sexual abuse. J Trauma Stress 8:691–716, 1995

Rubin D, Kozin M: Vivid memories. Cognition 16:81–95, 1984

Russell DEH: The Secret Trauma: Incest in the Lives of Girls and Women. New York, Basic Books, 1986

Saywitz KJ, Goodman GS, Nicholas E, et al: Children's memories of a physical examination involving genital touch: implications for reports of child sexual abuse. J Consult Clin Psychol 59:682–691, 1991

Schacter DL, Kagan J, Leichtman MD: True and false memories in children and adults: a cognitive neuroscience perspective. Psychology, Public Policy, and Law 1:411–428, 1995

Siegel DJ: Memory, trauma, and psychotherapy. Journal of Psychotherapy Practice and Research 4:93–122, 1995

Spence DP: Narrative Truth and Historical Truth. New York, WW Norton, 1984

Spiegel D: Dissociating damage. Am J Clin Hypn 29:123–131, 1986

Spiegel D: Functional disorders with memory aspects: impact of acute vs. chronic and recurrent trauma on memory. Conference on Memories of Trauma, Clark University, Worcester, MA, December 1993

Squire LR: On the course of forgetting in very long-term memory. J Exp Psychol 15:241–245, 1989

Terr L: What happens to early memories of trauma? A study of twenty children under age five at the time of documented traumatic events. J Am Acad Child Adolesc Psychiatry 27:96–104, 1988

Terr LC: Too Scared to Cry. New York, Harper & Row, 1990

Terr LC: Childhood traumas: an outline and overview. Am J Psychiatry 148:10–20, 1991

Tromp S, Koss MP, Figueredo AJ, et al: Are rape memories different? A comparison of rape, other unpleasant, and pleasant memories among employed women. J Trauma Stress 8:607–628, 1995

Usher JA, Neisser U: Childhood amnesia and the beginnings of memory for four early life events. J Exp Psychol Gen 122:155–165, 1993

van der Kolk BA: Biological considerations about emotions, trauma, memory, and the brain, in Human Feelings: Explorations Affect Development and Meaning. Edited by Brown A, Khantzian M. (in press)

van der Kolk BA, Fisler R: Dissociation and the fragmentary nature of traumatic memories: overview and exploratory study. J Trauma Stress 8:505–526, 1995

van der Kolk BA, van der Hart O: The intrusive past: the flexibility of memory and the engraving of trauma. American Image 48:425–454, 1991

Wakefield H, Underwager R: Recovered memories of alleged sexual abuse: lawsuits against parents. Behavioral Sciences and the Law 10:483–507, 1991

Williams LM: Recall of childhood trauma: a prospective study of women's memories of child sexual abuse. J Consult Clin Psychol 62:1167–1176, 1994

Williams LM: Recovered memories of abuse in women with documented child sexual victimization histories. J Trauma Stress 8:649–673, 1995

Williams LM, Banyard VL: Consequences of remembering for adult adjustment in female survivors of sexual abuse: a prospective study. Paper presented at the 4th International Family Violence Research Conference, Durham, NH, July 1995

Williams LM, Banyard VL: Childhood trauma: men's memories of child sexual abuse. Paper presented at the NATO Advanced Scientific Institute on Trauma and Memory, Port de Bourgenay, France, June 1996

Williams LM, Finkelhor D: Paternal caregiving and incest: a test of a biosocial model. Am J Orthopsychiatry 65:101–113, 1995

Winograd E, Neisser U: Affect and Accuracy in Recall: Studies of "Flashbulb" Memories. New York, Cambridge University Press, 1992

Yapko M: Suggestions of Abuse: True and False Memories of Childhood Sexual Trauma. New York, Simon & Schuster, 1994

Chapter 10

Repressed Memories in Patients With Dissociative Disorder: Literature Review, Controlled Study, and Treatment Recommendations

Philip M. Coons, M.D., Elizabeth S. Bowman, M.D., and Victor Milstein, Ph.D.

Whereas some doctors never trouble their heads about traumatic memories and do not even know that these exist, and whereas others fancy them everywhere, there is a place for persons who take a middle course and who believe they are able to detect the existence of traumatic memories in specific cases. The doctors comprising the last group need diagnostic rules.

Janet (1925), quoted in Powell and Boer (1995, p. 1296)

Currently, a heated controversy is raging among mental health professionals over whether memories of traumatic events can be forgotten and, if so, whether the process of forgetting should be called "repression," as has been the tradition since the time of Freud. Mental health professionals have become polarized into two groups. At one extreme are experimental psychologists (Ceci and Bruck 1993; Kihlstrom 1995; Lindsay and Read 1994; Loftus 1993; Spanos et al. 1994; Usher and Neisser 1993; Wakefield and Underwager 1992, 1994; Yapko 1994) and a few academic psychiatrists (Frankel 1994; McHugh and Butterfield 1993; Orne et al. 1988; Pope and Hudson 1995), who stress pseudomemory formation through the use of suggestive interview techniques, social pressure from self-help groups or overzealous therapists, hypnosis, dream analysis, and guided imagery. Experimental research in this area, unfortunately, has largely ignored the traumatized clinical population, and conclusions have been unfairly extrapolated from a largely non-clinical population of children and college students.

It is clear from this research, however, that memory is a reconstruc-

---

tive process (Spence 1995) and that many factors impinge on its accuracy. In a review of the literature on flashbacks, Frankel (1994) found that posttraumatic flashbacks may be considerably distorted compared with the actual traumatic event. Ceci and Bruck's review (1993) of the child literature indicates that the memory of children, especially young children, may be modified through suggestion, however subtle. Research on hypnotic recall indicates that memories may be created or distorted by the use of suggestive interview techniques and that individuals who have such "memories" may be extremely confident about their accuracy even after being told the truth (Orne et al. 1988).

At the other extreme are practicing mental health clinicians with years of clinical experience in treating victims of trauma. Until recently, many have been largely ignorant of the nature of memory and how the process of suggestion can distort memory retrieval. It is also unfortunate that until recently, neither group has paid sufficient attention to the other's scientific literature.

A large factor in creating the dispute over memories of abuse was the revision of many state laws to lengthen the statute of limitations for the recovery of damages due to childhood abuse. Many states now allow civil suits to be filed for damages when memories of childhood abuse finally surface, even if the victim is in her or his third, fourth, or fifth decade of life. This legal process has torn asunder many families and has been instrumental in the formation of the False Memory Syndrome Foundation, an organization composed of mostly parents who dispute their children's allegations of prior childhood abuse. This organization, which has many luminaries in the field of experimental memory research on its board of directors, has been behind an effort in several state legislatures to strictly limit how patients who allege memories of childhood abuse may be treated (Cronin 1995; Golston 1995).

The importance of this dispute cannot be underestimated. It essentially reiterates the same controversy that plagued Sigmund Freud and his colleagues and eventually led Freud to reverse his seduction hypothesis in favor of fantasy being responsible for the production of reports of sexual abuse in some of his patients (Powell and Boer 1995). This dispute has led seven journals to devote entire issues to the controversy (*Applied Cognitive Psychology* 1994; *Consciousness and Cognition* 1994, 1995; *Counseling Psychologist* 1995; *International Journal of Clinical and Experimental Hypnosis* 1994, 1995; *Journal of Psychohistory* 1995; *Journal of Traumatic Stress* 1995; *Psychiatric Annals* 1995) and several major organizations and prominent individuals to issue statements (American Medical Association, Council on Scientific Affairs 1994; American Psychiatric Association, Board of Trustees 1994; American Society of Clinical Hypnosis 1995; British Psychological Society 1995) and treatment guidelines (Allen 1995; Bloom 1994; Fowler 1994; Gutheil 1993;

Hammond 1995; Lynn and Nash 1994; van der Hart and Nijenhuis 1995; Watkins 1993; Yapko 1994) on the issue of memory and repression. Members of the American Psychological Association have become so mired in the dispute that their official statement is not expected until 1996. Conclusions of these major mental health organizations have been tempered by the relative lack of research in this important area. Most statements concur that memories of traumatic events can be forgotten but that pseudomemory formation is also possible. At present, the only way to determine whether a specific traumatic memory is genuine is with outside corroboration.

Review of Studies of Posttraumatic Memories

Studies Involving Predominantly Nonsexual Trauma

It is clear, even from the older literature, that memories of trauma can be forgotten and later retrieved. During World War II, several studies of amnesia for combat-related trauma were done (Table 10–1). Sargant and Slater (1941) found that 14% of 1,000 soldiers hospitalized for neuroses had amnesia. Torrie (1944) found a 9% incidence of amnesia and fugue in 1,000 cases of anxiety neuroses and hysteria among troops in North Africa. Henderson and Moore (1944) found a 5% incidence of amnesia among 200 neuropsychiatric patients in the South Pacific. Fisher (1944) observed and treated 20 sailors with fugue states. Although these studies had problems (i.e., neuropsychological causes for the amnesias were not ruled out in a consistent manner), it is remark-

Table 10–1. Studies of amnesia associated with combat during World War II

Study	Nature of population	Number in series	Percentage with amnesia	Confirmation of trauma
Sargant and Slater 1941	Soldiers hospitalized with neuroses	1,000	14	No
Torrie 1944	Soldiers with anxiety/hysteria	1,000	9	No
Henderson and Moore 1944	Soldiers with neuropsychiatric illness	200	5	No
Fisher 1944	Sailors with fugue	20	100	No

able that many amnesias cleared dramatically with the use of hypnosis, a result one would not expect if the cause were organic. Other major case reports of amnesia for trauma stem from other wars, including World War I (Thom and Fenton 1920), the Korean War (Archibald and Tuddenham 1956), the Vietnam War (Hendin et al. 1984; Sonneberg et al. 1985), and the Middle Eastern war between Israel and Egypt (Kalman 1977).

Both Jaffe (1968) and Niederland (1968) reported cases of amnesia among survivors of concentration camps, and Modai (1994) reported a case of amnesia in a Holocaust survivor who was not interned in a concentration camp. More recently, Kinzie (1993) reported amnesia in Southeast Asian war refugees.

Goldfield et al. (1988) reported on amnesia as a sequelae of torture. The experience of dissociative symptoms such as depersonalization, derealization, and even partial amnesia has become so well known among rape victims and survivors of natural disasters (Herman 1992; Madakasira and O'Brian 1987; Spiegel 1990; Wilkinson 1983) that these symptoms have been incorporated as DSM-IV diagnostic criteria for posttraumatic stress disorder (American Psychiatric Association 1994, pp. 424–429) and acute stress disorder (pp. 429–432).

Even more recently, investigators (Coons 1992; Coons and Milstein 1992; Coons et al. 1988; Putnam et al. 1986; Ross et al. 1989) have found that the amnesia characteristic of most of the dissociative disorders is linked to childhood trauma. The incidence of childhood trauma in dissociative identity disorder (DID) (formerly multiple personality disorder) varies from 85% to 98%, and the incidence of amnesia is virtually 100% (Coons et al. 1988; Putnam et al. 1986; Ross et al. 1989). In the studies involving DID, it is unclear whether the memories are merely dissociated into another personality state and available just to that personality state or whether the memories are totally forgotten or repressed and unavailable to any personality state. Of course, both mechanisms may be at work.

Studies Involving Predominantly Sexual Trauma

The most recent literature on recovered memories primarily involves memories of childhood sexual abuse. With one exception, all of these studies have been published since 1993 (Table 10–2).

Herman and Schatzow (1987) studied 53 female outpatients who had participated in short-term group psychotherapy for incest survivors and found that 74% of the patients had been able to corroborate their abuse experiences from perpetrator admissions, observations of other family members, physical evidence, or the discovery that another sibling had also been sexually abused. Onset of abuse ranged from ages 2 to 19 years, with an average age of 8. Abuse that began in or continued

Table 10–2.   Studies involving amnesia associated primarily with sexual trauma

Study	Nature of population	Number in series	Percent with amnesia (full or partial)	Confirmation of trauma
Herman and Schatzow (1987)	Female incest victims	53	64	74%
Briere and Conte (1993)	Adult psychiatric patients (mostly female)	450	59	No
Albach (1993)	Women reporting childhood incest	97	88	No
Binder et al. (1994)	Women with childhood sexual abuse	30	43	No
Burgess (1994)	Female military dependents sexually abused in day care	19	42	100%
Cameron (1994)	Women with childhood sexual abuse	60	65	No
Roesler and Wind (1994)	Female incest victims	228	28	No
Loftus et al. (1994)	Women with childhood sexual abuse	57	31	No
Feldman-Summers and Pope (1994)	Psychologists	79	40	46%
Williams (1994, 1995)	Women with childhood sexual abuse	129	48	100%
Elliott and Briere (1995)	Victims of childhood sexual abuse (55% female)	505	42	No
van der Kolk and Fisler (1995)	Men and women with childhood trauma (primarily sexual abuse)	36	42	75%
Tromp et al. (1995)	Employed women	1,037	—	No

into adolescence was never completely forgotten, and the most severe memory deficits were associated with either violent/sadistic abuse or abuse that began in early childhood and ended before adolescence.

Briere and Conte (1993) studied 450 adult psychiatric patients who reported sexual abuse histories and found that 59% had experienced amnesia for the abuse at some point in their lives before age 18. Predictors of amnesia included earlier age at onset of sexual abuse, longer abuse duration, larger number of abusers, greater current psychiatric symptomatology, and more violent abuse. Interestingly, guilt or shame was found not to be related to amnesia. No attempt was made to verify abuse histories in this study.

Albach (1993) studied 97 women who reported childhood incest and compared them with 65 female control subjects, matched for age and educational level, who denied childhood incest. The control subjects were asked to describe memories of other unpleasant childhood events. Of the women who were sexually abused, the duration was longer than 1 year in 90%. Violence was used in 43%. The mean duration of sexual abuse was 15 years. Amnesia was not correlated to age at onset of abuse, duration or frequency of abuse, or use of violence. Triggers for memory recovery included discovering that their own daughters had been abused, personal revictimization, illness or death of the perpetrator, and sensory cues (tactile, olfactory, visual, or auditory). Significantly more sexually abused subjects had either complete (29%) or partial amnesia (59%) for the abuse than the control group had for their experiences of unpleasant events.

Binder et al. (1994) studied 30 women who had been sexually abused as children and found that 43% had some amnesia for the abuse. In contrast to Briere and Conte's (1993) study, they found no relation in age at onset of abuse, length of abuse, number of abusers, and violence between their amnesic and nonamnesic samples. They did not attempt to independently verify sexual abuse histories. Interestingly, eight patients' conditions were described in detail, including how their memories were recovered. In three of these patients, memories were recovered through questionable memory enhancement techniques such as hypnosis ($n = 2$) and dreaming ($n = 1$). Burgess (1994, reported in Whitfield 1995, p. 72) followed up 19 military-dependent children with sexual abuse corroborated by day-care-center staff. At 10-year follow-up, 42% had either partially or completely forgotten the trauma. The abuse had occurred at a mean age of 2.5 years. Cameron (1994) interviewed and followed up, during a 6-year period, 60 women who had been sexually abused in childhood; 23% had partially forgotten and 42% had completely forgotten that they were sexually abused in childhood.

Roesler and Wind (1994) studied 228 adult women who reported incestuous experiences before age 18. The mean age at onset of abuse was 6.0 years, and the mean duration of abuse was 7.6 years. Twenty-eight percent had repressed memories of their abuse. The investigators did not seek to independently verify abuse histories in this study.

Loftus et al. (1994) studied 105 women in outpatient therapy for substance abuse, 54% of whom reported childhood sexual abuse. Of the sexually abused patients, 19% had completely forgotten and 12% had partially forgotten the abuse. The forgetting of abuse was not related to the number of abusers, frequency of abuse, or violent nature of the abuse, but it was associated with more intense feelings at the time of the abuse. As in most of the other studies, the investigators did not attempt to independently verify that the abuse had occurred.

Feldman-Summers and Pope (1994) administered a questionnaire to a national sample of psychologists. Of the respondents, 79 (24%) reported childhood abuse, 40% of whom had once been unable to remember the abuse. Those who reported being abused by more than one person were more likely to have amnesia than those who reported only one abuser, but amnesia was not correlated with severity of abuse. Both physical and sexual abuse were subject to periods of forgetting. Triggers for remembering abuse included reading a book or watching television or a movie (25.0%), being reminded about the abuse by an observer of the abuse (18.8%), engaging in psychotherapy (56.2%) or a self-help group (6.2%), and having an experience such as caring for others who were abused or making love (28.1%); no particular triggers for remembering abuse were found in 9.4% of the sample. Half of those who reported amnesia indicated that they had corroboration of the abuse. These types of corroboration included acknowledgment by the abuser (15.6%), acknowledgment by an observer (21.9%), notation in a diary by the victim (6.2%), reports of someone else being abused by the same perpetrator (15.6%), and evidence from medical records (6.2%).

Elliott and Briere (1995) studied 505 individuals (55% female) who had been sexually abused; 42% described full or partial amnesia for the experience. Delayed recall of the abuse was associated with the use of threats by the perpetrator at the time of the abuse and their perception of the abuse as very distressing. Factors not related to recall included age at the time of abuse, frequency of abuse, duration of abuse, use of actual physical force, and presence of sexual penetration.

Two recent studies provide data that traumatic memories are different from other types of memory. van der Kolk and Fisler (1995) studied 46 subjects (36 women and 10 men) with posttraumatic stress disorder who had endured a variety of traumas in both childhood and adulthood. However, the majority of the traumas (55%) consisted of childhood sexual abuse or assault. Of the 36 subjects with childhood trauma, 42% had either partial or total amnesia for the trauma, and 75% reported confirmation of the trauma through family members or court or hospital records. The initial return of their memories consisted of sensory (visual, olfactory, auditory, and kinesthetic) and affective experiences that emerged prior to a coherent narrative. Tromp et al. (1995) studied memories among 1,037 employed women and found that memories of rape experiences were less clear and vivid, less well remembered, and less talked about than other types of memories, both pleasant and unpleasant.

In the most sophisticated studies to date, Williams (1994, 1995) obtained follow-up data on 129 of 206 women who had documented evidence from a hospital emergency department for childhood sexual assault. Thirty-eight percent had no memory of the incident of sexual assault, and an additional 10% had forgotten the assault at one time but had subsequently remembered it. Amnesia was not associated with violence or repeated abuse; however, it was correlated with younger age at onset of the abuse and abuse by someone familiar. In the five case histories described in detail in the second paper (1995), it appears that memories of sexual assault were not immediately forgotten. These women stated that they began forgetting anywhere from 2 to 16 years after the assault and did not begin remembering the assault until their early 20s.

Although not related to recovered memories, Terr's studies (1988, 1991) of 20 children who had documented trauma prior to age 5 are instructive. These children were interviewed about the trauma an average of 4.4 years after it had occurred. She found that verbal recall of trauma was rare before age 36 months but that behavioral memories consisting of precise reenactments of the trauma were virtually universal and accurately conveyed the details of the trauma. Also, single episodes of trauma were more easily remembered than multiple episodes, and traumas of short duration were more easily remembered than traumas of long duration. Terr established that before age 28–36 months, full verbal memories of traumas did not occur.

Only two studies have confirmed trauma, consisting primarily of childhood physical and sexual abuse, in patients with DID and dissociative disorder not otherwise specified. In the first (Coons and Milstein 1986), 85% of 20 patients with DID had histories of childhood abuse, which were verified by either family members or emergency room reports. In the second study (Coons 1994a), a retrospective chart review of 19 cases of child and adolescent DID and dissociative disorder not otherwise specified, 8 of 9 patients with DID and 9 of 10 patients with dissociative disorder not otherwise specified had child abuse, which was verified by various family members and by medical, psychiatric, and police reports.

In contrast to the considerable confirmation of childhood physical and sexual abuse memories in the Feldman-Summers and Pope (1994) and Herman and Schatzow (1987) studies, reports of satanic ritual abuse have not received significant confirmation. These reports of multigenerational abuse include bizarre rituals of torture, perverted sex, human and animal sacrifice, cannibalism, and the breeding of babies for human sacrifice. Four studies of subjects reporting such practices (Bottoms et al. 1996; Coons 1994b; J. S. LaFontaine, "The extent and nature of organized and ritual abuse: a report to the department of health," unpublished manuscript, London, 1994; Weir and Wheatcroft 1995) found no corroboration of such horrific practices, and law enforcement agencies have not been able to find corroboration (Lanning 1992). However, evidence has been found that some individuals, usually acting alone, use paraphernalia, such as altars and candles, during their ritualistic abuse of children.

Present Study

Purpose

The purpose of the present study was to assess whether memories of reported trauma had been forgotten in patients with dissociative disorders and, if so, how the memories returned. The experiences of forgetting and remembering in patients with dissociative disorders were compared with the experiences of a control group of subjects with affective disorders but not dissociative disorders.

Methods

Subjects
The subjects were 50 consecutive patients in whom we (P. M. C. and E. S. B.) diagnosed dissociative disorders based on DSM-IV criteria. These patients included 28 with DID (3 were in remission), 20 with dissociative disorder not otherwise specified, and 1 each with dissociative amnesia and dissociative fugue. The control group consisted of 25 consecutive patients with various DSM-IV affective disorders, including 11 with major depression; 4 with schizoaffective disorder (depressed, in remission); 3 each with dysthymia, adjustment disorder with depression, and depression not otherwise specified; and 1 with organic affective disorder (depressed) secondary to hypothyroidism.

Of the 50 dissociative disorder patients, 46 (92%) were women and 48 (96%) were white. Mean age was 34.9 years (range, 16–63 years). Marital status was 23 (46%) single, 11 (22%) married, and 16 (32%) separated or divorced. Mean educational level was 13.8 years. Occupations included 14 (28%) professional or managerial, 7 (14%) skilled or semi-skilled, 2 (4%) unskilled, 14 (28%) disabled or unemployed, 6 (12%) homemakers, 6 (12%) students, and 1 (2%) retired. Religious affiliation was predominantly Protestant (52%), with 7 (14%) Catholic, 2 (4%) Jewish, and 15 (30%) who professed no religious affiliation.

Of the 25 affective disorder patients, 20 (80%) were women; all except 1 patient were white. Mean age was 33.2 years (range, 19–59 years). Marital status was 12 (48%) single, 8 (32%) married, and 5 (20%) separated or divorced. Mean educational level was 15.3 years. Occupations included 12 (48%) professional or managerial, 6 (24%) skilled or semiskilled, 3 (12%) unemployed or disabled, 2 (8%) homemakers, and 2 (8%) students. Religious affiliation was primarily Protestant (80%), with 1 (4%) Catholic and 4 (16%) who professed no religious affiliation.

Procedures

During their psychiatric examination, outpatients were given a trauma questionnaire to assess demographic data, types of trauma experienced both in childhood and in adulthood, whether the trauma was forgotten, circumstances under which the memory returned (fully awake, flashbacks, dreams, hypnosis, guided imagery, or relaxation), triggers for memory return, and the therapist's attitude toward memories. Statistical comparison between the dissociative disorder and affective disorder groups was calculated with a Yates-corrected χ^2.

Results

No significant differences in age, sex, race, marital status, or religious affiliation were found between the dissociative disorder and affective disorder groups. However, significantly more patients in the affective disorder group (12%) compared with the dissociative disorder group (4%) had 20 or more years of education ($\chi^2 = 7.150$, df = 1, $P = .006$). In addition, the number of subjects in the dissociative disorder group (24%) compared with the affective disorder group (4%) who were disabled tended toward significance ($\chi^2 = 3.362$, df = 1, $P = .067$).

Traumatic Experiences

A greater incidence of all types of child abuse (i.e., physical, sexual, or verbal abuse; abandonment; and neglect), rape in adulthood, and spouse abuse was reported by the dissociative disorder group. In the dissociative disorder and affective disorder groups, 96% and 56%, respectively, reported the incidence of any type of childhood abuse (see Table 10–3).

Only 17 (34%) of the dissociative disorder patients and 4 (16%) of the affective disorder patients had ever discussed their child abuse experiences directly with their abuser. None had ever filed a lawsuit against their abusers. Interestingly, half of the dissociative disorder group felt that their therapist believed fully or partially all of their traumatic experiences, whereas the other half felt that their therapists were neutral and encouraged them to discover for themselves whether the reported traumatic experiences did, in fact, happen.

Table 10–3. Experiences of trauma in patients with dissociative and affective disorders

Type of trauma	Dissociative disorder group (N = 50) n (%)	Affective disorder group (N = 25) n (%)	P value[a]
Child abuse			
Physical	39 (78)	5 (20)	<.001
Sexual	42 (84)	5 (20)	<.001
Verbal	41 (82)	5 (20)	<.001
Neglect	26 (52)	2 (8)	<.001
Abandonment	23 (46)	3 (12)	.008
None	2 (4)	11 (44)	<.001
Natural disaster			
Tornado	9 (18)	2 (8)	ID
Flood	3 (6)	0	ID
Earthquake	4 (8)	0	NS
Hurricane	4 (8)	3 (12)	NS
Fire	10 (20)	1 (4)	ID
Other			
Accident	13 (26)	2 (8)	NS
Rape	24 (48)	4 (16)	.014
Spouse abuse	20 (40)	3 (12)	.027

Note. ID = insufficient data; NS = not significant ($P > .05$).
[a]df = 1 for all values.

Memory Return

Loss of memory for trauma. In the dissociative disorder group, 96% of subjects reported that they had forgotten, either partially or fully, various forms of trauma compared with only 24% of the control group. Of the patients in the dissociative disorder group, 56%–86% forgot, either partially or fully, their childhood abuse experiences; 25%–66% forgot natural disasters; and 30%–45% forgot other types of trauma, including rape, accidents, and spouse abuse. Although the patients in the affective disorder group reported forgetting traumatic experiences at a much lower rate, they reported forgetting instances of verbal and sexual abuse, rape, and tornadoes. Although dissociative disorder patients reported higher instances of trauma in most cases, insufficient data from the affective disorder group prevented statistical comparisons for most types of trauma between the two groups. Of the three types of trauma for which the data were sufficient, only the difference in forgetting physical abuse was statistically significant (see Table 10–4).

Table 10–4.   Loss of memory (either full or partial) for trauma

Type of trauma	Dissociative disorder group (N = 50) n	Affective disorder group (N = 25) n	P value[a]
Child abuse			
Physical	28	0	.008
Sexual	36	3	ID
Verbal	24	1	ID
Neglect	17	0	NS
Abandonment	17	0	NS
Natural disaster			
Tornado	4	2	ID
Flood	2	0	ID
Earthquake	1	0	ID
Hurricane	2	0	ID
Fire	4	0	ID
Other			
Accident	4	0	ID
Rape	11	2	ID
Spouse abuse	6	0	ID

Note.   ID = insufficient data; NS = not significant (*P* > .05).
[a]df = 1 for all values.

Method of memory return.   Most instances of memory return in affective disorder patients occurred when they were fully awake. In contrast, among the dissociative disorder patients, memories returned in a variety of both awake and altered states of consciousness. In many instances, their memories returned in the form of flashbacks. Many memories returned in the form of dreams, while under hypnosis, during twilight states, or during therapeutic relaxation or guided imagery (see Table 10–5).

Triggers for memory return.   Return of memories in both groups was triggered by a wide variety of experiences including visual and auditory stimuli, retraumatization, hearing about someone else's trauma, reading, or group therapy sessions (Table 10–6). While the dissociative disorder patients were in treatment, their memories were as likely to return outside of the therapeutic situation as within. In half of the dissociative disorder patients, memories returned prior to the initiation of their treatment.

Table 10–5. Method of memory return

Method of return	Dissociative disorder group (N = 48) n (%)	Affective disorder group (N = 6) n (%)	P value[a]
Flashbacks	38 (79)	0	<.001
Awake	36 (75)	5 (83)	NS
Dreams	24 (50)	2 (33)	NS
Twilight states	19 (40)	0	NS
Relaxation	13 (27)	0	NS
Guided imagery	7 (15)	0	NS
Hypnosis	10 (21)	0	NS

Note. NS = not significant (P > .05).
[a]df = 1.

Table 10–6. Triggers for memory return

Triggers	Dissociative disorder group (N = 48) n (%)	Affective disorder group (N = 6) n (%)	P value[a]
Visual stimuli	34 (71)	4 (67)	ID
Auditory stimuli	27 (56)	2 (33)	ID
Another trauma	23 (48)	1 (17)	ID
Someone else's trauma	18 (38)	4 (67)	ID
Reading	17 (35)	3 (50)	ID
Group therapy	10 (21)	2 (33)	ID
No particular trigger	6 (13)	0	NS

Note. ID = insufficient data; NS = not significant (P > .05).
[a]df = 1 for all values.

Discussion and Conclusion

Summary of Studies of Traumatic Memory

To summarize the studies on traumatic memory to date, it is clear that memories of trauma can be partially or completely forgotten by 18%–59% of victims. Traumatic memories can be repressed for all types of trauma, including physical and sexual childhood abuse, rape, concentration camp or hostage experiences, combat, and natural disasters, but memory loss for childhood abuse appears to be the most common. Complete loss of memories of trauma usually occurs when the trauma takes place before adolescence. Amnesia for trauma is correlated with earlier onset of trauma and multiple types of trauma. In most of the studies reviewed, the trauma occurred after the usual period of infantile amnesia (birth to age 2.5–3 years). Traumatic memories may not be immediately forgotten. Repression may occur several years after the trauma has occurred. Repressed memories of child abuse can be corroborated in 50%–75% of cases. It is becoming more clear that traumatic memory is quite different from other forms of memory.

Amnesia for traumatic events can occur in several psychiatric illnesses. Amnesia is a diagnostic criterion for posttraumatic stress disorder, acute stress disorder, dissociative amnesia and fugue, and DID.

Traumatic events that occurred during childhood may not be remembered until the late teens and, most often, not until the third and fourth decades of life. The return of traumatic memories can be triggered by many events, including visual and auditory stimuli, hearing or reading about someone else's trauma, retraumatization, and group or individual psychotherapy.

Pseudomemories of traumatic events can definitely occur. Examples of pseudomemories include memories of infancy, many satanic ritual abuse reports, past-life experiences, and UFO abductions. The use of hypnosis, suggestive interview techniques, dream analysis, guided imagery, and fantasy predispose toward pseudomemory formation.

The existence of verbal childhood memories before age 1 year is impossible, and the veracity of verbal memories between ages 1 and 2 years should be highly suspect. The veracity of satanic ritual abuse memories is highly suspect. The reliability of adult memories of childhood abuse beginning before age 2 years is also highly suspect. At present, outside corroboration is the only way to determine whether a particular memory is reliable.

Comparison of Results With Those of Previous Studies

Our study confirmed and extended the results of previous studies on the forgetting of traumatic memories. We found that traumatic memories can be forgotten for childhood abuse, natural disasters, rape, and spouse abuse. We confirmed that there are many different types of triggers for traumatic memory return, including visual and auditory stimuli, retraumatization, hearing or reading about someone else's trauma, and group psychotherapy. Trauma occurs more often in DID and dissociative disorder not otherwise specified than in affective disorders. Forgetting of trauma appears to occur more in those with dissociative disorders than in those with affective disorders.

In dissociative disorder patients, we found that memories could return in the context of highly questionable therapeutic practices for memory retrieval, including dream analysis, hypnosis, and guided imagery. However, the return of traumatic memories was not necessarily related to therapy but could occur during relaxation or twilight states outside of therapy.

Limitations of This Study

One of the difficulties with our study was the small sample size, especially of the affective disorder patients. We were not always able to make statistical comparisons between the dissociative disorder and affective disorder groups. In future studies, investigators who want to compare the differences in traumatic forgetting between those with dissociative disorder and other diagnostic groups must use larger sample sizes (very much larger if items with low frequency of reporting are included). In this study, we did not confirm that the traumatic events had actually taken place. This and most of the other studies were self-reports of memory loss and later recovery, which might not be accurate. However, some of the previously cited studies on traumatic forgetting found considerable confirmation of trauma, lending some credibility to reports of trauma among psychiatric outpatients. In addition, in past studies on dissociative disorder, confirmation of trauma has been very high (Coons 1994a; Coons and Milstein 1986).

Treatment Recommendations

At present, clinicians should follow published treatment guidelines for patients with recovered memories of trauma. The following is our advice to clinicians who treat dissociative disorders:

Use psychodynamic psychotherapy. Although medication is often useful in the treatment of dissociative disorders and comorbid post-traumatic stress disorder (Davidson 1992; Loewenstein 1991), psychodynamic psychotherapy should be the primary mode of treatment for most of these patients (Kluft 1995). To avoid a worsening of the patient's symptomatology, the clinician should be careful to respect the patient's dissociative defenses by ensuring safety, proceeding slowly, and not overusing abreaction (Kluft 1995; Segall 1995). In addition, to avoid regression, clinicians should not utilize fringe therapies such as exorcism (Bowman 1993) or reparenting (Greaves 1988).

Maintain therapeutic neutrality. If patients ask whether the clinician believes that they were abused, the clinician should respond that abuse is possible, but the clinician cannot confirm that the abuse occurred because he or she was not an observer. It is important to explore why patients focus on belief. Were they not believed as children? Do they have a problem with trust? Lawsuits against abusers should not be encouraged, and, if a lawsuit is filed, the clinician should not involve himself or herself in a dual relationship by being both the patient's therapist and expert witness.

Educate both yourself and your patient about memory and enhancement procedures. The clinician should obtain collateral information to assess accuracy of memory. Hypnosis and Amytal sodium should be used rarely for memory retrieval. However, if either technique is used, the clinician should obtain informed consent and should adhere to guidelines for treatment (American Society of Clinical Hypnosis 1995) or use in forensic contexts (American Medical Association 1985). Suggestive interview techniques in memory retrieval should not be used. Suggestive questions should be avoided if hypnosis is utilized. The use of guided imagery or dream analysis for memory retrieval should be avoided altogether.

Stay within the limits of your clinical competence. If the clinician is not trained in psychodynamic therapy, the patient should be referred to someone well trained in this therapy. Consultations should be obtained when the clinician is treating difficult patients. If the clinician contemplates using hypnosis, he or she should have received proper training in its use from an accredited organization.

Maintain good records. The clinician should document the symptoms and memories with which patients initially present, the use of informed consent, the gathering of collateral information, whether memories are retrieved inside or outside of treatment, the triggers for memories, and any methods used to retrieve memories. The clinician should adequately document that he or she followed current guidelines for the treatment of DID (International Society for the Study of Dissociation 1994) and the use of memory enhancement procedures to aid in defending against malpractice lawsuits regarding false memories.

A Possible Biological Basis for Traumatic Forgetting

Recently, Bremner et al. (1995a) reviewed the neuroanatomical correlates of the effects of stress on memory. It has previously been shown that the limbic regions of the brain mediate memory function, fear-related behaviors, and the stress response. More specifically, recent research has shown that the hippocampal volume of patients with posttraumatic stress disorder is decreased as compared with those without posttraumatic stress disorder (Bremner et al. 1995b). The constant outpouring of glucocorticosteroids that occurs with chronic stress or trauma may somehow damage the hippocampus. If this is so, a mechanism may exist to explain not only why traumatic memories may be forgotten but also why they may not be remembered correctly.

Directions for Future Research

Many questions remain about traumatic memory. How and why are memories forgotten? Are shame or guilt involved in forgetting? Is damage to the hippocampus involved in patients with dissociative disorders and in others who have been traumatized and forgotten their trauma? Does damage to the hippocampus affect the accuracy of remembering in those who have been traumatized? Does the use of secrecy or threats by the perpetrators of child abuse affect whether the abuse is forgotten? Are clinical methods available to distinguish accurate from inaccurate memories? For those therapeutic techniques believed to distort accurate recall, how severely are memories distorted for each of these? For example, are memories retrieved from dreams ever accurate, or are most memories derived from flashbacks accurate? Most of all, as Janet implied in 1925, rules for discerning the accuracy of traumatic memories and for proper treatment are urgently needed. The answers to these and other questions await further research in this significant area.

References

Albach F: Freud's Verleidingstheorie: Incest, Trauma, and Hysterie [Freud's Seduction Hypothesis: Incest, Trauma, and Hysteria]. Amsterdam, Academisch Proefschrift, de Universiteit van Amsterdam, 1993

Allen JG: The spectrum of accuracy in memories of childhood trauma. Harvard Review of Psychiatry 3:84–95, 1995

American Medical Association, Council on Scientific Affairs: The status of refreshing recollection by the use of hypnosis. JAMA 253:1918–1923, 1985

American Medical Association, Council on Scientific Affairs: Report 5-A-94: Memories of Childhood Abuse. Chicago, IL, American Medical Association, 1994

American Psychiatric Association: Diagnostic and Statistical Manual of Mental Disorders, 4th Edition. Washington, DC, American Psychiatric Association, 1994

American Psychiatric Association, Board of Trustees: Statement on memories of sexual abuse. Int J Clin Exp Hypn 42:261–264, 1994

American Society of Clinical Hypnosis: Clinical Hypnosis and Memory: Guidelines for Clinicians and for Forensic Hypnosis. Chicago, IL, American Society of Clinical Hypnosis, 1995

Applied Cognitive Psychology 8:281–435, 1994

Archibald HC, Tuddenham RD: Persistent stress reaction after combat. Arch Gen Psychiatry 12:475–481, 1956

Binder RL, McNiel DE, Goldstone RL: Patterns of recall of childhood sexual abuse as described by adult survivors. Bull Am Acad Psychiatry Law 22:357–366, 1994

Bloom P: Clinical guidelines in using hypnosis in uncovering memories of sexual abuse: a master class commentary. Int J Clin Exp Hypn 42:173–178, 1994

Bottoms BL, Goodman GS, Shauer PR: An analysis of ritualistic and religion-related child abuse allegations. Law and Human Behavior 20:1–34, 1996

Bowman ES: Clinical and spiritual effects of exorcism in fifteen patients with multiple personality disorder. Dissociation 6:222–238, 1993

Bremner JD, Krystal JH, Southwick SM, et al: Functional neuroanatomical correlates of the effects of stress on memory. J Trauma Stress 8:527–553, 1995a

Bremner JD, Randall P, Scott TM, et al: MRI-based measurement of hippocampal volume in combat-related posttraumatic stress disorder. Am J Psychiatry 152:973–981, 1995b

Briere J, Conte J: Self-reported amnesia in adults molested as children. J Trauma Stress 6:21–31, 1993

British Psychological Society: Recovered memories. Psychologist 8:507–508, 1995

Cameron C: Women survivors confronting their abusers: issues, decisions, and outcomes. Journal of Child Sexual Abuse 3:7–35, 1994

Ceci SJ, Bruck M: Suggestibility of the child witness: a historical review and synthesis. Psychol Bull 113:413–439, 1993

Consciousness Cognition 3(3–4):265–469, 1994

Consciousness Cognition 4(1):63–134, 1995

Coons PM: Dissociative disorder not otherwise specified: a clinical investigation of 50 cases with suggestions for treatment. Dissociation 5:187–195, 1992

Coons PM: Confirmation of childhood abuse in child and adolescent cases of multiple personality disorder and dissociative disorder not otherwise specified. J Nerv Ment Dis 182:461–464, 1994a

Coons PM: Reports of satanic ritual abuse: further implications of pseudomemories. Percept Mot Skills 78:1376–1378, 1994b

Coons PM, Milstein V: Psychosexual differences in multiple personality: characteristics, etiology, and treatment. J Clin Psychiatry 47:106–110, 1986

Coons PM, Milstein V: Psychogenic amnesia: a clinical investigation of 25 cases. Dissociation 5:73–79, 1992

Coons PM, Bowman ES, Milstein V: Multiple personality disorder: a clinical investigation of 50 cases. J Nerv Ment Dis 176:519–527, 1988

Counseling Psychologist 23(2):181–363, 1995

Cronin JA: Science and the admissibility of evidence: the latest FMSF tactics. Treating Abuse Today 5(1):30–37, 1995

Davidson J: Drug therapy of post-traumatic stress disorder. Br J Psychiatry 160:309–314, 1992

Elliott DM, Briere J: Posttraumatic stress associated with delayed recall of sexual abuse: a general population study. J Trauma Stress 8:629–647, 1995

Feldman-Summers S, Pope KS: The experience of forgetting childhood abuse: a national survey of psychologists. J Consult Clin Psychol 62:636–639, 1994

Fisher C: Amnesic states in war neuroses: the psychogenesis of fugues. Psychoanal Q 14:437–458, 1944

Fowler C: A pragmatic approach to early childhood memories: shifting the focus from truth to clinical utility. Psychotherapy 31:676–686, 1994

Frankel FH: The concept of flashbacks in historical perspective. Int J Clin Exp Hypn 42:321–336, 1994

Goldfield AE, Mollica RF, Pesanvento BH: The psychical and psychological sequelae of torture: symptomatology and diagnosis. JAMA 25:2725–2729, 1988

Golston JC: A false memory syndrome conference: activist accused and their professional allies talk about science, law, and family reconciliation. Treating Abuse Today 5(1):24–30, 1995

Greaves GB: Common errors in the treatment of multiple personality disorder. Dissociation 1:61–66, 1988

Gutheil TG: True or false memories of sexual abuse? A forensic psychiatric view. Psychiatric Annals 23:527–531, 1993

Hammond DC: Clinical hypnosis and memory: guidelines for clinicians. Newsletter of the International Society for the Study of Dissociation 13(4):1,9, 1995

Henderson JL, Moore M: The psychoneuroses of war. N Engl J Med 230:274–278, 1944

Hendin H, Hags AP, Singer P: The reliving experience in Vietnam veterans with posttraumatic stress disorder. Compr Psychiatry 23:163–173, 1984

Herman JL: Trauma and Recovery. New York, Basic Books, 1992

Herman JL, Schatzow E: Recovery and verification of memories of childhood sexual trauma. Psychoanalytic Psychology 4:1–14, 1987

Int J Clin Exp Hypn 42(4):258–455, 1994

Int J Clin Exp Hypn 43(2):109–248, 1995

International Society for the Study of Dissociation: ISSD Guidelines for Treating Dissociative Identity Disorder (Multiple Personality Disorder) in Adults. Skokie, IL, International Society for the Study of Dissociation, 1994

Jaffe R: Dissociative phenomena in former concentration camp inmates. Int J Psychoanal 49:310–312, 1968

Janet P: Psychological Healing: A Historical and Clinical Study, Vol 1. New York, Macmillan, 1925, p 670

Journal of Psychohistory 23(2):119–190, 1995

J Trauma Stress 8(4):501–726, 1995

Kalman G: On combat-neurosis. Int J Soc Psychiatry 23:195–203, 1977

Kihlstrom JF: The trauma-memory argument. Consciousness Cognition 4:63–67, 1995

Kinzie JD: Posttraumatic effects and their treatment among Southeast Asia refugees, in International Handbook of Traumatic Stress Syndromes. Edited by Wilson JP, Raphael B. New York, Plenum, 1993, pp 311–319

Kluft RP: Dissociative identity disorder, part II: treatment. Directions in Psychiatry 15(24):1–7, 1995

Lanning KV: A law enforcement perspective on allegations of ritual abuse, in Out of Darkness: Exploring Satanism and Ritual Abuse. Edited by Sakheim DK, Levine SE. New York, Lexington Books, 1992, pp 109–144

Lindsay DS, Read JD: Psychotherapy and memories of childhood sexual abuse: a cognitive perspective. Applied Cognitive Psychology 8:281–338, 1994

Loewenstein RJ: Rational psychopharmacotherapy in the treatment of multiple personality disorder. Psychiatr Clin North Am 14:721–740, 1991

Loftus EF: The reality of repressed memories. Am Psychol 48:517–537, 1993

Loftus EF, Polonsky S, Fullilove MT: Memories of childhood sexual abuse: remembering and repressing. Psychology of Women Quarterly 18:67–84, 1994

Lynn SJ, Nash MR: Truth in memory: ramifications for psychotherapy and hypnotherapy. Am J Clin Hypn 36:194–208, 1994

Madakasira S, O'Brian K: Acute posttraumatic stress disorder in victims of natural disaster. J Nerv Ment Dis 175:286–290, 1987

McHugh PR, Butterfield MI: Do patients' recovered memories of sexual abuse constitute a "false memory syndrome"? Psychiatric News 28(23):18, 1993

Modai I: Forgetting childhood: a defense mechanism against psychosis in a holocaust survivor. Clinical Gerontologist 14(3):61–67, 1994

Niederland WG: Clinical observations on the "survivor syndrome." Int J Psychoanal 49:313–315, 1968

Orne MT, Whitehouse WC, Dinges DF, et al: Reconstructing memory through hypnosis: forensic and clinical implications, in Hypnosis and Memory. Edited by Pettinati HM. New York, Guilford, 1988, pp 21–63

Pope HG, Hudson JL: Can memories of childhood sexual abuse be repressed? Psychol Med 25:121–126, 1995

Powell RA, Boer DP: Did Freud mislead patients to confabulate memories of abuse? Psychol Rep 74:1283–1298, 1995

Psychiatric Annals 25(12):713–735, 1995

Putnam FW, Guroff JJ, Silberman EK, et al: The clinical phenomenology of multiple personality disorder: a review of 100 recent cases. J Clin Psychiatry 47:285–293, 1986

Roesler TA, Wind TW: Telling the secret: adult women describe their disclosures of incest. Journal of Interpersonal Violence 9:327–338, 1994

Ross CA, Norton G, Wozney K: Multiple personality disorder: an analysis of 236 cases. Can J Psychiatry 34:413–418, 1989

Sargant W, Slater E: Amnesic syndromes of war. Proceedings of the Royal Society of Medicine 34:757–764, 1941

Segall SR: Misalliances and misadventures in the treatment of dissociative disorders, in Dissociative Identity Disorder: Theoretical and Treatment Controversies. Edited by Cohen LM, Berzoff JN, Elin MR. Northvale, NJ, Jason Aronson, 1995, pp 379–412

Sonneberg SM, Blank AS, Talbott JA: The Traumas of War: Stress and Recovery in Vietnam Veterans. Washington, DC, American Psychiatric Press, 1985

Spanos NP, Burgess CA, Burgess MF: Past-life identities, UFO abductions, and satanic ritual abuse: a social construction of memories. Int J Clin Exp Hypn 42:433–446, 1994

Spence DP: Narrative truth and putative child abuse. Int J Clin Exp Hypn 42:289–303, 1995

Spiegel D: Trauma, dissociation, and hypnosis, in Incest-Related Syndromes of Adult Psychopathology. Edited by Kluft RP. Washington, DC, American Psychiatric Press, 1990, pp 247–261

Terr L: What happens to early memories of old trauma? A study of twenty children under age five at the time of documented traumatic events. J Am Acad Child Adolesc Psychiatry 27:96–104, 1988

Terr L: Childhood traumas: an outline and overview. Am J Psychiatry 148:10–20, 1991

Thom DA, Fenton N: Amnesias in war cases. American Journal of Insanity 7:437–448, 1920

Torrie A: Psychosomatic casualties in the Middle East. Lancet 1:139–143, 1944

Tromp S, Koss MP, Figuredo AJ, et al: Are rape memories different: a comparison of rape, other unpleasant, and pleasant memories among employed women. J Trauma Stress 8:607–627, 1995

Usher JA, Neisser U: Childhood amnesia in the beginnings of memory for four early life events. J Exp Psychol Gen 2:155–165, 1993

van der Hart O, Nijenhuis E: Amnesia for traumatic experiences. Hypnos 22:73–86, 1995

van der Kolk BA, Fisler R: Dissociation and the fragmentary nature of traumatic memories: overview and exploratory study. J Trauma Stress 8:505–525, 1995

Wakefield H, Underwager R: Uncovering memories of alleged sexual abuse: the therapists who do it. Issues in Child Abuse Accusations 4:197–213, 1992

Wakefield H, Underwager R: Return of the Furies: An Investigation Into Recovered Memory Therapy. Chicago, IL, Open Court, 1994

Watkins JG: Dealing with the problem of "false memory" in clinic and court. Journal of Psychiatry and the Law 21:297–317, 1993

Weir IK, Wheatcroft MS: Allegations of children's involvement in ritual sexual abuse: clinical experience in 20 cases. Child Abuse Negl 19:491–505, 1995

Whitfield CL: Memory and Abuse: Remembering and Healing the Effects of Trauma. Dearfield Beach, FL, Heath Communications, 1995

Wilkinson CB: Aftermath of a disaster: collapse of the Hyatt Regency Hotel skywalks. Am J Psychiatry 140:1134–1139, 1983

Williams LM: Recall of childhood trauma: a prospective study of women's memories of child sexual abuse. J Consult Clin Psychol 62:1167–1176, 1994

Williams LM: Recovered memories of abuse in women with documented child sexual victimization histories. J Trauma Stress 8:649–673, 1995

Yapko MD: Suggestions of Abuse: True and False Memories of Childhood Sexual Traumas. New York, Simon & Schuster, 1994

Afterword to Section II

David Spiegel, M.D., Section Editor

In the chapters in Section II, a sizable body of research and systematic clinical observation is reviewed. Despite disparate professional interests and orientations, common ground is found. The authors generally agree that memory of any event is a reconstructive process, a matching of schema with memory trace, subject to suggestive influence and the need for affect regulation. At the same time, memory defects, including traumatic amnesia, are observed commonly after traumatic stressors, consistent with the alteration in cognitive function that commonly occurs during trauma. The evidence that suggestion can alter memory retrieval does not prove that memory, even recovered memory, is inherently unreliable. Rather, it provides further evidence that memory of real traumatic events can be repressed with suggestion, just as false memories can be suggested. Indeed, some research indicates that people vulnerable to suggestion effects are more likely to have real memories of events similar to those suggested: the schema exists even though the event did not.

The guidelines suggested by the authors in this section are similar in content and spirit to the American Psychiatric Association's recommendations listed at the end of the foreword. Memories of trauma, especially those that were repressed, should be taken seriously but not at face value. Distortion of memory is not uncommon, but error in some areas does not imply error in all. Research is needed to link what is known about memory processing to the effects of trauma on memory. Also, the role of memory retrieval and working through in the psychotherapy of trauma requires further empirical exploration: must one remember in order to forget? These chapters combine the cold light of investigation with the empathic warmth of clinical care. Sullivan defined psychotherapy as "participant observation." The therapist must participate in a real and caring relationship but always be able to step back and observe what is happening in it. Therapists must be neither credulous nor calculating: don't forget.

III

Obsessive-Compulsive Disorder Across the Life Cycle

III

Obsessive-Compulsive Disorder Across the Life Cycle

Contents

Section III

Obsessive-Compulsive Disorder Across the Life Cycle

Foreword

Michele T. Pato, M.D., and Gail Steketee, Ph.D.,
Section Editors

It is particularly relevant to study obsessive-compulsive disorder (OCD) throughout the life cycle, because for many suffering with OCD, it is a chronic illness beginning in childhood and continuing into later life.

In reading Chapters 11 through 13 of this section—OCD in Children and Adolescents (Drs. Penn, March, and Leonard), in Adults (Drs. Pato and Pato), and in Later Life (Drs. Pollard, Carmin, and Ownby)—the reader should be struck most by the persistence and similarity of symptoms, as well as the comparable prevalences of the disorder, across the life cycle. In addition, the same treatments are effective in different age groups. With regard to pharmacological treatment in particular, it is notable that although dosage adjustments are needed depending on age, a relatively long treatment duration—beginning with 10–12 weeks in the initial treatment phase—seems to be indicated at all stages of the life cycle.

It is generally believed that any stress can cause an exacerbation of OCD symptoms. Thus, it is not surprising to find, in Chapter 15 (by Diaz, Grush, Sichel, and Cohen), that pregnancy and the puerperium—life-cycle events of particular importance for many women—can be a time of worsening obsessive-compulsive symptoms. This finding runs counter to the traditional belief that pregnancy is a period of relative mental well-being.

Chapter 14 (Drs. Eisen and Steketee) reinforces and extends the notion established by the other chapters in this section—namely, that OCD is a lifelong illness and that relatively few patients experience a total disappearance of symptoms over time. More than anything, this chapter highlights the work that still needs to be done to identify factors that contribute to and predict OCD course and outcome.

Chapter 11

Obsessive-Compulsive Disorder in Children and Adolescents

Joseph V. Penn, M.D., John March, M.D., M.P.H., and Henrietta L. Leonard, M.D.

Only 10 years ago, the perception existed that obsessive-compulsive disorder (OCD) was rare in childhood. Psychiatrists saw few patients, perhaps because of the secretive nature of the disorder or the reluctance of patients, or because OCD symptoms were not appropriately recognized or treated. It is now estimated that perhaps as many as 1 million children and adolescents in this country may suffer from OCD. Similar to adults, children with OCD often have their symptoms for quite a while before they receive assessment and treatment. Families may turn first to nonpsychiatric specialists, who have varying degrees of experience with the disorder, which may further delay recognition and treatment. With increasing professional and media interest in this disorder and greater sensitivity to its diagnosis, many people with OCD are now receiving accurate diagnoses and effective treatments. In this chapter we review the phenomenology, diagnosis, etiology, and treatment issues of OCD in children and adolescents. Pediatric pharmacological treatment and cognitive-behavior therapy of OCD is emphasized. Also presented is recent evidence for a subtype of pediatric-onset OCD.

Phenomenology

Symptoms

In DSM-IV (American Psychiatric Association 1994), as in DSM-III-R (American Psychiatric Association 1987), OCD is characterized by recurrent obsessions and/or compulsions that are severe enough to "cause marked distress or significant impairment" (American Psychiatric Association 1994, p. 417). An affected child or adolescent must have either obsessions or compulsions, although the majority seem to have both. DSM-IV specifies that affected individuals must recognize at some point in the illness that their obsessions are not simply excessive worries about real problems; and, similarly, compulsions must be seen as

---

excessive or unreasonable, although this condition may not always hold true for young children. A change in the DSM-IV criteria from those in DSM-III-R specifies that persons of all ages who lack insight receive the added specification *poor insight type.* The specific content of the obsessions cannot be related to another Axis I diagnosis, such as preoccupations about food resulting from an eating disorder or guilty thoughts (ruminations) from major depressive disorder.

Children and adolescents with OCD typically have both obsessions and compulsions (Flament et al. 1988; Judd 1965; Riddle et al. 1990b; Swedo et al. 1989b). An individual typically attempts to ignore, suppress, or neutralize the intrusive obsessive thoughts. Generally, compulsions are carried out to dispel anxiety and/or in response to an obsession (e.g., to ward off harm to someone). Berkowitz and Rothman (1960) described obsessions in children that varied greatly, ranging from an ideational wish that misfortune or death would befall a parent to bizarre, unrealistic, persistent thoughts. The most commonly reported obsessions focus on concerns about germs and contamination, fears about harm or danger, worries about right and wrong, or having a "tune in the head" (Swedo et al. 1989b). The major presenting ritual symptoms include (in order of decreasing frequency) excessive "cleaning" (hand washing, showering, bathing, or tooth brushing); repeating rituals (going in and out doors, getting up from and sitting down on chairs, restating phrases, or rereading); checking behaviors (making sure that doors and windows are locked, that appliances are turned off, or that homework is done "right"); counting; ordering/arranging; touching; and hoarding (Flament et al. 1988; Judd 1965; Rettew et al. 1992; Riddle et al. 1990b; Swedo et al. 1989b). Some of the obsessions and rituals involve an internal sense that "it doesn't feel right" until the thought or action is completed.

In contrast to other forms of psychopathology, the specific symptoms of OCD are essentially identical in children and adults (Hanna 1995; Rapoport 1986; Rettew et al. 1992; Swedo et al. 1989b). The individual types of obsessions and compulsions have been reported to be numerous although of a finite type and to change in both content and severity over time in most individuals (Rapoport 1989; Swedo et al. 1989b). Rettew and colleagues (1992) studied the individual OCD symptoms of 79 children and adolescents with severe OCD over an average of 7.9 years (range 2–16 years) and found no significant relationships with either the number or the type of OCD symptoms and age. Despite a diversity in symptoms, the symptom "pool" was remarkably finite and very similar to that seen in adults. Most OCD patients simultaneously experience several OCD symptoms, which change over time. This finding would argue against a unique, specific symptom content (e.g., obsessions versus rituals, washing versus checking) being representative of a subgroup (phenotype) of OCD.

Age and Gender Effects

Seventy consecutive child and adolescent patients were prospectively examined at the National Institute of Mental Health (NIMH) (Swedo et al. 1989b). These 47 boys and 23 girls met diagnostic criteria for primary severe OCD, and had a mean age at onset of illness of 10 years of age. Seven of the patients had the onset of their illness prior to age 7. Boys tended to have an earlier (prepubertal) onset, usually around age 9, whereas girls were more likely to have a later (pubertal) illness onset, around age 11. Interestingly, the children with an earlier onset of OCD were more likely to be male and to have a family member with OCD or a tic disorder. Patients with a very early onset of OCD (less than 6 years old) were more likely to have compulsions than obsessions, and their symptoms (such as blinking and breathing rituals) tended to be more unusual than the classic OCD symptoms.

There is some disagreement regarding the gender distribution of children and adolescents with OCD. Although a preponderance of males is seen in most studies of children and adolescents with OCD, two epidemiological studies of OCD in adolescents and two studies of referred children and adolescents with OCD found an approximately equal number of males and females with OCD (for a review, see Hanna 1995). This finding is most likely explained by the fact that in the prepubertal years, there is a higher male-to-female ratio for the disorder, whereas postpubertally this ratio is reversed. At least one-third of adults with OCD have reported to have first developed the disorder in childhood (Black 1974), often at a very early age. Age at onset can range from 3 to 18 years (Riddle et al. 1990b) but is typically 9 to 11 years (Last and Strauss 1989), or 7 to 18 years with a mean age at onset of 12.8 years (Flament et al. 1988). Several studies suggest that boys have an earlier age at onset than girls (Flament et al. 1985; Last and Strauss 1989; Swedo et al. 1989b), that younger boys have more severe symptoms than younger girls (Flament et al. 1988), and that boys are more likely than girls to have a comorbid tic disorder (Leonard et al. 1992). It has been suggested that earlier onset of illness may be associated with increased genetic loading (Lenane et al. 1990; Leonard et al. 1992; Pauls et al. 1995).

OCD is characterized by a waxing and waning course, often with worsening related to psychosocial stressors. Children will often initially disguise their rituals (Swedo et al. 1989b). Severely incapacitated children and adolescents with hallmark OCD symptoms will be more readily diagnosed. Less severely ill patients, and those attempting to hide symptoms, are more difficult to recognize. "Red flags" for OCD may include lengthy, unproductive hours spent on homework, holes erased into test papers and homework, or retracing over letters or words. Unexplained high utility bills, a dramatic increase in laundry, an insistence on wearing clothes or using a towel only once, or toilets being stopped up from too much paper may alert the family to an obsession about germs and contamination. Behaviors suspicious for OCD include lengthy bedtime rituals; exaggerated requests for reassurance; difficulty leaving the house; peculiar patterns for walking, breathing, or sitting; requests for family members to repeat phrases; a recurring fear of harm coming to oneself or others; or a persistent fear that one has an illness. Finally, hoarding seemingly useless objects such as magazine subscription coupons, empty juice cans, or street garbage requires differentiation from normal childhood behavior of collecting rocks, sticks, or other sentimental "treasures."

Few rating scales are available to assess OCD severity in children or adolescents. The Children's Yale-Brown Obsessive Compulsive Scale (CY-BOCS; Goodman et al. 1992) has been specifically adapted for children and is the most widely used. The CY-BOCS can document baseline severity of symptoms and changes over time that otherwise might not be reported unless specifically assessed. Part of this scale, the Y-BOCS Symptom Checklist, is particularly useful in a clinical interview to elicit all the symptoms, including more "minor" and more secretive ones that might go unnoticed or undisclosed.

Epidemiology

Initial estimates of the incidence of childhood OCD were derived from psychiatric clinic populations. Berman (1942) reported "obsessive-compulsive phenomena" in 6 of 2,800 (0.2%) patients. Hollingsworth and colleagues (1980) found 17 cases of OCD in 8,367 (0.2%) child and adolescent inpatient and outpatient records. Judd (1965) conducted a retrospective chart review study that revealed 5 cases in 425 (1.2%) pediatric records.

The first epidemiological study, the Isle of Wight study, reported "mixed obsessional/anxiety disorders" in 7 of 2,199 (0.3%) 10- and 11-year-old children surveyed (Rutter et al. 1970). Flament and colleagues (1988) found a (weighted point) prevalence rate of 0.8% and a lifetime prevalence of 1.9% in a whole-population adolescent epidemiology study. These data suggest that OCD is a relatively common disorder in adolescence. Furthermore, this is compatible with both the estimated prevalence in the general population (Karno et al. 1988) and the finding that at least one-third to one-half of adult OCD patients first developed the illness in childhood (Black 1974).

Differential Diagnosis

The differential diagnosis of OCD is broad and includes the depressive and anxiety disorders (separation anxiety, simple phobia, social phobia, panic disorder, and generalized anxiety disorder) with obsessional features; stereotypies seen in mental retardation, pervasive developmental disorders (PDDs), autism, and brain damage syndromes; obsessive-compulsive personality disorder (OCPD); anorexia and bulimia; tic disorders; and, more rarely, childhood schizophrenia. Obsessive brooding and ruminating may be demonstrated in major depressive disorder, but the thoughts are usually more content specific and are not seen as senseless. Fear of harm coming to oneself or others can be found in separation anxiety disorder, but in OCD this specific thought usually results in the need to perform compulsive rituals. Similarly, the excessive and unrealistic worry in generalized anxiety disorder is not accompanied by classic compulsive rituals. Avoidance secondary to simple phobia does not usually involve germs as a primary object of avoidance; and the phobic person's fear usually decreases when he or she is not confronted with the stimuli, unlike the case in OCD. The relationship between OCPD and OCD remains unclear for children as well as for adults, and merits more study.

Although repetitive, formalized behaviors such as the stereotypies seen in children and adolescents with autism, mental retardation, PDD, or organic brain damage may superficially resemble OCD rituals, OCD rituals are typically well organized, complex, and ego-dystonic. In autism, the rituals seem reassuring, lack ego-dystonicity, and are not associated with an obsession. Other features of autism, such as peculiar speech patterns and severely impaired interpersonal relationships, are not seen in OCD (Swedo and Rapoport 1989). Rigid and repetitive behaviors of Asperger's syndrome may appear to resemble those seen in OCD. A careful assessment of developmental history, clinical presentation, social relationships, and symptoms may be helpful in making the distinction between stereotypies and OCD rituals.

The anorexic or bulimic patient's consuming or "obsessive" interest in calories, exercise, and food and "compulsive" avoidance, measuring, and monitoring of food may certainly bear a resemblance to symptoms of OCD. Although OCD and eating disorders may coexist, the distinction can usually be made between OCD and a primary eating disorder, because when considered in context, the focus of the obsessions and compulsions in eating disorders are all related to food and body image.

Associated Disorders

Disorders most commonly associated with childhood OCD follow patterns somewhat similar to those reported in adults, with affective and anxiety disorders most common (Swedo et al. 1989b). However, attention-deficit/hyperactivity disorder (ADHD) and behavioral disorders may be more prevalent in children. In the 70 consecutive children studied at the NIMH, comorbidity was common, with only 18 (26%) having no other psychiatric diagnosis (Swedo et al. 1989b). At initial presentation, the children and adolescents had the following concurrent diagnoses: tic disorder (30%), major depression (26%), specific developmental disability (24%), simple phobia (17%), overanxious disorder (16%), adjustment disorder with depressed mood (13%), oppositional disorder (11%), attention-deficit disorder (10%), conduct disorder (7%), separation anxiety disorder (7%), enuresis (4%), alcohol abuse (4%), and encopresis (3%) (Swedo et al. 1989b).

Hanna (1995) found that lifetime rates of depressive, anxiety, disruptive behavior, and tic disorders ranged from 26% to 32%. Depression is frequently associated with OCD, with secondary depression developing in response to distress and interference from OCD. Phobias and anxiety disorders may also occur concurrently with OCD. Riddle and colleagues (1990b) found that among children without preexisting major neuropsychiatric disorders, the rates of comorbid anxiety and mood disorder diagnoses were relatively high.

Patients with Tourette's syndrome (TS) often have associated obsessive-compulsive symptomatology and/or meet full DSM-IV OCD criteria (Cohen and Leckman 1994; Frankel et al. 1986; Leckman et al. 1993; Leonard et al. 1992; Pauls et al. 1986). It is important to carefully distinguish between rituals and tics, as each requires different treatments. In general, OCD patients' rituals are more complex and occur in response to an obsession. Thus, if an action is preceded by a specific cognition and is performed to "undo" or "dispel" the thought, it is considered to be a compulsive ritual. Some complex motor tics may be preceded by tension, a sensation, or an "urge"; however, they are not typically initiated by a thought or accompanied by anxiety. On rare occasions, a complex motor tic preceded by a cognition, sensation, or urge may be difficult to distinguish from a compulsive ritual (Leckman et al. 1994). These experiences may include premonitory feelings or urges that are relieved with the performance of the act and a need to perform tics or compulsions until they are felt to be "just right." For a more detailed discussion, readers are referred to Leckman et al. (1993, 1994).

ADHD may also occur concurrently with OCD, and appears to have a higher frequency in male patients (Hanna 1995; Riddle et al. 1990b; Swedo et al. 1989b). Hanna (1995) found that one-third of 31 children and adolescents with OCD also had a current disruptive behavior disorder (DBD). The ADHD arose before the OCD, whereas the oppositional defiant and conduct disorders tended to develop in conjunction with the OCD. Geller and colleagues (1995) found that DBDs were among the most common comorbid diagnoses in their sample of 38 patients with OCD. In addition to the greater severity of OCD illness in patients with a prepubertal onset, increased rates of comorbid DBD are seen, although DBDs are generally more common in boys than in girls (Anderson et al. 1987).

Etiology

The etiology of OCD is unknown, but research suggests frontal lobe–limbic–basal ganglia dysfunction (Insel 1992; Wise and Rapoport 1989). Additionally, neurotransmitter dysregulation, genetic susceptibility, and environmental triggers appear to have roles in the pathogenesis of the illness. The demonstration that serotonin reuptake inhibitors (SRIs) are specifically efficacious in the treatment of OCD has led to the "serotonin hypothesis" of OCD. However, it is unlikely that neurotransmitter dysregulation can be attributed to only one system, given that others (e.g., dopamine) have also been implicated. For an excellent review, the reader is referred to Insel (1992).

Additional evidence supports a neurobiological etiology of OCD, which includes neuroanatomical, neurophysiological, and neuroimmunological associations and metabolic abnormalities. Head injury, brain tumors, carbon monoxide poisoning, and other brain insults resulting in basal ganglia damage have been reported to be related to the onset of OCD symptomatology (Insel 1992). Basal ganglia diseases, such as postencephalitic Parkinson's disease (von Economo 1931) and Huntington's chorea (Cummings and Cunningham 1992), also have an increased rate of OCD. Neuroimaging studies in adult OCD patients with a childhood onset of symptoms compared with nonimpaired control subjects have shown decreased caudate size on computed tomography (CT) scans (Luxenberg et al. 1988) and abnormal patterns of regional glucose metabolism on positron-emission tomography (PET) scans (Swedo et al. 1989c, 1992).

Generally, pediatric OCD probands do not appear to have either gross or clinically impairing neurological or neuropsychological abnormalities, although "soft signs" may be present. Minor perinatal or premorbid developmental problems were reported for several children and adolescents in Riddle and colleagues' phenomenology study (1990b); however, none of the children had a major perinatal or developmental problem that appeared to have an obvious relationship to the onset or course of OCD. In general, the children with OCD performed comparably with the control subjects on neuropsychological measures; however, increased errors produced on a select subset of tests were interpreted to be consistent with frontal lobe or caudate lesions or both (Cox et al. 1989). On stressed neurological examination of 54 pediatric OCD patients, more than 80% had some positive "soft" neurological finding (Denckla 1989). The subtle findings on stressed neurological examination and on complete neuropsychological testing are suggestive of underlying abnormalities. Children with OCD who show specific abnormalities in visual-spatial-organizational information processing are at risk for specific learning problems, such as dysgraphia, arithmetic and expressive written-language deficiencies, and slow processing speed and efficiency (J. March and C. K. Conners, unpublished data). When poor social skills resulting from weaknesses in the nonverbal processing of social-emotional communication are also present (J. March, unpublished data), OCD may overlap Asperger's syndrome. These subtle neuropsychological and academic impairments may be missed and may contribute clinically to "treatment-resistant" cases.

Intriguing links have also been found among TS, tic disorders, and OCD. Patients with TS frequently have obsessive-compulsive features, and OCD patients have an increased incidence of tic disorders (Leonard et al. 1992; Pauls et al. 1986). Since the initial systematic family study of probands with TS (Pauls et al. 1986), other studies have demonstrated increased rates of OCD in families of probands with TS and increased rates of tic disorders in families of probands with OCD (Leonard et al. 1992). A number of studies have demonstrated familial links among OCD, tic disorders, and TS (see Pauls et al. 1986, 1995), suggesting a genetic vulnerability for OCD and tic disorders. Pauls and colleagues (1986) hypothesized that OCD and TS may be different manifestations of the same gene(s). Walkup and colleagues (1995) recently proposed a mixed model of inheritance. OCD probands often have a family history of tic disorders and OCD, and TS probands often have a family history of tic disorders and OCD. Lenane and colleagues (1990) found that 20% of personally interviewed first-degree relatives of children and adolescents with OCD also met lifetime history criteria for OCD. Of note, the primary OCD symptom in the affected family member was usually different from that in the proband, a finding arguing against both a modeling theory for OCD and familial symptom subtypes.

Holzer and colleagues (1994) compared the phenomenological features of 35 adult OCD patients with a lifetime history of tics and those of age- and sex-matched OCD patients without tics. They found that the OCD patients with tics had more touching, tapping, rubbing, blinking, and staring—and fewer cleaning—rituals but did not differ from the non-tic OCD patients on obsessions. Continued studies of OCD symptom phenomenology may reveal that those with a lifetime history of a chronic tic disorder represent a potential subtype (Goodman et al. 1990). Similarly, McDougle and colleagues (1994) also described a possible subtype of OCD. They studied the efficacy of adding haloperidol to the treatment regimens of OCD patients with or without a comorbid chronic tic disorder who were refractory to adequate treatment with the selective serotonin reuptake inhibitor (SSRI) fluvoxamine. Their study suggested that OCD patients with a comorbid tic disorder constitute a subtype of OCD that might require conjoint SSRI and dopamine-blocking-agent therapy for effective symptom reduction.

Pauls and colleagues' (1995) family study described OCD as being a heterogeneous disorder with some cases being genetically mediated. They found that rates of OCD and subthreshold OCD were significantly greater among the relatives of the probands with OCD than among comparison subjects. They also found that children with onset of OCD between 5 and 9 years of age had a much higher rate of family members with tics, suggesting an increased genetic loading. Their study supported a previous hypothesis that earlier-onset cases of OCD represent more severe forms of disease (at least in terms of risk to relatives) (Leonard et al. 1992).

Heterogeneity of pediatric OCD has been described, and a large phenomenological study showed that some children have an abrupt onset, some have a dramatic and episodic course, and some exhibit coexisting choreiform movements. In recent years, parallel studies of Sydenham's chorea (SC) (Allen et al. 1995; Swedo et al. 1989a, 1993, 1994) and OCD have been conducted; these have demonstrated that a subgroup of OCD children first developed their OCD symptoms after a Group A beta-hemolytic streptococcal infection (GABHS) (Swedo 1994). There have been exciting research developments regarding the relationship between OCD and SC. SC is the neurological variant of rheumatic fever and is characterized by an autoimmune response in the region of the basal ganglia caused by misdirected antibodies from a streptococcal infection (Swedo et al. 1989a, 1993). There is an increased incidence of OCD in pediatric patients with SC, and it has been hypothesized that SC serves as a medical model for OCD (Swedo et al. 1989a). Recently, a subgroup of children with a pediatric onset of either OCD or a tic disorder has been described (pediatric autoimmune neuropsychiatric disorders associated with streptococcal infection [PANDAS]). These patients are characterized by an abrupt prepubertal onset of their symptoms after a GABHS and by a course of illness characterized by alternating periods of remission and dramatic, acute worsening of symptoms. This group likely represents a genetic vulnerability different from that associated with later-onset OCD. PANDAS children often have neurological signs such as choreiform movements and tics. These children appear to have an underlying pathophysiology similar to that seen in SC, although they do not have SC.

It is critical to delineate this prepubertal pediatric subtype, as these patients require a different assessment and treatment. A child presenting with an acute onset of OCD with or without tics, or a significant deterioration, requires a thorough assessment and evaluation of recent or concomitant medical illnesses, including seemingly benign upper-respiratory-tract infections. Laboratory analyses such as a throat culture, an antistreptolysin O (ASO) titer, and an antinuclear antibody test (which may be nonspecifically positive) may be helpful in diagnosing GABHS infections.

Thus, evidence suggests that early (prepubertal)-onset OCD may represent a meaningful OCD subtype. Interestingly, Ackerman and colleagues (1994) found age at OCD onset to be a strong predictor of response to clomipramine in adults. People who develop OCD later in life appear to have a better chance of responding than do those who become ill earlier, independent of length of illness, again providing indirect evidence that early onset may represent a more severe and less responsive form of the illness. The association between age at the time of onset and response to clomipramine may indicate a basic difference in the pathology of the disorder.

The successful integration of these neuroanatomical and neurophysiological hypotheses of childhood OCD with theories of genetic susceptibility and environmental stressors will generate additional research questions.

Treatment

Selection of Treatment(s)

Children and adolescents with OCD vary significantly with respect to the specific nature of the OCD and its impact. Thus, each child or adolescent requires a comprehensive individualized assessment of symptoms, comorbidity, and psychosocial factors. For an excellent reference on the general clinical assessment of the child, the reader is referred to King (1995). The individualized treatment plan should take into consideration the unique psychosocial and family issues that may influence compliance and treatment response. Whenever possible, both the patient and his or her family should participate in the development of treatment plans.

Psychodynamic Psychotherapy

Whether particular OCD symptoms represent specific intrapsychic conflicts is debatable. Esman (1990) eloquently described how OCD can be understood as having both biological and psychodynamic components. Jenike (1990) reviewed psychotherapeutic interventions available for OCD and concluded that "the traditional psychodynamic psychotherapy is not an effective treatment for patients with OCD as defined in DSM-III-R, as there are no reports in the psychiatric literature of patients who stopped ritualizing when treated with this method alone" (p. 113). Psychodynamic psychotherapy may play an important role by addressing specific issues in a patient's life—for example, the impact of the illness on the patient's self-esteem, relationships, and other psychosocial conflicts—and by improving compliance with the behavioral or pharmacological treatments that deal more directly with OCD symptomatology.

Individual and Family Therapy

Psychotherapy may play an important role in teaching coping skills, addressing comorbid diagnoses and family issues, treating the accompanying anxiety and depressive symptoms of OCD, and helping to improve peer and family relationships. Because families affect and are affected by OCD, family members often need assistance and direction in how to effectively participate in pharmacological and behavioral treatment. Thus, a thorough family assessment is necessary as part of the initial diagnostic evaluation of every child or adolescent with OCD. Family therapy is an important treatment consideration for pediatric OCD patients because family discord, marital difficulties, problems with a specific family member, or inappropriate roles or boundaries will interfere with the family's and the individual's functioning, and therefore will ultimately affect the long-term outcome of the identified patient (Hafner et al. 1981; Hoover and Insel 1984; Lenane 1991). Specific family therapy and/or marital therapy may be appropriate when family dysfunction or marital discord impedes OCD treatment. Lenane (1989) described the goals of family therapy as involving the whole family in treatment, getting all behaviors "out in the open," obtaining full and accurate understanding of how everyone in the family participates in the OCD behavior, and also reframing less-than-positive behavior. The end result of this process is that the family is better able to participate in the treatment plan of the identified OCD patient in a more positive and constructive manner.

Behavioral Treatment

Cognitive-behavior therapy (CBT)—in particular, in the form of exposure and response prevention (ERP)—has been well developed and studied in adults with OCD (Baer 1992; Foa and Emmelkamp 1983; Greist 1992; Marks 1987) but has not been systematically studied in children and adolescents with OCD. Original pediatric case reports suggested that behavioral techniques employed with adults (Marks 1987) were also appropriate for children (Berg et al. 1989; March et al. 1994; Wolfe and Wolfe 1991). CBT is used clinically with much success, although its efficacy is based predominantly on empirically supported and open trials (March 1995). Available reports suggest that techniques employed with adults (Marks 1987) are also generally applicable to and can be modified for children (for reviews, see Berg et al. 1989; March 1995; Wolff and Rapoport 1988; Wolfe and Wolfe 1991). In adults diagnosed with OCD, ERP is considered the behavior treatment of choice (Dar and Greist 1992). In the largest single pediatric behavioral study to date, Bolton and colleagues (1983) used ERP for 15 adolescents with OCD and achieved good treatment results in 11. In addition to ERP, other specific behavioral treatment techniques (e.g., anxiety management training and relaxation techniques) should be considered, with overall modification of these behavioral treatments for children (March et al. 1994).

There appears to be a shortage of mental health practitioners experienced in the behavioral treatment of OCD (March et al. 1994). Some clinicians may have misconceptions regarding CBT and ERP in children and adolescents with OCD, including those about time, effort, expense, and associated patient anxiety. Clinicians may complain that child patients do not comply with behavioral treatments, and parents may complain that clinicians are not specifically trained in CBT for OCD (March et al. 1994). The involvement of family members is paramount in the behavioral treatment of OCD. Familial overinvolvement, marital stress, and psychopathology can interfere with the success of behavior modification. There may be premature discontinuation of behavioral treatment.

Based on clinical reports, cognitive-behavioral psychotherapy, using ERP, appears to be an important behavioral treatment intervention to consider in children and adolescents with OCD. Exposure-based treatments include gradual (sometimes termed *graded*) exposure or flooding, with the exposure targets under patient and/or therapist control. For example, a child with contamination fears must come into and remain in contact with a particular OCD phobic stimulus. Dar and Greist (1992) have postulated that response prevention operates under the principle that adequate exposure depends on blocking rituals or avoidance behaviors. Thus, aside from touching "contaminated" objects, the patient must refrain from rituals to dispel the anxiety. Together, the patient and therapist develop a "tolerable" hierarchy of anxiety-producing stimuli, and these stimuli are assigned Subjective Units of Disturbance Scale (SUDS; Wolpe 1973) scores to quantify the increasing exposure. Through repeated exposure and response prevention, a substantial reduction eventually occurs in previously incapacitating anxiety on confrontation with the stimulus.

Other CBT techniques include anxiety management training, which consists of relaxation and breathing control training, and cognitive restructuring. Additional cognitive therapies are available (e.g., satiation, thought stopping, habit reversal) that may supplement ERP (for reviews, see March 1995; March et al. 1994). Habit reversal may play a role in the treatment of the more repetitive "complex tic-like rituals" (Vitulano et al. 1992).

Successful behavioral treatment of OCD requires developmental sensitivity and careful attention to unique issues in each age group. Children and adolescents with OCD may often view symptoms or experience distress and interference very differently from their parents (Berg et al. 1989). Thus, it is paramount for the CBT therapist to gain the child's cooperation, to individualize treatment, to attempt to instill in the child a sense of mastery and accomplishment, and to minimize massive initial anxiety (such as in flooding). Unlike CBT in adults with OCD, in which the therapist selects the treatment plan, hierarchy of exposure targets, and SUDS items, these tasks must be established by the child and therapist in collaboration. March and Mulle (1993) recently developed a protocol-driven treatment manual ("How I Ran OCD Off My Land") based on a framework of cognitive interventions and ERP (available on request from authors; see references). It is designed to facilitate patient and parental compliance, exportability to other clinicians, and empirical evaluation (March et al. 1994). For example, the child is in charge of choosing exposure targets and selecting metaphors. This manualized treatment protocol appears to be practical to implement and effective for treatment.

It should be reemphasized that empirical evidence for the efficacy of CBT in child subjects with OCD remains limited, especially in contrast to the literature on pharmacotherapy (Rapoport et al. 1992). March (1995) reviewed 32 investigations, most of them single case reports with varying degrees of terminology, theoretical framework, and methodological limitations (i.e., outcomes by self-report) and found that all but one found benefit for CBT interventions. Because most of these reports were not designed to test the specific effects of one behavioral protocol, it was difficult to draw generalizable conclusions. In most of these investigations, behavioral treatment was only one part of a multimodal approach and sometimes had only a secondary role. Future research in this area will use controlled trials—with standardized diagnostic definitions, baseline observations, established treatment time courses, and objective rating scales—and follow-up studies to compare medications, behavior therapy, and combination treatment (March 1995).

Several prognostic indicators for successful response to behavioral treatment of OCD include a motivated patient, the presence of overt rituals and compulsions, an ability to monitor and report symptoms, an absence of complicating comorbid illnesses, and a willingness to cooperate with treatment (Foa and Emmelkamp 1983). Behavior modification therapy may be less successful for patients with obsessions only (as opposed to both obsessions and compulsions), for very young patients, for uncooperative patients, or for those with obsessional slowness. Children with primary obsessional slowness generally respond poorly to both behavioral and medication treatment (Wolff and Rapoport 1988). Because ERP has not demonstrated significant benefit in obsessional slowness, modeling and shaping procedures may be the CBT treatment(s) of choice with this OCD subtype (Ratnasuriya et al. 1991). Future investigations with diverging subjects and clinical settings will be necessary to determine whether children and adolescents with difficult-to-manage OCD respond to manualized CBT.

Systematic comparisons of drug versus behavioral therapy in children and adolescents with OCD are limited, as are such studies in adults. There are few clinical guidelines for selecting initial treatment; thus, clinicians must carefully evaluate available behavioral treatments, patient cooperation, and constellation or specific symptom pattern. Baer and Minichiello (1990) suggest that medication and behavior therapy actually complement each other and that the use of antiobsessional agents may help improve compliance with behavioral treatment. Potential advantages of using behavioral therapy alone may include the avoidance of adverse medication side effects. March et al. (1994) hypothesized that booster behavior therapy may prevent relapse when medications are discontinued. Patients treated with medication and concurrent CBT (including booster treatments during medication discontinuation), as well as those for whom ongoing pharmacotherapy proves necessary, may exhibit both short- and long-term improvement in medication responsiveness (March 1995). In conclusion, CBT and pharmacotherapy appear to work well together, and many children with OCD require or would benefit from both CBT and pharmacotherapy (Piacentini et al. 1992).

Abundant clinical and emerging empirical evidence exists that CBT—alone or in combination with pharmacotherapy—is an important, safe, acceptable, and effective treatment for OCD in children and adolescents (March 1995; March et al. 1994). A proposed trial of CBT should be presented to and discussed with the child and family. As long as the patient is motivated and able to understand directions, he or she is an appropriate candidate for behavior treatment.

Pharmacological Treatment

SRIs such as clomipramine, fluoxetine, sertraline, and fluvoxamine have shown efficacy in controlled trials of adults with OCD (for a review, see March et al. 1995b). They may also prove to be effective treatments for children and adolescents with OCD. Early studies showed that children and adolescents with OCD responded well to the tricyclic antidepressant (TCA) and potent SRI clomipramine (Flament et al. 1985, 1988; Leonard et al. 1989). The first study consisted of 23 pediatric patients who participated in a 10-week double-blind, placebo-controlled crossover (Flament et al. 1985). Dosages of clomipramine targeting 3 mg/kg were used, with a mean dose of 141 mg/day. In the 19 OCD patients who completed the trial, clomipramine was significantly superior to placebo in decreasing obsessive-compulsive symptomatology at week 5, an improvement in symptoms could usually be seen as early as week 3, and 75% had moderate to marked improvement. In a large multicenter study, DeVeaugh-Geiss and colleagues (1992) reported that clomipramine was superior to placebo for the treatment of OCD in adolescents. This finding led to the U.S. Food and Drug Administration's (FDA) approval of clomipramine for the treatment of OCD in children and adolescents (10 years or older).

Clomipramine is unique among the TCAs in that it significantly inhibits serotonin reuptake. Its primary metabolite, desmethylclomipramine, is a potent noradrenergic reuptake inhibitor; thus, clomipramine has both noradrenergic and serotoninergic action. To assess the specificity of this agent, a double-blind, crossover comparison of clomipramine and desipramine (a selective noradrenergic-blocking TCA) was conducted in 48 children and adolescents with OCD (Leonard et al. 1989). Clomipramine was clearly superior to desipramine in ameliorating OCD symptoms at week 5, and some improvement could be seen as early as the third week of treatment. Desipramine was no more effective in improving obsessive-compulsive symptoms than placebo had been in the Flament and colleagues (1985) study. In fact, when desipramine was given as the second active medication, 64% of the patients had some degree of relapse within several weeks of crossover. Clomipramine was generally well tolerated in these studies, as it has been in clinical experience. Long-term clomipramine maintenance has not revealed any unexpected adverse reactions (DeVeaugh-Geiss et al. 1992; Leonard et al. 1991, 1995).

Anticholinergic, antihistaminic, and alpha-blocking side effects are associated with clomipramine. The most common side effects reported in children and adolescents include (in order of decreasing frequency) dry mouth, somnolence, dizziness, fatigue, tremor, headache, constipation, anorexia, abdominal pain, dyspepsia, and insomnia; these effects are comparable to (but anecdotally are reported as milder than) those reported in adults (DeVeaugh-Geiss et al. 1992; Leonard et al. 1989). Although no defined indications exist for electrocardiogram (ECG) or plasma-level monitoring, Leonard and colleagues (1995) suggest that baseline and periodic ECG monitoring are advisable. Several adolescents who discontinued clomipramine abruptly (during long-term maintenance) experienced withdrawal symptoms of gastrointestinal distress, which appeared to represent a cholinergic rebound syndrome, as has been reported with other antidepressants (Leonard et al. 1989). Thus, abrupt discontinuation of clomipramine is not recommended.

The SSRIs (e.g., fluoxetine, sertraline, paroxetine, fluvoxamine) are considered *selective* inhibitors of serotonin because of their limited effect on other monoamines (Warrington 1992). They represent a new class of agents with distinct advantages in their side-effect profiles and their broad therapeutic index over those of the TCAs. Riddle and colleagues (1990a, 1992) concluded that fluoxetine, FDA-approved for the treatment of depression and OCD in adults, appeared to be safe, effective, and well tolerated at dosages of 10–40 mg/day in children and adolescents with primary OCD or TS and OCD. Geller and colleagues (1995) found that fluoxetine may be effective in the treatment of OCD in prepubertal children and that the effect can be sustained over time. Dosages used in children may be as low as 5 mg/day. Fluoxetine and other SSRIs have less anticholinergic side effects than TCAs, but common side effects include nervousness, insomnia, activation, and restlessness. The majority of the side effects reported for SSRIs are from adult studies, and include complaints of nausea, headache, nervousness, insomnia, diarrhea, and drowsiness (Stokes 1993). The reader is referred to March and colleagues (1995a) for specific issues of dosage and monitoring in children and adolescents.

Systematic studies of the SSRIs are ongoing for the treatment of childhood and adolescent OCD. Evidence suggests that the drugs are well tolerated and effective. The advantage of the SSRIs' few anticholinergic side effects and limited cardiovascular toxicities are particularly relevant for the pediatric population (Leonard et al. 1995). The specific choice of SRI/SSRI should involve consideration of risk–benefit ratio, side-effect profile, pharmacokinetics (long versus short half-life), route of metabolism with other concomitant medications, comorbid diagnoses, and individual response (for a review of pediatric psychopharmacological treatment studies of OCD, see March and colleagues (1995a). Clinicians should inquire about all over-the-counter and recreational drugs and all prescription medications, especially terfenadine and astemizole (particularly in combination with certain medications; for example, ketoconazole), which have been shown to prolong the QT interval (Leonard et al. 1995). Additionally, it has been established that the combination of clomipramine and an SSRI may result in unexpectedly high clomipramine levels as a result of competitive inhibition by hepatic microenzyme systems.

Generally, a 12-week trial of an SRI/SSRI at an adequate dosage is considered necessary. Clinicians should be aware that many patients do not experience symptom relief until 6–10 weeks of receiving these agents, and that during early treatment (i.e., the first 1–10 days) with SSRIs, some patients may actually develop a worsening of their OCD symptoms or experience particularly annoying side effects (e.g., insomnia, increased psychomotor activity). This has been referred to as an "agitated syndrome" and has been well described in patients at certain doses and particularly in panic disorder patients. Typically, the exacerbation subsides and a positive clinical response ensues. Thus, the patient and the family should be educated and encouraged to report worsening or problematic side effects to the clinician. Initial worsening during the first week usually is not a reason in and of itself to discontinue the medication. For patients who exhibit a partial response to an SRI, augmentation strategies may be considered. Clonazepam is occasionally used, or a neuroleptic if a comorbid tic or schizotypal personality disorder is present (Leonard et al. 1994). Behavioral treatments should be considered as an adjunct to pharmacotherapy.

Many patients will continue to experience some OCD symptoms that vary ien severity over time, because of OCD's tendency to wax and wane. Although periodically decreasing the dosage should be considered, long-term maintenance may be required for some patients. Leonard and colleagues (1991) conducted a double-blind desipramine-substitution study of long-term clomipramine–maintained patients, and found that 8 of the 9 desipramine-substitution patients, but only 2 of the 11 nonsubstitution patients, relapsed. This result might argue for consideration of concomitant behavioral treatment. March and colleagues (1994) found greater improvement and lower relapse rates in patients treated with both medications and CBT. This issue clearly merits further study.

Although many patients respond early to one of the SRIs or SSRIs, a substantial minority do not respond until 8 or even 12 weeks of treatment (with therapeutic doses toward the end of this period). Thus, it is important for the clinician to be patient, to target a therapeutic dosage, and to wait at least 10–12 weeks before changing agents or undertaking augmentation regimens. If no clinical response has occurred after 12 weeks, switching to another SSRI would be reasonable.

Although various agents have been studied as augmentation strategies in adults and children with OCD, only clonazepam and haloperidol have been proven effective in controlled trials in adults (McDougle et al. 1994; Pigott and Rubenstein 1992). Clonazepam is a potential choice, but the clinician must also consider issues such as long-term dependency, cognitive effects, and possible side effects of paradoxical disinhibition. Thus, if only a partial response occurs after 12 weeks, the clinician might augment with clonazepam. Haloperidol should be used cautiously, and only if a comorbid tic-spectrum disorder or schizotypal personality disorder is present. A more systematic study of the use of augmentation medications in children and adolescents is indicated. Generally, augmentation strategies are started when there has been only a partial response to an SSRI, whereas an alternative SSRI is tried when there has been no response.

Summary

It is estimated that perhaps as many as 1 million children and adolescents in this country may have OCD. Childhood OCD presents in a form essentially identical to that seen in adults, and one-third of adult patients first developed the illness in childhood. Boys seem to have an earlier age at onset of OCD (prepuberty), whereas girls are more likely to develop OCD around puberty. Washing, repeating, checking, touching, counting, arranging, hoarding, and scrupulosity are the most commonly seen rituals. Almost all patients have reported a change in their principal symptoms over time. Increasing evidence supports a neuro-biological theory for the etiology of OCD—specifically, a frontal lobe–basal ganglia dysfunction.

Most recent studies suggest that early (prepubertal)–occurring OCD and/or tic disorders characterized by abrupt onset and acute exacerbations may represent a subtype of pediatric OCD. Patients with this sub-type typically have a comorbid tic disorder and an increased family loading. Identification of a new subtype of pediatric-onset OCD with abrupt onset and dramatic exacerbations may lead to new assessment and treatment interventions.

Childhood OCD and adult OCD appear to respond similarly to treat-ment. Although behavioral treatment has not been systematically stud-ied in children and adolescents, reports suggest that ERP techniques are useful. In children and adolescents, clomipramine was superior to placebo and to desipramine at week 5 in a double-blind, crossover com-parison (Leonard et al. 1989). Fluoxetine has been reported to be safe and well tolerated in the pediatric population, although systematic studies are still ongoing. Follow-up studies indicate that at least 50% of patients with pediatric-onset OCD are still symptomatic as adults (Ber-man 1942; Hollingsworth et al. 1980). These findings suggest that al-though the majority of OCD patients can expect improvement with the new treatments available, there remains a small group of patients who continue to have a chronic and debilitating course.

A number of important research issues exist for childhood-onset OCD. For example, it is not known which children will respond prefer-entially to behavioral or pharmacological treatments. The identification of children at risk for OCD, through genetic or biological studies, is a research priority. It is hoped that new treatment modalities and combi-nations of available treatments will improve the long-term outcome.

References

Ackerman D, Greenland S, Bystritsky A, et al: Predictors of treatment response in obses-sive-compulsive disorder: multivariate analyses from a multicenter trial of clomipra-mine. J Clin Psychopharmacol 14:247–254, 1994

Allen AJ, Leonard HL, Swedo SE: Case study: a new infection-triggered, autoimmune subtype of pediatric OCD and Tourette's syndrome. Am Acad Child Adolesc Psychia-try 34:307–311, 1995

American Psychiatric Association: Diagnostic and Statistical Manual of Mental Disorders, 3rd Edition, Revised. Washington, DC, American Psychiatric Association, 1987

American Psychiatric Association: Diagnostic and Statistical Manual of Mental Disorders, 4th Edition. Washington, DC, American Psychiatric Association, 1994

Anderson JC, Williams S, McGee R, et al: DSM-III disorders in preadolescent children. Arch Gen Psychiatry 44:69–76, 1987

Baer L: Behavior therapy for obsessive-compulsive disorder and trichotillomania: impli-cations for Tourette's syndrome. Adv Neurol 58:333–340, 1992

Baer L, Minichiello WE: Behavior therapy for obsessive-compulsive disorder, in Obsessive Compulsive Disorders: Theory and Management. Edited by Jenike M, Baer L, Minichiello W. Chicago, IL, Year Book Medical, 1990, pp 203–232

Berg CZ, Rapoport JL, Wolff RP: Behavioral treatment for obsessive-compulsive disorder in childhood, in Obsessive-Compulsive Disorder in Children and Adolescents. Edited by Rapoport JL. Washington, DC, American Psychiatric Press, 1989, pp 169–185

Berkowitz PH, Rothman EP: The Disturbed Child: Recognition and Psychoeducational Therapy in the Classroom. New York, New York University Press, 1960, pp 61–65

Berman L: Obsessive-compulsive neurosis in children. J Nerv Ment Dis 95:26–39, 1942

Black A: The natural history of obsessional neurosis, in Obsessional States. Edited by Beech HR. London, Methuen, 1974

Bolton D, Collins S, Steinberg D: The treatment of obsessive-compulsive disorder in adolescence: a report of fifteen cases. Br J Psychiatry 142:456–464, 1983

Cohen D, Leckman JF: Developmental psychopathology and neurobiology of Tourette's syndrome. J Am Acad Child Adolesc Psychiatry 33:2–15, 1994

Cox CS, Fedio P, Rapoport JL: Neuropsychological testing of obsessive compulsive adolescents, in Obsessive-Compulsive Disorder in Children and Adolescents. Edited by Rapoport JL. Washington, DC, American Psychiatric Press, 1989, pp 73–86

Cummings JL, Cunningham K: Obsessive-compulsive disorder in Huntington's disease. Biol Psychiatry 31:263–270, 1992

Dar R, Greist J: Behavior therapy for obsessive compulsive disorder. Psychiatr Clin North Am 15:885–894, 1992

Denckla MB: The neurological examination, in Obsessive-Compulsive Disorder in Children and Adolescents. Edited by Rapoport JL. Washington, DC, American Psychiatric Press, 1989, pp 107–118

DeVeaugh-Geiss GJ, Moroz G, Biederman J, et al: Clomipramine hydrochloride in childhood and adolescent obsessive-compulsive disorder: a multicenter trial. J Am Acad Child Adolesc Psychiatry 31:45–49, 1992

Esman A: Psychoanalysis in general psychiatry: obsessive-compulsive disorder as a paradigm. J Am Psychoanal Assoc 37:316–319, 1990

Flament MF, Rapoport JL, Berg C, et al: Clomipramine treatment of childhood obsessive-compulsive disorder. Arch Gen Psychiatry 42:977–983, 1985

Flament MF, Whitaker A, Rapoport JL, et al: Obsessive compulsive disorder in adolescence: an epidemiological study. J Am Acad Child Adolesc Psychiatry 27:764–771, 1988

Foa E, Emmelkamp P: Failures in Behavior Therapy. New York, Wiley & Sons, 1983

Frankel M, Cummings JL, Robertson MM, et al: Obsessions and compulsions in Gilles de la Tourette's syndrome. Neurology 36:378–382, 1986

Geller DA, Biederman J, Reed ED, et al: Similarities in response to fluoxetine in the treatment of children and adolescents with obsessive-compulsive disorder. J Am Acad Child Adolesc Psychiatry 34:36–44, 1995

Goodman WK, McDougle CJ, Price LH, et al: Beyond the serotonin hypothesis: a role for dopamine in some forms of obsessive compulsive disorder? J Clin Psychiatry 51 (suppl):36–43, 1990

Goodman WK, Price LH, Rasmussen SA, et al: The Yale-Brown Obsessive Compulsive Scale, Vol 2: Validity. Arch Gen Psychiatry 46:1012–1016, 1992

Greist JH: An integrated approach to treatment of obsessive compulsive disorder. J Clin Psychiatry 53 (suppl):38–41, 1992

Hafner RJ, Gilchrist P, Bowling J, et al: The treatment of obsessional neurosis in a family setting. Aust N Z J Psychiatry 15:145–151, 1981

Hanna GL: Demographic and clinical features of obsessive-compulsive disorder in children and adolescents. J Am Acad Child Adolesc Psychiatry 34:19–27, 1995

Hollingsworth C, Tanguay P, Grossman L, et al: Long-term outcome of obsessive compulsive disorder in childhood. J Am Acad Child Psychiatry 19:134–144, 1980

Holzer JC, Goodman WK, McDougle CJ, et al: Obsessive-compulsive disorder with and without a chronic tic disorder: a comparison of symptoms in 70 patients. Br J Psychiatry 164:469–473, 1994

Hoover CF, Insel TR: Families of origin in obsessive compulsive disorder. J Nerv Ment Dis 172:207–215, 1984

Insel TR: Toward a neuroanatomy of obsessive-compulsive disorder. Arch Gen Psychiatry 49:739–744, 1992

Jenike MA: Psychotherapy of Obsessive-Compulsive Personality Disorder. Chicago, IL, Year Book Medical, 1990

Judd LL: Obsessive compulsive neurosis in children. Arch Gen Psychiatry 12:136–143, 1965

Karno B, Golding J, Sorenson S, et al: The epidemiology of obsessive compulsive disorder in five U.S. communities. Arch Gen Psychiatry 45:1094–1099, 1988

King RA: Practice parameters for the psychiatric assessment of children and adolescents. J Am Acad Child Adolesc Psychiatry 34:1386–1402, 1995

Last CG, Strauss CC: Obsessive-compulsive disorder in childhood. Journal of Anxiety Disorders 3:295–302, 1989

Leckman JF, Walker DE, Cohen DJ: Premonitory urges in Tourette's Syndrome. Am J Psychiatry 150:98–102, 1993

Leckman JF, Walker DE, Goodman WK, et al: Just right perceptions associated with compulsive behavior in Tourette's syndrome. Am J Psychiatry 151:675–680, 1994

Lenane M: Families and obsessive-compulsive disorder, in Obsessive-Compulsive Disorder in Children and Adolescents. Edited by Rapoport JL. Washington, DC, American Psychiatric Press, 1989, pp 237–252

Lenane M: Family therapy for children with obsessive compulsive disorder, in Current Treatments of Obsessive-Compulsive Disorder. Edited by Pato MT, Zohar M. Washington, DC, American Psychiatric Press, 1991, pp 103–113

Lenane M, Swedo S, Leonard H, et al: Psychiatric disorders in first degree relatives of children and adolescents with obsessive compulsive disorder. J Am Acad Child Adolesc Psychiatry 29:407–412, 1990

Leonard HL, Swedo S, Rapoport JL, et al: Treatment of obsessive compulsive disorder with clomipramine and desipramine in children and adolescents: a double-blind crossover comparison. Arch Gen Psychiatry 46:1088–1092, 1989

Leonard HL, Swedo SE, Lenane MC, et al: A double-blind desipramine substitution during long-term clomipramine treatment in children and adolescents with obsessive-compulsive disorder. Arch Gen Psychiatry 48:922–926, 1991

Leonard HL, Lenane MC, Swedo SE, et al: Tics and Tourette's syndrome: a 2- to 7-year follow-up study of 54 obsessive-compulsive children. Am J Psychiatry 149:1244–1251, 1992

Leonard HL, Topol D, Bukstein O, et al: Clonazepam as an augmenting agent in the treatment of childhood-onset obsessive-compulsive disorder. J Am Acad Child Adolesc Psychiatry 33:792–794, 1994

Leonard H, Swedo S, March J, et al: Obsessive-compulsive disorder, in Treatments of Psychiatric Disorders, 2nd Edition. Edited by Gabbard G. Washington, DC, American Psychiatric Press, 1995, pp 301–313

Luxenberg JS, Swedo SE, Flament MF, et al: Neuroanatomical abnormalities in obsessive-compulsive disorder detected with quantitative X-ray computed tomography. Am J Psychiatry 145:1089–1093, 1988

March J: Cognitive-behavioral psychotherapy for children and adolescents with OCD: a review and recommendations for treatment. J Am Acad Child Adolesc Psychiatry 34:7–18, 1995

March J, Mulle K: How I ran OCD off my land: a cognitive-behavioral program for the treatment of obsessive-compulsive disorder in children and adolescents. Durham, NC, Duke University, Department of Child Psychiatry, 1993[1]

---

[1] Available from the Obsessive-Compulsive Foundation (OCF), P.O. Box 70, Milford, CT 06460; (203) 878-5669.

March J, Mulle K, Herbel B: Behavioral psychotherapy for children and adolescents with obsessive-compulsive disorder: an open trial of a new protocol-driven treatment package. J Am Acad Child Adolesc Psychiatry 33:333–341, 1994

March J, Leonard HL, Swedo SE: Obsessive compulsive disorder, in Anxiety Disorders in Children and Adolescents. Edited by March J. New York, Guilford, 1995a, pp 251–275

March JS, Leonard HL, Swedo SE: Pharmacotherapy of obsessive-compulsive disorder. Child Adolesc Psychiatr Clin North Am 4:217–236, 1995b

Marks IM: Fears, Phobias and Rituals, Panic Anxiety and Their Disorders. Oxford, England, Oxford University Press, 1987

McDougle C, Goodman W, Leckman JJ, et al: Haloperidol addition in fluvoxamine-refractory obsessive compulsive disorder. Arch Gen Psychiatry 51:302–308, 1994

Pauls DL, Towbin K, Leckman J, et al: Gilles de la Tourette syndrome and obsessive-compulsive disorder: evidence supporting a genetic relationship. Arch Gen Psychiatry 43:1180–1182, 1986

Pauls DL, Alsobrook JP, Goodman W, et al: A family study of obsessive-compulsive disorder. Am J Psychiatry 152:76–84, 1995

Piacentini J, Jaffer M, Gitow A, et al: Psychopharmacologic treatment of child and adolescent obsessive compulsive disorder. Psychiatr Clin North Am 15:87–107, 1992

Pigott T, Rubenstein C: A controlled trial of clonazepam augmentation in OCD patients treated with clomipramine or fluoxetine. Paper presented at the 145th Annual Meeting of the American Psychiatric Association, Washington, DC, May 2–7, 1992

Rapoport JL: Annotation: child obsessive-compulsive disorder. J Child Psychol Psychiatry 27:285–289, 1986

Rapoport JL (ed): Obsessive-Compulsive Disorder in Children and Adolescents. Washington, DC, American Psychiatric Press, 1989

Rapoport J, Swedo S, Leonard H: Childhood obsessive compulsive disorder. J Clin Psychiatry 53 (suppl):6–11, 1992

Ratnasuriya R, Marks IM, Forshaw D, et al: Obsessional slowness revisited. Br J Psychiatry 159:273–274, 1991

Rettew DC, Swedo SE, Leonard HL, et al: Obsessions and compulsions across time in 79 children and adolescents with obsessive compulsive disorder. J Am Acad Child Adolesc Psychiatry 29:766–772, 1992

Riddle MA, Hardin M, King R, et al: Fluoxetine treatment of children and adolescents with Tourette's and obsessive compulsive disorders: preliminary clinical experience. J Am Acad Child Adolesc Psychiatry 29:45–48, 1990a

Riddle MA, Scahill L, King R, et al: Obsessive compulsive disorder in children and adolescents: phenomenology and family history. J Am Acad Child Adolesc Psychiatry 29:766–772, 1990b

Riddle MA, Scahill L, King R, et al: Double-blind, crossover trial of fluoxetine and placebo in children and adolescents with obsessive-compulsive disorder. J Am Acad Child Adolesc Psychiatry 31:1062–1069, 1992

Rutter M, Tizard J, Whitmore K: Education, Health and Behavior. London, Longmans, 1970

Stokes PE: Fluoxetine: a five-year review. Clin Ther 15:216–243, 1993

Swedo SE: Sydenham's chorea: a model for childhood autoimmune neuropsychiatric disorders. JAMA 272:1788–1791, 1994

Swedo SE, Rapoport JL: Phenomenology and differential diagnosis of obsessive-compulsive disorder in children and adolescents, in Obsessive-Compulsive Disorder in Children and Adolescents. Edited by Rapoport JL. Washington, DC, American Psychiatric Press, 1989, pp 13–33

Swedo SE, Rapoport JL, Cheslow DL, et al: High prevalence of obsessive-compulsive symptoms in patients with Sydenham's chorea. Am J Psychiatry 146:246–249, 1989a

Swedo SE, Rapoport JL, Leonard HL, et al: Obsessive-compulsive disorder in children and adolescents: clinical phenomenology of 70 consecutive cases. Arch Gen Psychiatry 46:335–344, 1989b

Swedo SE, Shapiro ME, Grady CL, et al: Cerebral glucose metabolism in childhood-onset obsessive compulsive disorder. Arch Gen Psychiatry 46:518–523, 1989c

Swedo SE, Pietrini P, Leonard HL, et al: Cerebral glucose metabolism in childhood-onset obsessive-compulsive disorder. Arch Gen Psychiatry 49:690–694, 1992

Swedo SE, Leonard HL, Schapiro MB, et al: Sydenham's chorea: physical and psychological symptoms of St. Vitus's Dance. Pediatrics 91:706–713, 1993

Swedo SE, Leonard HL, Kiessling LS: Speculations on antineuronal antibody-mediated neuropsychiatric disorders of childhood: commentaries. Pediatrics 93:323–326, 1994

Vitulano LA, King RA, Scahill L, et al. Behavioral treatment of children and adolescents with trichotillomania. J Am Acad Child Adolesc Psychiatry 31:139–146, 1992

Von Economo C: Encephalitis Lethargica: Its Sequelae and Treatment. Translated by Neuman KO. New York, Oxford University Press, 1931

Walkup JT, LaBuda MJ, Hurko O, et al: Evidence for a mixed model of inheritance in Tourette's syndrome. Paper presented at the 42nd Annual Meeting of the American Academy of Child and Adolescent Psychiatry, New Orleans, LA, October 21, 1995

Warrington SJ: Clinical implications of the pharmacology of serotonin reuptake inhibitors. Int Clin Psychopharmacol 7:13–19, 1992

Wise SP, Rapoport JL: Obsessive-compulsive disorder: is it basal ganglia dysfunction? in Obsessive Compulsive Disorder in Children and Adolescents. Edited by Rapoport JL. Washington, DC, American Psychiatric Press, 1989, pp 327–344

Wolff R, Rapoport JL: Behavioral treatment of childhood obsessive compulsive disorder. Behav Modif 12:252–266, 1988

Wolfe RP, Wolfe LS: Assessment and treatment of obsessive-compulsive disorder in children. Behav Modif 15:372–393, 1991

Wolpe J: The Practice of Behavior Therapy, 2nd Edition. New York, Pergamon, 1973

Chapter 12

Obsessive-Compulsive Disorder in Adults

Michele T. Pato, M.D., and Carlos N. Pato, M.D.

Clinical Characteristics

Although obsessive-compulsive disorder (OCD) has finally been recognized as an important illness in childhood, there are still a large number of individuals with OCD who do not experience significant symptoms until adulthood. However, as we look at the symptoms of OCD throughout the life cycle, it is important to note that patients are usually stricken at a relatively young age even in adulthood, with a mean age at onset of 19.8 ± 9.6 years, and that fewer than 15% of patients date the onset of their symptoms after age 35 (Rasmussen and Eisen 1991).

Clinically, patients with OCD present with many different types of obsessions and compulsions. The symptom checklist of the Yale-Brown Obsessive Compulsive Scale (Y-BOCS; Goodman et al. 1989b) is one of the most clinically useful methods for assessing OCD. The value of elucidating the specific obsessions and compulsions with which a patient presents is twofold. First, given the secretive nature of and the sense of embarrassment many patients feel about their symptoms, the act of divulging these symptoms to the clinician often represents a critical step in the establishment of clinician-patient rapport—one that will ultimately affect patient compliance. Second, the identification of specific symptoms is important for the designing of individualized treatment. In the case of behavioral therapy in particular, the challenges and hierarchies developed must be specifically related to the symptoms present.

Obsessions are usually described as recurrent, intrusive, unwanted ideas. They often consist of disturbing thoughts or impulses that are difficult to dismiss. Compulsions are behaviors that are often, but not always, repetitive and can be either observable or mental. The compulsive behaviors are intended to reduce the anxiety engendered by obsessions. Many people, even those without OCD, may perform certain behaviors in a ritualistic way, repeating, checking, or washing things over and over out of habit or concern. What distinguishes OCD as a psychiatric disorder is that the experience of obsessions, and the performance of rituals, reaches such an intensity or frequency that it causes significant psychological distress or interferes in a significant way with psychosocial functioning. The guideline of at least 1 hour expended on symptoms per day (American Psychiatric Association 1994; Goodman et al. 1989b) has been presented as a measure for "significant interference." However, in patients who often avoid situations that bring on rituals, the actual symptoms may not consume an hour, yet the amount of "time lost" from having to avoid objects or situations would surely be defined as interfering with functioning. Consider, for instance, the single mother of three on welfare who throws out more than $100 of groceries a week because of contamination fears. Although such behavior surely has an impact on socioeconomic functioning, one may be hard pressed to demonstrate that it consumes 1 hour per day.

Historically, individuals with OCD were distinguished from those with psychotic disorders by the maintenance of insight into the irrational and senseless nature of their symptoms. However, as more and more patients have sought treatment and more careful longitudinal assessments have been conducted, it has become apparent that patients can exhibit a full range of insight about their symptoms, from complete awareness (excellent insight) to delusional insight (poor insight) (Eisen and Rasmussen 1993; Foa and Kozak 1995; Insel and Akiskal 1986; Kozak and Foa 1994; Lelliott et al. 1988). Given this clearer clinical picture of OCD, DSM-IV (American Psychiatric Association 1994), unlike previous DSM editions, includes a new specifier for OCD: "with poor insight." Such specification is important because this factor seems to have some bearing on treatment choice and outcome (Foa 1979). Specifically, patients with poor insight that reaches psychotic proportions can have comorbid schizoid or schizotypal personality disorder or schizophrenia and tend to be more treatment resistant. These psychotic or delusional patients may benefit from the addition of an antipsychotic medication (Eisen and Rasmussen 1993; McDougle et al. 1990).

The typical pattern for obsessions and compulsions is for the obsessions to cause a mounting sense of anxiety or concern that can be nullified only by either performing a compulsion or avoiding the situation that brings on the obsessional thinking. Thus, the obsessions and compulsions often occur together—for example, obsessional fear of dirt, germs, or contaminants leading to excessive washing of hands, sanitizing of objects, or avoidance of touching anything that might be contaminated. Based on the DSM-IV field trials, the most common obsessions are contamination and fear of harming oneself or others. The most common compulsions are checking and cleaning/washing (Foa and Kozak 1995). The presence of obsessions without compulsions is rare. Often, adult patients who appear to have only obsessions actually have subtle compulsions such as repeated asking for reassurance that they did something correctly or that something did happen. Others may have difficult-to-observe mental rituals such as counting in their head or saying things over and over again, be it a prayer, a nonsense phrase, or a short rhyme. The presence of compulsions without obsessions also appears to be quite rare but has been noted in young children 6–8 years of age (Swedo et al. 1989a). One is left to wonder whether some obsessions have evolved as a way of rationalizing the irrational compulsive behaviors that OCD patients feel driven to perform.

Some typical examples of such obsession/compulsion pairs are described below. Contamination fears are usually characterized by a fear of dirt or germs but may also involve toxins or environmental hazards (e.g., asbestos, lead) or bodily waste or secretions. Patients usually describe a fear that harm will come to them or others by contact with the feared contaminants. For instance, a 33-year-old mother of a 5-year-old would not allow her son outside to play if she saw a Chemlawn truck on the street, fearing that he might somehow become contaminated. As her symptoms evolved, she could no longer buy groceries except in an organic supermarket because of her fear of chemical contaminants. Eventually, she stopped cooking for her family completely, forcing them to go for meals to relatives, out of fear she could not prepare food that was not contaminated. Another middle-aged woman with Crohn's disease spent hours in the shower washing herself in a special sequence and needed to have her adolescent children available to hand her a towel directly from the dryer to ensure that it had not been contaminated by touching the towel rack or floor of the bathroom.

Pathological doubt and compulsions such as checking, counting, and asking for reassurance is another obsessive-compulsive pairing often seen in OCD patients. Patients with pathological doubt are often concerned that as a result of their carelessness, harm will come to themselves or someone else. This concern has often been described as a "sense of overresponsibility." Patients with these symptoms often tend to "catastrophize," or see the worst possible outcome, no matter how unlikely. Often, OCD patients with these symptoms find it difficult to take medications. Not only is it hard for them to take risks or to feel out of control, but they are also convinced that they will experience every side effect, no matter how rare. This pathological doubt may lead to compulsive avoidance to the point of being housebound. Such a presentation can be difficult to distinguish from severe agoraphobia. A careful history will usually reveal that the avoidance is precipitated by obsessive thoughts rather than a fear of open spaces, crowds, or panic attacks.

Pathological doubt can also appear in conjunction with aggressive obsessions that are often described as a fear of doing violent harm to others. For instance, an adoring aunt refused to babysit her nieces and nephews, fearing that she might take a knife and stab them while they were sleeping. A man in his 40s could not take the subway to work for fear that he would act on his obsessive thought of pushing someone off the platform into an oncoming train. No amount of reassurance that they were not violent people by nature could convince these patients that they would not do these things. However, through behavioral therapy with exposure and response prevention (ERP), which included not avoiding these situations, the obsessive thoughts and the compulsive avoidance were treated.

Somatic obsessions are worries that one will contract or has contracted an illness or disease. Common somatic obsessions include a fear of cancer, venereal disease, or acquired immunodeficiency syndrome (AIDS). Checking compulsions consisting of checking and rechecking the body part of concern, as well as reassurance seeking, are commonly associated with this fear. The difference between the somatic obsessions of OCD and the somatic obsessions of hypochondriasis may be unclear, but there are several distinguishing features. Patients with OCD usually have a history of other "classic" OCD obsessions (e.g., checking, reassurance seeking). They are more likely to engage in these classic OCD compulsions and may not experience somatic symptoms of illness.

Comorbidity and Differential Diagnosis

It is sometimes difficult to determine, on the basis of a single symptom, whether the problem requiring treatment is OCD or another disorder. At times, a symptom may be shared by a number of different disorders, thus making it difficult to perform a differential diagnosis. At other times, the symptom may be shared by OCD and another comorbid disorder. Nonetheless, this distinction between a comorbid disorder with OCD and a distinct disorder that is not OCD can have a significant bearing on treatment decisions, as the following example illustrates. Patient 1, a young man who presents with a swinging of his glance from side to side in what looked like a motor tic, may on further questioning report that the entire behavior was motivated by a need for symmetry (diagnosis: OCD). Patient 2, another young man demonstrating the same motor behavior, might describe a motor tic to the right with a compulsion to the left to balance out the behavior symmetrically (diagnosis: OCD and tic disorder). Finally, patient 3 may have no explanation at all for his motor behavior other than an involuntary urge to perform it (diagnosis: tic disorder). Treatment of these three patients would vary, with patient 1 receiving a selective serotonin reuptake inhibitor (SSRI), patient 2 receiving both an SSRI and a high-potency neuroleptic (e.g., haloperidol, pimozide), and patient 3 receiving haloperidol or pimozide alone.

Tourette's syndrome and complex motor tics are often comorbid with OCD. Other potentially comorbid disorders include psychotic disorders (especially when insight is an issue), major depression (especially with excessive rumination), other anxiety disorders (specific phobias, social phobia, agoraphobia), hypochondriasis, body dysmorphic disorder, impulse-control disorder, and obsessive-compulsive personality disorder. In trying to differentiate among potential alternative diagnoses, it is often helpful to consider content of the person's thoughts (obsessions) or behaviors (compulsions). If the content is limited in its focus—for instance, a concern about the hopelessness of life (as in depressive ruminations), about bodily appearance (as in body dysmorphic disorder), about pulling hair (as in trichotillomania, an impulse-control disorder), or about thinness and food (as in anorexia nervosa), it is better to diagnose and treat these disorders. However, if these more focused symptoms appear along with more typical obsessions and compulsions and cause significant functional impairment and distress, a diagnosis of OCD may be more appropriate. Finally, in cases in which two distinct illnesses are present that seem to have different severity and/or different time courses or responses to treatment, comorbid disorders should be diagnosed and treated. For instance, there is a relatively high comorbidity between anorexia nervosa and OCD (Rubenstein et al. 1992). In one study, 17% of 100 OCD subjects were found to have a lifetime history of an eating disorder (Rasmussen and Eisen 1991). In another series of 93 subjects with an eating disorder, 37% met criteria for comorbid OCD (Thiel et al. 1995).

OCD and Other Anxiety Disorders

In DSM-IV, OCD is classified as an anxiety disorder because of the features it shares with other anxiety disorders—namely, the evocation of anxiety and the management of anxiety by means of avoidance. At times, patients will present complaining of a specific "phobia" such as "I'm phobic about dirt." At first glance, this complaint might appear to represent a simple phobia, in which patients avoid anything dirty, use gloves, and experience extreme anxiety or even panic attacks if they feel they have dirt on them. However, on further exploration, the clinician may find that the symptoms are based on contamination concerns and might even involve rituals or ritualistic avoidance of certain objects or things. Examples may include never entering certain rooms in the house or touching certain objects without using a tissue. In such cases, OCD may be a more accurate diagnosis.

A critical distinction must be made with respect to treatment, given that the treatment of panic disorder is relatively nonspecific, making use of a number of different antidepressants and benzodiazepines. In contrast, the treatment of OCD is quite specific, and a SSRI is commonly indicated. This specificity in treatment has prompted some to argue against including OCD as an anxiety disorder. The European symptom classification (*International Classification of Diseases*, 10th Revision [ICD-10; World Health Organization 1992]) does not classify OCD as an anxiety disorder, but instead places it in a separate group (Montgomery

1994). Anxiety disorders frequently coexist with OCD. Relatively high lifetime rates of social phobia (18%), panic disorder (12%), and specific phobia (22%) are reported in patients with OCD (Rasmussen and Eisen 1991).

OCD and Body Dysmorphic Disorder

Like patients with OCD, patients with body dysmorphic disorder (BDD) can experience obsessional thinking around their supposed defect in appearance and will often engage in rituals such as mirror checking, reassurance seeking, and avoidance (Phillips 1991). In addition, the existing data seem to indicate that, as in OCD, SSRIs have some treatment efficacy in BDD (Phillips et al. 1995). Although more data are needed on differentiating these two disorders, if obsessions and compulsions concern only bodily appearance, a diagnosis of BDD should be made. However, if obsessions and compulsions unrelated to appearance issues are also present, the OCD diagnosis should be given.

OCD and Tourette's Syndrome

There is compelling evidence of the relationship between Tourette's syndrome (TS) and OCD. Of particular note is that 7% of OCD patients also meet criteria for TS (Rasmussen and Eisen 1991), and patients with TS have a high rate of OCD symptoms. The combined prevalence of TS symptoms plus OCD is about 30%–40% (Lees et al. 1984; Robertson et al. 1988). Differentiating the intrusive urge to perform a tic from an obsessional drive to perform a compulsion is not always easy. The patient will often describe a muscle tension or a physical urge rather than the obsessional thought and anxiety that precede compulsive motor behaviors. Most important, then, is the patient's explanation about why he or she performs the behavior.

OCD Versus Obsessive-Compulsive Personality Disorder

Research on the coexistence of OCD and personality disorders has been hampered by some methodological concerns, including relatively poor interrater reliability for Axis II disorders. In a study of 96 subjects with OCD in which a structured interview with adequate interrater reliability (the Structured Interview for DSM-III Personality Disorders [SID-P; Stangl et al. 1985]) was used, 36% met criteria for one or more DSM-III (American Psychiatric Association 1984) personality disorders (Baer et al. 1990). Dependent (12%), histrionic (9%), and obsessive-compulsive (6%) personality disorders were diagnosed most frequently, but other comorbid personality disorders (schizotypal [5%], paranoid [5%], and avoidant [5%]) were also noted. A higher rate of obsessive-compulsive personality disorder (OCPD) was found with DSM-III-R (American Psychiatric Association 1987) criteria (25% of 59 OCD probands), which may reflect changes in the criteria set between DSM-III and DSM-III-R. The comorbidity of OCD and OCPD appears relatively low, a finding that is at odds with earlier literature, which postulated that OCD and OCPD are closely related disorders on a continuum of severity. Although personality disorders are considered to be stable over time, a recent study found that among 17 OCD patients with a personality disorder, 9 of 10 treatment responders no longer met criteria for a personality disorder after successful pharmacotherapy, thus raising the question of whether the apparent personality disorder was actually a manifestation of, or a result of, chronic OCD (Ricciardi et al. 1992).

OCD Versus Psychotic and Impulse-Control Disorders

Although it is easy to provide specific examples of obsessions and compulsions that help to distinguish them from other behaviors that might be part of a more psychotic picture or an impulse-control disorder, in real life these distinctions are often hard to make. It may be preferable to think of the mental phenomena of obsessions on a continuum from normal worry to ruminations to overvalued ideas and delusions. In addition, OCD patients rarely stay in one place along this continuum. Eisen and Rasmussen (1993) and Insel and Akiskal (1986) have noted that individuals with OCD can develop a transient delusional certainty about their thoughts or rituals. In a similar vein, how can one explain behaviors as varied as compulsive gambling or shopping, hair pulling, and hand washing over which a patient feels little control yet is compelled to perform? One framework that has been offered to deal with this broad spectrum of thoughts and behaviors posits continua along the dimensions of "uncertainty–certainty" and "risk aversion–risk seeking" (Hollander 1993). In such a framework, patients with OCD occupy a position at the uncertainty and the risk-avoidance ends of the continua—often ridden with doubt about the need to perform their rituals, yet uncertain enough about the risk of harm that "to be safe," they ritualize. Within such a framework, a whole spectrum of disorders that share some common features (e.g., clinical symptoms, family history, comorbidity, genetic transmission, treatment response, etiology) can be viewed as related. These "OC-related disorders" include BDD, depersonalization disorder, anorexia nervosa, hypochondriasis, trichotillomania, TS, sexual compulsions, pathological gambling, impulse-control disorders, and delusional disorders.

Etiology and Pathophysiology

The evidence regarding the etiology and pathophysiology of OCD is by no means definitive. Factors contributing to OCD can be broadly categorized into neurochemical, neuroanatomical, neuroimmunological, genetic, ethological, learning theory, and psychodynamic.

Neurochemical Contributions

Serotonin plays an important role but does not appear to be the sole factor involved in OCD. Exploration of the role of serotonin in OCD is based on three types of studies: 1) direct measurements of concentrations of central and peripheral neurotransmitters and their metabolites, 2) pharmacological challenge studies measuring the immediate behavioral and neuroendocrinological effects of certain pharmacological agents, and 3) treatment trials measuring the response of patients to chronic administration of medications that differentially affect specific neurotransmitters (Pigott 1996). To date, the most consistent data supporting the serotonin hypothesis have come from treatment trials. More specifically, the most effective agents all seem to be serotonin reuptake inhibitors. Treatment trials with drugs having other 5-hydroxytryptamine (5-HT) mechanisms of action (trazodone and m-chlorophenylpiperazine [m-CPP]) have not been effective (Pigott et al. 1992b). A correlation between relative affinity for reuptake sites and relative efficacy has not been borne out. Such a correlation would imply that fluvoxamine would have the greatest antiobsessional effect, since it is the most potent inhibitor of reuptake, followed by sertraline, paroxetine, fluoxetine, and clomipramine. However, clomipramine may be superior to the more selective agents, which are probably about equal in efficacy (DeVane 1992; Greist et al. 1995c; Pigott 1996). (See "Treatment" section for more details.)

Findings from direct measurement of cerebrospinal 5-hydroxyindoleacetic acid (5-HIAA) (Thorén et al. 1980) and platelet serotonin levels (Flament et al. 1987) have not always been consistent but have supported the notion that perturbations in the serotonin system are more common in OCD patients than in control subjects. Similarly, challenge studies with agents that specifically affect the functional integrity of the serotonin system, such as tryptophan (Barr et al. 1994), fenfluramine (Hewlett and Martin 1993), metergoline (Pigott et al. 1991), and m-CPP (Hollander et al. 1992; Zohar et al. 1987), have at times suggested that serotonergic—but not dopaminergic or adrenergic—dysregulation plays the major role in OCD (for a review, see Pigott 1996).

In an attempt to further explore the neurochemistry of OCD and how it relates to the serotonin system, studies have measured serum metabolites of various effective medications. Again, results have been unhelpful in that most studies have not identified any specific correlation between serum levels of parent compounds or metabolites and overall efficacy (Flament et al. 1987; Insel et al. 1983; Thorén et al. 1980). However, one study (Mavissakalian et al. 1990) has provided at least some support for the serotonin hypothesis. In this study, the concentration of the serotonergic parent compound clomipramine, but not of its noradrenergic metabolite N-desmethylclomipramine, correlated positively with symptom improvement. Compared with nonresponders, responders tended to have higher clomipramine levels and lower ratios of *N*-desmethylclomipramine to clomipramine (Mavissakalian et al. 1990).

Augmentation studies with dopamine antagonists such as haloperidol, pimozide, and, most recently, risperidone (Jacobsen 1995) in patients with comorbid tics and psychotic symptoms have contributed to the belief that the dopamine system may also be involved in the pathophysiology of OCD (Goodman et al. 1990). Neuroimmunological factors may also play a role (see Chapter 11 in this volume). However, despite the many pharmacological manipulations conducted, the interplay among the various neurotransmitters, their contribution to the etiology of OCD, and their implications for treatment of the illness remain unclear.

Neuroanatomical Contributions

Anecdotal and historical evidence of insults to basal ganglion structures leading to OCD had already implicated these structures in the etiology of the disorder (Insel 1992; Insel and Winslow 1992). However, some of the most compelling work comes from brain-imaging studies. Various imaging techniques have been used, including static measures such as computed tomography (CT) as well as functional measures such as positron-emission tomography (PET) and functional magnetic resonance imaging (MRI). The latter techniques have been particularly exciting because they afford the investigator the opportunity to "watch" the obsessions evolve in the brain as the patient in the scanner is "challenged" with stimuli that bring on his or her obsessions and compulsions (Rauch et al. 1994). These various techniques have implicated areas of the brain that—not surprisingly—are often rich in serotonin connections and, in addition, seem to play a role in behaviors related to process and procedural learning and approach and avoidance behaviors (Schwartz et al. 1996). More specifically, PET studies have shown increased glucose metabolism in the caudate nucleus and orbitofrontal cortex in untreated OCD patients compared with control subjects (Baxter et al. 1988; Nordahl et al. 1989; Swedo et al. 1989b). When the OCD patients were challenged with feared stimuli, changes in the caudate, cingulate cortex, and orbitofrontal cortex were noted (Rauch et al. 1994). Studies comparing PET scans pre- and posttreatment showed a correlation between treatment response and normalization of the increased activity of the caudate nucleus (Baxter et al. 1992; Benkelfat et al. 1990; Hoehn-Saric et al. 1991; Schwartz et al. 1996; Swedo et al. 1992).

Genetic Contributions

The two basic approaches that have been used to explore genetic factors in OCD have been twin studies and family studies. Twin studies have revealed a concordance rate among monozygotic twins of 63%. This finding obviously supports a genetic contribution to OCD but is not the 100% concordance that one would expect in a simple dominantly inherited disorder (Rasmussen and Tsuang 1986).

The family-study work has also lent support to a genetic component in the transmission of OCD. Whereas early studies had indicated increased frequencies of OCD in families (McKeon and Murray 1987), the most accurate data come from more recent studies (Black et al. 1992; Lenane et al. 1990; Pauls et al. 1995; Riddle et al. 1990) that have used more rigorous methodologies, including structured interviews, systematic diagnostic criteria, control groups, and direct interviews of relatives. In the Pauls et al. (1995) study, which included 100 OCD patients and direct interviews with 446 first-degree relatives, 10.3% of the relatives met criteria for OCD and an additional 7.9% had "subthreshold" OCD. This represented a significantly higher rate than that found in a comparison control group in which 1.9% of relatives had OCD and 2.0% of relatives had subthreshold OCD. In another family study, age at onset was shown to have some significance, with an increased frequency of OCD within the family when the patient's age at onset was younger than 14 years (Bellodi et al. 1992).

Given the comorbidity between TS and OCD, it is not surprising that family studies of TS have also contributed to the supporting data on a role for genetics in OCD. First-degree relatives of patients with TS had a much higher rate of OCD as well as tics and TS. The overall risk was higher for males than for females; in addition, females were more likely to have OCD and males to have tics or TS (Pauls et al. 1991). In terms of OCD prevalence among first-degree relatives, 13% had OCD alone and 10% had OCD and tics or TS, for a total of 23% with OCD (Pauls et al. 1986). These rates of OCD are much higher than the approximate 2% prevalence of OCD that has been found in epidemiological studies (Robins et al. 1984). The child literature also supports increased frequencies of TS and tics among first-degree relatives in child patients with OCD (Leonard et al. 1992).

Ethological (Animal) Contributions

One of the more compelling animal models is a kind of compulsive grooming behavior seen in dogs, called *canine acral lick syndrome.* In this condition, dogs (and cats) cause cutaneous lesions to the skin and hair loss secondary to excessive grooming (Rapoport et al. 1992). Interestingly, not only does the condition worsen with stress, but it has been treated successfully with the same serotonin reuptake inhibitors used in OCD: clomipramine, fluoxetine, and sertraline. However, other animal models have not been so straightforward. Many of the repetitive and grooming animal behaviors that are likened to compulsions seen in OCD seem to be precipitated or exacerbated by drugs that manipulate the dopamine rather than the serotonin system (Pitman 1991).

Learning Theory Contributions

The contributions of learning theory to understanding OCD have been more in the area of how the symptoms are perpetuated than in how they actually arise. However, this understanding has allowed for important breakthroughs in developing effective nonpharmacological treatments. The underlying tenets of learning theory regarding OCD are based on a model of conditioning, tension reduction, and lack of habituation. According to the theory, the compulsions are conditioned responses to anxiety. This anxiety is brought on by obsessive thoughts about contamination, doubt, fear of self-harm, and the like. The performance of a compulsive behavior, such as hand washing, is the conditioned response that temporarily reduces the stress brought on by the obsessive thought. However, by performing the compulsive behavior, the subject never actually receives a chance to habituate to the anxiety caused by the obsessional thought, but only transiently avoids feeling more anxious. Thus, this compulsion actually reinforces the obsession (Rachman and Hodgson 1980). For OCD symptoms to be treated, the patient must habituate to the anxiety provoked by his or her obsessions instead of performing compulsions. As anxiety decreases and compulsions are prevented, the urge to ritualize declines. The type of treatment employing this model is called ERP and is elaborated in the "Treatment" section below.

Psychodynamic Theory

The contributions of psychodynamic theory have been in the understanding of the etiology of OCD more from a psychodynamic than a neurobiological formulation. Although such psychodynamic understanding alone rarely contributes to significant reduction in symptoms, it can play a role in the overall understanding and treatment of the patient, especially in cases where prominent or excessive doubt, poor insight, and fear of losing control, all features of treatment resistance, are part of the clinical picture.

Freud's model for understanding OCD postulates that obsessions and compulsions develop through fixation on or regression to the anal-sadistic stage of development. Prominent features of this stage of development are issues relating to control, aggression, and autonomy. Management of impulses and conflicts that develop at this stage is accomplished through the defense mechanisms of reaction formation, isolation, and undoing. The repetitive rituals and compulsions seen in OCD patients exemplify this doing and undoing behavior. In addition, issues around control often contribute to patients' willingness to take medications or change compulsive behaviors.

Treatment

General Considerations

Before the 1980s, it was believed that OCD was a rare and treatment-resistant disorder. However, the epidemiological and treatment data collected since the 1980s have changed this clinical picture, so that most clinicians view OCD as a common disorder with approximately a 2%–3% prevalence (Karno et al. 1988; Robins et al. 1984) in which the majority of patients (60%–80%) exhibit some response to treatment—pharmacological, behavioral, or both (Jenike 1992). However, the key features of OCD, as already discussed, include obsessional doubt, a need to feel in control, and risk aversion, and these features have a significant bearing on the successful application of both pharmacological and behavioral treatments.

Obsessional doubt and risk aversion are often initial barriers to treatment. The clinician may often find him- or herself with a patient who doubts that treatment will be successful and who is unwilling to deal with the risk of side effects or the anxiety that behavioral treatment will evoke. Often, the clinician must take extra time to explain the benefits of treatment that make it worth the risk.

In addition, the OCD patient's cognitive misperceptions often lead to beliefs that he or she will experience each and every side effect to the most severe degree or that the anxiety evoked by the ERP will be totally unbearable. This cognitive distortion leads the patient to see everything in extremes. Again, the clinician must take extra time to inform without provoking irrational concerns, thus providing a corrective cognitive experience. Giving accurate data on side effects also includes correcting cognitive distortions. In this regard, it is important to identify for patients that their OCD and fear of risk may be contributing to their trepidation about medications and that although there are many side effects, especially with clomipramine, they will not get every one, or even experience the side effects at an intensity that is unbearable. In the case of fear about overwhelming anxiety from behavioral interventions, it can be helpful to have patients actually write down their worst fears in a scripted imagery and read them over and over. Often, simply writing them down helps patients to see the irrational nature of their fears, and by reading the script over and over, they can begin to habituate to the anxiety.

Fear of losing control can also manifest itself throughout treatment. In the case of behavioral treatment, patients may feel, based on the anxiety provoked, that they are moving too quickly. However, by setting up their own hierarchy of behaviors, patients can feel in control of the pace and rate at which they move forward. Because treatment response to pharmacological agents for OCD usually requires 6–10 weeks, patients have plenty of time to get accustomed to the medicine, and, therefore, the issue of control of the pace during medication trials is less prominent. However, the issue of control often arises in the long duration of treatment required before any treatment effect is usually seen. Issues around doubt can enter the treatment as the patient becomes frustrated by an absence of symptom improvement in the face of significant side effects. For this reason, preparing the patient in the early stages of treatment for what to anticipate over the course of treatment is very helpful in maintaining treatment compliance.

When insight is poor, as in more delusional OCD, or severe anxiety is a comorbid symptom, the patient may be unable or unwilling to engage in behavioral treatment. In such cases, it may be better to start with medication and achieve some initial reduction in symptoms or improvement in insight before engaging in behavioral treatment.

Assessment

The most widely used measure in treatment outcome studies is the Y-BOCS. This scale was developed on the basis of clinical interviews with OCD subjects in the 1980s. Unlike instruments that preceded it, the Y-BOCS measures severity rather than types of symptoms, and its 10 questions can be divided into two parallel subscales, one for obsessions and one for compulsions, each with a potential score of 20, adding up to an overall total score of 40. In general, patients scoring at least 16–18 are considered ill enough to require treatment, and those scoring over 30 are considered severely ill (Pato et al. 1994). In terms of treatment outcome, a 25%–35% reduction is felt to represent significant improvement in symptoms (Goodman et al. 1993). It can be helpful to use the Y-BOCS in everyday clinical practice as well as in the research setting as a measure of symptom improvement and, as such, a justification for remaining on a given medication or switching to another. The key to obtaining a valid measure of symptom severity with the Y-BOCS is eliciting a careful history of the patient's specific symptoms, both obsessions and compulsions. This can be done with the help of the Y-BOCS symptom checklist. The patient version of this checklist can actually be given to the patient to complete; it contains a list of symptoms with easy-to-understand explanations of what each symptom is.

Pharmacological Treatments

As previously discussed in the section on etiology and pathophysiology, the serotonin system and, more specifically, serotonin reuptake inhibitors have been found to be an integral part of the pharmacological treatment of OCD. These agents include clomipramine, fluoxetine, sertraline, paroxetine, and fluvoxamine. All are currently available in the United States, and all have OCD among their indications. Clomipramine (Anafranil) was the first agent to receive U.S. Food and Drug Administration (FDA) approval for the treatment of OCD and thus was the first to have large multicenter placebo-controlled data available (Clomipramine Collaborative Study Group 1991). Other agents have followed with similar placebo-controlled multicenter studies: fluoxetine (Prozac; Tollefson et al. 1994a, 1994b; Wood et al. 1993), sertraline (Zoloft; Greist et al. 1995c), paroxetine (Paxil; Wheadon et al. 1993), and fluvoxamine (Luvox; Greist et al. 1995a; Rasmussen et al., in press). Ideally, the choice of a pharmacological agent for treating OCD would be based on comparative efficacy of the different serotonin reuptake–inhibiting agents available. However, the choice of treatment is difficult for two major reasons: 1) lack of large comparative efficacy trials (although some small trials have studied clomipramine versus fluoxetine [Pigott et al. 1990] and clomipramine versus fluvoxamine [Freeman et al. 1994; Koran et al. 1996]), and 2) differences in side-effect profiles.

Despite the lack of head-to-head comparison data, comparative efficacies have been gleaned from meta-analyses of these large, controlled studies on individual drugs (Greist et al. 1995b; Jenike et al. 1990a). However, such analyses are not without their problems. These include differences in dosing strategies, differences in illness severity of those treated, and heterogeneity of subject pools. The latter issue reflects the 10-year time course over which these clinical trials have been conducted. In the beginning of this decade, during which clomipramine was tested, most patients who sought treatment had never been treated for their OCD. In the later portion of the period, during which trials of sertraline, paroxetine, and fluvoxamine were conducted, many of the subjects entering the studies had already received trials of clomipramine or fluoxetine, which were readily available. Several authors have attributed the smaller effect sizes of newer agents, as well as the larger placebo response rates seen with these agents, to this factor (Greist et al. 1995b; Jenike et al. 1990b).

Given these limitations, the following conclusions can be drawn. The overall effect size seen with clomipramine has been consistently higher than that with the SSRIs, although fluoxetine, sertraline, fluvoxamine, and paroxetine all have shown good efficacy compared with placebo in the treatment of OCD (Freeman et al. 1994; Jefferson and Greist 1996; Koran et al. 1996; Pigott 1996). Comparative tolerability has been a mixed picture. In terms of side effects (see Table 12–1), clomipramine clearly has more than any of the SSRIs. A number of studies have reported that a greater number of patients experience some side effects with clomipramine (between 80% and 97%) than with either fluoxetine or paroxetine (Greist et al. 1995c; Jenike et al. 1990a; Pigott et al. 1990; Tollefson et al. 1994b; Wheadon et al. 1993; Wood et al. 1993), whereas others have shown similarly high side-effect frequencies with other SSRIs, including sertraline and fluvoxamine (Freeman et al. 1994; Greist et al. 1995b; Koran et al. 1996). However, such findings must be viewed with caution, since it is not always easy to measure the severity—or rather, the significance—of side effects. For instance, is "very dry mouth" as big a problem as "mild impotency"? Such a judgment would depend on the patient's interpretation of the symptoms. Thus, many clinicians and researchers have turned to comparative dropout rates rather than number or intensity of side effects to provide an indirect measure of the tolerability of a medication. The results in this regard have been mixed but interesting. In comparative studies of fluvoxamine and clomipramine (Freeman et al. 1994; Koran et al. 1996), dropout rates were virtually identical for both medications, around 15%. However, in a meta-analysis, Greist et al. (1995c) noted that analysis of the pooled multicenter studies revealed the lowest rates of dropout in the clomipramine group (12%), followed by fluoxetine (23%), fluvoxamine (24%), and sertraline (27%).

Another important consideration in treatment is cross-responsivity. *Cross-responsivity* refers to the probability of a patient's responding to a second antiobsessional agent if he or she has already responded to one antiobsessional agent—or, on a more pessimistic note, whether a patient will respond to a second or third agent if he or she has failed to respond to previous agents. Although data are sparse in this regard, those available are hopeful. In a multicenter trial of fluvoxamine (Rasmussen et al., in press), 19% of patients who had failed to respond to previous trials with clomipramine or fluoxetine responded to fluvoxamine. In an analysis of a small trial comparing fluoxetine and clomipramine, Pigott (1996) noted that only 65% of patients who responded to clomipramine also responded to fluoxetine, whereas 80% of patients who responded to fluoxetine also responded to clomipramine. On the negative side, patients who had not responded to clomipramine had only a 20% chance of responding to fluoxetine. Thus, it would appear that if an initial agent is unsuccessful, it is reasonable to pursue a trial with other agents, and that response to clomipramine is the best harbinger of responsivity to other agents.

Duration of Treatment

Clinical recommendations for duration of treatment differ significantly from the 2–4 weeks recommended for depression. Numerous trials with various antiobsessional agents have demonstrated that most patients do not begin to respond until 4–6 weeks of treatment and that a full 10-week trial at an adequate dose (see "Dosing," below) is needed before a trial can be deemed sufficient (Goodman et al. 1989a; Greist et al. 1995a, 1995b; Jefferson and Greist 1996; Jenike et al. 1990a; Ras-

Table 12–1. Common side effects of serotonergic medications (occurring in more than 10% of individuals)

Clomipramine[a,b]	Fluoxetine[c]	Fluvoxamine[a,d]	Sertraline[e]	Paroxetine[f]
abnormal vision	decreased libido	asthenia	anorexia	asthenia
anorexia	dry mouth	dyspepsia[a]	decreased libido	decreased appetite
constipation[a]	nausea	headache[a]	diarrhea	dry mouth
dizziness	somnolence	insomnia[a]	headache	insomnia
dry mouth[a]		nausea	insomnia	nausea
fatigue		nervousness[a]	nausea	sexual dysfunction
insomnia		somnolence		somnolence
micturition disorder				tremor
myoclonus				
nausea				
nervousness				
postural hypotension[a]				
sexual dysfunction				
somnolence				
sweating				
tremor				

[a] Koran 1996; Freeman 1994 (clomipramine vs. fluvoxamine); Koran found that dry mouth, constipation, and postural hypotension were more common with clomipramine, whereas insomnia, nervousness, dyspepsia, and headache were more common with fluvoxamine.
[b] Clomipramine Collaborative Study Group 1991 (clomipramine vs. placebo).
[c] Tollefson 1994 (fluoxetine vs. placebo).
[d] Greist 1995a (fluvoxamine vs. placebo).
[e] Greist 1995b (sertraline vs. placebo).
[f] Wheadon 1993 (paroxetine vs. placebo).

mussen et al. 1993; Rasmussen et al., in press). This long treatment trial can raise some significant issues in terms of compliance, as already noted. However, given that the typical patient with OCD has experienced symptoms for many years, most are willing to endure this long treatment trial if its necessity is explained.

Dosing

The issue of how much medication to give a patient has recently received more systematic study. Clinical wisdom still maintains that maximal doses of each of the antiobsessional agents be given. For clomipramine, the maximum dose is 250 mg/day; doses higher than this significantly increase the risk of seizures (DeVeaugh-Geiss et al. 1989). For fluoxetine, the maximum dose is 80 mg/day, although fluoxetine's exceptionally long half-life may complicate washout (DeVane 1994; Pato et al. 1991). For sertraline, the maximum dose is 200 mg/day, and for fluvoxamine and paroxetine, 300 mg/day and 60 mg/day, respectively. A trial of 10–12 weeks should still be pursued with any one of these medications before abandoning its use.

The results of recent fixed-dose studies of three agents—fluoxetine (Tollefson et al. 1994a, 1994b; Wood et al. 1993), sertraline (Greist et al. 1995a), and paroxetine (Wheadon et al. 1993)—should cause clinicians to reconsider the steps in dosing for initial treatment, keeping in mind that fixed-dose studies of clomipramine and fluvoxamine have not yet been reported. The fluoxetine fixed-dose studies are noteworthy because they showed effectiveness at all three doses studied—20, 40, and 60 mg (Tollefson et al. 1994a, 1994b; Wood et al. 1993). However, there was a trend toward 60 mg being more effective, and in a follow-up study in which patients were allowed to increase their dose from that used in the initial trial, patients demonstrated increased improvement at higher doses. Furthermore, this improvement was either maintained or increased further over the 5–6 months of follow-up (Levine et al. 1989; Tollefson et al. 1994a). In the paroxetine fixed-dose study (Wheadon et al. 1993), patients did not respond to the lower dose of 20 mg but needed higher doses of 40 or 60 mg to show improvement in their obsessive-compulsive symptoms. Perhaps the most interesting, if problematic, data have come from the sertraline trials (Greist et al. 1995b). In this study, 50 mg and 200 mg showed therapeutic benefit in all four measures of improvement (Y-BOCS, National Institute of Mental Health Global Obsessive-Compulsive [NIMH-GOC], and Clinical Global Impression [CGI] Severity and Improvement) but the 100-mg dose showed improvement only in one global measure (NIMH-GOC). Such results are not easy to explain, except perhaps by noting that patients who do not respond at 50 mg may need to be tried at 200 mg before they are considered nonresponders to sertraline.

Jefferson and Greist (1996) note that although these different doses are effective, higher doses are associated with more frequent and more severe side effects. Thus, it seems advisable to ask patients to tolerate the wait of using a lower dose of medication for 10 weeks before trying a higher one. Clinically, a compromise might be struck by the clinician. Whereas most researchers recommend 10 weeks for an adequate trial, many have noted some response beginning at 4 weeks (Greist et al. 1995b, 1995c). Thus, the clinician could start a patient at a low dose and then switch him or her to a higher dose in 4–6 weeks if no response is seen at the lesser dose. Although such a strategy might miss some "late responders" (Rasmussen et al., in press) to the lower dose, it could reduce the overall duration of a treatment trial of two different doses from 20 weeks to 14 weeks.

It is worth noting that the SSRIs, via their effect on the cytochrome P450 system, can inhibit the metabolism of certain other drugs. This effect is best documented for fluoxetine, which has been shown to elevate blood levels of a variety of coadministered drugs, including various tricyclics (e.g., clomipramine), carbamazepine, phenytoin, and trazodone (DeVane 1994). However, other SSRIs may cause similar elevations. Thus, the clinician may have to base the choice of medication on what the patient is already taking or adjust the dose of other medications when these SSRIs are used.

Recommendations

Taking into consideration comparative efficacy and comparative tolerability data, general recommendations for pharmacological treatment are that an adequate pharmacological trial must consider the use of multiple agents, including clomipramine. High doses (up to the manufacturer's recommended maximums) should be used if lower doses are not effective. Finally, whereas some benefit may be seen as early as 4 weeks, an adequate duration of pharmacological treatment for OCD is considered to be 10–12 weeks at maximum tolerated doses (Rasmussen et al. 1993). Although it is reassuring to know that continued medication administration will afford many patients continued improvement, patients often wish to stop medication for a variety of reasons, including cost, a desire to become pregnant, or unwanted side effects such as weight gain or sexual dysfunction. The only double-blind, controlled discontinuation trials have involved clomipramine. There have been three such studies, one with adults (Pato et al. 1988) and two with children (Leonard et al. 1989, 1991). All three of these reports, as well as anecdotal ones, have shown that approximately 90% of patients experience a return of symptoms within 4 to 7 weeks of discontinuing treatment or, in the case of the child studies, of substituting desipramine for clomipramine.

As noted by Jefferson and Greist (1996), these recommendations for medication regimens are based on clinical research. How a medication performs in the clinical arena of private practice is often quite different from how it performs in a carefully controlled research study. For this reason, some helpful clinical algorithms have been developed (Jefferson and Greist 1996; see Figure 12–1) to provide a flexible framework for the clinician in treating OCD patients.

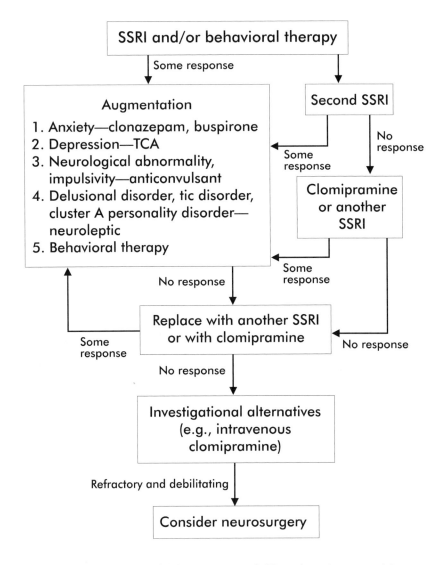

Figure 12–1. Algorithm of OCD treatment. OCD = obsessive-compulsive disorder; SSRI = selective serotonin reuptake inhibitor; TCA = tricyclic antidepressant.

Resistance to Treatment and Augmentation Strategies

Some data provide information about the characteristics of patients who are more resistant to treatment. In particular, patients with schizotypal personality disorder, borderline personality disorder, avoidant personality disorder, and obsessive-compulsive personality disorder have shown poorer response to pharmacotherapy in some studies. Thus, accurate diagnosis is a crucial aspect of assessing treatment resistance. However, perhaps more importantly, before giving a patient the label of treatment-resistant, one needs to assess the adequacy of each medication trial from the point of both dose (was it high enough?) and duration (was it long enough?). In addition, given the data on cross-responsivity, one should note which medications have been tried and whether one of them has been clomipramine. Finally, if adequate doses of primary medications have been given, the clinician should explore whether augmenting agents were given, especially in cases of partial response to monotherapy (Goodman et al. 1993; Jenike 1993; Jenike et al. 1986).

Although the use of an augmenting agent should be considered, clinical wisdom suggests that if there has been no response at all to the initial agent, it is probably better to simply switch medications rather than add an augmenting agent (Jefferson and Greist 1996). If augmenting agents are used, a trial of 2 weeks or, in some cases (e.g., buspirone), up to 8 weeks may be warranted (Goodman et al. 1993; Jenike 1993; Jenike et al. 1991). Overall, most augmenting agents have not performed well in systematic trials, although a number of anecdotal reports have shown them to be effective in some patients.

Another potential guideline for choosing an augmenting agent is the presence of comorbid symptoms in the patient. For instance, if poor insight or psychosis is present, one might add an antipsychotic such as pimozide (McDougle et al. 1990) or risperidone (Jacobsen 1995). With prominent anxiety features, one might consider buspirone (Jenike et al. 1991; Markovitz et al. 1990; McDougle et al. 1993; Pigott et al. 1992a), trazodone (Pigott et al. 1992b), or clonazepam, and, with mood lability, lithium (McDougle et al. 1991).

Psychosurgery

In recent years, psychosurgical techniques have been examined for their potential benefit in extremely severe cases of OCD that have been unresponsive to two to three adequate medication trials with augmentation and to adequate trials of behavioral therapy. Small studies with very well-defined samples have showed success rates of 55%–67% without significant side effects (Mindus and Jenike 1992). Techniques have included surgical procedures such as anterior capsulotomy, cingulotomy, and limbic leukotomy. Noninvasive surgical techniques such as gamma knife procedures are also being explored.

Behavioral Therapy

Behavioral therapy—specifically, ERP—has been successfully used for the treatment of OCD since the late 1970s (Foa et al. 1985; Greist 1994; Marks et al. 1980, 1988). Recent studies that used PET scans before and after behavioral and pharmacological treatment (Baxter et al. 1992; Schwartz et al. 1996) have further reinforced these positive assessments of the efficacy of behavioral therapy. These studies have shown that pharmacotherapy and behavioral therapy produce similar decreases in brain activity. In addition, the areas of the brain that are affected by behavioral treatment have, in many cases, also been identified as areas of brain abnormality from other imaging techniques (Breiter et al. 1996; Rauch et al. 1994; Swedo et al. 1992).

The basic principles underlying ERP are that compulsions provide only a temporary reduction of the anxiety produced by obsessions. Furthermore, the only way to experience more permanent relief is to habituate to the anxiety caused by the obsession without performing the compulsion. Habituation is the key factor, and clinicians proceed by first identifying triggers and situations that bring on obsessional thoughts and compulsive behaviors and then developing a graduated hierarchy of anxiety based on the patient's report. The patient "challenges" him- or herself with the least anxiety-provoking items first and then moves up the hierarchy. In addition to exposure, the patient is instructed to refrain from carrying out the associated rituals. These techniques have shown particular success with washing rituals (Jenike 1993) but can be adapted to almost any type of compulsions, including mental rituals, with some creativity. For instance, traditional wisdom held that mental rituals were difficult to treat because the lack of observable behavior (compulsions) created an obstacle to response prevention. However, effective ERP has been accomplished with scripted imagery and continuous-loop tapes in which patients record their obsessional fears and mental compulsions and then expose themselves to these materials over and over again until they have habituated. Another recent innovation in behavioral treatment is treatment in a group setting with and without family members (Fals-Stewart et al. 1993; Livingston–Van Noppen et al. 1991). Not only is group treatment equally effective and more cost efficient than individual treatment, but the group cohesion lends mutual support and encouragement to the participants in behavioral treatment. In addition, as Calvocoressi et al. (1995) and others have demonstrated, families are often directly or indirectly affected by the patient's OCD, so including family members in treatment is often critical to optimizing recovery.

An added benefit of behavioral treatment is its long-term efficacy. Unlike pharmacotherapy, whose palliative effects do not persist in the great majority of patients after medication is discontinued (Pato et al. 1988), behavioral therapy has shown continued efficacy in follow-up studies ranging from 1 to 6 years, although booster sessions may be needed (O'Sullivan and Marks 1991).

Yet despite its benefits, behavioral treatment is not for everyone. About 15%–25% of patients refuse, at least initially, to engage in behavioral therapy because of its anxiety-provoking nature (Greist 1994), and another 25% fail to benefit from treatment (Foa et al. 1983; Greist 1994), leaving only about 50%–70% of patients initially responsive to this treatment. These statistics may improve, however, in a comprehensive program that includes behavioral, pharmacological, and other support networks for patients and family members. Integrated programs encourage patients, over time, to stay in treatment and to pursue modalities that they initially were unwilling to consider or unsuccessful in sustaining.

Conclusions

OCD is a prevalent illness in adulthood that often presents comorbidly with other disorders. Increasingly, it appears to have a strong biological and genetic basis. OCD is quite responsive to treatment, especially combined treatment with medications that have some impact on the serotonin system and behavioral therapy that specifically includes ERP. These modalities produce symptom improvement in up to 85% of patients. However, unlike the case for other illnesses such as depressive and anxiety disorders, few OCD patients achieve total remission (i.e., "cure") of their symptoms. Yet for most patients, even a modest improvement of 15%–25% can make a significant difference in their overall functioning.

References

American Psychiatric Association: Diagnostic and Statistical Manual of Mental Disorders, 3rd Edition. Washington, DC, American Psychiatric Association, 1984

American Psychiatric Association: Diagnostic and Statistical Manual of Mental Disorders, 3rd Edition, Revised. Washington, DC, American Psychiatric Association, 1987

American Psychiatric Association: Diagnostic and Statistical Manual of Mental Disorders, 4th Edition. Washington, DC, American Psychiatric Association, 1994

Baer L, Jenike MA, Ricciardi JN, et al: Standardized assessment of personality disorders in obsessive-compulsive disorder. Arch Gen Psychiatry 47:826–830, 1990

Barr LL, Goodman WK, McDougle LJ, et al: Tryptophan depletion in patients with obsessive-compulsive disorder who respond to serotonin reuptake inhibitors. Arch Gen Psychiatry 51:309–317, 1994

Baxter LR, Schwartz JM, Mazziotta JC, et al: Cerebral glucose metabolic rates in nondepressed patients with obsessive-compulsive disorder. Am J Psychiatry 145:1560–1563,
1988

Baxter LR, Schwartz JM, Bergman KS, et al: Caudate glucose metabolic rate changes with
both drug and behavior therapy for obsessive-compulsive disorder. Arch Gen Psychiatry 49:681–689, 1992

Bellodi L, Sciuto G, Diaferia G, et al: Psychiatric disorders in the families of patients with
obsessive-compulsive disorder. Psychiatry Res 42:111–120, 1992

Benkelfat C, Nordahl TE, Semple WE, et al: Local cerebral glucose metabolic rates in obsessive-compulsive disorder: patients treated with clomipramine. Arch Gen Psychiatry 47:840–848, 1990

Black DW, Noyes R, Goldstein RB, et al: A family study of obsessive compulsive disorder.
Arch Gen Psychiatry 49:362–368, 1992

Breiter HC, Rauch SL, Kwong KK, et al: Functional magnetic resonance imaging of symptom provocation in obsessive compulsive disorder. Arch Gen Psychiatry 53:595–606,
1996

Calvocoressi LC, Lewis B, Harris M, et al: Family accommodation in obsessive-compulsive disorder. Am J Psychiatry 152:441–443, 1995

Clomipramine Collaborative Study Group: Efficacy of clomipramine in OCD: results of a
multicenter double-blind trial. Arch Gen Psychiatry 48:730–738, 1991

DeVane CL: Pharmacokinetics of the selective serotonin reuptake inhibitors. J Clin Psychiatry 53 (2, suppl):13–20, 1992

DeVane CL: Pharmacogenetics and drug metabolism of newer antidepressant agents.
J Clin Psychiatry 55 (12, suppl):38–45, 1994

DeVeaugh-Geiss J, Landau P, Katz R: Treatment of obsessive-compulsive disorder with
clomipramine. Psychiatric Annals 19:97–101, 1989

Eisen JL, Rasmussen SA: Obsessive-compulsive disorder with psychotic features. J Clin
Psychiatry 54:373–379, 1993

Fals-Stewart W, Marks AP, Schafer J: A comparison of behavioral group therapy and individual behavioral therapy in treating obsessive compulsive disorder. J Nerv Ment Dis
18:189–193, 1993

Flament MF, Rapoport JL, Murphy DL, et al: Biochemical changes during clomipramine
treatment of childhood obsessive-compulsive disorder. Arch Gen Psychiatry 44:219–
225, 1987

Foa EB: Failure in treating obsessive-compulsives. Behav Res Ther 17:169–176, 1979

Foa EB, Kozak MJ: DSM-IV field trial: obsessive-compulsive disorder. Am J Psychiatry
152:90–96, 1995

Foa EB, Grayson JB, Steketee GS, et al: Success and failure in the behavioral treatment of
obsessive-compulsives. J Consult Clin Psychol 51:287–297, 1983

Foa EB, Steketee GS, Ozarow BJ: Behavior therapy with obsessive-compulsives: from theory to treatment, in Obsessive-Compulsive Disorder: Psychological and Pharmacological Treatment. Edited by Mavissakalian M, Turner SM, Michelson L. New York,
Plenum, 1985, pp 49–129

Freeman CPL, Trimble MR, Deakin JFW, et al: Fluvoxamine versus clomipramine in the
treatment of obsessive-compulsive disorder: a multicenter randomized, double-blind,
parallel group comparison. J Clin Psychiatry 55:301–305, 1994

Goodman WK, Price LH, Rasmussen SA, et al: Efficacy of fluvoxamine in obsessive compulsive disorder: a double-blind comparison with placebo. Arch Gen Psychiatry 46:36–
44, 1989a

Goodman WK, Price LH, Rasmussen SA, et al: The Yale-Brown Obsessive Compulsive
Scale, I: development, use, and reliability. Arch Gen Psychiatry 46:1006–1011, 1989b

Goodman WK, McDougle CJ, Lawrence HP, et al: Beyond the serotonin hypothesis: a role
for dopamine in some forms of obsessive-compulsive disorder. J Clin Psychopharmacol 51 (8, suppl):36–43, 1990

Goodman WK, McDougle CJ, Barr LC, et al: Biological approaches to treatment-resistant
obsessive-compulsive disorder. J Clin Psychiatry 54 (6, suppl):16–26, 1993

Greist JH: Behavior therapy for obsessive compulsive disorder. J Clin Psychiatry 55 (10, suppl):60–68, 1994

Greist JH, Charnard G, Duboff E, et al: Double-blind parallel comparison of three dosages of sertraline and placebo in outpatients with obsessive-compulsive disorder. Arch Gen Psychiatry 52:53–60, 1995a

Greist JH, Jefferson JW, Kobak KA, et al: Efficacy and tolerability of serotonin transport inhibitors in obsessive-compulsive disorder. Arch Gen Psychiatry 52:53–60, 1995b

Greist JH, Jenike MA, Robinson D, et al: Efficacy of fluvoxamine in obsessive compulsive disorder: results of a multicentre, double-blind placebo-controlled trial. European Journal of Clinical Research __:195–204, 1995c

Hewlett WA, Martin K: Fenfluramine challenges and serotonergic functioning in obsessive compulsive disorder. Paper presented at the First International Obsessive-Compulsive Disorder Congress, Capri, Italy, March 12–13, 1993

Hoehn-Saric R, Pearlson G, Harris G, et al: Effects of fluoxetine on regional cerebral blood flow in obsessive-compulsive patients. Am J Psychiatry 148:1243–1245, 1991

Hollander E: Introduction, in Obsessive-Compulsive Related Disorders. Edited by Hollander E. Washington, DC, American Psychiatric Press, 1993, pp 1–16

Hollander E, DeCaria C, Nitescu A, et al: Serotonergic function in obsessive-compulsive disorder: behavioral and neuroendocrine responses to oral *m*-chlorophenylpiperazine and fenfluramine in patients and healthy volunteers. Arch Gen Psychiatry 49:21–28, 1992

Insel TR: Toward a neuroanatomy of obsessive-compulsive disorder. Arch Gen Psychiatry 49:739–744, 1992

Insel TR, Akiskal HS: Obsessive-compulsive disorder with psychotic features: a phenomenological analysis. Am J Psychiatry 143:1527–1533, 1986

Insel TR, Winslow JT: Neurobiology of obsessive-compulsive disorder. Psychiatr Clin North Am 15:813–824, 1992

Insel T, Murphy D, Cohen R, et al: Obsessive-compulsive disorder: a double-blind study of clomipramine and clorgyline. Arch Gen Psychiatry 40:605–612, 1983

Jacobsen FM: Risperidone in the treatment of affective illness and obsessive-compulsive disorder. J Clin Psychiatry 56:423–429, 1995

Jefferson JQ, Greist JH: The pharmacotherapy of obsessive-compulsive disorder. Psychiatric Annals 26:202–209, 1996

Jenike MA: Pharmacologic treatment of obsessive-compulsive disorders. Psychiatr Clin North Am 15:895–919, 1992

Jenike MA: Augmentation strategies for treatment-resistant obsessive compulsive disorder. Harvard Review of Psychiatry 1:17–26, 1993

Jenike MA, Baer L, Minichiello WE, et al: Concomitant obsessive-compulsive disorder and schizotypal personality disorder. Am J Psychiatry 143:530–532, 1986

Jenike MA, Baer L, Greist JH: Clomipramine versus fluoxetine in obsessive-compulsive disorder: a retrospective comparison of side effects and efficacy. J Clin Psychopharmacol 10:122–124, 1990a

Jenike MA, Hyman SE, Baer L, et al: A controlled trial of fluvoxamine for obsessive-compulsive disorder: implications for a serotonergic theory. Am J Psychiatry 147:1209–1215, 1990b

Jenike MA, Baer L, Buttolph L: Buspirone augmentation of fluoxetine in patients with obsessive compulsive disorder. J Clin Psychiatry 1:13–14, 1991

Karno M, Golding JM, Sorenson SB, et al: The epidemiology of obsessive compulsive disorder in five U.S. communities. Arch Gen Psychiatry 45:1094–1099, 1988

Koran LM, McElroy SL, Davidson JRT, et al: Fluvoxamine vs clomipramine for obsessive-compulsive disorder: a double-blind comparison. J Clin Psychopharmacol 16:121–129, 1996

Kozak MJ, Foa EB: Obsessions, overvalued ideas, and delusions in obsessive-compulsive disorder. Behavior Res Ther 32:343–353, 1994

Lees AJ, Robertson M, Trimble MR, et al: A clinical study of Gilles de la Tourette syndrome in the United Kingdom. J Neurol Neurosurg Psychiatry 47:1–8, 1984

Lelliott PT, Noshirvani HF, Basoglu M, et al: Obsessive-compulsive beliefs and treatment outcome. Psychol Med 18:697–702, 1988

Lenane MC, Swedo SE, Leonard H, et al: Psychiatric disorders in first-degree relatives of children and adolescents with obsessive compulsive disorder. J Am Acad Child Adolesc Psychiatry 29:407–412, 1990

Leonard HL, Swedo SE, Rapport JL, et al: Treatment of childhood obsessive-compulsive disorders with clomipramine and desipramine: a double-blind crossover comparison. Arch Gen Psychiatry 46:1088–1092, 1989

Leonard HL, Swedo SE, Lenane MD, et al: A double-blind desipramine substitution during long-term clomipramine treatment in children and adolescents with obsessive compulsive disorder. Arch Gen Psychiatry 922–927, 1991

Leonard HL, Lenane MC, Swedo SE, et al: Tics and Tourette's disorder: a 2- to 7-year follow-up of 54 obsessive-compulsive children. Am J Psychiatry 149:1244–1251, 1992

Levine R, Hoffman JS, Knepple ED, et al: Long-term fluoxetine treatment of a large number of obsessive compulsive patients. J Clin Psychopharmacol 9:281–283, 1989

Livingston–Van Noppen B, Rasmussen SA, McCartney L, et al: A multi-family group approach as an adjunct to treatment of obsessive compulsive disorders, in Current Treatments of Obsessive-Compulsive Disorder. Edited by Pato MT, Zohar J. Washington, DC, American Psychiatric Press, 1991, pp 115–134

Mavissakalian M, Jones B, Olson S, et al: Clomipramine in obsessive-compulsive disorder: clinical response and plasma levels. J Clin Psychopharmacology 10:261–268, 1990

Markovitz PJ, Stagnos J, Calabresa JR: Buspirone augmentation of fluoxetine on obsessive compulsive disorder. Am J Psychiatry 147:798–800, 1990

Marks I, Stern A, Mawson D, et al: Clomipramine and exposure for obsessive-compulsive rituals. Br J Psychiatry 136:1–25, 1980

Marks I, Lelliott P, Basoglu M, et al: Clomipramine, self-exposure and therapist-added exposure in obsessive-compulsive ritualizers. Br J Psychiatry 152:522–534, 1988

McDougle CJ, Goodman WK, Price LH, et al: Neuroleptic addition in fluvoxamine refractory obsessive compulsive disorder. Am J Psychiatry 147:652–654, 1990

McDougle CJ, Price LH, Goodman WK, et al: A controlled trial of lithium augmentation in fluvoxamine refractory obsessive compulsive disorder: lack of efficacy. J Clin Psychopharmacol 11:175–184, 1991

McDougle CJ, Goodman WK, Leckman JF, et al: Limited therapeutic effect of addition of buspirone in fluvoxamine refractory obsessive compulsive disorder. Am J Psychiatry 150:647–649, 1993

McKeon P, Murray R: Familial aspects of obsessive compulsive neurosis. Br J Psychiatry 51:528–534, 1987

Mindus P, Jenike MA: Neurosurgical treatment of malignant obsessive compulsive disorder. Psychiatr Clin North Am 15:921–938, 1992

Montgomery SA: Pharmacological treatment of obsessive-compulsive disorder, in Current Insights in Obsessive-Compulsive Disorder. Edited by Hollander E, Zohar J, Marazziti D, et al. West Sussex, UK, John Wiley & Sons, 1994, pp 214–225

Nordahl TE, Benkelfat C, Semple WE, et al: Cerebral glucose metabolic rates in obsessive compulsive disorder. Neuropsychopharmacology 2:23–28, 1989

O'Sullivan G, Marks I: Follow-up studies of behavioral treatment of phobia and obsessive compulsive neurosis. Psychiatric Annals 21:368–373, 1991

Pato MT, Zohar-Kadouch R, Zohar J, et al: Return of symptoms after discontinuation of clomipramine in patients with obsessive compulsive disorder. Am J Psychiatry 145:1521–1525, 1988

Pato MT, Murphy DL, DeVane CL: Sustained plasma concentrations of fluoxetine and/or norfluoxetine 4 and 8 weeks after fluoxetine discontinuation. J Clin Psychopharmacol 11:224–225, 1991

Pato MT, Eisen JL, Pato CN: Rating scales for obsessive-compulsive disorder, in Current Insights in Obsessive-Compulsive Disorder. Edited by Hollander E, Zohar J, Marazziti D, et al. West Sussex, UK, John Wiley & Sons, 1994, pp 77–92

Pauls DL, Towbin KE, Leckman JF, et al: Gilles de la Tourette's syndrome and obsessive-compulsive disorder: evidence supporting a genetic relationship. Arch Gen Psychiatry 43:1180–1182, 1986

Pauls DL, Raymond CL, Stevenson JF, et al: A family study of Gilles de la Tourette's syndrome. Am J Hum Genet 48:154–163, 1991

Pauls DL, Alsobrook MP, Goodman W, et al: A family study of obsessive compulsive disorder. Am J Psychiatry 152:76–84, 1995

Phillips KA: Body dysmorphic disorder: the distress of imagined ugliness. Am J Psychiatry 148:1138–1149, 1991

Phillips KA, McElroy SL, Hudson JI, et al: Body dysmorphic disorder: an OCD spectrum disorder, a form of affective spectrum disorder, or both? J Clin Psychiatry 56 (4, suppl):41–51, 1995

Pigott TA: OCD: where the serotonin selective story begins. J Clin Psychiatry 57 (6, suppl):11–20, 1996

Pigott TA, Pato MT, Bernstein SE, et al: Controlled comparison of clomipramine and fluoxetine in the treatment of obsessive-compulsive disorder. Arch Gen Psychiatry 47:926–932, 1990

Pigott TA, Zohar J, Hill JL, et al: Metergoline blocks the behavioral and neuroendocrine effects of orally administered *m*-chlorophenylpiperazine in patients with obsessive-compulsive disorder. Biol Psychiatry 29:418–426, 1991

Pigott TA, L'Hereux F, Hill JL, et al: A double-blind study of adjuvant buspirone hydrochloride in clomipramine-treated patients with obsessive compulsive disorder. J Clin Psychopharmacol 12:11–18, 1992a

Pigott TA, Littenfer XF, Rubenstein CS, et al: A double-blind, placebo-controlled study of trazodone in patients with obsessive compulsive disorder. J Clin Psychopharmacol 12:156–162, 1992b

Pitman RK: Historical considerations, in Psychobiology of Obsessive Compulsive Disorder. Edited by Zohar J, Insel T, Rasmussen S. New York, Springer-Verlag, 1991, pp 1–12

Rachman SJ, Hodgson RJ: Obsessions and Compulsions. Englewood Cliffs, NJ, Prentice-Hall, 1980

Rapoport JL, Ryland D, Kriete M: Drug treatment of canine acral lick: an animal model of obsessive-compulsive disorder. Arch Gen Psychiatry 49:517–521, 1992

Rasmussen SA, Eisen JL: Phenomenology of obsessive compulsive disorder, in Psychobiology of Obsessive-Compulsive Disorder. Edited by Insel J, Rasmussen S. New York, Springer-Verlag, 1991, pp 743–758

Rasmussen SA, Tsuang MT: Clinical characteristics and family history in DSM-III obsessive-compulsive disorder. Am J Psychiatry 143:317–322, 1986

Rasmussen SA, Eisen JL, Pato MT: Current issues in the pharmacologic management of obsessive-compulsive disorder. J Clin Psychiatry 54 (6, suppl):4–9, 1993

Rasmussen SA, Goodman WK, Greist JH, et al: Fluvoxamine in the treatment of obsessive compulsive disorder: a multicenter, double-blind placebo-controlled study in outpatients. Am J Psychiatry (in press)

Rauch SL, Jenike MA, Alpert NM, et al: Regional cerebral blood flow measured during symptom provocation in obsessive-compulsive disorder using oxygen 15-labeled carbon dioxide and positron emission tomography. Arch Gen Psychiatry 51:62–70, 1994

Ricciardi JN, Baer L, Jenike MA, et al: Changes in DSM-III-R Axis II diagnoses following treatment of obsessive-compulsive disorder. Am J Psychiatry 149:829–831, 1992

Riddle MA, Scahill L, King R, et al: Obsessive compulsive disorder in children and adolescents: phenomenology and family history. J Am Acad Child Adolesc Psychiatry 29:766–772, 1990

Robertson MM, Trimble MR, Lees AJ: The psychopathology of the Gilles de la Tourette syndrome: a phenomenological analysis. Br J Psychiatry 152:283–390, 1988

Robins LN, Helzer JE, Weissman MM, et al: Lifetime prevalence of specific psychiatric disorders in three sites. Arch Gen Psychiatry 41:958–967, 1984

Rubenstein CS, Pigott TA, L'Heureux F, et al: A preliminary investigation of the lifetime prevalence of anorexia and bulimia nervosa in patients with obsessive compulsive disorder. J Clin Psychiatry 53:309–314, 1992

Schwartz JM, Stoessel PW, Baxter LR, et al: Systematic changes in cerebral glucose metabolic rate after successful behavior modification treatment of obsessive-compulsive disorder. Arch Gen Psychiatry 53:109–113, 1996

Stangl D, Pfohl B, Zimmerman M, et al: A structured interview for the DSM-III personality disorders: preliminary report. Arch Gen Psychiatry 42:591–596, 1985

Swedo SE, Rapoport JL, Leonard H, et al: Obsessive-compulsive disorder in children and adolescents: clinical phenomenology of 70 consecutive cases. Arch Gen Psychiatry 46:335–341, 1989a

Swedo SE, Schapiro MB, Grady CL, et al: Cerebral glucose metabolism in childhood-onset obsessive compulsive disorder. Arch Gen Psychiatry 46:518–523, 1989b

Swedo SE, Pietrini P, Leonard HL, et al: Cerebral glucose metabolism in childhood onset obsessive-compulsive disorder: revisualization during pharmacology. Arch Gen Psychiatry 49:690–694, 1992

Thiel A, Broocks A, Ohlmeier M, et al: Obsessive-compulsive disorder among patients with anorexia nervosa and bulimia nervosa. Am J Psychiatry 152:72–75, 1995

Thorén P, Åsberg M, Bertilsson L, et al: Clomipramine treatment of obsessive compulsive disorder, II: biochemical aspects. Arch Gen Psychiatry 37:1289–1294, 1980

Tollefson GD, Birkett M, Koran L, et al: Continuation treatment of OCD: double-blind and open-label experience with fluoxetine. J Clin Psychiatry 55 (10, suppl):69–76, 1994a

Tollefson GD, Rampey AH, Potvin JH, et al: A multicenter investigation of fixed dose fluoxetine in the treatment of obsessive-compulsive disorder. Arch Gen Psychiatry 51:559–567, 1994b

Wheadon D, Bushnell W, Steiner M: A fixed-dose comparison of 20, 40, or 60 mg paroxetine to placebo in the treatment of obsessive-compulsive disorder. ACNP Annual Meeting, Honolulu, Hawaii, December 1993

Wood A, Tollefson GD, Birkett M: Pharmacotherapy of obsessive compulsive disorder: experience with fluoxetine. Int Clin Psychopharmacol 8:301–306, 1993

World Health Organization: International Classification of Diseases, 10th Revision. Geneva, Switzerland, World Health Organization, 1992

Zohar J, Mueller E, Insel T et al: Serotonergic responsivity in obsessive-compulsive disorder: comparison of patients and healthy controls. Arch Gen Psychiatry 44:946–951, 1987

Chapter 13

Obsessive-Compulsive Disorder in Later Life

C. Alec Pollard, Ph.D., Cheryl N. Carmin, Ph.D., and
Raymond Ownby, M.D., Ph.D.

The past decade has witnessed phenomenal growth in the clinical and research literature on obsessive-compulsive disorder (OCD). However, until recently, very little has been written about OCD in the elderly. Although general knowledge about the nature and treatment of OCD has no doubt assisted clinicians working with elderly patients, the applicability of this information to older adults has not been clearly established. Furthermore, information relevant to the elderly is scattered throughout a variety of different sources. In this chapter we review the literature and discuss clinical issues concerning the epidemiology, diagnosis, and treatment of OCD in later life.

Epidemiology and Demographics

It has been more than a decade since large-scale epidemiological studies revealed that OCD affects a significantly larger portion of the general population than was previously assumed (Myers et al. 1984; Robins et al. 1984). Subsequently, more-specific information regarding the prevalence of OCD in the elderly has become available. Although initial onset of OCD is less common in later life (Blazer et al. 1991; Flint 1994), 1- and 6-month prevalence rates of 0.8% (Regier et al. 1988) and 1.5% (Bland et al. 1988; Kolada et al. 1994), respectively, have been reported for OCD in samples of the general population over 65 years old. Somewhat lower OCD rates of 0.0%–0.6% were found in one study that used a different diagnostic method (Copeland et al. 1987a, 1987b). The prevalence of OCD in those who live in institutions, such as nursing homes, is several times greater than that in other elderly persons (Bland et al. 1988; Junginger et al. 1993).

Data regarding the relative morbidity risk of OCD in elderly men and women are inconsistent. Findings from five sites in the United States suggest that elderly men and women are at equal risk for OCD

The authors wish to express their appreciation to Roberto A. Dominguez, M.D., for his comments on an earlier version of this chapter.

(Regier et al. 1988). However, another study conducted in Edmonton, Canada, found prevalence rates of 0.9% and 1.9%, respectively, in elderly males and females, suggesting that morbidity risk is higher for women (Bland et al. 1988). Evidence of a clear association between OCD and other demographic variables in older adult samples has not been reported.

Diagnosis

Diagnostic Criteria and Clinical Presentation

At present there is no reason to believe that DSM-IV (American Psychiatric Association 1994) criteria are not equally applicable to the elderly. To meet criteria for OCD, individuals must have either obsessions or compulsions that cause marked distress or that significantly interfere with their lives. Obsessions are recurrent and persistent thoughts, impulses, or ideas that are experienced as intrusive and inappropriate and that cause marked anxiety or distress. Common themes of obsessions include contamination, harm to oneself or others, sex, and blasphemy. Compulsions are the repetitive behaviors (e.g., hand washing, checking, straightening) or mental acts (e.g., replacing "bad" thoughts with "good" thoughts, praying, counting) a person performs to reduce or otherwise neutralize an obsession or the discomfort associated with it.

It has been suggested that certain specific presentations of OCD are more likely to occur in the elderly. Examples reported by clinicians include obsessions and compulsions related to fear of forgetting names (Jenike 1991), OCD accompanied by bipolar illness (Gordon and Rasmussen 1988), and pronounced ego-syntonic scrupulosity (Fallon et al. 1990). Despite these case examples, there is currently no convincing evidence that particular constellations of obsessions and compulsions are unique to older adults. Typical presentations of OCD, such as contamination fears with washing rituals and fears of harming others accompanied by checking compulsions, are also commonly found in elderly patients (Calamari et al. 1994).

Differential Diagnosis of Medical Disorders

Because of the prominence of anxiety in OCD, consideration should be given during assessment to medical illnesses common in the elderly that can produce or exacerbate anxiety-like symptoms (Gurian and Miner 1991; Markovitz 1993; Shader et al. 1987). The association between anxiety symptoms and disease in almost any organ system is well known but not always well appreciated. Cardiovascular disease, especially such conditions as cardiac arrhythmias or congestive heart failure resulting in shortness of breath, can produce anxiety-like symptoms such as tachycardia and chest pain. Diseases of the respiratory system such as pneumonia or chronic obstructive pulmonary disease (COPD) may manifest as symptoms resembling anxiety, such as difficulty breathing or lightheadedness. Other conditions that can produce symptoms difficult to distinguish from anxiety include endocrinological diseases such as hyper- or hypothyroidism and diabetes mellitus, neurological diseases such as stroke or the degenerative dementias, and use or abuse of certain substances (e.g., alcohol). The myriad illnesses that may mimic or be accompanied by anxiety symptoms make accurate evaluation of the elderly OCD patient imperative. At a minimum, such an evaluation should include a complete medical and psychiatric history, a physical examination that includes a meticulous neurological assessment, and appropriate laboratory studies.

Although these diseases are always important to consider, few of them can be expected to produce the full syndrome of OCD, with the possible exception of a cerebrovascular accident in the area of the basal ganglia (Simpson and Baldwin 1995). It may be best to view OCD in the elderly from a biopsychosocial perspective, wherein medical illnesses, developmental stressors, and social stressors each function in varying degrees as predisposing or exacerbating factors that then interact in combination with premorbid personality, social functioning, and the larger psychosocial environment. From this perspective, the stress of a medical illness may elevate a subclinical pattern of functioning to clinical prominence for the first time in old age. Similarly, removal of an important social support, as may happen with the death of a spouse, might bring an already extant disorder to clinical attention. Following the general principle of trying to maximize functioning in all systems, clinicians treating an older adult with OCD should be concerned with obtaining optimal treatment for all presenting problems. For example, this objective might encompass optimizing treatment for a patient's COPD, providing pharmacological and behavioral treatments for the OCD, intervening in marital discord, and arranging social service support to help the patient deal with third-party payers and other practical issues.

Differential Diagnosis of Psychiatric Disorders

Psychiatric comorbidity in elderly OCD patients does not appear to be substantially different from that found in younger adults. Conditions most commonly accompanying OCD include depression, other anxiety disorders, and DSM Axis II disorders (Steketee et al., in press). Identification of psychiatric comorbidity can have clear implications for treatment. In some cases, for example, treatment of the OCD may need to be delayed until the comorbid condition has been addressed. A severely depressed patient may lack the energy and motivation needed to engage in behavior therapy (Foa et al. 1983). Remediation of the depression can help prepare the patient to begin addressing his or her OCD.

In addition to assessing comorbidity, it is also important to consider psychiatric conditions that sometimes include symptoms appearing to be obsessive-compulsive in nature. Depression, delusional disorders, degenerative dementias, and schizophrenia can all develop late in life, and each can produce persistent obsessive thoughts that resemble OCD. Repetitive behavior that has the appearance of a compulsion can also occur in disorders other than OCD. Stereotyped movements and checking behaviors, for example, are not uncommon in schizophrenia (Berman et al. 1995).

Careful history taking, with information obtained from collateral sources, is critical in understanding the patient's presentation. With adequate information, the clinician can determine whether a patient's excessive concern about having things stolen from his or her home is a symptom of OCD, a continuation of a lifelong pattern of suspiciousness, or the first manifestation of a degenerative dementia. True OCD symptoms can usually be distinguished by their typical presentation (e.g., contamination fears), their long-standing character (with onset early in life), and the relative preservation of reality testing in other areas of the patient's life. Conversely, persistent, unrealistic beliefs characteristic of late-life schizophrenia or delusional disorder are more likely to focus on persecutory themes, whereas such beliefs in depression are usually related to themes of loss.

It is important to keep in mind that OCD may develop de novo late in life, and that any individual elderly patient can present with an unusual pattern of symptoms. There are no inviolable rules for differentiating obsessions or compulsions from similar phenomena in other disorders. The final determination regarding differential diagnosis rests on the skill and thoroughness of the evaluating clinician. Accurate diagnosis requires a clear understanding of the range of presentations of OCD possible in the elderly (Calamari et al. 1994).

Treatment

Pharmacological Intervention

Serotonergic medications such as clomipramine, fluoxetine, fluvoxamine, sertraline, and paroxetine have been effective in improving OCD symptoms (Greist et al. 1995; Piccinelli et al. 1995; Stein et al. 1995). Although controlled trials with older adults are currently not available to guide clinical practice, case reports suggest that these same medications are likely to be as effective in the elderly as they are in younger adults (Austin et al. 1991; Bajulaiye and Addonizio 1993; Shader et al. 1987; Sheikh and Salzman 1995; Stoudemire and Moran 1993). Selection of the appropriate medication for an elderly person with OCD, however, should be based on history of response, adverse side-effect profile, and likely efficacy. For example, although clomipramine is effective in treating OCD in younger persons, its adverse sedative and anticholinergic effects makes it less desirable for use in the elderly.

The clinician initiating pharmacological treatment with geriatric OCD patients must take into account several factors that affect amount and scheduling of dose. Ability to metabolize drugs may diminish with increasing age due to changes in enzyme activity in the liver and reduced clearance of drugs by the kidneys. Body composition also can change with increased age, resulting in a decrease in the ratio of lean muscle to fat. Lipophilic drugs may thus have higher volumes of distribution and slower elimination, so that the activity of some medications may be prolonged. In addition, perhaps due to decreased cognitive reserve, some elderly individuals are more sensitive to the cognitive side effects of medications. Older adults are also more susceptible to adverse drug interactions, a vulnerability compounded by the larger number of medications they are likely to be taking. These facts warrant an approach to pharmacotherapy that begins with careful evaluation of the patient's medical and psychiatric status. The physician should initiate treatment with low doses of medication, maintain vigilance for the emergence of adverse effects, and increase doses slowly.

Considering a medication's potential for adverse effects is extremely important when initiating therapy with the elderly, and the OCD patient is no exception. Assessment of a patient's susceptibility to other anxiety-producing agents, such as caffeine or the pseudoephedrine contained in many cold medications, may help guide the clinician in prescribing low doses of medication and in alerting the patient to possible adverse effects. Although some physicians have expressed concern about increasing an already vigilant patient's awareness of side effects, forewarning patients more often serves as an inoculation procedure. Informed patients are less likely to be surprised by side effects and may be more willing to endure the protracted pharmacological treatment sometimes necessary with OCD.

Although studies have shown that all five of the serotonergic medications available in the United States are effective in treating OCD, a comparison of treatment effect sizes suggests an inverse relationship between serotonergic specificity and amount of symptom improvement (Jenike et al. 1990). Studies thus favor the less serotonin-specific agents such as clomipramine, fluoxetine, and fluvoxamine over the more specific agent sertraline.

Thus, the first-choice treatment for OCD in the elderly might be a low dose of fluoxetine. The dose should then be increased gradually.

Because fluoxetine may initially increase anxiety, therapy with this agent should begin at a low dose (as low as 10 mg/day or lower if needed) that is increased gradually. OCD treatment sometimes requires higher doses of medication than are needed for managing depression. Although doses should be increased cautiously in the elderly, many older persons may ultimately require doses similar to those used to treat younger adults with OCD. Age and health of the person, of course, should also affect dosage decisions. The initial dose of medication for a healthy 65-year-old man might be substantially different from that prescribed for a frail 80-year-old woman. As therapy progresses, dosage changes should be individualized according to clinical response and tolerance of adverse effects.

As is true in the treatment of younger OCD patients, an extended period of therapy may be required. Patients should receive an adequate dose (maximized with respect to treatment response and adverse effects) of medication for at least 10 weeks before a particular drug is determined ineffective. It is useful to supplement a patient's report of therapeutic response to medication with a standardized self-report measure such as the Modified Maudsley Obsessive-Compulsive Inventory (MMOCI; Dominguez et al. 1989) or a therapist rating scale such as the Yale-Brown Obsessive Compulsive Scale (Y-BOCS; Goodman et al. 1989a; Goodman et al. 1989b). If possible, assessment of treatment response should also include reports from family members and other collateral sources familiar with the patient's day-to-day functioning.

Data on alternative strategies for elderly patients with inadequate response to serotonergic monotherapy are virtually nonexistent. Augmentation is one option, but other steps should be considered first. If response to one serotonergic medication is inadequate, it is reasonable to try another. It may even be worthwhile to try a third serotonergic medication before investigating strategies that combine several medications (Dominguez and Mestre 1994). Furthermore, before initiating augmentation, it is useful to thoroughly review the diagnosis, the patient's compliance with therapy, the adequacy of dosing (via blood levels when available), the potential impact of family functioning and life stressors, and the status of the patient's participation in behavior therapy. The importance of participation in behavior therapy cannot be overemphasized. Consideration of the patient's status in behavioral treatment should be an integral part of evaluating response to medication.

After first-line treatments have been fully explored, augmentation with one of the serotonergic medications can be considered. Each augmentation strategy has advantages and disadvantages, and choice of strategy should involve consideration of patient characteristics such as frailty, susceptibility to falls, ability to metabolize the various medications available, and sensitivity to cholinergic effects.

Augmentation strategies targeting serotonergic pathways, such as the use of lithium or buspirone, have been disappointing in small controlled trials. Although lithium is undoubtedly an effective augmentation agent in treating depression, there is little evidence of its effectiveness in augmenting the antiobsessional effects of other serotonergic medications. Because of the risk of toxicity and potential interactions with medications (e.g., antihypertensive and nonsteroidal antiinflammatory drugs) commonly used by the elderly, lithium augmentation should be viewed in most cases as an undesirable approach to augmentation with this population.

An augmentation strategy with minimal risk is to add buspirone to one of the monotherapy agents. The anxiolytic effect of buspirone may improve some patients' functioning even if it does not directly affect OCD symptoms. Buspirone has few adverse effects and is unlikely to impair cognitive or motor functioning in the elderly. It thus appears to be a safe choice for augmentation, although its efficacy with OCD needs to be more clearly demonstrated.

Although clonazepam has been used as an effective augmentation strategy (Dominguez and Mestre 1994), enthusiasm for its use with the elderly must be tempered by its potential to cause excessive sedation and to accumulate in the patient's system over time. Because benzodiazepine use is a risk factor for falls in the elderly, clonazepam should not be prescribed for persons who are frail or who already have gait disturbances. If augmentation with clonazepam is attempted, the clinician should carefully monitor the elderly person's cognitive and motor functioning.

The addition of low doses of a high-potency neuroleptic, such as haloperidol, to a serotonergic medication can be considered with the elderly because of the low likelihood of adverse effects. However, this augmentation strategy is probably most likely to be successful in patients with comorbid tic disorder. Several authors have also described the use of newer atypical neuroleptics alone or in combinations as therapy for OCD (Jacobsen 1995; McDougle et al. 1995). Preliminary data suggest that risperidone may be a useful agent for augmenting the effects of other serotonergic agents (Jacobsen 1995), whereas clozapine is probably not effective as a single-agent treatment for OCD (McDougle et al. 1995). Clinicians treating OCD with clozapine or risperidone should also consider reports suggesting both drugs can exacerbate OCD symptoms (Patel and Tandon 1993; Patil 1992; Remington and Adams 1994).

Very limited evidence exists to support the use of medical interventions other than pharmacotherapy to treat OCD in the elderly. One exception may be the use of cingulotomy and related psychosurgery procedures, which could play a role in the treatment of some highly refractory cases of OCD (Jenike et al. 1991), although data on older adults have not been published. There is one report of the successful use of electroconvulsive therapy (ECT) to treat an 84-year-old woman with a long history of OCD (Casey and Davis 1994). However, both psychosurgery and ECT need to be studied further, specifically with elderly OCD patients.

Psychosocial Intervention

Psychosocial treatment of elderly OCD patients is based largely on research with the general adult population. By far the most consistently effective and well-studied psychological intervention for OCD has been the behavioral treatment known as exposure and response prevention (ERP) (Baer and Minichiello 1990; Dar and Greist 1992; Stanley and Turner 1995; Steketee and Foa 1985). With this procedure, patients are systematically exposed to their obsessions (e.g., contamination) while attempting to resist engaging in compulsions (e.g., washing).

Although ERP is well established as a treatment for OCD in young adults, little has been written on the specific application of this procedure to the elderly (Calamari et al. 1994). King and Barrowclough (1991) have reported success with cognitive-behavioral interventions in a sample of older patients with various anxiety disorders, thus challenging the notion that cognitive deficits of normal aging preclude benefit from psychosocial treatment. Applying behavioral treatments specifically to OCD, several case studies have provided more direct evidence that ERP is effective with elderly patients (Calamari et al. 1994; Junginger and Ditto 1984; Rowan et al. 1984; Turner et al. 1979). Results of one study indicate that older persons with OCD may derive as much benefit from behavioral treatment as do younger OCD patients (Carmin et al. 1995). Ten OCD patients aged 60 and older and 10 younger adult OCD patients matched for sex and clinical severity received ERP. At the end of treatment, both groups had improved, and no significant differences in outcome were found between the older and younger patients. This finding is particularly noteworthy given that the duration of illness reported by the older patients was more than twice that reported by their younger counterparts. Although these reports are promising, more research is needed to clearly establish the exportability of behavioral treatment to the elderly (Hersen and Van Hasselt 1992; McCarthy et al. 1991).

No controlled studies have evaluated modifications of behavior therapy that might be necessary to successfully address the needs of elderly OCD patients. However, the clinical literature and our experience suggest that certain adaptations of treatment are sometimes needed. One important clinical consideration is how physical illness, which is more prevalent in older adults, affects treatment planning and implementation. For example, patients whose treatment for contamination fears could involve touching objects outdoors may be unable to do so during hot, cold, or windy weather if they suffer from severe or poorly controlled angina. Similarly, the pace of exposure will need to be reduced for patients with emphysema who require supplemental oxygen and are unable to engage in more than limited physical exertion. Clinicians treating the medically compromised elderly must be adept at suspending, reinitiating, and modifying behavior therapy as needed in response to medical complications.

Nonphysician behavior therapists working with elderly OCD patients should familiarize themselves with side-effect and drug-interaction profiles of medications such as the serotonin reuptake inhibitors. Age-related changes in response to some medications and increased medical comorbidity mean greater potential for drug interactions. Behavior therapists often see patients more frequently than do other clinicians and should thus be observant for medication problems that need to be communicated to the patient's physician. When patients are seen by multiple specialists, collaborative case management is even more important. To begin with, it is crucial that elderly patients are medically cleared for behavioral treatment and that the physician understands what this form of therapy involves. A collaborative approach provides a safeguard for the therapist in terms of the interaction of treatment strategies with the patient's medical condition and helps prevent patients from inappropriately using their medical problems as a reason to avoid behavioral interventions. In turn, the therapist may be able to assist physicians in addressing behavioral problems that complicate the patient's medical treatment.

In addition to increased medical comorbidity, normal aging is associated with some limitations in physical and cognitive agility that can affect treatment. ERP, for example, may need to be modified. This intervention ordinarily involves experiencing modest to high levels of anxiety, and the attenuated stamina of some older patients can dissuade them from pursuing behavior therapy. Pacing treatment judiciously helps prevent some patients from becoming overwhelmed. On the other hand, some patients will resist pacing because they perceive it as a concession to their advancing age. The speed at which treatment progresses and the level of difficulty of the ERP regimen need to be discussed regularly in therapy to help prevent patients from becoming unnecessarily discouraged or overwhelmed.

Just as reduced stamina presents a challenge to treatment, so, too, can the presence of physical disability. Treatment strategies sometimes need to be tailored to accommodate sensory or motor impairment. It is also important to differentiate OCD symptoms from compensatory behaviors related to impairment. For example, a patient who repeatedly asks if a chair looks clean enough to sit on could be compulsively seeking reassurance or might simply be compensating for poor vision. Sometimes interventions like a hearing aid, glasses, or cataract surgery clarify the nature of the behavior. Non-OCD impairments that interfere with treatment but cannot be corrected may still need to be addressed in order to administer therapy successfully. For example, using audio-taped descriptions of exposure scenes to administer imaginal flooding will be of little value to a patient who is hearing impaired. In this situation, creative use of written or videotaped material may be necessary for adequate exposure.

Elderly individuals are also more vulnerable to decline in cognitive functions such as memory (Lindesay et al. 1989), which presents an assessment challenge similar to that involved in evaluating sensory and motor impairment. The clinician needs to discern whether ritualistic behavior is, in fact, a compulsion or an adaptation to offset cognitive deficits. Repetitive checking, placement, and list-making behaviors can all serve as memory aids in certain individuals. Although the presence of mild to moderate memory deficits in addition to OCD symptoms does not obviate behavioral treatment, adaptations sometimes need to be made. For example, failure to remember the principles of response prevention will seriously threaten the success of behavior therapy in OCD. However, written reminders to resist rituals can be strategically placed within the patient's environment as aids to help ensure proper adherence to the response prevention protocol.

General Treatment Considerations

In addition to factors specifically related to pharmacological or behavioral treatment, other general clinical issues and practical obstacles exist that can complicate the management of OCD in elderly patients. In this section we discuss additional treatment considerations relevant to the geriatric OCD patient.

Circumventing resistance to treatment.   Although the stigma of having OCD has certainly not vanished, older adults grew up in a society in which having a psychiatric condition was considered more shameful than it is today. Not surprisingly, many elderly patients are reluctant to acknowledge their problem and to seek help (German et al. 1985; Himmelfarb and Murrell 1984). Extra time may need to be devoted to preparing older patients to engage in treatment. For the elder who refuses help altogether, family counseling is sometimes the first step. Whether working with patients or their families, it is important that clinicians respect the values and cultural background of their older patients.

Sometimes reluctance to engage in treatment comes from a culture-bound belief that, unlike medical disorders, psychiatric problems reflect a weakness in intelligence or moral character. It is therefore not unusual for patients to focus on some other illness or the "medical" aspects of their OCD. Rather than attempting to persuade the patient to assume a biopsychosocial model of OCD, the clinician may find it more helpful initially to adopt the patient's model and then to gradually introduce the importance of managing behavioral aspects of disease. Management of medical conditions such as diabetes and hypertension can be used as an illustration of the role behavioral interventions can play in the treatment of OCD.

Resistance may also be reflected in a patient's reluctance to use contemporary mental health language. In such cases, the clinician can adopt language meaningful to the patient. For example, some older patients do not like the word *anxiety*, either because its meaning is less familiar or because the word has a negative connotation for them. Use of another word, such as "nervous" or "distressed," might be more readily accepted. Some patients are unable or reluctant to rate their distress levels with numeric scales like the Subjective Units of Disturbance Scale (SUDS; Wolpe 1973). In such cases, it is sometimes helpful to adopt a more acceptable alternative method by asking patients simply to rate their anxiety level as high, medium, or low.

Dealing with family issues. Although family intervention is not always necessary, it is usually helpful. Recent evidence that family behavior is related to level of functioning in OCD patients (Calvocoressi et al. 1995) has confirmed what many clinicians have long suspected. The more OCD patients interact with or are dependent upon spouses, children, and other relatives, the greater the need for family intervention. In many ways, the goals of intervening with families of older individuals are similar to those of dealing with families of younger adults. The aim is to correct misinformation and negative stereotypes about OCD, teach ways to support the patient's recovery, and help family members reduce behavior that can impede the patient's progress. The therapist tries to help them learn that responding to the patient by being overly critical, accommodating rituals, or providing repeated reassurances will only exacerbate the patient's condition.

There are a few family-related issues that clinicians working with older individuals are especially likely to encounter. In many instances, the therapist is working with the patient's adult children, who may be grappling with a shift in the nature of their relationship to the OCD patient. Because of limitations in the patient's functioning imposed by OCD or other infirmities associated with aging, the adult children may have assumed more of a parental or custodial role. Extra attention may need to be devoted in family sessions to facilitation of this often awkward and uncomfortable reversal of roles. Under these circumstances, issues of patient confidentiality and family boundaries are in many ways similar to those involved in working with the families of children and adolescents.

Consulting to residential and home healthcare personnel. Although many older OCD patients are otherwise physically and mentally healthy, some require regular contact with caregivers such as nursing home staff or home healthcare providers. To the extent that these individuals interact with and thus have the opportunity to influence the behavior of the OCD patient, it is important to involve them in treatment. Objectives of involving caregivers in treatment are largely the same as those of including family members. For practical and therapeutic reasons, it may be necessary for the therapist to consult with caregivers at the patient's residence, a practice that is admittedly not routine for many clinicians. However, the positive impact of involving key individuals in therapy is worth the extra effort of coordinating a home visit with that of the home healthcare professional. When the patient lives in a nursing home, it is helpful to meet with as many of the relevant staff as possible. The change of shift, usually occurring in the late afternoon, is often a good time to catch day and evening personnel together. Although it is beneficial to educate as many staff members as possible, it also helps to identify a primary individual to serve as liaison with the rest of the staff.

Addressing stressors and fears common in later life. Each developmental stage has its own unique challenges for obsessive-compulsive individuals (Francis and Borden 1993). Although there is little evidence of an OCD presentation unique to older adults, clinicians should be aware of stressors and fears common in later life that could influence the course of the disorder (Patterson 1988). Certain major life events, such as death of a spouse, onset or development of physical illness or disability, or relocation to a retirement or nursing home, are more likely to occur in later life. Such stressors can contribute to relapse in recovered individuals, and may also play a role in the development of late-life-onset OCD. Assisting patients to address life stressors can have a positive effect on OCD symptoms. At the very least, it is helpful for patients to understand the factors that exacerbate their condition.

Some fears are more common than others in later life. On the one hand, the elderly are often less worried than younger adults about social threats such as rejection or criticism (Wisocki 1994). However, infirmity, loss of mobility and independence, and becoming a burden to loved ones are common worries during this phase of life (Wisocki 1994). The elderly are also more prone to fears of falling. Typically, a fall may involve surgical intervention with all of the attendant concerns that hospitalization and recovery imply. The emergence of such fears can add to the patient's overall anxiety and can indirectly exacerbate OCD symptoms or interfere with treatment. Each case must be considered individually, but it is sometimes necessary to treat significant comorbid fears along with or before treating OCD symptoms.

Monitoring relapse. Cognitive decline can be confounded with the symptoms of relapse. The first evidence of memory problems associated with dementia, for example, might appear to be compulsive reassurance-seeking. Alternatively, OCD-related behaviors should not be dismissed as age-related when, in fact, they could be signaling impending relapse. The therapist working with an elderly patient must be sensitive to both sides of this complex issue. It is generally advisable to set up a regular schedule of maintenance visits after the patient has completed therapy. The patient, family members, and caregivers should also be informed of the principles of relapse prevention.

Conclusions

There is preliminary evidence that established pharmacological and behavioral treatments for OCD are beneficial for older adults with this disorder. Nonetheless, guidelines for the clinical management of OCD in elderly patients are still based in large part on research conducted in samples of younger adults. Practitioners providing care to older individuals with OCD are encouraged to be cognizant of clinical issues particularly relevant to this phase of adulthood. Diagnostic and treatment procedures may need to be modified to attend to the physical, psychological, and social complications that can emerge in later life. Further research is needed to fully establish the safety and efficacy of serotonergic medications, ERP, and other interventions used to treat late-life OCD. It will also be important to determine when and how to adapt these interventions to effectively address clinical challenges associated with treating OCD in the elderly.

References

American Psychiatric Association: Diagnostic and Statistical Manual of Mental Disorders, 4th Edition. Washington, DC, American Psychiatric Association, 1994

Austin LS, Zealberg JJ, Lydiard RB: Three cases of pharmacotherapy of obsessive-compulsive disorder in the elderly. J Nerv Ment Dis 179:634–635, 1991

Baer L, Minichiello WE: Behavior therapy for obsessive-compulsive disorder, in Obsessive-Compulsive Disorders: Theory and Management, 2nd Edition. Edited by Jenike MA, Baer L, Minichiello WE. Chicago, IL, Year Book Medical, 1990, pp 203–232

Bajulaiye R, Addonizio G: Obsessive-compulsive disorder arising in a 75-year-old woman. International Journal of Geriatric Psychiatry 7:139–142, 1993

Berman I, Kalinowski A, Berman SM, et al: Obsessive and compulsive symptoms in chronic schizophrenia. Compr Psychiatry 36:6–10, 1995

Bland RC, Newman SC, Orn H: Prevalence of psychiatric disorders in the elderly in Edmonton. Acta Psychiatric Scand Suppl 338:57–63, 1988

Blazer D, George LK, Hughes D: The epidemiology of anxiety disorders: an age comparison, in Anxiety in the Elderly: Treatment and Research. Edited by Salzman C, Lebowitz BD. New York, Springer, 1991, pp 17–30

Calamari JE, Faber SD, Hitsman BL, et al: Treatment of obsessive compulsive disorder in the elderly: a review and case example. Journal of Behavior Therapy and Experimental Psychiatry 25:95–104, 1994

Calvocoressi L, Lewis BL, Harris J, et al: Family accommodations in obsessive-compulsive disorder. Am J Psychiatry 152:441–443, 1995

Carmin CN, Pollard CA, Ownby RL: Effects of cognitive behavioral treatment of obsessive-compulsive disorder in geriatric vs. younger adult patients. Paper presented at the 29th annual convention of the Association for the Advancement of Behavior Therapy, Washington, DC, November 1995

Casey DA, Davis MH: Obsessive-compulsive disorder responsive to electroconvulsive therapy in an elderly woman. Southern Medical Journal 87:862–864, 1994

Copeland JRM, Dewey ME, Wood N, et al: Range of mental illness among the elderly in the community: prevalence in Liverpool using the GMS-AGECAT package. Br J Psychiatry 150:815–823, 1987a

Copeland JRM, Garland BJ, Dewey ME, et al: Is there more dementia, depression and neurosis in New York? a comparative study of the elderly in New York and London using the computer diagnosis AGECAT. Br J Psychiatry 151:466–473, 1987b

Dar R, Greist JH: Behavior therapy for obsessive compulsive disorder. Psychiatr Clin North Am 15:885–894, 1992

Dominguez RA, Mestre SM: Management of treatment-refractory obsessive compulsive disorder patients. J Clin Psychiatry 55 (suppl):86–92, 1994

Dominguez RA, Jacobson AF, Del Gandra J, et al: Drug response assessed by the Modified Maudsley Obsessive-Compulsive Inventory. Psychopharmacol Bull 25:215–218, 1989

Fallon BA, Liebowitz MR, Hollander E, et al: The pharmacotherapy of moral or religious scrupulosity. J Clin Psychiatry 51:517–521, 1990

Flint AJ: Epidemiology and comorbidity of anxiety disorders in the elderly. Am J Psychiatry 151:640–649, 1994

Foa EB, Steketee GS, Grayson JB, et al: Treatment of obsessive-compulsives: when do we fail? in Failures in Behavior Therapy. Edited by Emmelkamp PMG. New York, Wiley, 1983, pp 10–34

Francis G, Borden J: Expression and treatment of obsessive-compulsive disorder in childhood, adolescence, and adulthood, in Anxiety Across the Lifespan: A Developmental Perspective. Edited by Last C. New York, Springer, 1993, pp 148–166

German PS, Shapiro S, Skinner EA: Mental health of the elderly: use of health and mental health services. J Am Geriatr Soc 33:246–252, 1985

Goodman WK, Price L, Rasmussen S, et al: The Yale-Brown Obsessive Compulsive Scale, I: development, use, and reliability. Arch Gen Psychiatry 46:1006–1011, 1989a

Goodman, WK, Price L, Rasmussen S, et al: The Yale-Brown Obsessive Compulsive Scale, II: validity. Arch Gen Psychiatry 46:1012–1016, 1989b

Gordon A, Rasmussen SA: Mood-related obsessive compulsive symptoms in a patient with bipolar affective disorder. J Clin Psychiatry 49:27–28, 1988

Greist JM, Jefferson JW, Kobak KH, et al: Efficacy and tolerability of serotonin transport inhibitors in obsessive-compulsive disorder: a meta-analysis. Arch Gen Psychiatry 52:53–60, 1995

Gurian BS, Miner JH: Clinical presentation of anxiety in the elderly, in Anxiety in the Elderly: Treatment and Research. Edited by Salzman C, Lebowitz BD. New York, Springer, 1991, pp 31–44

Hersen M, Van Hasselt VB: Behavioral assessment and treatment of anxiety in the elderly. Clinical Psychology Review 12:619–640, 1992

Himmelfarb S, Murrell SA: The prevalence and correlation of anxiety symptoms in older adults. J Psychology 116:159–167, 1984

Jacobsen FM: Risperidone in the treatment of affective illness and obsessive-compulsive disorder. J Clin Psychiatry 56:423–429, 1995

Jenike MA: Geriatric obsessive compulsive disorder. Geriatric Psychiatry and Neurology 4:34–39, 1991

Jenike MA, Baer L, Ballentine HT, et al: Cingulotomy for refractory obsessive-compulsive disorder. Arch Gen Psychiatry 48:548–555, 1991

Jenike MA, Hyman S, Baer L, et al: A controlled trial of fluvoxamine in obsessive-compulsive disorder: implications for serotonergic theory. Am J Psychiatry 147:1209–1215, 1990

Junginger J, Ditto B: Multitreatment of obsessive-compulsive checking in a geriatric patient. Behavior Modification 8:379–390, 1984

Junginger J, Phelan E, Cherry K, et al: Prevalence of psychopathology in elderly persons in nursing homes and in the community. Hospital and Community Psychiatry 44:381–383, 1993

King P, Barrowclough C: A clinical pilot study of cognitive-behavioral therapy for anxiety disorders in the elderly. Behavioral Psychotherapy 19:337–345, 1991

Kolada JL, Bland RC, Newman SC: Obsessive-compulsive disorder. Acta Psychiatr Scand 376 (suppl):24–35, 1994

Lindesay J, Briggs K, Murphy E: The Guys/Age Concern Survey: prevalence rates of cognitive impairment, depression, and anxiety in an urban elderly community. Br J Psychiatry 155:317–329, 1989

Markovitz PJ: Treatment of anxiety in the elderly. J Clin Psychiatry 54 (suppl):64–68, 1993

McCarthy PR, Katz IR, Foa EB: Cognitive-behavioral treatment of anxiety in the elderly: a proposed model, in Anxiety in the Elderly: Treatment and Research. Edited by Salzman C, Lebowitz BD. New York, Springer, 1991, pp 197–214

McDougle CJ, Barr LC, Goodman WK, et al: Lack of efficacy of clozapine monotherapy in refractory obsessive-compulsive disorder. Am J Psychiatry 152:1812–1814, 1995

Myers JK, Weisman MM, Tischler GL, et al: Six-month prevalence of psychiatric disorders in three communities. Arch Gen Psychiatry 41:959–967, 1984

Patel B, Tandon R: Development of obsessive-compulsive symptoms during clozapine treatment (letter). Am J Psychiatry 150:836, 1993

Patil VJ: Development of transient obsessive-compulsive symptoms during treatment with clozapine (letter). Am J Psychiatry 149:272, 1992

Patterson RL: Anxiety in the elderly, in Handbook of Anxiety Disorders. Edited by Last CG, Hersen M. Elmsford, NY, Pergamon, 1988, pp 541–551

Piccinelli M, Pini S, Bellantuono C, et al: Efficacy of drug treatment in obsessive-compulsive disorder: a meta-analytic review. Br J Psychiatry 36:6–10, 1995

Regier DA, Boyd JH, Burke JD, et al: One-month prevalence of mental disorder in the United States. Arch Gen Psychiatry 45:977–986, 1988

Remington D, Adams M: Risperidone and obsessive compulsive symptoms. J Clin Psychopharmacol 14:358–359, 1994

Robins LN, Helzer JE, Weissman MM, et al: Lifetime prevalence of specific psychiatric disorders in three sites. Arch Gen Psychiatry 41:958–967, 1984

Rowan VC, Holburn W, Walker JR, et al: A rapid multi-component treatment for an obsessive-compulsive disorder. Journal of Behavior Therapy and Experimental Psychiatry 15:347–352, 1984

Shader RI, Kennedy JS, Greenblatt DJ: Treatment of anxiety in the elderly, in Psychopharmacology: The Third Generation of Progress. Edited by Meltzer HY. New York, Raven, 1987, pp 1141–1147

Sheikh JL, Salzman C: Anxiety in the elderly. Psychiatr Clin North Am 18:871–883, 1995

Simpson S, Baldwin B: Neuropsychiatry and SPECT of an acute obsessive-compulsive syndrome patient. Br J Psychiatry 166:390–392, 1995

Stanley MA, Turner SM: Current status of pharmacological and behavioral treatment of obsessive-compulsive disorder. Behavior Therapy 26:163–186, 1995

Stein DJ, Spadacini E, Hollander E: Meta-analysis of pharmacotherapy trials for obsessive-compulsive disorder. Int Clin Psychopharmacol 10:11–18, 1995

Steketee G, Foa EB: Obsessive-compulsive disorder, in Handbook of Clinical Disorders. Edited by Barlow DH. New York, Guilford, 1985, pp 69–144

Steketee G, Heninger N, Pollard CA: Predicting treatment outcome for OCD: effects of comorbidity, in Treatment-Refractory Obsessive-Compulsive Disorder. Edited by Goodman WK, Maser J, Rudorfer M. Mahwah, NJ, Lawrence Erlbaum (in press)

Stoudemire A, Moran MG: Psychopharmacologic treatment of anxiety in the medically ill elderly patient: special considerations. J Clin Psychiatry 54 (suppl):27–33, 1993

Turner SM, Hersen M, Bellack AS, et al: Behavioral treatment of obsessive compulsive neurosis. Behaviour Research and Therapy 17:95–106, 1979

Wisocki PA: The experience of worry among the elderly, in Worrying: Perspectives on Theory, Assessment and Treatment. Edited by Davey GCL, Tallis F. New York, Wiley, 1994, pp 247–261

Wolpe J: The Practice of Behavior Therapy, 2nd Edition. New York, Pergamon, 1973

Chapter 14

Course of Illness in Obsessive-Compulsive Disorder

Jane Eisen, M.D., and Gail Steketee, Ph.D.

Until the mid-1980s, obsessive-compulsive disorder (OCD) was thought to be a rare psychiatric illness. With the use of more sophisticated epidemiological techniques to determine prevalence, OCD is now considered to be a common psychiatric disorder with a lifetime prevalence of 2.5% (Karno et al. 1988). Demographic, epidemiologic, and clinical features of OCD have been well characterized (Rasmussen and Eisen 1992). However, little is known about the course of the disorder over time in terms of patterns of remission and relapse or about factors that may affect illness course, such as age at onset, severity of illness, treatment, comorbidity with Axis I and/or II disorders, and symptom subtypes.

DSM-IV (American Psychiatric Association 1994) describes the course of OCD as typically chronic with some fluctuation in the severity of symptoms over time. Although terminology and definitions vary from study to study, overall, this chronic fluctuating course appears to be supported both retrospectively before treatment and in follow-up after treatment. Early phenomenological and follow-up studies of OCD suffered from a number of methodological limitations, including retrospective study design; small sample sizes; lack of standardized criteria for determining diagnosis; use of hospital-based samples not representative of the spectrum of the disorder found in the population as a whole; biases in inclusion and exclusion criteria; use of chart review rather than personal interview, absence of structured interviews, and lack of consensus on the definition of relapse, remission, and recovery. Because of these flaws in study design, the earlier studies of OCD may have included subjects who would not meet today's criteria. In particular, clear distinctions between OCD and obsessive-compulsive personality disorder (OCPD) were often not made, and obsessions and compulsions occurring in the context of other disorders (e.g., major depression, psychosis, eating disorders) may have been included as OCD.

More recent studies using a prospective design and standardized criteria have also shown that episodicity in this disorder (with clear periods of complete remission off medication) is uncommon. Once established, obsessions and compulsions usually persist, although the content, intensity, and frequency of these symptoms change over time.

In this chapter we review early and more recent findings regarding the course of OCD and then turn our attention to predictors of course. Because data on course inevitably overlap with treatment outcome findings, we also review factors that predict medication and behavioral treatment outcome.

Retrospective Follow-Up Studies

In retrospective studies, fluctuations in the severity of psychiatric symptoms and their impact on functioning over time are ascertained based on subjects' recall. Several investigators have identified patterns of course of illness in OCD as falling into the following categories: complete remission of obsessions and compulsions, symptoms much improved, minimal improvement with poor functioning, and symptoms unchanged or worsening. In these studies, it is often unclear whether patients described as "much improved" would nevertheless still meet criteria for the disorder. Another approach has been to determine the episodicity of a patient's OCD—that is, whether the OCD is characterized by distinct periods of illness and remission, similar to major depressive disorder. Such follow-up studies are compared in Table 14–1, although readers should bear in mind that different measures were used to assign patients into categories of course of illness. For the sake of comparison in Table 14–1, subjects considered to be mildly improved but with poor functioning were combined with subjects whose symptoms were classified as minimally improved, unchanged, or worse.

In the majority of studies described in this section, patients were selected based on chart review and were subsequently assessed at the time of the study either in person or through questionnaires. In the earliest longitudinal study of OCD, a relatively good outcome was observed by Lewis (1936), who followed 50 OCD patients (most of whom received some psychotherapy) at least 5 years after initial assessment. Among this group, 32% were symptom-free, 14% were "much improved," and 44% were minimally improved, unchanged, or worse. Only 10% had followed an episodic course marked by later recurrence after remission. When Pollitt (1957) followed 67 nonleucotomized individuals for a mean of 3.4 years, 24% were symptom-free (similar to the results with psychotherapy), 36% had mild symptoms and were functioning well, and 12% were improved but had impaired functioning. Only 25% reported no change or more severe symptoms than at baseline. This study was somewhat unusual because the majority of patients were selected from an outpatient practice. This selection may explain the better outcome in this study in comparison with other studies that assessed only inpatients. Longer duration of illness at initial evaluation was associated with poorer outcome with respect to severity of symp-

Table 14–1. Retrospective follow-up studies of obsessive-compulsive disorder (OCD)

Author	N	Mean follow-up (years)	Well (%)	Much improved (%)	Minimally improved, unchanged, or worse (%)	Comments
Lewis (1936)	50	>5	32	14	44	10% episodic course
Pollitt (1957)	67[a]	3.4	24	36	37	Mostly outpatients
Ingram (1961)	29	5.9	7	21[b]	72	Inpatients
Kringlen (1965)	80	13–20	0	24	76	Inpatients
Grimshaw (1965)	100	5	40	24	35	Inpatients
Lo (1967)	88	3.9	23	50	27	In- and outpatients, diagnostic heterogeneity
Coryell (1981)	44	0.5+	8	20	8	Inpatients
Thomsen (1995)	47	6–22	28	47[c]	25	Childhood OCD

[a] nonleucotomized. [b] 1 patient nonleucotomized; 5 patients leucotomized. [c] 26% had subclinical OCD at follow-up, and 21% had episodic course with partial or complete remission between episodes.

toms at follow-up, as might be expected. Duration of illness was also a predictor of course of illness in a study of 29 inpatients with obsessional symptoms whom Ingram (1961) followed for 6 years. In this study, only 21% of the patients were much improved; 72% were minimally improved but functioning poorly, unchanged, or worse. Seven of the 8 patients with much improvement or complete remission of symptoms received leucotomies.

In a study characterized by a long follow-up period, Kringlen (1965) found that at 13–20 years after initial contact, only 24% of the subjects were much improved, whereas 34% described slight improvement in obsessive-compulsive (OC) symptoms, and the largest group, 42%, were unimproved or worse. The patients included in this study were all hospitalized for the first time and may have had severe symptoms, thus contributing to poorer outcome in this study. Somewhat better results were reported in another retrospective follow-up study of inpatients: Grimshaw (1965) assessed 100 inpatients an average of 5 years after discharge. 40% were recovered or only slightly symptomatic, 24% had improved moderately, and 35% remained unchanged or had worsened. Improvements were not associated with any particular treatment.

Lo (1967), in a study conducted in China, also had more optimistic results. He followed 88 patients diagnosed with OCD for a mean of 3.9 years and found 23% symptom-free and 50% with symptoms much improved. This study also followed both in- and outpatients. Patients followed for more than 4 years after initially presenting for treatment were more often found symptom-free (14 of 52, 40%) than were those followed for shorter intervals (4 of 35, 8%). There was clearly some diagnostic heterogeneity in this cohort of patients. More than half the patients had distinct obsessions and compulsions. However, 10% had prominent affective symptoms, and 31% were described as having "phobic and ruminative symptoms" with minimal compulsions. It appears, then, that some of the patients who were in remission at follow-up may have had major depression with obsessional or ruminative thinking during their index episode.

The subsequent occurrence of other psychiatric disorders following onset of OCD has been evaluated. Several investigators have found a relatively high rate of development of schizophrenia, ranging from 6% to 8% (Ingram 1961; Kringlen 1965). By contrast, schizophrenia was seen less frequently in several other studies (Lo 1967; Pollitt 1957; Rosenberg 1968). Lack of standardized diagnostic criteria, leading to the inclusion of depression with psychotic features as schizophrenia, may have contributed to the range of schizophrenia found in these earlier studies. Another factor involved may have been patients' degree of insight regarding their obsessions and compulsions. Patients described as having periods of losing insight into the irrationality of their obsessions and as losing resistance were characterized as being "doubtfully schizophrenic" in several studies. The inclusion of these patients may also have led to a higher frequency of schizophrenia in follow-up studies.

In reviewing these follow-up studies, Goodwin et al. (1969) concluded that the course of OCD is usually chronic but variable, with fluctuations in severity of symptoms. He described depression as being the most common psychiatric disorder to develop after the onset of OCD, and noted that subsequent development of schizophrenia is rare if that disorder is adequately excluded at baseline. In follow-up studies conducted since 1980, criteria used to evaluate course of illness have been different from those used in the earlier studies described previously. Patients have been retrospectively assigned to categories such as "continuous," "waxing and waning," "deteriorative," and "episodic with full remissions between episodes." Rasmussen and Tsuang (1986) conducted a study in which patients were selected based on current enrollment in an outpatient OCD clinic. OCD course among the 44 patients in the study was described as chronic or "continuous" for the vast majority (84%), deteriorating for a few (14%), and episodic for only 1 (2%). The average duration of illness at time of assessment was more than 15 years, again suggesting the chronicity of this disorder. Because these subjects were selected through the process of clinic referral and prospective follow-up was not conducted, no former OCD patients who had already recovered and remained well were included. Patients who developed other major psychiatric disorders such as schizophrenia were also unlikely to be represented in this cohort of clinic patients. In a more recent study of 53 OCD outpatients, Gojer and associates (1987) found a primarily deteriorating course in a surprising 66%, with only 11% remaining the same, 17% fluctuating, 2% improving, and 4% not identifiable.

Two studies have compared control groups with an OCD cohort. Coryell (1981) compared course of illness following hospitalization in 44 patients with OCD versus inpatients with major depression. He observed that although 56% of the patients with OCD demonstrated some improvement at follow-up, this cohort was significantly less likely to experience remission after discharge (22%) than was the comparison cohort of depressed patients (64%). However, suicide occurred significantly less frequently in the cohort of patients with OCD compared with patients with depression.

In a cross-sectional follow-up study, Thomsen (1995) interviewed 47 patients with OCD 6–22 years after they had been treated for OCD as children and compared their characteristics with those of a group of non-OCD psychiatric control subjects. All subjects were at least 18 years old at the time of the follow-up interview. The majority of subjects had either no OCD symptoms (28%) or only subclinical OC symptoms (26%)

at follow-up. Ten subjects (21%) had a chronic course of OCD. This study also assessed outcome by using the Global Assessment Scale (GAS; Endicott et al. 1976). Although findings were not statistically significant, males with childhood-onset OCD appeared to have a poorer outcome than females: 9 of the 10 subjects with GAS scores below 50 at follow-up were males.

More recently, studies have used the Yale-Brown Obsessive Compulsive Scale (Y-BOCS; Goodman et al. 1989)—a scale designed to measure the severity of OC symptoms—to assign patients into groups by percentage of improvement. A recent follow-up study conducted in Austria used structured interviews to assess 62 inpatients who met *International Classification of Diseases,* Ninth Revision (ICD-9; World Health Organization 1977) criteria for OCD (Demal et al. 1993) (see Table 14–2). This study's findings were consistent with those of earlier studies: episodic course with complete remission (11%), episodic with partial remission (24%), deteriorative (10%), continuous and unchanging (27%), and continuous with improvement (24%). The authors found that 29% of the patients had Y-BOCS scores in the normal range, 21% had scores in the "subclinical" range (8–15), and 50% had scores in the clinical range (16–40).

Synthesizing methodologically varied studies, some of which present an optimistic picture and others a pessimistic one, may require more careful examination of reported outcomes. It may be important to separate the best possible outcomes ("full remission" or "symptom free") from those described as "much improved" or "improved," which may indicate persistent symptoms in the abatement phase of a chronic waxing and waning illness. The episodic pattern of full remission (and sometimes later recurrence) appears to occur in about 10%–15% of OCD patients, although this proportion may increase somewhat as follow-up is extended for several years and may also be greater in childhood OCD (Apter and Tyano 1988), in which improvement can be rapid even without treatment (Berman 1942). In most studies, with the notable exception of Gojer et al. (1987), a smaller proportion of OCD patients (6%–14%) seem to follow a deteriorating course. The majority presumably have a course marked by chronicity, with some symptom fluctuation over time but without clear-cut remissions or deterioration.

Several studies in both adults and children with OCD have observed that patients typically have multiple obsessions and compulsions at any given time and that the content of their concerns changes over time (Hanna 1995; Rasmussen and Eisen 1992; Rettew et al. 1992; Swedo et al. 1989). In their study of childhood OCD, Rettew et al. (1992) reported that 85% of their subjects had experienced some change in symptom patterns over time, and usually had more than one type of obsession and compulsion concurrently. Content of obsessions did not seem to be related to developmental stage. In subjects with very early-onset

Table 14–2. Obsessive-compulsive disorder follow-up studies using the Yale-Brown Obsessive Compulsive Scale (Y-BOCS) as the outcome measure

Author	N	Normal range Y-BOCS 0–7 (%)	Subclinical range Y-BOCS 8–15 (%)	Clinical range Y-BOCS 16–40 (%)	Methodology
Demal et al. 1993	62	29.1	20.9	50	Cross-sectional
Orloff et al. 1994	85				Percentage improvement did not allow estimates
Eisen et al. 1995b	65	16.9	35.4	47.7	Prospective

illness (before age 6), symptoms often started with a solitary ritual without associated obsessive thoughts. New symptoms arose that would sometimes become predominant over earlier ones. The factors involved in changes in focus of OC symptoms over time have yet to be delineated. Thus far, symptom subtype has not been found to be a predictor of either illness course or treatment response (see "Predictors of Course," later in this chapter).

Prospective Studies

Over the past decade, several studies of course of illness in childhood-onset OCD have used a prospective design. In one of these studies, all students in a high school were screened for the presence of obsessions and/or compulsions (Flament et al. 1988). Fifty-nine adolescents out of 5,596 high school students screened (1%) were identified as having OCD, subclinical OCD, other psychiatric disorders with OC symptoms, or OCPD. This subgroup was subsequently reinterviewed 2 years after the initial interview by raters blind to the baseline diagnosis (Berg et al. 1989). Of the 12 subjects initially diagnosed with OCD, only 5 still met full criteria for the disorder; 2 had developed OCPD and 3 had other disorders with some obsessional features. The 1 subject who was diagnosed with OCD at baseline but with subclinical OCD at the 2-year interview can be considered analogous to subjects described in other studies as much improved or in partial remission (see Table 14–3). Only 1 subject originally diagnosed with OCD had no diagnosis after 2 years. Of interest is the development of psychiatric symptoms in the 15 students who had subclinical OCD at baseline: at follow-up, 4 met full criteria for OCD, 4 continued to have subclinical OCD, 4 developed other psychiatric disorders with OC features, 1 had OCPD, and only 1 subject had no diagnosis.

Another study prospectively assessed 25 children with OCD 2–7 years after initial evaluation (Flament et al. 1990). Although the majority of subjects (68%) still met criteria for OCD at follow-up, 28% were considered completely well, with no obsessions or compulsions. More than half of the subjects had a lifetime history of major depression, and 44% had another anxiety disorder in addition to OCD, such as social phobia or separation anxiety. Five patients had OCPD, and two patients developed psychotic symptoms (diagnosed as atypical psychosis or schizophreniform disorder).

Over the past few years, several longitudinal naturalistic studies have also been conducted in which adults with OCD were followed prospectively. In one such study, data were collected on course of illness in 68 subjects over a 2-year period (Eisen et al. 1995a). Two instruments were used to evaluate severity of symptoms: the Y-BOCS and the Psy-

Table 14–3. Prospective follow-up studies of obsessive-compulsive disorder (OCD)

Author	Treatments	N	Mean follow-up (years)	Remained in episode (%)	Partial remission (%)	Full remission (%)	Comments
Children and adolescents							
Berg et al. 1989		12	2	42	17[a]	8	17% had compulsive personality or traits
Leonard et al. 1993	SSRIs, BT, psychotherapy, family therapy	54	3.4	43	46	11[b]	70% on medication at follow-up
Adults							
Orloff et al. 1994[c]	SSRIs, BT	85	2.1			33	
Eisen et al. 1995b	SSRIs, BT	51	2	57	31	12	
G. Steketee, J. Eisen, I. Dyck, M. Warshaw, S. Rasmussen, "Predictors of Course of OCD" (submitted for publication)	SSRIs, BT	107	0.5–5	47	31	22	Mainly outpatients

Note. BT = behavior therapy; SSRIs = selective serotonin reuptake inhibitors; Y-BOCS = Yale-Brown Obsessive Compulsive Scale.
[a] Subjects had subclinical OCD at follow-up (i.e., obsessions/compulsions present but not at full criteria). [b] Three of the six subjects in remission (i.e., symptom free) were receiving medication. [c] Course assessed by percentage change in Y-BOCS score only.

chiatric Rating Scale (PSR; Keller et al. 1987) for OCD. The PSR rates symptom severity on a 6-point scale ranging from a high of 6 (severely symptomatic and unable to function at work and socially) to a low of 0 (no OC symptoms or avoidance). Follow-up measures were obtained at 3 months, 6 months, 1 year, and 2 years after baseline assessment.

Course of illness was assessed both descriptively and with survival analysis to determine probability of remission and relapse. Of the 51 subjects who started the study meeting full criteria for OCD (Y-BOCS score greater than 16), 57% still met full criteria after 2 years. Although some of these subjects had considerable improvement in the severity of their OC symptoms, they nonetheless continued to experience significant impairment because of obsessions and/or compulsions. Twelve percent had minimal or no symptoms (Y-BOCS scores below 8). The remainder of the subjects (31%) had obsessions and compulsions that persisted but did not meet full criteria, and thus might be classified as being in partial remission or much improved.

Statistical analysis with survival analysis revealed a 47% probability of achieving at least partial remission during the 2-year study period. However, if more stringent criteria were used to define remission, in which patients must have had only occasional or no obsessions and compulsions for 8 consecutive weeks (Y-BOCS score below 8), there was only a 12% probability of achieving remission. Once in remission, the probability of subsequent relapse (returning to a Y-BOCS score greater than 16) was 48%. Of the 22 patients who achieved partial remission, 10 patients relapsed and 12 patients remained in partial remission throughout the study.

Another prospective study examined 107 clinic patients with OCD followed up to 5 years after intake (G. Steketee, J. Eisen, I. Dyck, M. Warshaw, and S. Rasmussen, "Predictors of Course of OCD" [submitted for publication]). The probability of full remission for at least a 2-month period was .22 at 5 years, with a probability of .53 for partial remission. Interestingly, the likelihood of improvement increased substantially with time, doubling from the 6-month point (.27) to the 5-year point (.53). Although outcome in this study was assessed with only a 3-point rating scale, the study findings are very similar to those reported by Eisen and colleagues (1995b), who, as previously noted, used the PSR and the Y-BOCS.

These findings are in keeping with those of most of the retrospective and prospective studies of OCD, which demonstrate that the majority of people who meet full criteria for this disorder continue to suffer from obsessions and compulsions, although they may experience considerable improvement in both the intensity of their symptoms and the corresponding degree of impairment. Those fortunate subjects who experience complete remission of their OC symptoms are very much in the minority.

Effect of Treatment on Course of Illness

A follow-up study of children with OCD was conducted by Leonard et al. (1993) to determine outcome after standardized short-term treatment with clomipramine (a medication known to be effective in OCD). Fifty-four children and adolescents were reinterviewed 2–7 years after participation in a controlled trial of clomipramine and a variety of interim interventions. At follow-up the majority of patients were only mildly symptomatic, and OC symptoms were more severe in only 10 subjects at reassessment, so that, as a whole, the cohort had improved. However, only 3 subjects (6%) were considered to be in true remission (defined as experiencing no obsessions or compulsions and receiving no medication), whereas 23 subjects (43%) still met full criteria for OCD (see Table 14–2). In addition, the majority of patients were taking medication at follow-up, which suggests that maintenance of improvement in OCD may require ongoing pharmacological intervention.

In a 1994 study conducted by Orloff et al., findings were more optimistic than those in the studies described above. Of 85 subjects assessed 1–3 years after baseline evaluation, 64% had a greater than 50% decrease in Y-BOCS score and 33% had a greater than 75% decrease in Y-BOCS score. The mean follow-up Y-BOCS score (10.1 ± 7.0) showed mild to minimal obsessions and compulsions that did not interfere with functioning. This improvement in OC symptoms may be the result of the availability of current, effective behavioral and pharmacological treatments for OCD that use exposure and response prevention techniques· and selective serotonin reuptake inhibitors (SSRIs). In fact, nearly all subjects had received at least a 10-week trial of an SSRI, and almost half had received some behavior therapy (BT) (although only 16% had received at least 20 hours of BT). Of note are the findings that most patients were still taking medication at follow-up and that there were clear relapses in those patients who had discontinued their medication. Again, maintenance of improvement of OC symptoms over time appeared to require continued treatment.

The effect of treatment on course of illness in OCD was also evaluated in the previously described prospective 2-year follow-up of 68 subjects conducted by Eisen et al. (1995b). Among this group, a large percentage had received at least 12 weeks of a serotonergic medication: 49% received clomipramine, 29%, fluvoxamine, and 15%, fluoxetine, and some had received more than one SSRI. Patients took medication for 70 weeks on average. Thus, 84% of the total sample received an adequate trial of at least one SSRI during the study period. Patients were considered to have received adequate BT if their therapist had used exposure and response prevention and they had spent at least 20 hours practicing homework assignments. According to this definition, only 18% of patients had received adequate BT.

The mean GAS and Y-BOCS scores at intake and at 2 years were similar for subjects who had and who had not received adequate trials of an SSRI. However, patients who subsequently received adequate BT over the course of the study had worse initial functioning than those without BT, and they had improved more at 2 years. In effect, these patients "caught up" and functioned as well as those who did not have BT at the end of the trial.

If Orloff et al.'s (1994) method is used to assess outcome, the results of this study are not as optimistic about the course of illness in OCD. Only 9% of the subjects had more than a 75% decrease in Y-BOCS scores over the 2 years, whereas 26% reported 50%–75% improvement, 23% had 25%–49% improvement, and 35% improved less than 25%. For 7%, OC symptoms worsened. However, the results again support the findings of most previous studies that even with adequate pharmacotherapy, course of illness in OCD is usually continuous, with fluctuations in severity. Few people (only about 10%–12%) achieve true remission of symptoms.

Predictors of Course

Demographic and Clinical Features

Other retrospective studies found that improvement in OCD course was associated with shorter duration of illness (Goodwin et al. 1969; Ingram 1961; Kringlen 1965; Pollitt 1957). Findings concerning whether age at onset (or presence/absence of childhood symptoms) was predictive of subsequent course were inconsistent, as were findings regarding the predictive value of marital status or of obsessional premorbid personality. However, a recent study of a large clinical sample indicated that those who were married and who had better general functioning were more likely to show symptom improvement up to 5 years later (G. Steketee, J. Eisen, I. Dyck, M. Warshaw, and S. Rasmussen, "Predictors of Course of OCD" [submitted for publication]). Type of symptoms consistently did not appear to influence course across studies (Ingram 1961; Kringlen 1965; Pollitt 1957). Summarizing these studies, Goodwin et al. (1969) concluded that short duration of symptoms prior to treatment and good premorbid personality were both associated with better prognosis. The content of obsessions did not influence outcome.

More recent studies have identified a number of factors that may influence outcome or course of illness in OCD. In one follow-up study of childhood-onset OCD, the presence of signs of puberty in males at the time of referral indicated a better prognosis (Thomsen 1995). Several studies consistently found that severity of symptoms at baseline, family history of affective or anxiety disorders, and baseline demographic variables (gender, age at onset, duration of illness at baseline, age at initial assessment) did not predict severity of OCD at follow-up (Flament et al. 1990; Leonard et al. 1993). Inconsistent results have been reported regarding the predictive value of initial good response to clomipramine and presence of neurological symptoms: Flament et al. (1990) found no effect from these factors, whereas Leonard et al. (1993) found that severity of OC symptoms after 5 weeks of clomipramine treatment was a strong predictor both of severity of OCD and of functioning at follow-up. (Similar findings have been reported for behavioral treatment of adults [e.g., Foa et al. 1983; Steketee 1993].) Interestingly, the presence of a tic disorder predicted more severe OC symptoms at follow-up in children.

In the recent studies of factors influencing course of illness in adults with OCD, some findings are consistent with those of studies of OCD in children discussed above. Several studies found that the following variables did not affect outcome: severity of depression at baseline, age at onset, duration of follow-up, presence of a personality disorder, total number of personality disorders diagnosed, adequacy of pharmacotherapy or behavioral therapy, and presence of a current affective or anxiety disorder (Eisen et al. 1995b; Orloff et al. 1994; G. Steketee, J. Eisen, I. Dyck, M. Warshaw, and S. Rasmussen, "Predictors of Course of OCD" [submitted for publication]). Eisen et al. (1995b) found a trend for subjects whose OC symptoms were improved at 3 months (25% decrease in Y-BOCS score) to be significantly more likely to achieve remission 2 years later. In that study, probability of remission was not different for OCD patients with or without comorbid tic disorders, perhaps because of the small number of patients with OCD plus tics.

Insight is another clinical feature that has been assessed as a potential predictor of course of illness in OCD. An awareness of the senselessness or unreasonableness of obsessions (often referred to as "insight") and the accompanying struggle against the obsessions (referred to as "resistance") have been generally accepted as fundamental to the diagnosis of OCD. However, numerous descriptions of OCD patients who are completely convinced of the reasonableness of their obsessions and who need to enact compulsions have appeared in the psychiatric literature during the past century. In 1986, Insel and Akiskal described several such patients and presented the hypothesis that patients with OCD have varying degrees of insight and resistance, with "obsessive-compulsive psychosis" at one extreme of a hypothesized continuum. They also noted a fluidity between "neurotic" (i.e., associated with insight) and psychotic states in these patients.

To reflect these clinical observations and research findings, which have established that a range of insight exists in OCD (Foa and Kozak 1995; Kozak and Foa 1994; Lelliott et al. 1988), DSM-IV designated a new OCD specifier—"with poor insight," applying to individuals who generally fail to recognize their obsessions and compulsions as excessive or irrational. Eisen and Rasmussen (1993) retrospectively assessed course of illness in four categories of patients: those with OCD and schizophrenia (*n* = 18), OCD and schizotypal personality disorder (*n* = 14), OCD with poor insight (*n* = 27), and OCD without psychotic features (*n* = 408). High percentages of both the schizophrenia (82%) and the schizotypal (69%) groups had a deteriorative course. In contrast, very few of the OCD patients with poor insight (17%) and without psychotic features (8%) had a worsening course. Although these results need to be replicated with more rigorous methodology, the findings suggest that lack of insight does not significantly affect course of illness.

Axis I and II Comorbidity

The presence of other concurrent anxiety disorders has been examined in only one prospective study of course in clinic patients (G. Steketee, J. Eisen, I. Dyck, M. Warshaw, and S. Rasmussen, "Predictors of Course of OCD" [submitted for publication]). Surprisingly, having another anxiety disorder was actually protective; those with more comorbid anxiety disorders were more likely to improve. Perhaps the presence of other anxiety disorders, which may have been predominant over OCD symptoms in these patients, signaled a general vulnerability to anxiety that could change focus to other content, reducing obsessive and compulsive complaints.

Welner et al. (1976) compared the clinical pictures via chart review before, during, and after hospitalization of 150 patients with OCD. Their sample was divided into five subgroups: 1) OCD only (20%), 2) OCD followed by depression (developing an average of 14 years later) (38%), 3) concurrent onset of OCD and depression (13%), 4) primary depression with subsequent development of OCD (11%), and 5) OCD associated with other disorders. Clearly, depressive symptoms developing long after OCD onset was the predominant pattern. Patients with this history had an earlier age at OCD onset, a longer duration of illness, and less frequent and shorter remissions than patients in other groups. Patients with OCD only also had an earlier onset of OCD than did those in the concurrent depression onset group. The "primacy" of OCD over depression thus seemed associated with earlier onset and greater chronicity, a finding in agreement with the results of several other studies (see also Coryell 1981; Gittleson 1966b; Lion 1942; Stengel 1991). In contrast, the "primacy" of depression over OCD, which might include concurrent onset of both, was associated with a more episodic course, as one might predict given the seemingly different course characteristics of depression.

The co-occurrence of OCD with bipolar disorder is much less common than that with unipolar depression, no doubt in part because bipolar disorder is less common in general than unipolar depression. However, clinical reports (Keck et al. 1986; Gordon and Rasmussen 1988) have suggested that when bipolar disorder and OCD coexist, the OC symptoms may become exacerbated during depression but resolve completely during mania. This circumstance may contribute to some of the disparate results described below on the prognostic implications of OCD in the context of psychotic disorders, including alleged schizophrenia.

Several investigators have examined the prognostic implications of psychotic features in OCD. For schizophrenic individuals with OCD, both Stengel (1991) and Rosen (1957) determined that preexisting OCD symptoms predicted a more benign course for the schizophrenia. Interestingly, in the latter study, in no case did onset of schizophrenia precede onset of OCD, and in most cases OC symptoms persisted unchanged after onset of schizophrenia. However, the marked depressive symptoms present in most of the patients may have accounted for the better prognoses, given that such symptoms typically remit with time. In contradiction to these reports, Fenton and McGlashan (1986) found that the presence of OCD contributed to worse outcome in schizophrenic inpatients who were followed retrospectively 16 years after intake. Otherwise, the combined group resembled other schizophrenic patients at admission except for earlier onset of illness, an obvious contributor to chronicity. The authors were able to determine that OC symptoms came first in 13 of the 21 cases; in other cases, no determination regarding onset could be made. Thus, whether earlier onset of OC symptoms predicted a worse course is unclear. Given that diagnostic precision in this study is undoubtedly better than that in the earlier reports, these findings may be more accurate.

A few investigators have attempted to relate various personality traits to course of illness. Inconsistent results have been reported concerning the presence of compulsive personality traits: both positive and negative effects have been described. Kendell and Discipio (1970) characterized 45% of their 60 depressed inpatients as having premorbid "obsessional traits." These obsessional depressive patients did not show as much reduction in OC symptom scores after recovery from depression as did other depressed patients. On the other hand, Lo (1967) reported that premorbid obsessional personality predicted more favorable outcome of OCD at 4-year follow-up. This positive influence has also been reported in the behavioral treatment literature (Boulougouris 1977).

More consistent results have been found concerning schizotypal personality disorder. Its presence predicted a less favorable course of OCD in several studies (Orloff et al. 1994; Eisen and Rasmussen 1993) as well as a poorer treatment response.

Predictors of Behavioral and Pharmacological Treatment Outcome

Findings regarding variables that affect the long-term outcome of treatment, both behavioral and pharmacological, may have some bearing on the course of illness for this disorder.

Demographic and Clinical Features

Relatively few demographic variables have been found to influence treatment outcome. Current age did not predict the outcome of behavioral (e.g., Hoogduin and Duivenvoorden 1988; O'Sullivan et al. 1991; Rabavilas et al. 1976) or pharmacological treatment (e.g., Ackerman et al. 1994). In contrast to studies of course and findings for drug treatment trials (e.g., Ackerman et al. 1994; Ravizza et al. 1995), OCD patients with earlier symptom onset maintained their gains better after behavioral treatment than did those with later symptom onset (Emmelkamp et al. 1985; Foa et al. 1983). Gender did not affect OCD symptoms over time for behavioral or medication treatment (Ackerman et al. 1994; Boulougouris 1977; Drummond 1993; Hoogduin and Duivenvoorden 1988; O'Sullivan et al. 1991; Ravizza et al. 1995), although Basoglu et al. (1988) observed that women with washing rituals fared better than men with such rituals at follow-up. Unfortunately, gender in that study was confounded with symptom type and appeared to influence depressed mood more than OCD symptoms. Marital status was not related to pharmacological or behavioral treatment outcome (Foa et al. 1983; Hoogduin and Duivenvoorden 1988; Ravizza et al. 1995), nor were education level (Hoogduin and Duivenvoorden 1988) or whether patients lived alone or with others (Foa et al. 1983). Greater work satisfaction was related to more enduring gains (Mawson et al. 1982), but it is likely that this variable reflects better overall functioning. Not surprisingly, lower income was associated with poorer outcome (Steketee 1993; Steketee et al. 1985).

As in studies of course of OCD, symptom severity was not predictive of long-term outcome in most behavioral and drug studies (Ackerman et al. 1994; Basoglu et al. 1988; Foa et al. 1983; Hoogduin and Duivenvoorden 1988; Marks et al. 1980; O'Sullivan et al. 1991), indicating that severity alone does not necessarily signal a poor prognosis. However, it does seem likely that more severe symptoms will also be associated with more functional impairment—and perhaps with more comorbid conditions—and that this combination of factors will adversely affect treatment outcome. This hypothesis remains to be tested, although one study of response to SSRI medication showed that episodic course and no previous hospitalizations, which might be expected to signal better functioning and less severity, did indeed predict a good outcome

(Ravizza et al. 1995). However, in the only study we could locate that actually examined level of functioning in OCD, pretreatment functioning did not predict follow-up BT outcome (Steketee 1993). Surprisingly, the duration of symptoms was also not predictive in any study (Cottraux et al. 1993; Foa et al. 1983; Hoogduin and Duivenvoorden 1988; O'Sullivan et al. 1991), although again it is possible that chronicity accompanied by comorbidity may worsen prognosis. As was the case for studies of course, type of ritual (washing versus checking) was unrelated to outcome in most behavioral studies (Foa et al. 1983; Rachman et al. 1973) and medication trials (e.g., Ackerman et al. 1994). This factor had erratic predictive value in other behavioral studies (Basoglu et al. 1988; Drummond 1993), thus arguing against any consistent relationship of symptom type to outcome.

Mood State and Comorbid Conditions

Researchers have disagreed strongly over the role of depression in OCD. In some behavioral studies, patients who were more depressed before therapy had improved less at follow-up (Foa et al. 1983; Keijers et al. 1994) and were taking more medications 6 years later (Jenike 1990; O'Sullivan et al. 1991). Furthermore, better outcome was observed in depressed OCD patients who received medication (Cottraux et al. 1993; Marks et al. 1980). On the other hand, depression failed to predict outcome in many other behavioral studies (see Steketee and Shapiro 1995 for a review) as well as in pharmacological trials (e.g., Ravizza et al. 1995). Likewise, in a prospective study, Foa and colleagues (1992) found that neither baseline depression level nor implementation of effective antidepressant intervention predicted outcome at follow-up.

Interestingly, one study examined the predictive value of OCD patients' histories of mood fluctuations prior to treatment (Rabavilas and Boulougouris 1979). The absence of mood changes was associated with more improvement at follow-up, whereas the presence of mood fluctuations predicted relapse over time. In studies of the influence of diagnosed major depressive disorders on OCD outcome, no relationship was observed in outcome after BT (Steketee et al. 1995) or SSRI medication (e.g., Goodman et al. 1989; Pigott et al. 1991). Unfortunately, this body of research leaves considerable uncertainty regarding the importance of depressed mood in patients with OCD. Whether antidepressant medication should be used in such patients to manage the depression is far from clear, but such use might be advisable in severe cases.

Findings for pretreatment levels of anxious mood in OCD are somewhat consistent, although not entirely so. No significant association was observed in the majority of behavioral and medication studies of follow-up outcome (e.g., Emmelkamp et al. 1985; Orloff et al. 1994;

O'Sullivan et al. 1991; Ravizza et al. 1995; Steketee 1988). In contrast, both Foa et al. (1983) and Visser et al. (1992) found that greater initial anxiety predicted worse BT outcome. However, the path of this association was not direct in Foa's study, and the variance accounted for was quite small in the Visser et al. study. The effects of comorbid generalized anxiety disorder (GAD) on OCD outcome at 6-month follow-up were more negative. Steketee et al. (1995) noted that all four of their patients with this condition failed to benefit from BT. It seems, then, that whereas general anxious mood is unlikely to pose a problem, concurrent GAD may do so. Other anxiety comorbidity such as panic disorder has not been studied, but clinical experience suggests that concurrent treatment for panic symptoms that appear in response to obsessive focus will be needed, particularly during exposure treatment.

The presence of any personality disorder did not predict outcome for OCD patients after BT (Steketee 1991; Steketee et al. 1995) or SSRI medication (Orloff et al. 1994). However, Aubuchon and Malatesta (1994) found that OCD patients with comorbid personality disorders tended to drop out of and to be more difficult to manage during therapy. Furthermore, particular types of personality disorders, such as avoidant, borderline, and paranoid personality disorders (Cottraux et al. 1993; Jenike 1990), as well as passive-aggressive personality traits (Steketee 1991), have predicted poor outcome. Compliance was a problem for all eight of Hermesh et al.'s (1987) borderline personality disorder patients, who failed to respond to BT or clomipramine. Likewise, Rasmussen and Tsuang (1987) concurred that borderline, as well as histrionic, OCD patients responded poorly to treatment, although these authors provided no data to support their contention. Steketee et al. (1995) observed that dramatic-cluster traits were marginally correlated with 6-month outcome, but this association disappeared when other variables were considered. Jenike and colleagues (1986; Minichiello et al. 1987) reported that, in contrast to nonschizotypal patients, 90% of whom improved at least moderately with behavioral treatment or medications, only 7% of schizotypal patients showed lasting gains. Further, the number of schizotypal traits correlated strongly with negative outcome $(r = -.74)$. Ravizza et al. (1995) reported similar findings for response to clomipramine or fluoxetine. Overall, then, although a number of personality disorders appear to be benign accompaniments to OCD, others (e.g., borderline or schizotypal personality disorder) are likely to present problems for long-term OCD course.

Whether insight is an important predictor of prognosis and treatment response in OCD is an intriguing question that has received little investigation. The few available reports are conflicting. One study noted that patients with overvalued ideas did not respond as well to BT as did those with good insight (Foa 1979), but another study reported that patients with high conviction about their obsessions and the need to enact compulsions responded well to behavioral intervention (Lel-liott et al. 1988). This latter finding was also reported in a study that assessed insight as a potential predictor of response to sertraline (Eisen et al. 1995a). A rating scale developed to evaluate degree of insight and conviction, the Brown Assessment of Beliefs Scale (BABS; J. L. Eisen, K. A. Philips, D. Beer, S. A. Rasmussen, and L. Baer, unpublished, 1994), was administered to 38 OCD subjects before and after a 16-week open trial of sertraline. Poor insight did not predict response to medication. It is clear that more research will be needed to determine the effect of insight and of variables associated with poor insight on course.

Summary

In keeping with the older literature, several more recent studies using a prospective design, standardized criteria to assess diagnosis, and structured interviews with direct patient contact have shown that the majority of patients either continue to meet full criteria for the disorder or retain significant OC symptoms. This finding has also been supported in several prospective studies of children with OCD. In all these studies examining changes in severity of OC symptoms over time, the effect of treatment on the course of illness has not been firmly established. However, several recent prospective studies suggest that appropriate pharmacological treatment may improve outcome only while the patient continues to receive this treatment (Leonard et al. 1993; Orloff et al. 1994).

Factors that contribute to the course of illness severity in OCD have been assessed in many retrospective as well as prospective studies. Determining which variables influence the likelihood of remission or worsening of symptoms is clinically useful and may enhance our understanding of the underlying processes involved in OCD.

According to both course and treatment literature on predictors of follow-up outcome for OCD, surprisingly few demographic and clinical features, including severity and duration of symptoms, consistently predict outcome at follow-up. Even the role of age at onset is uncertain, given that early onset has been associated with poorer response in some studies and with better response in others. Onset age may interact with gender, so that boys/men with early-onset OCD fare worse than do girls/women, perhaps because of other associated features such as personality traits. More careful research to clarify these points are needed, especially if early intervention methods are to be guided by research findings.

The role of general functioning variables in long-term gains is less certain, since some studies suggest that poor adjustment negatively influences maintenance of gains. Neither depressed nor anxious mood have been found to be definitive predictors of outcome, although the former remains a question, and studies of OCD patients with comorbid major depressive disorder are needed. There is remarkably little information about the effect of comorbid anxiety disorders on outcome. Because OCD rarely occurs in the absence of other Axis I conditions, it is important to know whether any of these consistently affect treatment outcome. The predictive utility of comorbid personality disorders is far from established, given the paucity of research in this area. However, some personality styles appear to be potentially problematic, including schizotypal personality and possibly passive-aggressive, borderline, and paranoid personality disorder. Considerably more research on these comorbid conditions and their specific effects is needed.

References

Ackerman D, Greenland S, Bystritsky A, et al: Predictors of treatment response in obsessive-compulsive disorder: multivariate analyses from a multicenter trial of clomipramine. J Clin Psychopharmacol 14:247–254, 1994

American Psychiatric Association: Diagnostic and Statistical Manual of Mental Disorders, 3rd Edition, Revised. Washington, DC, American Psychiatric Association, 1987

American Psychiatric Association: Diagnostic and Statistical Manual of Mental Disorders, 4th Edition. Washington, DC, American Psychiatric Association, 1994

Apter A, Tyano S: Obsessive compulsive disorders in adolescence. Journal of Adolescence 11:183–194, 1988

Aubuchon PG, Malatesta VJ: Obsessive compulsive patients with comorbid personality disorder: associated problems and response to a comprehensive behavior therapy. J Clin Psychiatry 55:448–453, 1994

Basoglu M, Lax T, Kasvikis Y, et al: Predictors of improvement in obsessive-compulsive disorder. Journal of Anxiety Disorders 2:299–317, 1988

Berg CL, Rapoport JL, Whitaker A, et al: Childhood obsessive compulsive disorder: a two-year prospective follow-up of a community sample. J Am Acad Child Adolesc Psychiatry 28:528–533, 1989

Berman L: The obsessive-compulsive neurosis in children. J Nerv Ment Dis 95:26–39, 1942

Boulougouris J: Variables affecting the behavior of obsessive-compulsive patients treated by flooding, in Phobic and Obsessive Compulsive Disorders. Edited by Boulougouris JC, Rabavilas AD. New York, Pergamon, 1977, pp 73–84

Coryell W: Obsessive-compulsive disorder and primary unipolar depression: comparisons of background, family history, course, and mortality. J Nerv Ment Dis 169:220–224, 1981

Cottraux J, Messy P, Marks IM, et al: Predictive factors in the treatment of obsessive-compulsive disorders with fluvoxamine and/or behavior therapy. Behavioral Psychology 21:45–50, 1993

Demal U, Gerhard L, Mayrhofer A, et al: Obsessive-compulsive disorder and depression. Psychopathology 26:145–150, 1993

Drummond LM: The treatment of severe, chronic, resistant obsessive-compulsive disorder. Br J Psychiatry 163:223–229, 1993

Eisen JL, Rasmussen SA: Obsessive-compulsive disorder with psychotic features. J Clin Psychiatry 54:373–379, 1993

Eisen JL, Rasmussen SA, Goodman W: Does insight predict response to SSRIs in OCD? Poster presented at the American Psychiatric Association Annual Meeting, Miami, FL, May 1995a

Eisen JL, Rasmussen SA, Goodman W, et al: Patterns of remission and relapse: a 2-year prospective study of OCD. Poster presented at the American Psychiatric Association Annual Meeting, Miami, FL, May 1995b

Emmelkamp PMG, Hoekstra RJ, Visser A: The behavioral treatment of obsessive-compulsive disorder: prediction of outcome at 3.5-year follow-up, in Psychiatry: The State of the Art. Edited by Pichot P, Berner R, Wolf R, et al. New York, Plenum, 1985, pp 265–270

Endicott J, Spitzer RL, Fleiss JL: The Global Assessment Scale: a procedure for measuring overall severity of psychiatric disturbance. Arch Gen Psychiatry 33:766–771, 1976

Fenton WS, McGlashan TH: The prognostic significance of obsessive-compulsive symptoms in schizophrenia. Am J Psychiatry 143:437–441, 1986

Flament MF, Whitaker A, Rapoport JL, et al: Obsessive compulsive disorder in adolescence. J Am Acad Child Adolesc Psychiatry 27:764–771, 1988

Flament MF, Koby E, Rapoport JL, et al: Childhood obsessive-compulsive disorder: a prospective follow-up study. J Child Psychol Psychiatry 31:363–380, 1990

Foa EB: Failure in treating obsessive-compulsives. Behav Res Ther 17:169–176, 1979

Foa EB, Kozak MJ: DSM-IV field trial: obsessive-compulsive disorder. Am J Psychiatry 152:90–96, 1995

Foa EB, Grayson JB, Steketee GS, et al: Success and failure in the behavioral treatment of obsessive-compulsives. J Consult Clin Psychol 51:287–297, 1983

Foa EB, Kozak MJ, Steketee GS, et al: Treatment of depressive and obsessive-compulsive symptoms in OCD by imipramine and behavior therapy. J Clin Psychiatry 31:279–292, 1992

Gittleson NL: Depressive psychosis in the obsessional neurotic. Br J Psychiatry 112:883–887, 1966

Gojer J, Khanna S, Channabasaranna S, et al: Obsessive compulsive disorder, anxiety and depression. Indian Journal of Psychological Medicine 10:25–30, 1987

Goodman WK, Lawrence HP, Rasmussen SA, et al: The Yale-Brown Obsessive Compulsive Scale, I: development, use, and reliability. Arch Gen Psychiatry 46:1006–1011, 1989

Goodwin DW, Guze SB, Robins E: Follow-up studies in obsessional neurosis. Arch Gen Psychiatry 20:182–187, 1969

Gordon A, Rasmussen S: Mood-related obsessive-compulsive symptoms in a patient with bipolar affective disorder. J Clin Psychiatry 49:27–28, 1988

Grimshaw L: The outcome of obsessional disorder: a follow-up study of 100 cases. Br J Psychiatry 111:1051–1056, 1965

Hanna GL: Demographic and clinical features of obsessive-compulsive disorder in children and adolescents. J Am Acad Child Adolesc Psychiatry 34:19–27, 1995

Hermesh H, Shahar A, Munitz H: Obsessive-compulsive disorder and borderline personality disorder. Am J Psychiatry 144:120–121, 1987

Hoogduin CAL, Duivenvoorden HJ: A decision model in the treatment of obsessive-compulsive neurosis. Br J Psychiatry 144:516–521, 1988

Ingram IM: Obsessional illness in mental hospital patients. J Ment Sci 107:382–402, 1961

Insel TR, Akiskal HS: Obsessive-compulsive disorder with psychotic features: a phenomenological analysis. Am J Psychiatry 143:1527–1533, 1986

Jenike MA: Predictors of treatment failure, in Obsessive-Compulsive Disorders: Theory and Management. Edited by Jenike MA, Baer L, Minichiello WE. Chicago, IL, Year Book Medical, 1990, pp 306–311

Jenike MA, Baer L, Minichiello WE, et al: Concomitant obsessive-compulsive disorder and schizotypal personality disorders. Am J Psychiatry 143:306–311, 1986

Karno M, Golding J, Sorenson S, et al: The epidemiology of obsessive compulsive disorder in five U.S. communities. Arch Gen Psychiatry 45:1094–1099, 1988

Keck PE, Lipinski JF, White K: An inverse relationship between mania and obsessive-compulsive disorder. J Clin Psychopharmacol 6:123–124, 1986

Keijers GP, Hoogduin AL, Schaap CPDR: Predictors of treatment outcome in the behavioral treatment of obsessive-compulsive disorder. Br J Psychiatry 165:781–786, 1994

Keller MB, Lavori PW, Friedman B, et al: The Longitudinal Interval Follow-Up Evaluation: a comprehensive method for assessing outcome in prospective longitudinal studies. Arch Gen Psychiatry 44:540–548, 1987

Kendell RE, Discipio WJ: Obsessional symptoms and obsessional personality traits in patients with depressive illnesses. Psychol Med 1:65–72, 1970

Kozak MJ, Foa EB: Obsessions, overvalued ideas, and delusions in obsessive-compulsive disorder. Behavior Res Ther 32:343–353, 1994

Kringlen E: Obsessional neurotics: a long-term follow-up. Br J Psychiatry 111:709–722, 1965

Lelliott PT, Noshirvani HF, Basoglu M, et al: Obsessive-compulsive beliefs and treatment outcome. Psychol Med 18:697–702, 1988

Leonard HL, Swedo SE, Lenane MC, et al: A two- to seven-year follow-up study of 54 obsessive compulsive children and adolescents. Arch Gen Psychiatry 50:429–439, 1993

Lewis A: Problems of obsessional illness. Proc Royal Soc Medicine 29:325–336, 1936

Lion EG: Anancastic depressions: obsessive-compulsive symptoms occurring during depressions. J Nerv Ment Dis 95:730–738, 1942

Lo WH: A follow-up study of obsessional neurotics in Hong Kong Chinese. Br J Psychiatry 113:823–832, 1967

Marks IM, Stern RS, Mawson D, et al: Clomipramine and exposure for obsessive-compulsive rituals, I. Br J Psychiatry 136:1–25, 1980

Mawson D, Marks IM, Ramm L, et al: Clomipramine and exposure for chronic obsessive-compulsive rituals: two-year follow-up and further findings. Br J Psychiatry 140:11–18, 1982

Minichiello W, Baer L, Jenike MA: Schizotypal personality disorder: a poor prognostic indicator for behavior therapy in the treatment of obsessive-compulsive disorder. Journal of Anxiety Disorders 1:273–276, 1987

Orloff LM, Battle MA, Baer L, et al: Long-term follow-up of 85 patients with obsessive-compulsive disorder. Am J Psychiatry 151:441–442, 1994

O'Sullivan G, Noshirvani H, Marks I, et al: Six-year follow-up after exposure and clomipramine therapy for obsessive compulsive disorder. J Clin Psychiatry 52:150–155, 1991

Pato MT, Eisen JL, Pato CN: Rating scales for obsessive-compulsive disorder, in Current Insights in Obsessive-Compulsive Disorder. Edited by Hollander E, Zohar J, Marazziti D, et al. West Sussex, UK, John Wiley & Sons, 1994, pp 77–92

Pigott TA, Pato MT, L'Heureux F, et al: A controlled comparison of adjuvant lithium carbonate or thyroid hormone in clomipramine-treated patients with obsessive-compulsive disorder. J Clin Psychopharmacol 11:242–248, 1991

Pollitt J: Natural history of obsessional states: a study of 150 cases. BMJ 1:194–198, 1957

Rabavilas AD, Boulougouris JC: Mood changes and flooding outcome in obsessive-compulsive patients: report of a 2-year follow-up. J Nerv Ment Dis 167:495–496, 1979

Rabavilas AD, Boulougouris JC, Stefanis C: Duration of flooding sessions in the treatment of obsessive-compulsive patients. Behav Res Ther 14:349–355, 1976

Rachman S, Marks IM, Hodgson R: The treatment of obsessive-compulsive neurotics by modelling and flooding in vivo. Behav Res Ther 14:349–355, 1973

Rasmussen SA, Eisen JL: The epidemiology and clinical features of OCD. Psychiatr Clin North Am 15:743–758, 1992

Rasmussen SA, Tsuang MT: Clinical characteristics and family history in DSM-III obsessive-compulsive disorder. Am J Psychiatry 143:317–322, 1986

Rasmussen SA, Tsuang MT: Obsessive-compulsive disorder and borderline personality disorder. Am J Psychiatry 144:121–122, 1987

Ravizza L, Barzega G, Bellino S, et al: Predictors of drug treatment response in obsessive-compulsive disorder. J Clin Psychiatry 56:368–373, 1995

Rettew DC, Swedo SE, Leonard HL, et al: Obsessions and compulsions across time in 79 children and adolescents with obsessive-compulsive disorder. J Am Acad Child Adolesc Psychiatry 31:1050–1056, 1992

Rosen I: The clinical significance of obsessions in schizophrenia. J Ment Sci 103:773–785, 1957

Rosenberg CM: Complications of obsessional neurosis. Br J Psychiatry 114:477–478, 1968

Steketee G: Intra- and interpersonal characteristics predictive of long-term outcome following behavioral treatment of obsessive-compulsive disorder, in Panic and Phobias II. Edited by Hand I, Wittchen HU. Berlin, Springer-Verlag, 1988, pp 221–232

Steketee G: Personality traits and disorders in obsessive-compulsives. Journal of Anxiety Disorders 4:351–364, 1991

Steketee G: Social support and treatment outcome of obsessive compulsive disorder at 9-month follow-up. Behavioral Psychotherapy 21:81–95, 1993

Steketee G, Shapiro L: Predicting behavioral treatment outcome for agoraphobia and obsessive compulsive disorder. Clinical Psychology Review 15:317–346, 1995

Steketee G, Kozak MJ, Foa SB: Predictors and outcome for obsessive-compulsives treated with exposure and response prevention. Paper presented at the European Association for Behavior Therapy, Munich, West Germany, September 1985

Steketee G, Chambless D, Tran G, et al: Comorbidity and outcome for behaviorally treated clients with OCD and agoraphobia. Paper presented at the World Congress of Behavioral and Cognitive Therapy, Copenhagen, Denmark, July 1995

Stengel E: A study on some clinical aspects of the relationship between obsessional neurosis and psychotic reaction types. J Ment Sci 166–187, 1991

Swedo SE, Rapoport JL, Leonard H, et al: Obsessive-compulsive disorder in children and adolescents: clinical phenomenology of 70 consecutive cases. Arch Gen Psychiatry 46:335–341, 1989

Thomsen PH: Obsessive-compulsive disorder in children and adolescents: a 6- to 22-year follow-up study of social outcome. European Child and Adolescent Psychiatry 4:112–122, 1995

Visser S, Hoekstra RJ, Emmelkamp PMG: Long-term follow-up study of obsessive-compulsive patients after exposure treatment, in Perspectives and Promises of Clinical Psychology. Edited by Ehlers A, Fiegenbaum W, Florin I, et al. New York, Plenum, 1992, pp 157–170

Welner A, Reich T, Robins E, et al: Obsessive-compulsive neurosis: record, follow-up, and family studies. Compr Psychiatry 17:527–539, 1976

World Health Organization: International Classification of Diseases, 9th Revision. Geneva, Switzerland, 1977

Chapter 15

Obsessive-Compulsive Disorder in Pregnancy and the Puerperium

Susan F. Diaz, M.D., Lynn R. Grush, M.D., Deborah A. Sichel, M.D., and Lee S. Cohen, M.D.

Pregnancy has traditionally been thought of as a time of mental well-being. However, recent studies have indicated that some women may not be protected from depression (Gotlib et al. 1989; O'Hara 1986) or panic disorder (Cohen et al. 1994a) during pregnancy. In contrast, the puerperium has generally been recognized as a period of increased risk for the development of psychiatric illness (Kendell et al. 1981; Paffenberg 1982). Reports describing postpartum depression (O'Hara 1986) and puerperal psychosis (Kendell et al. 1981) are predominant in the literature, and panic disorder in the postpartum period has more recently been described in the literature (Cohen et al. 1994b). Little is known, however, about the natural history of obsessive-compulsive disorder (OCD) in women during pregnancy and the puerperium.

In the general population, OCD has an estimated lifetime prevalence of roughly 2%, with men and women equally affected (Karno et al. 1988). The age at onset for women tends to be the early 20s, and the course is typically continuous, with waxing and waning symptoms (Rasmussen and Eisen 1991). Symptomatic periods will therefore coexist with reproductive events and persist throughout a woman's childbearing years. In this chapter we review the literature on OCD in pregnancy and the puerperium and discuss preliminary data from a naturalistic study that followed 19 women with OCD through their pregnancies.

Epidemiology

The existing literature on OCD in pregnancy and the puerperium includes epidemiological data on rates of patients who reported OCD onset during pregnancy, studies of postpartum illnesses including OCD, and case reports that specifically examined OCD in women during pregnancy and the puerperium.

In the 1950s and 1960s, several studies attempted to describe the natural history of obsessional illness by examining large groups of patients with this disorder. Each of these reports found a relationship between the onset of obsessional symptoms and pregnancy or childbirth in a subset of the patients studied. Pollitt (1957) evaluated 150 inpatients and outpatients (63 men and 87 women) with obsessional illness. He found that 93 patients (62%) identified an event that seemed to precipitate the onset of their illness. Three of these 93 patients (3%) identified pregnancy and 7 (7%) identified childbirth as the precipitant.

In a similar study of patients with obsessional illness, Ingram (1961) described several clinical features of 89 inpatients (55 women and 34 men). Among this sample, 61 (69%) identified an event occurring within 1 year of the onset of obsessional illness that was considered to be related to the onset. Pregnancy was the most common event identified. Fifteen of the 61 patients (25%) felt that the onset of their illness was related to pregnancy. The symptoms typically reported by these patients included fear of harming the child, as well as washing and avoidance rituals involving both the mother and the child. Lo (1967), in Hong Kong, studied 88 outpatients and inpatients (64 men and 24 women) with obsessional illness. Fifty-six patients (64%) identified an event occurring within 6 months of the onset of their obsessional illness that they considered significant in triggering the symptoms. Pregnancy or childbirth was identified by 3 of these 56 patients (5%). It is not clear from these studies by Politt, Ingram, and Lo whether the patients who reported perinatal onset of obsessional illness were exclusively female or included male patients as well.

Current investigators into the phenomenology of OCD continue to report an association between the acute onset of obsessive-compulsive symptoms and the perinatal period in a subset of patients. Rasmussen and Eisen have collected clinical information on 749 patients (410 women and 339 men) with DSM-III-R (American Psychiatric Association 1987)–defined OCD. Of the 410 women evaluated, 21 (5%) identified pregnancy and 12 (3%) identified childbirth as precipitants to their illness (S. Rasmussen and J. Eisen, personal communication, March 1996).

The wide range in incidence reported by these studies may be accounted for by several factors, including lack of uniform diagnostic criteria, varying severities of illness among the patient populations, and differing methods of data collection. Nonetheless, each descriptive series consistently identified a subgroup of patients whose illness onset coincided with pregnancy or the puerperium.

Several studies that identified groups of patients with postpartum illnesses also suggested vulnerability for the onset of obsessional illness in the puerperium. Button et al. (1972) reviewed the cases of 42 psychiatric patients in whom obsessions of infanticide were the central pathological feature. Diagnoses in these patients included schizophrenic reaction (40%), depression (26%), and obsessive-compulsive reaction (16%). This 16% stands in contrast to the 1 patient with obsessional illness that Davidson and Robertson (1985) reported in their review of 82 women with postpartum illness treated as inpatients between 1946 and 1971. This patient had obsessions of drowning the child and of stabbing the child with a kitchen knife, and she reported a prior postpartum exacerbation of a similar nature.

The literature contains case reports of new-onset OCD after abortion and childbirth as well as worsening of preexisting OCD during pregnancy. Lipper and Feigenbaum (1976) described a 19-year-old woman who developed disabling preoccupations with contamination, accompanied by ritualized hand washing, following a therapeutic abortion of a 20-week-old fetus.

Brandt and Mackenzie (1987) presented a case of a 26-year-old woman with a 3-year history of OCD who, after an uneventful first pregnancy at age 20, experienced an unprecedented worsening of her illness in her second pregnancy. Her symptoms included an obsessional fear of rat germs and compulsive cleaning that rendered her unable to eat or to care for her family. She required four successive hospitalizations during the pregnancy for worsening symptoms of OCD and the development of secondary major depression. Treatment during pregnancy included electroconvulsive therapy (ECT), alprazolam, and thioridazine, none of which effectively reduced her obsessive-compulsive symptoms. Her illness improved postpartum after several weeks of treatment with clomipramine.

Sichel et al. (1993a) described the onset of OCD during the puerperium in two women, aged 30 and 34 years, both with no past psychiatric history. Each woman's illness was characterized by recurrent, intrusive thoughts of harming the child by such means as stabbing it or throwing it down the stairs or out the window. In one patient the symptoms began within 3 days of the delivery, whereas the other patient developed symptoms at 4 weeks postpartum. Both women engaged in behaviors to avoid the infant, and both improved symptomatically after treatment with fluoxetine.

In the early 1990s, three groups of researchers began to more systematically review the relationship between OCD and childbearing. Buttolph and Holland (1990) sent a questionnaire to retrospectively probe for events that precipitated the onset or worsening of obsessive-compulsive symptoms to 180 consecutively evaluated patients with OCD. Of the 39 female respondents, a striking 69% ($n = 27$) related onset or worsening of OCD to pregnancy or childbirth. Within this group of 27 women, 6 (22%) reported a new onset of obsessive-compulsive symptoms during pregnancy, and 3 (11%) reported worsening of preexisting OCD during pregnancy. Eight (30%) of the 27 women reported an onset of OCD in the puerperium as they attempted to care for the child, and 6 (22%) reported worsening of preexisting OCD in the puerperium. Ten of the 14 women with postpartum exacerbations of OCD experienced symptoms after the birth of their first child, whereas 4 had puerperal exacerbations after the birth of subsequent children. Also included in this group of 27 women were 2 who reported that their OCD worsened after miscarriages and 2 who felt that the trigger for their OCD was an inability to conceive.

Neziroglu et al. (1992) conducted a similar retrospective study in a large sample of 106 women to test their hypothesis that pregnancy is a life event that may hasten the onset of OCD. These women with OCD responded to a questionnaire assessing parity and life events associated with the onset of their illness. Fifty-nine of the 106 respondents had children. Twenty-three of these 59 (39%)—still quite a large percentage but not the 69% reported by Buttolph and Holland (1990)—reported an onset of their illness during pregnancy. Of these 23 women, 12 reported onset during their first pregnancy and 11 during subsequent pregnancies. Five childless women in the sample had had first-trimester therapeutic abortions or miscarriages. Four of these 5 reported an onset or exacerbation of OCD while pregnant. This study also found that the women without children tended to first develop OCD during adolescence, whereas the women with children developed the illness later in their 20s, around the times of their pregnancies. This finding raises the possibility that patients with OCD exacerbations related to pregnancy may represent a subgroup of patients with distinct physiological contributions—possibly neurohormonal—to their illness.

Sichel et al. (1993b) retrospectively evaluated 15 women with puerperal onset of OCD. The mean age of this sample was 32 ± 6.2 years. The women presented for treatment an average of 2.2 ± 1.2 weeks after delivery, all reporting a rapid escalation of ego-alien obsessional thoughts of harming the newborn, accompanied by generalized anxiety and disruption of the mother-infant relationship. Eight of the 15 had no prior psychiatric history, whereas 5 had previous histories of panic disorder and 2 of generalized anxiety disorder. Each patient described intrusive thoughts about harming her infant as the original source of distress, but 9 women later developed depressive symptoms 2–3 weeks after the onset of their obsessional thoughts. On presentation, their Clinical Global Impression (CGI; Guy 1976) scores[1] ranged from 5 to 7, and 10 women were hospitalized for treatment. At 1-year follow-up, 12 patients remained on antiobsessional agents and reported mild symptoms (CGI scores ranging from 1 to 3). One patient discontinued treatment without recurrence of symptoms; 2 others attempted to taper their medication but became ill again. Interestingly, the symptoms of OCD in the entire sample, both at presentation and

---

[1]The CGI scale is a 7-point scale that rates severity of disease, with 1 = not at all ill and 7 = extremely ill patients.

at follow-up, were limited to intrusive obsessional thoughts without compulsions. This finding raises the possibility that puerperal OCD may be distinct from OCD affecting nongravid women.

Review of the literature reveals the absence of prospective studies following the course of OCD during pregnancy and the puerperium. A pilot study has been performed by Sichel, Cohen, and Grush of the Perinatal and Reproductive Psychiatry Clinical Research Program at Massachusetts General Hospital (D. A. Sichel, personal communication, May 1996). In this study, 19 women with a pregravid history of OCD were followed prospectively from the first trimester to 9 months postpartum. Data from the first trimester are available for 17 subjects. Fifty-nine percent (10/17) of these women met DSM-III-R criteria for OCD. By the third trimester, 74% (14/19) of the women met OCD criteria, and by 3 months postpartum, 84% (16/19) met OCD criteria.

Consistent with Rasmussen and Eisen's (1991) data on a 70% lifetime prevalence of comorbid major depression in patients with OCD, 18 of the 19 women in this sample had a lifetime history of comorbid depression. Development of major depression during the study period occurred most commonly in the first trimester ($n = 7$) and was associated with antidepressant discontinuation in the majority of these women.

Although the sample size is small, and some of the data from early pregnancy are not available, this pilot study, like much of the retrospective data, suggests that pregnancy does not confer a protective effect for women with a prior history of OCD. In addition, the third trimester and the puerperium may be times of heightened risk for the worsening of OCD.

Etiology and Pathophysiology

Compilation of the available data suggests that, in a subpopulation of vulnerable women, OCD may begin or worsen during pregnancy or in the puerperium. Women with pregravid OCD appear to be at risk for worsening during pregnancy, particularly in the third trimester or during the postpartum period. It is still not clear what factors might predict onset or worsening. Sichel et al. (1993b) and Buttolph and Holland (1990) both point out that, given the relatively high prevalence of OCD in the general population and the mean onset of illness in the childbearing years, it cannot yet be concluded that pregnancy and childbirth are causative in the development of OCD. It has been suggested that rates of affective disorder in postpartum women may not significantly differ from rates of affective disorder in nonpuerperal women (O'Hara et al. 1990); similarly, rates of puerperal OCD may reflect the prevalence of the disorder in the general population.

However, if an association between OCD and the complex events of pregnancy and childbirth exists in a subgroup of patients, it is interesting to speculate on the etiology of this association. A wide range of possible reasons for this association have been offered in the literature, including psychodynamic factors (Button et al. 1972), behavioral explanations (e.g., inability to engage in usual avoidance strategies while caring for the child) (Brandt and Mackenzie 1987; Buttolph and Holland 1990), environmental triggers (e.g., overwhelming psychosocial stress of childbirth triggering illness) (Lo 1967), and biological etiologies (Sichel et al. 1993b; Stein et al. 1993).

Understanding how biological factors affect psychiatric disorders is the focus of much research today. Several investigators have suggested that OCD may be neurohormonally modulated. There is strong evidence to suggest that the serotonin system plays a central role in OCD (Murphy et al. 1989) and some evidence that changes in estrogen can alter serotonergic binding sites (Biegor et al. 1983; Ehrenkranz 1976) and that serotonergic neurotransmission may be partially modulated by changes in estrogen and progesterone (Stockert and deRobertis 1985). The fluctuations in estrogen and progesterone during pregnancy and the puerperium may influence serotonergic function, resulting in the onset or exacerbation of obsessive-compulsive symptoms.

Oxytocin has also been hypothesized to play a role in the production of obsessive-compulsive symptoms (Altemus et al. 1994; Leckman et al. 1994; Swedo et al. 1992). Among children with OCD, Swedo et al. (1992) reported a positive correlation between cerebrospinal fluid (CSF) oxytocin levels and depressive symptoms, and in the same subjects, Altemus et al. (1994) found that treatment with clomipramine increased CSF levels of oxytocin. Leckman and colleagues (1994) found a marked elevation in CSF oxytocin levels in a subgroup of OCD patients who were medication-free, and correlated the severity of their obsessive-compulsive symptoms to the CSF oxytocin levels. Oxytocin is essential in late pregnancy and the postpartum period, as it promotes uterine contractions and lactation. One might speculate that increased concentrations of oxytocin late in pregnancy and in the postpartum period may be influential in the onset of perinatal OCD.

Prolactin is another neuropeptide whose levels rise throughout the course of pregnancy and remain elevated during lactation. Prolactin levels have been hypothesized to reflect pre- and postsynaptic serotonergic activity by Hanna et al. (1991). Their study of 18 children and adolescents with severe OCD found that prolactin levels prior to treatment with medication were negatively correlated with the duration and severity of obsessive-compulsive symptoms, whereas treatment with clomipramine significantly increased prolactin levels. The role of androgens in producing obsessive-compulsive symptoms has been questioned by Casas et al. (1986). They treated four OCD patients with cyproterone acetate, a potent antiandrogen, and noted a remission in symptoms.

In addition to research relating hormonal changes to obsessive-compulsive symptoms, several clinical observations have also pointed to hormonal fluctuations as one factor in the onset of obsessive-compulsive symptoms. Puberty is the time when girls who develop OCD typically experience symptoms for the first time. In children under the age of 10, boys with OCD outnumber girls 7 to 1; after puberty, the sex ratio shifts to 1 : 1.5 (Swedo et al. 1989). Among adults with OCD, Rasmussen and Eisen (1991) observed that 60% of the 138 women in their clinically derived sample reported worsening of their obsessive-compulsive symptoms premenstrually.

Research into the effects of hormones on OCD is quite preliminary at this time. However, these early observations raise the possibility that neurohormonal fluctuations, including those that occur during pregnancy and the puerperium, may affect neurotransmitter activity and result in the behavioral and psychic symptoms of OCD.

Treatment Recommendations

Women with OCD should be closely monitored throughout pregnancy and into the puerperium for exacerbations of obsessive-compulsive symptoms as well as symptoms of comorbid major depression. In addition, the clinician should be aware of the potential for onset of OCD in a previously healthy woman during pregnancy or the postpartum period. In this section we first present recommendations for the clinical management of women with OCD who wish to conceive or who present during pregnancy, and then provide some clinical examples of the use of these treatments.

Preconception Counseling

Women in their reproductive years who have a history of OCD should be informed that their disorder may worsen during pregnancy and the postpartum period. They should be encouraged to use adequate contraceptive methods until they are ready to conceive. Once ready to conceive, potential treatment options and psychosocial stressors and supports should be reviewed. Treatment plans may need to be modified to increase or add cognitive-behavioral therapy (CBT) and/or supportive psychotherapy. The risk of medication use during pregnancy, as well as the risk of its discontinuation, should be discussed.

Pregnancy

First-trimester worsening of OCD symptoms or comorbid depressive symptoms may occur, particularly if pharmacotherapy is discontinued just before conception or early in the pregnancy. This worsening may be a withdrawal effect from the medication or may reflect monoamine dysregulation secondary to the acute endocrinological changes of the first trimester. Unless symptoms are severe and incapacitating, other therapies should be maximized before pharmacotherapy is introduced in the first trimester. Our experience and preliminary data suggest that obsessive-compulsive symptoms and comorbid depressive symptoms often improve in the second trimester. Conversely, our experience and preliminary data suggest that the third trimester is a period of increased vulnerability for worsening of obsessive-compulsive symptoms, although perhaps not comorbid depressive symptoms. Patients may require pharmacotherapy at this time, in addition to psychotherapy.

Postpartum

Women with pregravid OCD or circumscribed postpartum OCD may demonstrate worsening of the disorder within the first 6 weeks postpartum. If pharmacotherapy has been deferred during pregnancy, reintroduction at this time is usually necessary to treat both worsening OCD and comorbid mood disorders. The selective serotonin reuptake inhibitor antidepressants and clomipramine are the mainstays of treatment. Doses have typically been higher than those used to treat postpartum affective disorders (see Chapter 12, "Obsessive-Compulsive Disorder in Adults," in this section).

Specific Treatments

Psychotherapy

Psychodynamic and supportive therapies have not been found to be efficacious in the treatment of OCD. However, given the psychosocial stress of pregnancy and the importance of psychosocial supports during this time, these therapies remain an important intervention, although not specifically to target obsessive-compulsive symptoms.

CBT is an effective treatment for OCD and may be the only treatment required for pregnant women with mild obsessive-compulsive symptoms. It should always be considered as part of the treatment for more severe cases of OCD in pregnancy. In the general population, CBT has been shown to be effective as an adjunct to treatment with pharmacotherapy and may permit lower doses of OCD-specific pharmacotherapy (Baer and Minichiello 1990). However, studies of CBT's efficacy during pregnancy have not been reported.

Pharmacotherapy

Identification of drugs that are effective against OCD has greatly improved the lives of many OCD sufferers. The mainstays of treatment are the serotonin reuptake inhibitors clomipramine and fluoxetine, with fluvoxamine a recent addition. The question of whether or not to continue medication during pregnancy remains a dilemma, one whose risks and benefits must be carefully weighed. The extent to which medication discontinuation may worsen maternal symptoms of OCD, potentially endangering the mother and fetus, must be weighed against the potential teratological effects of prenatal antidepressant exposure.

Altshuler et al. (1996) recently reviewed the literature on the use of psychotropic medication in pregnancy. In reviewing the data on first-trimester exposure to tricyclic antidepressants (TCAs), they report that there is not a significant association between fetal exposure to TCAs and high rates of congenital malformations. They note, however, that the data are largely retrospective and are available only on a relatively small number of subjects (*n* = 414). Except for clomipramine, the TCAs do not generally provide efficacy in the treatment of OCD. Similarly, retrospective reviews indicate that exposure to fluoxetine in the first trimester does not appear to increase the risk of congenital malformations (Goldstein 1995; Pastuszak et al. 1993; Shader 1992). No data exist regarding prenatal fluvoxamine exposure.

Data regarding neonatal toxicity after in utero exposure to antidepressant medication are sparse, relying mostly on case reports and retrospective reviews. Transient withdrawal syndromes have been described in infants exposed to imipramine and nortriptyline (Eggermont 1973; Shearer et al. 1972; Webster 1973). Prenatal clomipramine exposure has resulted in cases of infant hypothermia, respiratory acidosis, and seizures (Ben Musa and Smith 1979; Cowe et al. 1982; Schimmell et al. 1991; Zahle Ostergaard and Pedersen 1982).

There are minimal prospective data on the use of psychotropics in pregnancy. Misri and Sivertz (1991) prospectively studied women with pregravid major depression who were treated with TCAs during their pregnancies. Nine women conceived while taking a TCA. Of the nine infants born to these women, none displayed any physical malformations, but one exhibited transient hypotonia and mild irritability. Nine mothers took tricyclics from the second or third trimester until delivery. Eight of the nine infants born to these women displayed withdrawal symptoms, including irritability, transient cyanosis, hypotonia, poor sucking, and tachypnea. This study is limited by its small sample size, lack of suitable control subjects, and nonstandardized assessments of infant development.

Goldstein (1995) prospectively studied the outcomes of pregnancies reported to Eli Lilly in which exposure to fluoxetine had occurred in the third trimester. One hundred and fifteen infants were identified prenatally, 89 of which had been exposed to fluoxetine during all three trimesters. Among this latter group, the rate of congenital malformations was 3.5%, which is consistent with the rate seen in the general population. Among the entire sample, transient neonatal complications were reported in 15 infants and included irritability, hyperbilirubinemia, and somnolence. Limitations of this study included the facts that the outcome data were obtained from the initial reporter of the exposure, and that there were no suitable control subjects or standardized assessments of infant development.

Remarkably few data exist regarding long-term neurobehavioral effects in children after in utero exposure to antidepressants. One small group of children exposed to TCAs in utero demonstrated normal motor skills and behavioral development at age 3 (Misri and Sivertz 1991).

For the patient requiring pharmacological treatment for OCD during pregnancy, fluoxetine appears to be the safest choice. It must be made clear to the patient that although the rate of congenital malformations may not be increased with fluoxetine use in pregnancy, the neurobehavioral effects of prenatal exposure on the neonate and in the child over the long term have not been well studied. Given the case reports of clomipramine withdrawal syndromes, it seems prudent to avoid clomipramine exposure during pregnancy. If clomipramine is used in pregnancy, consideration should be given to a slow taper prior to delivery, and the pediatrician should be notified of the possibility of clomipramine withdrawal in the infant.

Clonazepam may be considered for treating pregnant women with OCD whose anxiety is disabling. In their review of the data on first-trimester exposure to benzodiazepines, Altshuler et al. (1996) note a small absolute risk (<1%) of oral clefts. One prospective study found no maternal or neonatal compromise in 39 subjects exposed to clonazepam during pregnancy (Weinstock et al. 1996). Our clinical experience with low doses of clonazepam in pregnancy (0.5–1.5 mg) supports this study finding; however, we have observed that higher doses of clonazepam (2.0–5.0 mg) have sometimes led to adverse neonatal outcomes, such as hypotonia, apnea, and failure to feed.

The treatment of OCD during pregnancy ultimately rests on a good understanding between the patient and her physician. Patients need to be informed of the potential risks to the fetus and to themselves. The ultimate decision is the patient's, guided by the information she has received.

Clinical Examples

Patients with OCD are often secretive about their symptoms, particularly during the perinatal period, when shame and fear about being perceived as an inadequate mother may accompany the distress of the illness. The following clinical examples are designed to familiarize the clinician with ways in which the illness may present during pregnancy and the puerperium. The cases also illustrate the variability in illness course and severity during pregnancy and the postpartum period.

OCD may present for the first time during pregnancy in women who have no past psychiatric histories.

> Ms. A. was a 32-year-old married woman with no prior psychiatric history. During the second trimester of her first pregnancy, she became obsessed with germs, paint, and disinfectants in her kitchen and started repeatedly washing her kitchen appliances. She would avoid going into the kitchen and using kitchen linen. Her anxiety and agitation worsened until, by 28 weeks' gestation, she avoided the kitchen altogether. Her obstetrician had reassured her that her symptoms were not of concern, and that everything would revert back to normal when she delivered. Eventually, Ms. A. presented for psychiatric treatment at 32 weeks' gestation in a highly agitated state. She had gained only 2 pounds during the pregnancy. She was not eating or sleeping well and was somewhat estranged from her husband, who could not understand her behavior. One week later, she went into premature labor and delivered a baby who required 3 weeks of treatment in the intensive care unit.
>
> By the tenth postpartum week, Ms. A. had responded to a regimen of fluoxetine 40 mg and nortriptyline 75 mg. She remained on these medications for a year before discontinuing them. She remained well and conceived again 2 years later. During the first trimester of this pregnancy, Ms. A. became mildly anxious and was treated with clonazepam 0.5 mg daily. She continued the clonazepam and supportive psychotherapy throughout the pregnancy. At 37 weeks' gestation, she delivered a healthy baby and resumed fluoxetine 20 mg daily. She remained well postpartum, with no further symptoms of OCD.

In this case, the patient experienced a new onset of OCD during her first pregnancy, with symptoms increasing to the point of incapacitation. One can speculate that the premature labor might have been precipitated by Ms. A.'s general state of agitation and poor weight gain. Failure to recognize her illness might have contributed to the infant's prematurity and its attendant complications. Ms. A.'s second pregnancy was notably different. She was aware of the possibility that her OCD might worsen, was treated for her anxiety, and received supportive therapy throughout the pregnancy. The outcome for mother and baby was significantly improved.

Women may be well during one or more pregnancies yet develop OCD de novo in a subsequent pregnancy.

> Ms. B. was a 30-year-old mother of a 2-year-old child. Premorbid psychiatric symptoms were limited to obsessional traits around making lists and tidiness, but these traits had never interfered with her functioning. Ms. B. conceived quadruplets after treatment for infertility. She was advised to have a selective reduction to improve the likelihood of a healthy fetal outcome. Although this option was contrary to her beliefs, she chose to have the reduction and continued the pregnancy to term with twins.

Soon after the reduction, she became increasingly obsessive about germs. She spent excessive amounts of time cleaning and would use only one room to avoid dirtying the rest of the house. Her obsessions and compulsions made it increasingly difficult to care for her son. She subsequently became severely depressed and suicidal. Although reluctant to expose the twins to medication in utero, she elected to start fluoxetine 10 mg daily in the third trimester, which improved her symptoms only slightly.

Postpartum, while receiving fluoxetine 40 mg daily, her depression improved, but she continued to have severe obsessive-compulsive symptoms. The fluoxetine was increased to 60 mg, but Ms. B. became hypomanic. The fluoxetine was stopped while lithium was started to target the hypomania. Once her mood was stabilized, the fluoxetine was restarted. On this regimen, Ms. B.'s obsessive-compulsive symptoms improved; however, they continue to impair her functioning.

The onset of OCD during Ms. B.'s second pregnancy coincided with the stress of a voluntary reduction, which was a traumatic event for this mother. Her OCD was complicated by affective instability, necessitating the introduction of medication during pregnancy and a mood stabilizer postpartum.

Women with pregravid OCD may experience worsening of their disorder during pregnancy.

Ms. C. was a 29-year-old mother of one with a history of OCD that was treated with clomipramine 75 mg daily. On discovering her pregnancy, Ms. C. discontinued her clomipramine during the first trimester. She soon noticed an increase in her OCD symptoms, including concerns about cleanliness and compulsive hand washing and checking. By the third trimester these symptoms had worsened, and she was unable to function at home or at work. She elected to restart clomipramine during the third trimester, with a plan to taper the medication before delivery to avoid a withdrawal syndrome in the newborn. On her previous dose, Ms. C.'s symptoms improved.

Women may develop a new onset of OCD in the postpartum period after an uneventful pregnancy.

Ms. D. was a 28-year-old woman with no previous psychiatric history who had an uneventful second pregnancy. At 3 weeks postpartum, she began to experience ego-dystonic, intrusive thoughts about harming her baby. These thoughts included sexually molesting the child, throwing him down the stairs, and stabbing him with a kitchen knife. She had no compulsive behaviors. She increasingly avoided the child and lay on the couch all day. She subsequently became severely depressed and suicidal, and was hospitalized for 2 weeks.

Ms. D. was treated with fluoxetine 60 mg daily, and by 4 months postpartum the obsessive thoughts and depression were much improved. Two years later, she was free of obsessive thoughts and was gradually tapered off the fluoxetine with no symptom recurrence. She remains well but has had no further pregnancies.

In multiparas, OCD exacerbations may occur following each pregnancy, with quiescence of the illness in between pregnancies.

> Ms. E. had no past psychiatric history, but presented early during the puerperium of her first pregnancy with an acute onset of intrusive, ego-dystonic thoughts of stabbing her infant. She was treated successfully with fluoxetine 60 mg, then tapered off medication after 1 year with no recurrence. Ms. E. subsequently had two pregnancies, during which she remained well. She developed similar intrusive thoughts after each delivery. Each postpartum episode was effectively treated with the same dose of fluoxetine. She has successfully tapered the medication without recurrence of obsessive thoughts or compulsive behaviors.

Conclusions

At present there is still much to be learned about the course of OCD in women during pregnancy and the puerperium. Controlled, prospective research is needed to clarify the rates of OCD in pregnancy and the puerperium, and to identify factors that make women more or less vulnerable to perinatal exacerbation of OCD. The extent to which a worsening of OCD in pregnancy or the postpartum period predicts a recurrence of the disorder in future pregnancies, implying a need for preventive measures in pregnancy or postpartum prophylaxis, also requires further study. Nonetheless, the clinician should be alerted to the possible emergence or exacerbation of OCD in women during pregnancy or the postpartum period.

Greater understanding is needed regarding the treatment of OCD during pregnancy and the puerperium, including the safety and efficacy of psychopharmacological treatments during pregnancy and breast feeding. Alternative modes of therapy for OCD (e.g., behavioral therapy) have not yet been studied in pregnancy and the puerperium but would likely be both efficacious and safe.

The effect of worsening obsessive-compulsive symptoms on early mother-infant relations is another unexplored area of study. Some research has shown that children of depressed mothers may develop maladaptive behaviors and experience emotional and cognitive deficits (Cogill et al. 1986; Zuckerman et al. 1990). It is possible that infants of mothers with anxiety disorders may also be vulnerable to these disturbances. If studies confirm such an association, the need for identification and intensive treatment of mothers with new or worsening OCD in the perinatal period is further underscored.

Finally, understanding the neurohormonal features that may trigger OCD in pregnancy and the puerperium could add to our understanding of the neurobiology of OCD. In addition, studies that examine the course of OCD during other times of hormonal change, such as puberty, the menstrual cycle, and menopause, would expand our knowledge and further address general issues of etiology. Taken together, this research may provide a fascinating medical model for the illness, possibly pointing toward new treatment options.

References

Altemus M, Swedo SE, Leonard HL, et al: Changes in CSF neurochemistry during treatment of OCD with clomipramine. Arch Gen Psychiatry 51:794–803, 1994

Altshuler LL, Cohen L, Szuba MP, et al: Pharmacological management of psychiatric illness during pregnancy: dilemmas and guidelines. Am J Psychiatry 153:592–606, 1996

American Psychiatric Association: Diagnostic and Statistical Manual of Mental Disorders, 3rd Edition, Revised. Washington, DC, American Psychiatric Association, 1987

Baer L, Minichiello WE: Behavioral therapy for obsessive compulsive disorder, in The Handbook of Anxiety, Vol 4. Edited by Burrows GD, Noyes R, Roth M. Amsterdam, Elsevier, 1990, pp 363–387

Ben Musa A, Smith CS: Neonatal effects of maternal clomipramine therapy (case report). Arch Dis Child 54:405, 1979

Biegor A, Reches A, Snyder L: Serotonergic and noradrenergic hormones. Life Sci 32:2015–2021, 1983

Brandt KR, Mackenzie TB: Obsessive compulsive disorder exacerbated during pregnancy: a case report. Int J Psychiatry Med 17:361–365, 1987

Buttolph ML, Holland AD: Obsessive compulsive disorders in pregnancy and childbirth, in Obsessive-Compulsive Disorders: Theory and Management. Edited by Jenike MA, Baer L, Minichiello WE. Chicago, IL, Year Book Medical, 1990, pp 89–97

Button JH, Reivich RS, Lawrence K: Obsessions of infanticide: a review of 42 cases. Arch Gen Psychiatry 27:235–240, 1972

Casas M, Alvarez E, Duro P, et al: Antiandrogenic treatment of obsessive-compulsive neurosis. Acta Psychiatr Scand 73:221–222, 1986

Cogill SR, Caplan HL, Alexandra H, et al: Impact of maternal depression on cognitive development of young children. BMJ 292:1165–1167, 1986

Cohen LS, Sichel DA, Dimmock JA, et al: Impact of pregnancy on panic disorder: a case series. J Clin Psychiatry 55:284–288, 1994a

Cohen LS, Sichel DA, Dimmock JA, et al: Postpartum course in women with preexisting panic disorder. J Clin Psychiatry 55:289–292, 1994b

Cowe L, Lloyd DJ, Dawling S: Neonatal convulsions caused by withdrawal from maternal clomipramine. BMJ 284:1837–1838, 1982

Davidson J, Robertson E: A follow-up study of postpartum illness, 1946–1978. Acta Psychiatr Scand 71:451–457, 1985

Eggermont E: Withdrawal symptoms associated with maternal imipramine therapy (case report). Lancet 2:680, 1973

Ehrenkranz JRL: Effects of sex steroids on serotonin uptake in blood platelets. Acta Endocrinol (Copenh) 83:420–428, 1976

Goldstein DJ: Effects of third trimester fluoxetine exposure on the newborn. J Clin Psychopharmacol 15:417–420, 1995

Gotlib IH, Whiffen VE, Mount JH, et al: Prevalence rates and demographic characteristics associated with depression in pregnancy and the postpartum. J Consult Clin Psychol 57:269–274, 1989

Guy W: ECDEU Assessment Manual for Psychopharmacology (DHEAW Publ No 76-338). Rockville, MD, National Institute of Mental Health, 1976

Hanna GL, McCracken JT, Cantwell DP: Prolactin in childhood OCD: clinical correlates and response to clomipramine. J Am Acad Child Adolesc Psychiatry 30:173–178, 1991

Ingram IM: Obsessional illness in mental hospital patients. J Ment Sci 107:382–402, 1961

Karno M, Goldin JM, Sorenson SB, et al: The epidemiology of OCD in five U.S. communities. Arch Gen Psychiatry 45:1094–1099, 1988

Kendell RE, McGuire RJ, Connor Y: Mood changes in the first 3 weeks after childbirth. J Affect Disord 3:317–326, 1981

Leckman JF, Goodman WK, North WG, et al: Elevated CSF levels of oxytocin in OCD. Arch Gen Psychiatry 51:782–792, 1994

Lipper S, Feigenbaum WM: Obsessive compulsive neurosis after viewing the fetus during therapeutic abortion. Am J Psychother 30:666–674, 1976

Lo WH: A follow-up study of obsessional neurotics in Hong Kong Chinese. Br J Psychiatry 113:823–832, 1967

Misri S, Sivertz K: Tricyclic drugs in pregnancy and lactation: a preliminary report. Int J Psychiatry Med 21:157–171, 1991

Murphy DL, Zohar J, Benkelfat MT, et al: OCD as a 5-HT subsystem–related behavioral disorder. Br J Psychiatry 155:15–24, 1989

Neziroglu F, Anemone R, Yaryara-Tobias JA: Onset of OCD in pregnancy. Am J Psychiatry 149:947–950, 1992

O'Hara MW: Social supports, life events and depression during pregnancy and the puerperium. Arch Gen Psychiatry 43:569–573, 1986

O'Hara MW, Zekoski EM, Philipps LK, et al: Controlled prospective study of postpartum mood disorders: comparison of childbearing and nonchildbearing women. J Abnorm Psychol 99:3–15, 1990

Paffenberg RA: Epidemiological aspects of mental illness associated with childbearing, in Motherhood and Mental Illness. Edited by Brockington IF, Kumar R. New York, Grune & Stratton, 1982, pp 19–36

Pastuszak A, Schick-Boschetto B, Zuber C, et al: Pregnancy outcome following first trimester exposure to fluoxetine (Prozac). JAMA 269:2246–2248, 1993

Pollitt J: Natural history of obsessional states: a study of 150 cases. BMJ 1:194–198, 1957

Rasmussen SA, Eisen JL: Phenomenology of OCD: clinical subtypes, heterogenicity and coexistence, in The Psychobiology of OCD. Edited by Zohar J, Insel T, Rasmussen S. New York, Springer, 1991, pp 13–43

Schimmell MS, Katz EZ, Shaag Y, et al: Toxic neonatal effects following maternal clomipramine therapy. Clin Toxicology 29:479–484, 1991

Shader RI: Does continuous use of fluoxetine during the first trimester of pregnancy present a high risk for malformation or abnormal development to the exposed fetus? J Clin Psychopharmacol 12:441, 1992

Shearer WT, Schreiner RL, Marshall RE: Urinary retention in a neonate secondary to maternal ingestion of nortriptyline. J Pediatr 81:570–572, 1972

Sichel DA, Cohen LS, Rosenbaum JF, et al: Postpartum onset of OCD. Psychosomatics 34:277–279, 1993a

Sichel DA, Cohen LS, Dimmock JA, et al: Postpartum OCD: a case series. J Clin Psychiatry 54:156–159, 1993b

Stein DJ, Hollander E, Simeon D, et al: Pregnancy and OCD. Am J Psychiatry 150:1131–1132, 1993

Stockert M, deRobertis E: Effect of ovariectomy and estrogen on [^{3}H]imipramine binding on different regions of the rat brain. Eur J Pharmacol 119:255–257, 1985

Swedo SE, Rapoport JL, Leonard H, et al: OCD in children and adolescents: clinical phenomenology of 70 consecutive cases. Arch Gen Psychiatry 46:335–341, 1989

Swedo SE, Leonard HL, Kruesi MJP, et al: CSF neurochemistry in children and adolescents with OCD. Arch Gen Psychiatry 49:29–36, 1992

Webster PAC: Withdrawal symptoms in neonates associated with maternal antidepressant therapy. Lancet 2:318–319, 1973

Weinstock LS, Cohen LS, Sichel DA, et al: Clonazepam use during pregnancy. Paper presented at the 149th Annual Meeting of the American Psychiatric Association, New York, NY, May 4–9, 1996

Zahle Ostergaard G, Pedersen SE: Neonatal effects of maternal clomipramine treatment. Pediatrics 69:233–234, 1982

Zuckerman B, Baucher H, Parker S, et al: Maternal depressive symptoms during pregnancy and newborn irritability. J Dev Behav Pediatr 11:190–194, 1990

Afterword to Section III

Michele T. Pato, M.D., and Gail Steketee, Ph.D.,
Section Editors

The diagnosis and treatment of obsessive-compulsive disorder (OCD) have come a long way in the past 20 years. OCD has gone from being a rare, untreatable illness to one that is understood to affect up to 2% of the population and that can be treated effectively—although not "cured"—from childhood through later life. However, there remain many gaps in our knowledge of the disorder, which, if filled, could play a critical role in improving treatment outcome and in identifying new methods for managing treatment-resistant and comorbid disorders. The most notable of these gaps is in our understanding of the etiology and pathophysiology of the disorder. However, new imaging techniques, genetic methods, and pharmacological probes not only promise an exciting future for investigating the causes of OCD, but also provide hope for treating individuals who are at risk for or who suffer from this debilitating illness.

IV

---

*Psychopharmacology
Across the Life Span*

IV

Psychopharmacology Across the Life Span

Contents

Section IV

Psychopharmacology Across the Life Span

Foreword

Susan L. McElroy, M.D., Section Editor

The psychopharmacological treatment of mental illness is a rapidly advancing area of medicine. An increasing number of psychiatric disorders in persons of all age groups have been found to be amenable to treatment with psychotropic medications. The number of agents effective in disorders with established medical treatments is also increasing. Thus, serotonin reuptake inhibitors may reduce obsessive-compulsive symptoms in autism, cholinergic agents may improve cognitive function in Alzheimer's disease, a growing number of antiepileptic drugs may be effective in bipolar disorder, and an increasing number of atypical antipsychotics are available for schizophrenia.

It has also been increasingly recognized that many psychiatric disorders amenable to psychopharmacological treatment are lifelong illnesses that persist and often progress over time and that effective lifelong psychopharmacological treatment may reduce symptoms as well as illness progression. Although some of these disorders tend to begin later in life (e.g., dementia, delusional disorder), many others begin in childhood, adolescence, and/or early adulthood (e.g., attention-deficit/hyperactivity disorder, mood disorders, and schizophrenia). It is therefore imperative that these illnesses be recognized as early in the life cycle as possible so that appropriate psychopharmacological treatment can be instituted and maintained.

In this section, the psychopharmacological treatment of mental illness across the life span, from childhood through old age, is addressed. The section begins with three chapters addressing the presentation and lifelong psychopharmacological treatment of three disorders that extend over the entire life span. In Chapter 16, Drs. Keck and Strakowski discuss the psychopharmacological treatment of psychotic disorders. In Chapter 17, Dr. Weller and I discuss the psychopharmacological treatment of bipolar disorder from childhood through old age. We also review preliminary data suggesting that some new antiepileptic drugs (e.g., lamotrigine and gabapentin) and atypical antipsychotics (especially clozapine) may have mood-stabilizing effects. In Chapter 18, Drs.

Spencer, Biederman, and Wilens discuss the many psychopharmacological treatments for children, adolescents, and adults with attention-deficit/hyperactivity disorder.

The last two chapters provide overviews of childhood, adolescent, and geriatric psychopharmacology. In Chapter 19, Dr. West reviews the psychopharmacological treatment of depressive and anxiety disorders in children and adolescents. In Chapter 20, Drs. Satlin and Wasserman review important principles regarding use of psychotropic agents in elderly patients, as well as the psychopharmacological treatment of depression, anxiety, psychosis, delirium, dementia, and sleep disorders in elders.

Chapter 16

Psychopharmacological Treatment of Psychotic Disorders Across the Life Span

Paul E. Keck, Jr., M.D., and Stephen M. Strakowski, M.D.

The psychopharmacological treatment of the DSM-IV (American Psychiatric Association 1994) psychotic disorders is well established for schizophrenia but is remarkably understudied for schizoaffective disorder, delusional disorder, brief psychotic disorder and shared psychotic disorder (Buckley and Meltzer 1995; Csernansky and Newcomer 1994; Janicak et al. 1993; Wirshing et al. 1994). Although the effectiveness of antipsychotics in adult patients with schizophrenia has been shown in more than 100 double-blind, randomized clinical trials (Davis et al. 1987), there are few such studies in adolescent or geriatric patients and none in children (Campbell and Spencer 1988). Furthermore, children, adolescents and older persons, compared with adults, respond to psychotropic medications in some distinctive ways that have implications for both efficacy and safety. In this chapter we review the available evidence supporting the psychopharmacological treatment of the DSM-IV psychotic disorders in children, adolescent, adult, and older patients with these illnesses.

Schizophrenia

Acute Treatment

Adults.   The goal of pharmacological treatment of an acute exacerbation of psychotic symptoms in patients with schizophrenia is to alleviate positive symptoms such as delusions, hallucinations, formal thought disorder, and agitation. However, an increase in negative symptoms, such as affective flattening, alogia, and avolition, may also occur during an acute exacerbation of psychosis. Several different chemical classes of antipsychotic drugs are available in the United States for the treatment of schizophrenia. With the exception of clozapine (Kane et al. 1988), there are no convincing data that any one drug or class of drugs is more effective than any other (Wirshing et al. 1994). Although all the available antipsychotic drugs reduce positive symptoms of psychosis, only clozapine (Kane et al. 1988) and risperidone (Marder and Meibach 1994) have been shown to have greater efficacy compared with other antipsychotics in reducing negative symptoms. Of note, placebo-controlled, double-blind studies of the new atypical antipsychotics—olanzapine, sertindole, and quetiapine—suggest that these agents may also have superior efficacy compared with standard antipsychotics in the reduction of negative symptoms (Beasley et al. 1996; Borison et al. 1996; van Kammen et al. 1996).

Because all standard antipsychotics are comparable in efficacy for the treatment of adult patients with schizophrenia, the most important clinical decisions about treatment involve drug choice, usually made on the basis of differences in side effects and dose (Janicak et al. 1993; Wirshing et al. 1994). In general, in comparison with high-potency antipsychotics (e.g., haloperidol, fluphenazine), low-potency agents (e.g., chlorpromazine, thioridazine) are associated with greater sedation and anticholinergic and cardiovascular side effects but fewer extrapyramidal side effects (EPS) (Buckley and Meltzer 1995). Thus, the choice of which standard antipsychotic to use for a given patient is usually based on deciding which side effects would be least harmful or most beneficial.

In recent years, a number of studies have examined the efficacy and safety of antipsychotics at different dosage ranges (Levinson et al. 1990; McEvoy et al. 1991; Rifkin et al. 1991; Van Putten et al. 1992).

In the first study, Levinson et al. (1990) compared 10, 20, and 30 mg/day of fluphenazine in 53 patients with acute exacerbations of schizophrenia or schizoaffective disorder. After 4 weeks of treatment, there was no significant difference in improvement among the three groups. However, among patients displaying greater than 40% improvement in positive symptoms, doses of 0.3 mg/kg/day were associated with the greatest improvement but also with a higher incidence of EPS.

Rifkin et al. (1991) treated 87 patients who had acute exacerbations of schizophrenia with 10, 30, or 80 mg/day of haloperidol for 6 weeks. In contrast to the method in the study by Levinson et al. (1990), in which patients received antiparkinsonian medications on a prn basis, Rifkin et al. administered benztropine prophylactically to all subjects. There were no significant differences in treatment response or EPS (probably because of the prophylactic benztropine) between the three groups. Thus, in this study, no advantage was found in treating patients with haloperidol at dosages greater than 10 mg/day.

McEvoy et al. (1991) used the neuroleptic threshold hypothesis (Haase 1961)—that the lowest antipsychotic dose producing EPS corresponds to the lowest dose producing maximal therapeutic effect—to determine optimal doses for 106 patients with acute exacerbations of schizophrenia or schizoaffective disorder. In this design, patients received 2 mg/day of haloperidol in titration and typically reached neuroleptic threshold by 10–12 days; nearly all patients displayed EPS at 10 mg/day. After reaching the neuroleptic threshold dose, patients were maintained at this dosage for 14 days, then randomized to receive the same dosage or a dosage increased from twofold to tenfold. At the completion of the double-blind comparison, there was no difference in response rates between the neuroleptic-threshold groups and the higher-dose comparison groups. The latter groups, however, displayed higher rates of EPS. Thus McEvoy et al. found comparable efficacy but greater tolerability for lower haloperidol doses.

Finally, Van Putten et al. (1992) treated 80 male patients with acute schizophrenia on an open-label basis with 5, 10, or 20 mg/day of halo-peridol for 4 weeks. The group receiving 20 mg/day showed a greater response rate by 2 weeks of treatment but also had a higher dropout rate, a higher incidence of akinesia and akathisia, and a worsening of emotional withdrawal and psychomotor retardation.

Overall, the results of these studies suggest that doses below 15–20 mg/day of haloperidol or fluphenazine are adequate for most patients, especially those without a history of treatment refractoriness to anti-psychotics. These studies also suggest that even at these doses, EPS are likely to occur and should be treated prophylactically (Wirshing et al. 1994).

Although standard antipsychotics have been the mainstay of the acute treatment of patients with schizophrenia for more than 35 years, a number of new, atypical antipsychotics will soon be available. The available evidence from double-blind, randomized, controlled trials suggests that these new medications have a low incidence of neurolog-ical side effects and may have greater efficacy in the treatment of nega-tive symptoms than do standard agents (Beasley et al. 1996; Borison et al. 1996; van Kammen et al. 1996). These new medications should offer substantial advantages in safety and efficacy compared with standard antipsychotics for patients with schizophrenia.

Children and adolescents.   Schizophrenia beginning in childhood or early adolescence has been the subject of rigorous scientific study only recently (Campbell and Cueva 1995). The presentation of schizophre-nia in childhood is rare: estimates indicate that only 0.1%–1.0% of pa-tients with schizophrenia have an age less than 10 at onset, and 4% less than 15 (Remschmidt et al. 1994). According to DSM-IV, the diagnosis of schizophrenia in children is made according to adult criteria. The preliminary results of the first placebo-controlled trial of antipsychotic treatment in children (ages 5.5–11.75 years) with schizophrenia have only recently been reported (Spencer et al. 1992). In this crossover study, haloperidol at a dosage of 0.5–3.5 mg/day (0.02–0.12 mg/kg/day) was superior to placebo in ameliorating delusions of reference and persecution, thought disorder, and hallucinations. Haloperidol treatment was also associated with a significant decrease in the total pathology scores on the Brief Psychiatric Rating Scale for Children (BPRS-C) (Spencer et al. 1992) compared with placebo. Furthermore, 9 of 12 children (75%) displayed a marked response while receiving haloperidol, compared with none while receiving placebo. Two children (16.7%) experienced acute dystonic reactions. In an earlier controlled study, Campbell et al. (1972) compared chlorpromazine with lithium in 10 severely disturbed hyperactive children, 6 of whom were diagnosed with schizophrenia. All 6 children responded to treatment with chlorpromazine, but only 1 was classified as displaying a marked response.

Two controlled trials have assessed the efficacy and safety of standard antipsychotics in adolescents with schizophrenia. In a 4-week, double-blind study of loxapine, haloperidol, and placebo in 75 adolescents with schizophrenia, these antipsychotic agents were comparable in efficacy and superior to placebo in reducing psychotic symptoms (Pool et al. 1976). However, EPS were common, occurring in 73% of patients receiving loxapine and 80% of patients receiving haloperidol. In the second study, whose subjects were 21 adolescent patients with schizophrenia, thiothixene was compared with thioridazine without a placebo control group (Realmuto et al. 1984). As measured by the BPRS and the Clinical Global Impression (CGI), both agents produced significant improvement. However, sedation was a common and clinically significant side effect with both agents.

Preliminary results of an ongoing double-blind study of haloperidol and clozapine in adolescents with treatment-refractory schizophrenia were also reported (Gordon et al. 1994). All eight patients randomized to clozapine and an additional four patients treated on an open basis (Frazier et al. 1994) displayed marked reductions in symptoms as measured by total BPRS scores. Two open trials of clozapine in adolescents with treatment-refractory schizophrenia have also been reported (Remschmidt et al. 1994; Siefen and Remschmidt 1986). In the first study, 11 of 21 patients (52%) displayed marked improvement with clozapine treatment (average maintenance dose, 415 mg/day; average follow-up, 4.4 months). In the second study, 31 of 41 adolescents (76%) with treatment-refractory schizophrenia displayed marked with clozapine; 3 (7%) had complete remission of symptoms. However, in 7 patients (17%), clozapine side effects required discontinuation of treatment. Overall, the results of these initial studies suggest that clozapine is a useful treatment for children and adolescents with treatment-refractory schizophrenia.

Risperidone, the first of a new class of atypical antipsychotics that block dopamine$_2$ receptors and serotonin$_2$ (5-HT$_2$) receptors, has been reported to be effective in the treatment of adolescent schizophrenia

(Cozza and Edison 1994) and childhood schizophrenia (Sternlicht and Wells 1995). These preliminary reports require confirmation in controlled trials. However, because of initial evidence that risperidone may have greater efficacy in the treatment of negative symptoms of schizophrenia and has a lower incidence of EPS compared with standard antipsychotics (Chouinard et al. 1993; Marder and Meibach 1994), risperidone may be a better-tolerated and more efficacious treatment for some patients with childhood or adolescent schizophrenia. The availability of new antipsychotics such as olanzapine, sertindole, quetiapine and ziprasidone in the near future should also expand the pharmacological options available for the treatment of schizophrenia in children and adolescents.

In comparison to adults, children and adolescents respond to antipsychotic medications in a number of different ways that have implications for both dosing strategies and safety (Vitiello and Jensen 1995). First, acute dystonic reactions occur more frequently in children and adolescents (Keepers and Casey 1987). Second, neuroleptic-withdrawal dyskinesias are more common in children (Campbell et al. 1988). This risk was recently reported to be greater in children with a history of pre- and perinatal complications (Armenteros et al. 1995). Third, akathisia appears to occur less commonly in younger patients (Keepers et al. 1983). Children and younger adolescents also have a greater body-weight–adjusted liver mass than adults. This greater mass results in a higher body clearance and a shorter elimination half-life for antipsychotic medications metabolized by the liver (Vitiello and Jensen 1995). This explains why higher weight-adjusted doses are sometimes needed in children in order to achieve the same response as in adults. Morselli et al. (1983) reported that steady-state haloperidol plasma concentrations in children varied up to 15-fold at a given mg/kg/day dose, but that intraindividual variance between dose and plasma concentration was minimal. In this study, as anticipated, most children had shorter haloperidol elimination half-lives than did adolescents and adults. However, Morselli et al. (1983) observed that these patients did not require proportionally higher doses, because they both responded to, and experienced side effects from, lower plasma haloperidol concentrations than did older adolescents and adults.

Older patients. An Epidemiologic Catchment Area study (Keith et al. 1991) reported a 1-year prevalence rate of schizophrenia of 0.2% and a lifetime prevalence rate of 0.3% in persons older than 65 years, with no significant racial or gender differences in this distribution. Why these rates were lower than in younger groups is not clear. However, it is likely that as the population ages, these percentages will increase. A limitation of this study is that it restricted the diagnosis of schizophrenia to people whose illness began prior to age 45—consistent with the

DSM-III (American Psychiatric Association 1980) criteria in use at that time—thereby eliminating late-onset cases. The incidence of new-onset cases in the geriatric population, then, remains essentially unknown. In the ECA study, nearly 95% of patients experienced the onset of illness before age 40; in another report, Lacro et al. (1993) observed that more than 90% of elderly patients with schizophrenia experienced the onset of the illness before age 45. Thus, when the treatment of schizophrenia in geriatric populations is discussed, it usually involves the management of a long-standing, established disorder rather than a new-onset illness.

Antipsychotic medication is the backbone of pharmacological management of schizophrenia in the elderly, as it is for younger patients. However, a number of concerns unique to elderly patients should be considered when instituting and maintaining pharmacological treatment. These include differences between elderly and younger patients in course of illness, prominent symptoms, drug metabolism and response, and drug side effects.

Historically, since the time of Kraepelin, it has been generally assumed that the course of schizophrenia was one of unrelenting, progressive deterioration. This suggests that elderly patients are more symptomatic, more impaired, and, perhaps, require more pharmacological intervention than their younger counterparts. Recent studies have challenged this assumption. Manfred Bleuler (1968; 1979) studied 208 patients between 55 and 69 years of age and observed that the majority experienced substantial improvement in function and symptomatology as they aged. Harding et al. (1987) reported that 56 (68%) of 82 patients with DSM-III schizophrenia exhibited no symptoms of schizophrenia 20–25 years after release from state hospital back wards. Ciompi (1980) evaluated 289 patients, aged 65–97 years, diagnosed with schizophrenia 30–40 years previously, and noted that 62% of the original presenting symptoms had disappeared and 49% of the patients had a "favorable outcome." Negative symptoms tended to predominate in these older patients. Finally, Winokur et al. (1987) examined 17 patients from the Iowa 500, who had been hospitalized between 1935 and 1945 and had reached age 60 or older. They observed that these patients were considerably less likely to exhibit persecutory delusions or auditory hallucinations than were younger patients but that problems with orientation, memory, and negative symptoms were common.

Taken together, these studies suggest that schizophrenia is not necessarily chronically deteriorating and that elderly patients with schizophrenia are often less functionally impaired and less likely to exhibit active, positive psychotic symptoms than younger patients. Indeed, in many elderly patients, the positive symptoms of schizophrenia seem to remit. Nonetheless, elderly patients often continue to exhibit prominent negative symptoms. These observations suggest that, compared with younger patients, elderly patients with schizophrenia may preferentially benefit from pharmacological agents that are effective in the treatment of negative symptoms and that they may be more likely to benefit from trials of being withdrawn from antipsychotic agents. This topic will be discussed in more detail later in this section.

Relatively few studies have examined whether antipsychotic medication has similar efficacy in elderly patients and in young adults. Honigfeld et al. (1965) investigated the role of phenothiazines in 308 men ages 54–74 who had schizophrenia. In a 24-week, double-blind, placebo-controlled study, Honigfeld et al. observed that acetophenazine and trifluoperazine were significantly more effective than placebo in the amelioration of psychosis. Tsuang et al. (1971) compared haloperidol to thioridazine in 50 geriatric patients with psychosis, the majority of whom had schizophrenia, and observed marked improvement in psychosis for both medication groups. Branchey et al. (1978) compared fluphenazine to thioridazine in chronic schizophrenia in patients ages 60–81 and observed modest improvement in BPRS ratings. Madhussodanan et al. (1995) reported a case series of 11 geriatric patients (6 of whom had schizophrenia) who received risperidone treatment for psychosis. Of these, 8 (73%) tolerated risperidone up to 3 mg bid and exhibited a positive treatment response. Berman et al. (1996) gave 10 elderly patients (ages 66–81) with schizophrenia dosages of 4–6 mg/day of risperidone for 7 days after a 1- to 7-day washout. Eight of the patients continued risperidone in an open-ended extension. Patients showed significant improvement in overall symptom ratings and negative symptom ratings after a mean of 4 weeks of taking risperidone. There were no significant adverse events during this trial. Finally, Jeste et al. (1993) reviewed a number of uncontrolled studies of elderly patients with psychosis and observed that most of these demonstrated a positive outcome to antipsychotic medication. Nevertheless, there is a general lack of recent double-blind, placebo-controlled studies of antipsychotic medications in geriatric patients who have been diagnosed with schizophrenia by modern criteria and techniques. This lack leaves the issue of treatment efficacy in this population uncertain.

In addition to current age, the age at onset of the schizophrenic disorder may influence the treatment of elderly patients. Specifically, Pearlson et al. (1989) compared 54 elderly patients who had late-onset (after age 45 years) schizophrenia to 22 elderly patients who had schizophrenia beginning before age 45 and to 54 young adult patients. Persecutory delusions were more common in the late-onset group than in the other two groups, with less affective flattening and less thought disorder. Hallucinations were also common in these late-onset patients. Response to standard neuroleptic therapy in these late-onset patients was good: 48% exhibited complete remission, and an additional 28%

experienced partial remission. Rabins et al. (1984) also reported that 30 (86%) of 35 late-onset patients improved while taking neuroleptics. In contrast to elderly patients with early-onset schizophrenia, late-onset patients may exhibit fewer negative symptoms and more positive psychotic symptoms—in particular, persecutory delusions and hallucinations. Like other patient groups with schizophrenia, this patient group appears to exhibit good response to antipsychotic medication, although controlled data are lacking.

In addition to these considerations related directly to schizophrenia in geriatric patients, a number of treatment considerations for general geriatric patients also apply to this schizophrenic population. First, there are a number of age-related changes in pharmacokinetics and pharmacodynamics that influence the treatment of elderly patients with schizophrenia. Increasing age is associated with an increased body-fat-to-muscle ratio, a decrease in plasma albumin, a decrease in hepatic metabolism (particularly demethylation and hydroxylation), a decrease in nigrostriatal dopamine, and a decrease in central nervous system (CNS) cholinergic function, all of which may alter the metabolism or action of antipsychotic drugs (Salzman 1982). Specifically, the increase in the fat-to-muscle ratio may prolong drug clearance, because all antipsychotic agents are highly lipophilic. It is unclear, however, whether this has any meaningful clinical effect in geriatric patients (Zaleon and Guthrie 1994). The decrease in plasma albumin and in hepatic metabolism may both contribute to increased plasma levels of some antipsychotic agents. The CNS changes in dopaminergic and cholinergic function contribute to an increased risk of extrapyramidal and anticholinergic side effects, respectively. Together, these age-related physiological changes result in an increased risk of drug toxicity in elderly patients taking antipsychotic doses that are well tolerated in younger patients. In particular, the frequency and severity of sedation, orthostatic hypotension, anticholinergic symptoms (especially anticholinergic delirium), and marked extrapyramidal symptoms are increased (Salzman 1982). These side effects can have a significant effect on the safety and outcome of antipsychotic trials in elderly patients.

Although the sedating effects of antipsychotic agents may be useful at times in calming agitated elderly patients or patients with insomnia, daytime sedation can impair function and aggravate nighttime insomnia. Moreover, sedation may increase confusion and disorientation in some patients, leading to increased agitation (Salzman 1982). Unfortunately, this increased agitation may be clinically interpreted as worsening psychosis, leading to an increase in the antipsychotic dose and thereby further compounding the problem and ultimately leading to delirium in some patients (Salzman 1982). This problem is further compounded when patients are taking other sedating medications (Sargenti et al. 1988).

Orthostatic hypotension is a very common medication side effect in the elderly, affecting up to 25% of older patients receiving medication therapy (Rosen et al. 1990). Blumenthal and Davie (1980) studied 100 geriatric psychiatric outpatients for orthostatic hypotension, dizziness, and falling. In these patients, a phenothiazine was prescribed for 42%. The combination of a phenothiazine or a tricyclic antidepressant (TCA) together or with other drugs was strongly associated with a systolic blood pressure drop of almost 20 mm Hg, and there was a strong correlation between the use of these drugs and the development of dizziness or falling.

Many of the antipsychotic agents, particularly low-potency drugs, produce anticholinergic side effects. In elderly patients in whom drug clearance may be slowed and the overall CNS cholinergic activity decreased, there is a significant risk of anticholinergic complications. Peripheral anticholinergic side effects, such as dry mouth, constipation, blurred vision, and urinary retention can be uncomfortable and annoying, although not typically life-threatening. However, dry mouth, causing increased water ingestion, coupled with the use of a diuretic, could impair free water excretion, thereby leading to water intoxication (Raskind and Eisdorfer 1976; Salzman 1982). More important, elderly patients are at higher risk for CNS anticholinergic toxicity than are young patients. Anticholinergic delirium can cause symptoms such as agitation, disorientation, confusion, hallucinations, and paranoia, which may be mistaken for worsening psychosis, again resulting in a vicious circle wherein more antipsychotic is prescribed to treat the presumed worsening psychosis, thereby worsening the delirium. Elderly patients taking multiple anticholinergic medications are at particular risk (Zaleon and Guthrie 1994), and although low-potency agents are more likely to cause anticholinergic side effects, the combination of a high-potency neuroleptic with an anticholinergic antiparkinsonian drug appears to present an even higher anticholinergic risk than do low doses of low-potency agents (Eimer 1992).

In elderly patients being treated with antipsychotic agents, EPS occur commonly (Kalish et al. 1995). Petrie et al. (1982) reported a 38% rate of EPS in elderly patients receiving loxapine, and previous studies have reported rates of EPS up to 50% (Hamilton 1966). In contrast to the situation in younger patients, neuroleptic-induced dystonias in elderly patients are relatively rare (Zaleon and Guthrie 1994). Instead, elderly patients frequently experience parkinsonism and akathisia (Salzman 1982; Zaleon and Guthrie 1994). Drug-induced parkinsonism can present diagnostic ambiguities as it mimics idiopathic Parkinson's disease, and patients' masklike faces, immobility, and motor retardation can be confused with depression (Rifkin et al. 1975). The latter can lead to prescription of antidepressant agents that may further confound the clinical picture as a result of additive anticholinergic side effects or drug-drug interactions.

Moreover, treatment for parkinsonism typically involves anticholinergic agents, which themselves increase the risk of anticholinergic syndromes, as previously noted. In fact, it is probably advisable to avoid anticholinergic antiparkinsonian agents in elderly patients. Instead, this side effect should be managed with dose reduction, a switch to a lower-potency drug, or perhaps amantadine. Akathisia is also common in the elderly (Ayd 1978; Ganzini et al. 1991; Sandyk and Kay 1990) and may be confused with worsening psychosis, leading, again, to increased antipsychotic medication and increased risk of neuroleptic toxicity. The only proven effective treatment for akathisia is decreased dosing or drug discontinuation. Other compounds, such as β-blockers (Ryan 1991), benzodiazepines (Michels and Marzuk 1993), anticholinergic agents (Eimer 1992), and amantadine (Ryan 1991), may also treat this bothersome side effect, but all these interventions can produce additional side effects (e.g., anticholinergic toxicity, orthostatic hypotension) that can be problematic in elderly patients.

Tardive dyskinesia (TD) occurs more commonly in elderly than in younger patients with schizophrenia (Jeste and Wyatt 1982). Saltz et al. (1991) observed a 31% incidence of TD following 43 weeks of treatment with neuroleptics in 160 elderly patients (mean age of 77 years). Recently, Jeste et al. (1993) reported a longitudinal study of the development of TD in 48 patients over age 45 who had schizophrenia and who were receiving low doses of neuroleptics (< 300 mg/day of chlorpromazine equivalents). Approximately one-quarter of these patients developed TD during a 12-month follow-up period. No effective treatment for TD has yet been identified, although most patients experience resolution of TD symptoms following drug discontinuation (Lacro et al. 1994). There is some evidence that clozapine may also improve TD (Lieberman et al. 1991), although whether this is true in geriatric patients is unknown.

Finally, elderly patients are the most common users of psychotropic medication (Sargenti et al. 1988) and are frequently prescribed multiple-medication regimens, which, for example, have been estimated to adversely affect 23%–52% of nursing home patients (Lamy 1986; Richelson 1984). Because of this, elderly patients are at particular risk of drug-drug interactions when taking antipsychotic medications. This topic has been reviewed previously (Sargenti et al. 1988), but a few common interactions are discussed here.

First, the sedative properties of, particularly, the low-potency neuroleptics can be potentiated by the addition of other sedating drugs, such as benzodiazepines or TCAs. This combination can contribute to the problems associated with sedation in this patient population discussed previously. Drugs with hypotensive action, such as β-blockers and calcium-channel blockers, magnify the orthostatic properties of neuroleptic agents. These combinations place elderly patients at higher risk of dizziness and falls. Anticholinergic compounds can produce significant side effects when given in conjunction with antipsychotic agents by additively increasing anticholinergic effects. Moreover, there have been studies suggesting that anticholinergic agents may inhibit antipsychotic efficacy, although these data are conflicting (Sargenti et al. 1988). Finally, a number of compounds that inhibit hepatic cytochrome P450 enzyme systems (e.g., selective serotonin reuptake inhibitor [SSRI] antidepressants, carbamazepine) may alter antipsychotic drug levels and may result in neuroleptic toxicity or loss of efficacy (Arana et al. 1986; Jan et al. 1985; Nemeroff et al. 1996). When adding neuroleptics to an existing drug regimen or when adding new medications for elderly patients already taking neuroleptics, caution must be exercised to prevent untoward pharmacokinetic and pharmacodynamic drug interactions.

It is clear that there is a significant lack of research analyzing treatment approaches to elderly patients with schizophrenia (Jeste et al. 1993). Nonetheless, from the previous considerations, a number of general guidelines are suggested.

First, because it appears from long-term outcome studies that the severity of psychotic symptoms in many patients with schizophrenia diminishes as they age, some of these patients may tolerate or even benefit from reduction in or withdrawal of antipsychotic medication. Jeste et al. (1993), in their review of the literature of neuroleptic withdrawal in elderly patients (over the age of 45) who had schizophrenia, identified only six papers addressing the issue. Nonetheless, their summary analysis demonstrated that the mean rate of relapse for neuroleptic-withdrawn patients was 40%, in contrast with 11% for neuroleptic-maintained patients. However, some of these reviewed studies found that younger age was associated with relapse (Hershon et al. 1972; Rassidakis et al. 1970; Ruskin and Nyman 1991); the relative risk of relapse in older patients, particularly in those over 65 years old, remains understudied. Jeste et al. (1993) examined short-term neuroleptic withdrawal, involving a 7-day taper followed by 2 weeks of placebo, which did not produce significant clinical changes in a sample of 20 patients with schizophrenia. They also observed no differences in changes in symptoms between patients who were older than 45 versus those younger than 45. This study, however, was limited by small patient numbers and the short period of neuroleptic withdrawal. Longer-term, prospective studies of the risks and benefits of neuroleptic withdrawal in stable geriatric patients with schizophrenia are clearly indicated, given the risk of TD and side effects that these patients experience with continued use of antipsychotics.

A second consideration in the treatment of elderly patients with schizophrenia is that, although many have a diminution in positive symptoms, they frequently continue to exhibit marked negative symptoms. As noted previously, this suggests that elderly patients might benefit from treatment that more specifically targets negative symptoms. Typical antipsychotic agents are relatively ineffective for alleviating negative symptoms, and the EPS produced by these drugs may mimic negative symptoms (Csernansky and Newcomer 1994). Recent evidence suggests that atypical agents, such as risperidone and clozapine, may be more effective for the treatment of negative symptoms, with a concurrent lower risk for EPS (Kane et al. 1988; Marder and Meibach 1994). Some elderly patients with schizophrenia, then, might benefit by changing treatment from typical to atypical antipsychotic agents. This is further supported by the presumed lower risk of TD with these agents. However, clozapine has a number of other side-effect risks that can be problematic in elderly patients—particularly orthostatic hypotension, anticholinergic effects, seizures, and agranulocytosis. Thus, it should be administered cautiously in this patient population. A number of new pharmacological agents that should be available in the next few years (e.g., olanzapine, ziprasidone, quetiapine, and sertindole) appear to have favorable side-effect profiles, with significant alleviation of both negative and positive symptoms in patients with schizophrenia (Beasley et al. 1996; Borison et al. 1996; van Kammen et al. 1996). Whether these drugs will have a unique role in the management of elderly patients, however, remains to be seen.

Finally, because geriatric patients are particularly prone to side effects, treatment with antipsychotic medication should be carefully tailored to the individual patient. Low starting doses are recommended for patients older than 65, corresponding to 0.25–0.5 mg/day of haloperidol or its equivalent (Zaleon and Guthrie 1994). These dosages should be adjusted slowly, allowing adequate time for full drug effect (i.e., development of therapeutic and adverse effects). Typically, this involves waiting at least 1–2 weeks, when possible, between dose increases. Agents with low anticholinergic activity are probably preferable, although, because these same drugs are typically potent dopamine antagonists, the risk of developing EPS requires vigilant monitoring. When patients respond to antipsychotic treatment with worsening agitation, confusion, or changes in mental status, strong consideration should be given to the possibility of drug-induced toxicity or side effects (e.g., anticholinergic delirium, akathisia) as the primary cause of clinical change, suggesting the need for dosage reduction. Finally, the use of concomitant agents to treat side effects should be avoided, whenever possible, by instead lowering the dose of the original offending agent. With careful use, however, antipsychotic agents still remain the primary treatment for elderly patients with schizophrenia.

Maintenance Treatment

Maintenance antipsychotic treatment is required for most patients with schizophrenia, because schizophrenia is a chronic illness and exacerbations of psychotic symptoms are associated with substantial morbidity and mortality. The primary goals of maintenance antipsychotic treatment in patients with schizophrenia are to prevent relapse and improve quality of life and functioning, with minimal side effects (Csernansky and Newcomer 1994). The efficacy of antipsychotics in preventing relapse has been well established by at least 35 randomized, double-blind, placebo-controlled studies (Janicak et al. 1993). In these studies, more than 50% of patients treated with placebo relapsed within 6 months, compared with 20% of patients treated with antipsychotic medications (Davis 1985).

A number of recent studies have examined the efficacy of varying antipsychotic maintenance-dosage strategies (Hogarty et al. 1988; Kane et al. 1983, 1993; Marder et al. 1987; Schooler 1991). The results of these studies suggest that minimum effective doses for the two commonly used depot antipsychotics are 50 mg every 4 weeks for haloperidol decanoate and 5–10 mg every 2 weeks for fluphenazine decanoate. However, antipsychotic maintenance-dose treatment requires individual adjustment, because some patients may have lower relapse rates at higher dosages.

As with most chronic medical illnesses, treatment compliance greatly affects relapse prevention in schizophrenia. Characteristics of the illness (e.g., impaired insight, thought disorder, and delusional ideation) and neurological side effects (Van Putten 1974, Van Putten et al. 1976) both contribute to noncompliance.

Use of depot neuroleptics and minimization of side effects significantly enhance compliance. Strategies for minimizing side effects include using the lowest effective maintenance antipsychotic dose; specific treatment interventions, such as anticholinergic agents for EPS and β-blockers for akathisia; and consideration of newer antipsychotic medications (e.g., risperidone, clozapine), which have a lower incidence and severity of neurological side effects. Minimizing antipsychotic side effects is important—in order not only to enhance compliance, but also to improve quality of life, reduce dysphoria, and prevent secondary negative symptoms from EPS and psychic akinesia (Csernansky and Newcomer 1994).

As discussed previously, standard antipsychotics have their greatest effect on reducing positive symptoms. There is increasing evidence that atypical antipsychotics may have greater efficacy than standard agents in the treatment of negative symptoms. Improvement in negative symptoms, in turn, may be associated with improved quality of life. In one of few available long-term studies, Meltzer et al. (1990) reported improvement in deficits in social, vocational, and interpersonal functioning in an open study of outpatients with schizophrenia treated with clozapine for 6 months. Although no data regarding the long-term effects on negative symptoms of risperidone or other new antipsychotics are available, these agents may be more effective than standard antipsychotics. Finally, adjunctive psychosocial approaches to pharmacological treatment may also decrease negative symptoms and enhance quality of life in patients with schizophrenia (Liberman et al. 1986).

There are no controlled studies of maintenance antipsychotic treatment of patients with childhood, adolescent, or geriatric schizophrenia. Treatment approaches for these patients are thus adapted from data in adult patients, but further research in this area is greatly needed (Campbell and Cueva 1995; Green 1995; Rosenberg et al. 1994).

Schizoaffective Disorder

Acute Treatment

Adults. In contrast to the extensive research done on the pharmacological treatment of schizophrenia, there are few controlled studies of the pharmacological treatment of schizoaffective disorder. Only 13 controlled studies have examined standard antipsychotics, lithium, or antidepressants in the acute treatment of patients with schizoaffective disorder (reviewed in Keck et al. 1994). Several impressions emerge from these studies. First, the total number of patients with schizoaffective disorder studied in controlled treatment trials is strikingly small ($N = 292$). Second, the number of patients studied cannot be pooled because of differences in operational criteria used to define the disorder and in study design. None of these 13 studies used modern diagnostic criteria to define schizoaffective disorder; indeed, the most recent study was published in 1984 (Goodnick and Meltzer 1984). Third, all studies examined the efficacy of thymoleptic agents (primarily lithium), working from the assumption that standard antipsychotic medications were devoid of significant thymoleptic properties.

Eight studies compared lithium with standard antipsychotic agents (Bigelow et al. 1981; Braden et al. 1982; Brockington et al. 1978; Goodnick and Meltzer 1984); Johnson et al. 1968, 1971; Prien et al. 1972; Shopsin et al. 1971). Three of these also compared these treatments with combination treatment (Bigelow et al. 1981; Brockington et al. 1978; Goodnick and Meltzer 1984). Overall, in patients with schizoaffective disorder displaying manic symptoms, these studies found no significant difference in response to lithium compared with response to antipsychotics. However, studies examining the efficacy of combination treatment generally found this treatment superior to lithium or antipsychotics alone (Keck et al. 1994). Notably, only one study (Brockington et al. 1978) examined the acute treatment of patients with schizoaffective disorder with depression. In this study, response to treatment with amitriptyline, chlorpromazine, or both was poor, with no significant differences between treatment groups.

Five studies comparing thymoleptic agents with placebo as adjunctive treatment to ongoing antipsychotic medication provided further support for the combined use of thymoleptics and antipsychotics in patients with schizoaffective disorder (Biederman et al. 1979; Carman et al. 1981; Growe et al. 1979; Prusoff et al. 1979; Small et al. 1975). In four of these five studies, combined thymoleptic and antipsychotic treatment was superior to placebo added to antipsychotics (Biederman et al. 1979; Carman et al. 1981; Prusoff et al. 1979; Small et al. 1975).

In summary, controlled studies of the acute treatment of patients with schizoaffective disorder, using diagnostic criteria that resemble modern criteria, are limited by the small number of patients studied. Their findings must therefore be considered preliminary. These studies suggested that for schizoaffective disorder, bipolar type (manic), lithium and antipsychotics produced comparable but incomplete amelioration of both affective and psychotic symptoms and that the combination of lithium and antipsychotics may be superior to monotherapy with either agent (Keck et al. 1994). In the only controlled study of patients with schizoaffective disorder, depressive type, the presumed superiority of combined antipsychotic and antidepressant treatment to antipsychotic agents alone was not proved (Brockington et al. 1978).

The antiepileptic and mood-stabilizing agent carbamazepine has also been studied in two controlled trials in patients with schizoaffective disorder. Okuma et al. (1989) found modest benefit when carbamazepine was added to antipsychotics. Placidi et al. (1986) reported a trend toward greater improvement with lithium than with carbamazepine in a cohort of schizoaffective and bipolar patients, but they did not separately report the response of the schizoaffective patients. There are no controlled studies of valproate in the treatment of patients with schizoaffective disorder, but one retrospective report suggested beneficial effects in some patients (McElroy et al. 1987). Thus, in contrast to the established efficacy of carbamazepine and valproate in the treatment of bipolar disorder (Keck et al. 1992), the data supporting the use of these agents in schizoaffective disorder are limited. However, because of the substantial overlap between bipolar disorder and schizoaffective disorder, bipolar type, it is likely that these medications will prove useful in patients with this subtype of schizoaffective disorder.

The atypical antipsychotics clozapine and risperidone have also been studied in the acute treatment of patients with schizoaffective disorder. Five open studies (Naber and Hippius 1990; Banov et al. 1994; Lindstrom 1984; McElroy et al. 1991; Stefanowicz 1990) found that patients with schizoaffective disorder displayed higher response rates (mean ± SD, 74 ± 15%) to clozapine than patients with schizophrenia (mean ± SD, 52 ± 9%). In the only controlled study, Malhotra et al. (1993) found comparable clozapine response rates in patients with schizoaffective disorder (36%) and schizophrenia (67%), although with a larger sample size, these differences may have become significant. Preliminary data suggested that, like clozapine, risperidone may exert thymoleptic as well as antipsychotic effects in patients with schizoaffective disorder (Ceskova and Svestka 1993; Dwight et al. 1994; Hillert et al. 1992; Keck et al. 1995). Overall, these preliminary studies also suggested that patients with schizoaffective disorder may display a greater response to risperidone than may patients with schizophrenia. Clearly, controlled studies of clozapine, risperidone, and other new antipsychotic agents are needed in the treatment of patients with schizoaffective disorder.

Children, adolescents, and the elderly. There are no treatment studies of schizoaffective disorder in children or adolescents. When schizoaffective disorder is studied in geriatric patients, it is usually in the context of studies of schizophrenia or psychosis in general that happen to include some schizoaffective patients (e.g., Madhussodanan et al. 1995). At this time, therefore, the treatment of schizoaffective disorder in young and elderly patients is generally similar to that in adults: various antipsychotic-thymoleptic combinations. Guidelines for the use of antipsychotic agents in young and elderly patients with schizoaffective disorder simply follow those for schizophrenia previously discussed. The use of mood-stabilizer and antidepressant agents in children, adolescents, and elderly persons has been reviewed elsewhere (McElroy and Weller, Chapter 17, this book; Salzman 1982; Schatzberg and Cole 1991; Shulman et al. 1996) and is beyond the scope of this chapter. Nevertheless, as with antipsychotic agents, careful use of low doses of these drugs—with slow dosage adjustments, awareness of potential drug-drug interactions, and a high index of suspicion for drug-induced side effects and clinical worsening in schizoaffective patients of all ages—will help ensure the maximal benefit with the fewest risks.

Maintenance Studies

Adults. Three controlled studies have examined the efficacy of lithium, antipsychotics, and imipramine in the prevention of recurrent mood and psychotic episodes in adults with schizoaffective disorder (Angst et al. 1969; Mattes and Nayak 1984; Prien et al. 1974). Angst et al. (1969) found lithium to be significantly more effective than imipramine. From a contemporary vantage point, this is not surprising, given imipramine's lack of antipsychotic and mood-stabilizing activity. Two other studies (Mattes and Nayak 1984; Prien et al. 1974) found lithium alone to be ineffective in preventing relapses, predominantly because of recurrent mood episodes. Although combined antipsychotic and thymoleptic treatment represents common maintenance treatment practice, the efficacy of this strategy has never been studied in controlled trials.

Children, adolescents, and the elderly. There are no pharmacological maintenance treatment studies of schizoaffective disorder in children, adolescents, or elderly persons. Thus, clinical treatment can only be extrapolated from the limited data in studies of adults.

Delusional Disorder

In contrast to schizophrenia and schizoaffective disorders, which typically begin in the late teens or early 20s, the mean age at onset of delusional disorder is probably later, occurring around age 35–45, and is highly unusual in children and adolescents (Opjordsmoen and Retterstol 1991). The somatic and erotomanic types of delusional disorder appear to have an earlier age at onset than other types and may present during adolescence. The epidemiology of delusional disorder is not well known, although it appears to be a relatively uncommon condition, being identified in 2%–4.5% of hospitalized geriatric patients (Varner and Gaitz 1982). The treatment of these patients is even less clear, because to our knowledge there are no controlled, double-blind, clinical trials of any pharmacological agent in delusional disorder in general, much less in geriatric, child, or adolescent populations. Uncontrolled and anecdotal evidence suggests that antipsychotic agents (e.g., pimozide) (Janicak 1993; Munro 1992) and thymoleptic agents (e.g., imipramine and SRIs) (Akiskal et al. 1983) may be effective in some adult patients. Serotonin-reuptake–inhibiting antidepressants (SRIs) may be particularly useful for some patients; there are reports of patients with apparent delusional disorder responding to SRIs after failing to respond to antipsychotics and TCAs (Lane 1990). This may reflect a possible relationship between delusional disorder and obsessive-compulsive disorder (OCD) and other OCD-spectrum disorders (e.g., body dysmorphic disorder), which are responsive to SRIs (McElroy et al. 1993a, 1993b; Phillips et al. 1993). Indeed, there is marked phenomenological similarity between a circumscribed delusion and a severe obsession with minimal insight. In elderly patients, there are no data identifying any specific treatment approach; therefore the general maxim of "starting low, going slow" and remaining vigilant about drug-induced side effects seem again to be warranted.

Brief Psychotic Disorder and Shared Psychotic Disorder

Brief psychotic disorder is one of the least validated and least studied forms of psychosis (Siris and Lavin 1995). No controlled studies are available to provide definitive guidance regarding pharmacological treatment. Anecdotal reports suggest therapeutic benefit from antipsychotics or benzodiazepines in adults (Siris and Lavin 1995). There are no data regarding the pharmacological treatment of children, adolescents, or elderly patients who have brief psychotic disorder.

Shared psychotic disorder (folie à deux) is thought to be rare. Cases described in the literature suggest that shared psychotic disorder is associated with old age, low intelligence, sensory impairment, cerebrovascular disease, and alcohol abuse (Siris and Lavin 1995). However, cases have been described in which children are the secondary individuals affected by the delusion (Fernando and Frieze 1985). Initial treatment recommendations are to separate individuals sharing the disorder and to attempt to identify the individual who first had the delusion. Although separation alone may facilitate remission of the delusion in the secondary individual, some reports suggest that this is not a uniform occurrence and that both individuals may require treatment with antipsychotic medications (Siris and Lavin 1995). Suggestions for the use of antipsychotic medications in patients with shared psychotic disorder are derived almost entirely from case reports or small case series, because the rarity of the syndrome makes controlled trials difficult to conduct.

References

Akiskal HS, Arana GW, Baldessarini RJ, et al: A clinical report of thymoleptic-responsive atypical paranoid psychoses. Am J Psychiatry 140:1187–1190, 1983

American Psychiatric Association: Diagnostic and Statistical Manual of Mental Disorders, 3rd Edition. Washington, DC, American Psychiatric Association, 1980

American Psychiatric Association: Diagnostic and Statistical Manual of Mental Disorders, 4th Edition. Washington, DC, American Psychiatric Association, 1994

Angst J, Dittrich A, Grof P: The course of endogenous affective psychosis and its modification by prophylactic treatment. International Pharmacopsychiatry 2:1–11, 1969

Arana GW, Goff DC, Friedman H, et al: Does carbamazepine induced reduction of plasma haloperidol levels worsen psychotic symptoms? Am J Psychiatry 143:650–651, 1986

Armenteros JL, Adams PB, Campbell M, et al: Haloperidol-related dyskinesias and pre- and perinatal complications in autistic children. Psychopharmacol Bull 31:363–369, 1995

Ayd FJ: Haloperidol: Twenty years' clinical experience. J Clin Psychiatry 39:807–814, 1978

Banov M, Zarate CA Jr, Tohen M, et al: Clozapine therapy in refractory affective disorders: polarity predicts response in long-term follow-up. J Clin Psychiatry 55:295–300, 1994

Beasley CM Jr, Tollefson G, Tran P, et al: Olanzapine versus placebo and haloperidol: acute phase results of the North American double-blind olanzapine trial. Neuropsychopharmacology 14:111–123, 1996

Berman I, Merson A, Rachov-Pavlov J, et al: Risperidone in elderly schizophrenic patients: an open-label trial. American Journal of Geriatric Psychiatry 4:173–179, 1996

Biederman J, Lerner Y, Belmaker RH: Combination of lithium carbonate and haloperidol in schizoaffective disorder. Arch Gen Psychiatry 36:327–333, 1979

Bigelow LB, Weinberger DR, Wyatt RJ: Synergism of combined lithium-neuroleptic therapy: a double-blind, placebo-controlled case study. Am J Psychiatry 138:81–83, 1981

Bleuler M: A 23-year longitudinal study of 208 schizophrenics and impressions in regard to the nature of schizophrenia, in The Transmission of Schizophrenia. Edited by Rosenthal D, Kety SS. New York, Pergamon, 1968, pp.3–12

Bleuler M: On schizophrenic psychoses. Am J Psychiatry 136:1403–1409, 1979

Blumenthal MD, Davie JW: Dizziness and falling in elderly psychiatric outpatients. Am J Psychiatry 137:203–206, 1980

Borison RL, Arvanitis LA, Miller BG, et al: ICI 204, 636, an atypical antipsychotic: efficacy and safety in a multicenter, placebo-controlled trial in patients with schizophrenia. J Clin Psychopharmacol 16:158–169, 1996

Braden W, Fink EB, Qualls CB, et al: Lithium and chlorpromazine in psychotic inpatients. Psychiatry Res 7:69–81, 1982

Branchey MH, Lee JH, Ramesh A: High- and low-potency neuroleptics in elderly psychiatric patients. JAMA 239:1860–1862, 1978

Brockington IF, Kendal RE, Kellet JM, et al: Trials of lithium, chlorpromazine and amitriptyline in schizoaffective patients. Br J Psychiatry 133:162–165, 1978

Buckley PF, Meltzer HY: Treatment of schizophrenia, in Textbook of Psychopharmacology. Edited by Schatzberg AS, Nemeroff CB. Washington, DC, American Psychiatric Press, 1995, pp 615–639

Campbell M, Cueva J: Psychopharmacology in child and adolescent psychiatry: a review of the past seven years, II. J Am Acad Child Adolesc Psychiatry 34:1262–1272, 1995

Campbell M, Spencer EK: Psychopharmacology in child and adolescent psychiatry: a review of the past five years. J Am Acad Child Adolesc Psychiatry 27:269–279, 1988

Campbell M, Fish B, Dorein J, et al: Lithium and chlorpromazine: a controlled crossover study of hyperactive severely disturbed young children. J Autism Child Schizophren 2:23–26, 1972

Campbell M, Adams P, Perry R, et al: Tardive and withdrawal dyskinesia in autistic children: a prospective study. Psychopharmacol Bull 24:251–255, 1988

Carman JS, Bigelow LB, Wyatt RJ: Lithium combined with neuroleptics in chronic schizophrenic and schizoaffective patients. J Clin Psychiatry 42:124–128, 1981

Ceskova AB, Svestka J: Double-blind comparison of risperidone and haloperidol in schizophrenic and schizoaffective psychoses. Pharmacopsychiatry 26:121–124, 1993

Chouinard G, Jones B, Remington G, et al: A Canadian multicenter placebo-controlled study of fixed doses of risperidone and haloperidol in the treatment of chronic schizophrenic patients. J Clin Psychopharmacol 13:25–40, 1993

Ciompi L: Catamnestic long-term study on the course of life and aging of schizophrenics. Schizophr Bull 6:606–618, 1980

Cozza SJ, Edison DL: Risperidone in adolescents (letter). J Am Acad Child Adolesc Psychiatry 33:1211, 1994

Csernansky JG, Newcomer JG: Maintenance treatment for schizophrenia, in Psychopharmacology: The Fourth Generation of Progress. Edited by Bloom FE, Kupfer DJ. New York, Raven, 1994, pp 1267–1275

Davis JM: Maintenance therapy and the natural course of schizophrenia. J Clin Psychiatry 11:18–21, 1985

Davis JM, Comaty JE, Janicak PG: The psychological effects of antipsychotic drugs, in Schizophrenia, Recent Biosocial Developments. Edited by Stefanis CV, Rabavilas AD. New York, Human Sciences Press, 1987, pp 165–181

Dwight MM, Keck PE Jr, Stanton SP, et al: Antidepressant activity and mania associated with risperidone treatment of schizoaffective disorder. Lancet 344:554–555, 1994

Eimer M: Considerations in the pharmacologic management of dementia-related behavioral symptoms. Consulting Pharmacy 7:921–933, 1992

Fernando FP, Frieze M: A relapsing folie à trois. Br J Psychiatry 146:315–324, 1985

Frazier JA, Gordon CT, McKenna K, et al: An open trial of clozapine in 11 adolescents with childhood-onset schizophrenia. J Am Acad Child Adolesc Psychiatry 33:658–663, 1994

Ganzini L, Heintz R, Hoffman WF, et al: Acute extrapyramidal syndromes in neuroleptic-treated elders: a pilot study. J Geratr Psychiatry Neurol 4:222–225, 1991

Goodnick PJ, Meltzer HY: Treatment of schizoaffective disorder. Schizophr Bull 10:30–48, 1984

Gordon CT, Frazer JA, McKenna K, et al: Childhood onset schizophrenia: an NIMH study in progress. Schizophr Bull 20:697–712, 1994

Green WH: Child and Adolescent Clinical Psychopharmacology. Baltimore, MD, Williams & Wilkins, 1995, pp 78–120

Growe GA, Crayton JW, Klass DB, et al: Lithium in chronic schizophrenia. Am J Psychiatry 136:454–455, 1979

Haase HJ: Extrapyramidal modification of fine movements—a "conditio sine qua non" of the fundamental therapeutic action of neuroleptic drugs, in Système Extrapyramidal et Neuroleptiques. Edited by Bordeleau JM. Montreal, Canada, Editions Psychiatriques, 1961, pp 329–353

Hamilton LD: Aged brain and the phenothiazines. Geriatrics 21:131–138, 1966

Harding CM, Brooks GW, Ashikaga T, et al: The Vermont longitudinal study of persons with severe mental illness, II: long-term outcome of subjects who retrospectively met DSM-III criteria for schizophrenia. Am J Psychiatry 144:727–735, 1987

Hershon HI, Kennedy PF, McGuire RJ: Persistence of extrapyramidal disorders and psychiatric relapse after withdrawal of long-term phenothiazine therapy. Br J Psychiatry 120:41–50, 1972

Hillert A, Maier W, Wetzel L, et al: Risperidone in the treatment of disorders with a combined psychotic and depressive syndrome: a functional approach. Pharmacopsychiatry 25:213–217, 1992

Hogarty GE, McEvoy JP, Munetz M, et al: Dose of fluphenazine, familial expressed emotion, and outcome in schizophrenia. Arch Gen Psychiatry 45:797–805, 1988

Honigfeld G, Rosenbaum MP, Blumenthal LJ, et al: Behavioral improvement in the older schizophrenic patient: drug and social therapies. J Am Geriatr Soc 13:57–71, 1965

Jan MW, Ereshefsky L, Saklad SR, et al: Effects of carbamazepine on haloperidol levels. J Clin Psychopharmacol 5:106–109, 1985

Janicak PG, Davis JM, Preskorn SH, et al: Indications for antipsychotics, in Principles and Practice of Psychopharmacotherapy. Edited by Janicak PG, Davis JM, Preskorn SH, et al. Baltimore, MD, Williams & Wilkins, 1993, pp 81–92

Jeste DV, Lacro JP, Gilbert PL, et al: Treatment of late-life schizophrenia with neuroleptics. Schizophr Bull 19:817–830, 1993

Jeste DV, Wyatt RJ: Understanding and Treating Tardive Dyskinesia. New York, Guilford, 1982

Johnson G, Gershon S, Burdock EI, et al: Comparative effects of lithium and chlorpromazine in the treatment of acute manic states. Br J Psychiatry 119:267–276, 1971

Johnson G, Gershon S, Hekiman LJ: Controlled evaluation of lithium and chlorpromazine in the treatment of manic states: an interim report. Compr Psychiatry 9:563–573, 1968

Kalish SC, Bohn RL, Mogun H, et al: Antipsychotic prescribing patterns and the treatment of extrapyramidal symptoms in older people. J Am Geriatr Soc 43:967–973, 1995

Kane JM, Rifkin A, Woerner M, et al: Low-dose neuroleptic treatment of outpatient schizophrenics, I: preliminary results for relapse rates. Arch Gen Psychiatry 40:893–896, 1983

Kane JM, Honigfeld G, Singer J, et al: Clozapine for the treatment-resistant schizophrenic: a double-blind comparison with chlorpromazine. Arch Gen Psychiatry 45:789–796, 1988

Kane JM, Davis JM, Schooler NR, et al: A one-year comparison of four dosages of haloperidol decanoate. Schizophr Res 9:239–240, 1993

Keck PE Jr, McElroy SL, Nemeroff CB: Anticonvulsants in the treatment of bipolar disorder. J Neuropsychiatry Clin Neurosci 4:395–405, 1992

Keck PE Jr, McElroy SL, Strakowski SM, et al: Pharmacologic treatment of schizoaffective disorder. Psychopharmacology (Berlin) 114:529–538, 1994

Keck PE Jr, Wilson DR, Strakowski SM, et al: Clinical predictors of acute risperidone response in schizophrenia, schizoaffective disorder, and psychotic mood disorders. J Clin Psychiatry 56:466–470, 1995

Keepers GA, Casey DE: Prediction of neuroleptic-induced dystonia. J Clin Psychopharmcol 7:342–345, 1987

Keepers GA, Cleppison VJ, Casey DE: Initial anticholinergic prophylaxis for neuroleptic-induced extrapyramidal syndromes. Arch Gen Psychiatry 40:1113–1117, 1983

Keith SJ, Regier DA, Rae DS: Schizophrenic disorders, in Psychiatric Disorders in America. Edited by Robins LN, Regier DA. New York, Free Press, 1991, pp 33–52

Lacro JP, Jarris MJ, Jeste DV: Late life psychosis. International Journal of Geriatric Psychiatry 6:845–852, 1993

Lacro JP, Gilbert PL, Paulsen JS, et al: Early course of new-onset tardive dyskinesia in older patients. Psychopharmacol Bull 30:187–191, 1994

Lamy PP: The elderly and drug interactions. J Am Geriatr Soc 34:586–592, 1986

Lane RD: Successful fluoxetine treatment of pathological jealousy. J Clin Psychiatry 51:345–346, 1990

Levinson DF, Simpson GM, Singh H, et al: Fluphenazine dose, clinical response, and extrapyramidal symptoms during acute treatment. Arch Gen Psychiatry 47:761–768, 1990

Liberman RP, Mueser RP, Mueser KT, et al: Social skills training for schizophrenic individuals at risk for relapse. Am J Psychiatry 143:523–526, 1986

Lieberman JA, Saltz BL, Johns CA, et al: The effects of clozapine on tardive dyskinesia. Br J Psychiatry 158:503–510, 1991

Lindstrom LH: A retrospective study of the long-term efficacy and safety of clozapine in 96 schizophrenic and schizoaffective patients during a 13-year period. Psychopharmacol 99 [suppl]:84–86, 1989

Madhussodanan S, Brenner R, Araujo L, et al: Efficacy of risperidone treatment of psychoses associated with schizophrenia, schizoaffective disorder, bipolar disorder, or senile dementia in 11 geriatric patients. J Clin Psychiatry 56:514–518, 1995

Malhotra A, Litman RE, Su TP, et al: Clozapine response in schizoaffective disorder. American Psychiatric Association New Research Program and Abstracts, Annual Meeting, 1993, Abstract NR53, p 73

Marder SR, Meibach RC: Risperidone in the treatment of schizophrenia. Am J Psychiatry 151:825–835, 1994

Marder SR, Van Putten T, Mintz J, et al: Low- and conventional-dose maintenance therapy with fluphenazine decanoate: two-year outcome. Arch Gen Psychiatry 44:518–521, 1987

Mattes JH, Nayak D: Lithium versus fluphenazine for prophylaxis in mainly schizophrenic schizoaffectives. Biol Psychiatry 19:445–449, 1984

McElroy SL, Keck PE Jr, Pope HG Jr: Sodium valproate: its use in primary psychiatric disorders. J Clin Psychopharmacol 7:16–24, 1987

McElroy SL, Dessain EC, Pope HG, et al: Clozapine in the treatment of psychotic mood disorders, schizoaffective disorder, and schizophrenia. J Clin Psychiatry 52:411–414, 1991

McElroy SL, Hudson JI, Phillips KA, et al: Obsessive-compulsive and impulse control disorders: clinical and theoretical implications of a potential link. Depression 1:121–132, 1993a

McElroy SL, Phillips KA, Keck PE Jr, et al: Body dysmorphic disorder: does it have a psychotic subtype? J Clin Psychiatry 54:389–395, 1993b

McEvoy JP, Hogarty G, Steingard S: Optimal dose of neuroleptic in acute schizophrenia: a controlled study of the neuroleptic threshold and higher haloperidol dose. Arch Gen Psychiatry 48:739–745, 1991

Meltzer HY, Burnett S, Bastani B, et al: Effects of six months of clozapine treatment on the quality of life of chronic schizophrenic patients. Hosp Community Psychiatry 41:892–897, 1990

Michels R, Marzuk PM: Progress in psychiatry, I. N Engl J Med 329:552–560, 1993

Morselli PL, Bianchetti G, Dugas M: Therapeutic drug monitoring of psychotropic drugs in children. Pediatric Pharmacology 3:149–156, 1983

Munro A: Psychiatric disorders characterized by delusions: Treatment in relation to specific types. Psychiatric Annals 22:232–238, 1992

Naber D, Hippius H: The European experience with use of clozapine. Hosp Comm Psychiatry 41:886–890, 1990

Nemeroff CB, DeVane CL, Pollock BG: Newer antidepressants and the cytochrome P-450 system. Am J Psychiatry 153:311–320, 1996

Okuma T, Yamashita I, Takahashi R, et al: A double-blind study of adjunctive carbamazepine versus placebo on excited states of schizophrenic and schizoaffective disorders. Acta Psychiatr Scand 80:250–259, 1989

Opjordsmoen S, Retterstol N: Delusional disorder: the predictive validity of the concept. Acta Psychiatr Scand 84:250–254, 1991

Pearlson GD, Kreger L, Rabins PV, et al: A chart review study of late-onset and early-onset schizophrenia. Am J Psychiatry 146:1568–1574, 1989

Petrie WM, Ban T, Berney S, et al: Loxapine in psychogeriatrics: a placebo- and standard-controlled clinical investigation. J Clin Psychopharmacol 2:122–128, 1982

Phillips KA, McElroy SL, Keck PE Jr, et al: Body dysmorphic disorder: a report of 30 cases. Am J Psychiatry 150:302–308, 1993

Placidi GF, Lenzi A, Lazzerini F, et al: The comparative efficacy and safety of carbamazepine versus lithium: a randomized double-blind 3-year trial in 83 patients. J Clin Psychiatry 47:490–494, 1986

Pool D, Bloom W, Mielke DH, et al: A controlled evaluation of loxitane in seventy-five adolescent schizophrenic patients. Current Therapeutic Research 19:99–104, 1976

Prien RF, Point P, Caffey EM, et al: A comparison of lithium carbonate and chlorpromazine in the treatment of excited schizoaffectives. Arch Gen Psychiatry 27:182–189, 1972

Prien RF, Caffey EM, Klett CJ: Factors associated with treatment success in lithium carbonate prophylaxis. Arch Gen Psychiatry 31:189–192, 1974

Prusoff BA, Williams DH, Weissman MM, et al: Treatment of secondary depression in schizophrenia. A double-blind, placebo-controlled trial of amitriptyline added to perphenazine. Arch Gen Psychiatry 36:569–575, 1979

Rabins PV, Pauker S, Thomas J: Can schizophrenia begin after age 44? Compr Psychiatry 25:290–295, 1984

Raskind M, Eisdorfer C: Psychopharmacology of the aged, in Drug Treatment of Mental Disorders. Edited by Simpson LL. New York, Raven, 1976, pp 42–58

Rassidakis NC, Kondakis X, Papanastassiou A, et al: Withdrawal of antipsychotic drugs from chronic psychiatric patients. Bull Menninger Clin 34:216–222, 1970

Realmuto GM, Erkson WD, Yellin AM, et al: Clinical comparison of thiothixene and thioridazine in schizophrenic adolescents. Am J Psychiatry 141:440–442, 1984

Remschmidt HE, Schulz E, Martin M, et al: Childhood-onset schizophrenia: history of the concept and recent studies. Schizophr Bull 20:727–745, 1994

Richelson E: Psychotropics and the elderly: interactions to watch for. Geriatrics 39:30–42, 1984

Rifkin A, Quitkin F, Klein DF: Akinesia: a poorly recognized drug-induced extrapyramidal behavioral disorder. Arch Gen Psychiatry 32:672–674, 1975

Rifkin A, Doddi S, Karagi B, et al: Dosage of haloperidol for schizophrenia. Arch Gen Psychiatry 48:166–170, 1991

Rosen J, Bohon S, Gershon S: Antipsychotics in the elderly. Acta Psychiatr Scand 82 (suppl 358):170–175, 1990

Rosenberg DR, Holtum J, Gersham S: Textbook of Pharmacotherapy for Child and Adolescent Psychiatric Disorders. New York, Brunner/Mazel, 1994, pp 192–238

Ruskin PE, Nyman G: Discontinuation of neuroleptic medication in older, outpatient schizophrenics: a placebo-controlled, double-blind trial. J Nerv Ment Dis 179:212–214, 1991

Ryan PM: Epidemiology, etiology, diagnosis, and treatment of schizophrenia. Am J Hosp Pharm 48:1271–1280, 1991

Saltz GL, Woerner MG, Kane JM, et al: Prospective study of tardive dyskinesia incidence in the elderly. JAMA 266:2402–2406, 1991

Salzman C: A primer on geriatric psychopharmacology. Am J Psychiatry 139:67–74, 1982

Sandyk R, Kay SR: Relationship of neuroleptic-induced akathisia to drug-induced parkinsonism. Ital J Neurol Sci 11:439–442, 1990

Sargenti CJ, Rizos AL, Jeste DV: Psychotropic drug interactions in the patient with late-onset psychosis and mood disorder. Psychiatric Clin North Am 11:235–252, 1988

Schatzberg AF, Cole JO: Manual of Clinical Pharmacology, 2nd Edition. Washington, DC, American Psychiatric Press, 1991

Schooler NR: Maintenance medication for schizophrenia: strategies for dose reduction. Schizophr Bull 17:311–324, 1991

Shopsin B, Kim SS, Gershon S: A controlled study of lithium vs. chlorpromazine in acute schizophrenics. Br J Psychiatry 119:435–440, 1971

Shulman KI, Tohen M, Kutcher SP (eds): Mood Disorders Across the Lifespan. New York, Wiley, 1996

Siefen G, Remschmidt HE: Results of treatment with cloazpine in schizophrenic adolescents. Z Kinder Jugenpsychiatr 14:245–257, 1986

Siris SG, Lavin MR: Other psychotic disorders, in Comprehensive Textbook of Psychiatry/VI, 6th Edition. Edited by Kaplan HI, Saddock BJ, Cancro R, et al. Baltimore, MD, Williams & Wilkins, 1995, pp 1019–1949

Small JG, Kellams JJ, Milstein V, et al: A placebo-controlled study of lithium combined with neuroleptics in chronic schizophrenic patients. Am J Psychiatry 132:1315–1317, 1975

Spencer EK, Kafantoris V, Padron-Gayol MV, et al: Haloperidol in schizophrenic children: early findings from a study in progress. Psychopharmacol Bull 28:183–186, 1992

Stefanowicz P: Initial results of clozapine and lithium carbonate treatment of manic syndrome in the course of schizoaffective psychosis. Psychiatr Pol 24:27–30, 1990

Sternlicht HC, Wells SR: Risperidone in childhood schizophrenia. J Am Acad Child Adolesc Psychiatry 34:540, 1995

Tsuang MM, Lu LM, Stotsky BA, et al: Haloperidol versus thioridazine for hospitalized psychogeriatric patients: double-blind study. J Am Geriatr Soc 19:593–600, 1971

van Kammen DP, McEvoy JP, Targum SD, et al: A randomized, dose-ranging trial of sertindole in patients with schizophrenia. Psychopharmacology (Berlin) 124:168–175, 1996

Van Putten T: Why do schizophrenic patients refuse to take their drugs? Arch Gen Psychiatry 31:67–72, 1974

Van Putten T, Crupton E, Yale C: Drug refusal in schizophrenia and the wish to be crazy. Arch Gen Psychiatry 33:1443–1446, 1976

Van Putten T, Marder SR, Mintz J, et al: Haloperidol plasma levels and clinical response: a therapeutic window relationship. Am J Psychiatry 49:500–505, 1992

Varner RV, Gaitz CM: Schizophrenic and paranoid disorders of the aged. Psychiatr Clin North Am 5:107–120, 1982

Vitiello B, Jensen PS: Developmental perspectives in pediatric psychopharmacology. Psychopharmacol Bull 31:75–81, 1995

Winokur G, Pfohl B, Tsuang M: A 40-year follow-up of hebephrenic-catatonic schizophrenia, in Schizophrenia and Aging. Edited by Miller N, Cohen G. New York, Guilford, 1987, pp 52–60

Wirshing WC, Marder SR, Van Putten T, et al: Acute treatment of schizophrenia, in Psychopharmacology: The Fourth Generation of Progress. Edited by Bloom FE, Kupfer DJ. New York, Raven Press, 1994, pp 1259–1266

Zaleon CR, Guthrie SK: Antipsychotic drug use in older adults. Am J Hosp Pharm 51:2917–2943, 1994

Chapter 17

Psychopharmacological Treatment of Bipolar Disorder Across the Life Span

Susan L. McElroy, M.D., and Elizabeth Weller, M.D.

Bipolar disorder is a common, lifelong, genetic disease that is associated with significant morbidity and mortality (Akiskal 1995a, 1995b; Goodwin and Jamison 1990; Kraepelin 1989; Schou 1997; Winokur et al. 1969). Two major surveys of the general population in the United States estimate that the lifetime prevalence of bipolar disorder is 1.0%– 1.6% among adults and 1.2% among children and adolescents (ages 9–17 years) (Kessler et al. 1994; Robins and Regier 1991; Weissman et al. 1988). These and other studies also suggest that bipolar disorder is becoming more common and beginning earlier in younger generations than in older ones (Akiskal 1995a; Goodwin and Jamison 1990).

Bipolar disorder typically begins early in life: adolescence and early adulthood are the most common periods of its onset. However, this illness can begin at any age, including prepubertal childhood and old age. At least 90% of patients who have an episode of mania will have one or more subsequent mood episodes. Moreover, recurrent mood episodes tend to occur closer together over time (with shortening of the interepisode euthymic periods), are associated with progressive deterioration in interepisode functioning and loss of brain tissue, and may adversely affect subsequent treatment response and prognosis (Altshuler et al. 1991; R. M. Post 1992). The mortality rate for untreated bipolar disorder is higher than for most types of heart disease and many types of cancer, and approximately 15% of untreated patients commit suicide (Goodwin and Jamison 1990; Müller-Oerlinghausen et al. 1992; Schou 1997). A study of the long-term effect of bipolar disorder, sponsored by the U.S. Department of Health, Education, and Welfare (1979), estimated that, without adequate treatment, an average woman experiencing the onset of bipolar disorder at age 25 can expect a 9-year reduction in life expectancy, 24 years of cumulative loss of productivity (vocational, scholastic, and parental), and 12 years of overt illness.

Because bipolar disorder is a lifelong illness that often begins early

Supported in part by a grant from the Theodore and Vada Stanley Foundation.

in life and worsens with age, it is imperative that it be diagnosed and treated as early as possible and that treatment be continued throughout the life span (Shulman et al. 1996). Fortunately, growing data indicate that long-term medical treatment reduces the morbidity and mortality of bipolar disorder, and the number of pharmacological agents available to treat this illness is expanding (American Psychiatric Association 1994b; Baldessarini et al. 1996; Goodwin and Jamison 1990; Hopkins and Gelenberg 1994; Janicak et al. 1993; McElroy and Keck 1995; R. M. Post 1995b; Schou 1997).

However, many individuals with bipolar disorder do not seek treatment. Of those that do, many are misdiagnosed and treated inadequately or inappropriately (Lish et al. 1994). Moreover, although this disorder is a lifelong illness that often begins in adolescence and sometimes in childhood, less is known about the presentation and treatment of bipolar disorder in children, adolescents, and elderly persons. Finally, not all patients with bipolar disorder who receive appropriate treatment comply with that treatment or respond adequately to it. Thus, the recognition of bipolar disorder, especially in young and elderly persons, needs to be enhanced, and new medical treatments for this illness need to be developed.

In this chapter, we present a practical overview of the diagnosis and psychopharmacological treatment of bipolar disorder, with attention to similarities and differences in the presentation and treatment of this illness in childhood, adolescence, adulthood, and old age. The chapter is divided into four parts.

- In the first, the diagnosis of bipolar disorder is briefly reviewed, with focuses on the limitations of the diagnostic criteria in DSM-IV (American Psychiatric Association 1994a) for bipolar disorder and on age-related and comorbidity issues that may contribute to the underrecognition and inadequate treatment of this illness.
- In the second, general considerations for the medical treatment of bipolar disorder are addressed.
- In the third, the psychopharmacological agents used to treat bipolar disorder are briefly reviewed.
- In the fourth, the medical management of each phase of bipolar disorder (acute mania and hypomania, acute mixed mania, acute bipolar depression, acute rapid cycling, and maintenance treatment) is discussed.

Diagnosis

The first step in the successful psychopharmacological treatment of bipolar disorder is early diagnosis. Considerable data indicate that for individuals of all ages with bipolar disorder, the following disorders have been and continue to be frequently misdiagnosed:

- Schizophrenia and other psychotic disorders (if psychotic symptoms are prominent or bizarre)
- Major depressive disorders (if depressive symptoms are prominent)
- Primary substance use disorders (if comorbid substance use is present)
- Cluster B personality disorders (if affective instability or impulsivity is prominent) (Akiskal 1995a; Akiskal and Weller 1989; Carlson et al. 1994; Goodwin and Jamison 1990; Pope and Lipinski 1978; Shulman et al. 1996)

Children and adolescents with bipolar disorder are also often misdiagnosed with attention-deficit and disruptive behavior disorders, including attention-deficit/hyperactivity disorder (ADHD), conduct disorder, and oppositional defiant disorder (Akiskal and Weller 1989; Bowring and Kovacs 1992; Carlson 1990; Faedda et al. 1995; Kovacs and Pollock 1995; Weller et al. 1995).

Elderly patients are misdiagnosed as having agitated depression, delirium, and even dementia with behavioral disturbance.

DSM-III, DSM-III-R, and DSM-IV (American Psychiatric Association 1980, 1987, 1994a) have advanced the recognition of bipolar disorder by providing operational criteria for its diagnosis. In brief, DSM-IV defines bipolar disorder as the presence (or history) of one or more manic, mixed, or hypomanic episodes not due to a psychotic disorder, a general medical condition, or a substance. The DSM-IV criteria for manic, depressive, mixed, and hypomanic episodes are provided in Table 17–1. DSM-IV stipulates that these criteria are to be used in children, adolescents, and adults.

According to the types and pattern of mood episodes, DSM-IV describes four subtypes of bipolar disorder: bipolar I disorder, bipolar II disorder, cyclothymic disorder, and bipolar disorder not otherwise specified (NOS). DSM-IV discusses these subtypes as follows:

- The criteria for bipolar I (BP I) disorder require the presence of at least one manic or mixed episode that is not better accounted for by schizoaffective disorder, is not superimposed on a psychotic disorder, and is not due to a general medical condition or a substance.
- The criteria for bipolar II (BP II) disorder require the presence of at least one hypomanic episode and at least one major depressive episode without the occurrence of a manic or mixed episode.
- The criteria for cyclothymic disorder require that there have been numerous periods of hypomanic and depressive symptoms for at least 2 years (in children and adolescents, for at least 1 year); that the

Table 17–1.   DSM-IV criteria for mood episodes occurring in bipolar disorders

Criteria for Manic Episode

A. A distinct period of abnormally and persistently elevated, expansive, or irritable mood, lasting at least 1 week (or any duration if hospitalization is necessary).

B. During the period of mood disturbance, three (or more) of the following symptoms have persisted (four if the mood is only irritable) and have been present to a significant degree:
   (1) inflated self-esteem or grandiosity
   (2) decreased need for sleep (e.g., feels rested after only 3 hours of sleep)
   (3) more talkative than usual or pressure to keep talking
   (4) flight of ideas or subjective experience that thoughts are racing
   (5) distractibility (i.e., attention too easily drawn to unimportant or irrelevant external stimuli)
   (6) increase in goal-directed activity (either socially, at work or school, or sexually) or psychomotor agitation
   (7) excessive involvement in pleasurable activities that have a high potential for painful consequences (e.g., engaging in unrestrained buying sprees, sexual indiscretions, or foolish business investments)

C. The symptoms do not meet criteria for a Mixed Episode.

D. The mood disturbance is sufficiently severe to cause marked impairment in occupational functioning or in usual social activities or relationships with others, or to necessitate hospitalization to prevent harm to self or others, or there are psychotic features.

E. The symptoms are not due to the direct physiological effects of a substance (e.g., a drug of abuse, a medication, or other treatment) or a general medical condition (e.g., hyperthyroidism).

Note: Manic-like episodes that are clearly caused by somatic antidepressant treatment (e.g., medication, electroconvulsive therapy, light therapy) should not count toward a diagnosis of Bipolar I Disorder.

Criteria for Major Depressive Episode

A. Five (or more) of the following symptoms have been present during the same 2-week period and represent a change from previous functioning; at least one of the symptoms is either (1) depressed mood or (2) loss of interest or pleasure.

(continued)

Note: Do not include symptoms that are clearly due to a general medical condition, or mood-incongruent delusions or hallucinations.

(1) depressed mood most of the day, nearly every day, as indicated by either subjective report (e.g., feels sad or empty) or observation made by others (e.g., appears tearful). **Note:** In children and adolescents, can be irritable mood.

(2) markedly diminished interest or pleasure in all, or almost all, activities most of the day, nearly every day (as indicated by either subjective account or observation made by others)

(3) significant weight loss when not dieting or weight gain (e.g., a change of more than 5% of body weight in a month), or decrease or increase in appetite nearly every day. **Note:** In children, consider failure to make expected weight gains.

(4) insomnia or hypersomnia nearly every day

(5) psychomotor agitation or retardation nearly every day (observable by others, not merely subjective feelings of restlessness or being slowed down)

(6) fatigue or loss of energy nearly every day

(7) feelings of worthlessness or excessive or inappropriate guilt (which may be delusional) nearly every day (not merely self-reproach or guilt about being sick)

(8) diminished ability to think or concentrate, or indecisiveness, nearly every day (either by subjective account or as observed by others)

(9) recurrent thoughts of death (not just fear of dying), recurrent suicidal ideation without a specific plan, or a suicide attempt or a specific plan for committing suicide

B. The symptoms do not meet criteria for a Mixed Episode.

C. The symptoms cause clinically significant distress or impairment in social, occupational, or other important areas of functioning.

D. The symptoms are not due to the direct physiological effects of a substance (e.g., a drug of abuse, a medication) or a general medical condition (e.g., hypothyroidism).

E. The symptoms are not better accounted for by Bereavement, i.e., after the loss of a loved one, the symptoms persist for longer than 2 months or are characterized by marked functional impairment, morbid preoccupation with worthlessness, suicidal ideation, psychotic symptoms, or psychomotor retardation.

(continued)

Table 17–1. DSM-IV criteria for mood episodes occurring in bipolar disorders *(continued)*

Criteria for Mixed Episode

A. The criteria are met both for a Manic Episode and for a Major Depressive Episode (except for duration) nearly every day during at least a 1-week period.

B. The mood disturbance is sufficiently severe to cause marked impairment in occupational functioning or in usual social activities or relationships with others, or to necessitate hospitalization to prevent harm to self or others, or there are psychotic features.

C. The symptoms are not due to the direct physiological effects of a substance (e.g., a drug of abuse, a medication, or other treatment) or a general medical condition (e.g., hyperthyroidism).

Note: Mixed-like episodes that are clearly caused by somatic antidepressant treatment (e.g., medication, electroconvulsive therapy, light therapy) should not count toward a diagnosis of Bipolar I Disorder.

Criteria for Hypomanic Episode

A. A distinct period of persistently elevated, expansive, or irritable mood, lasting throughout at least 4 days, that is clearly different from the usual nondepressed mood.

B. During the period of mood disturbance, three (or more) of the following symptoms have persisted (four if the mood is only irritable) and have been present to a significant degree:
(1) inflated self-esteem or grandiosity
(2) decreased need for sleep (e.g., feels rested after only 3 hours of sleep)
(3) more talkative than usual or pressure to keep talking
(4) flight of ideas or subjective experience that thoughts are racing
(5) distractibility (i.e., attention too easily drawn to unimportant or irrelevant external stimuli)
(6) increase in goal-directed activity (either socially, at work or school, or sexually) or psychomotor agitation
(7) excessive involvement in pleasurable activities that have a high potential for painful consequences (e.g., the person engages in unrestrained buying sprees, sexual indiscretions, or foolish business investments)

C. The episode is associated with an unequivocal change in functioning that is uncharacteristic of the person when not symptomatic.

(continued)

Table 17–1. DSM-IV criteria for mood episodes occurring in bipolar disorders *(continued)*

D. The disturbance in mood and the change in functioning are observable by others.

E. The episode is not severe enough to cause marked impairment in social or occupational functioning, or to necessitate hospitalization, and there are no psychotic features.

F. The symptoms are not due to the direct physiological effects of a substance (e.g., a drug of abuse, a medication, or other treatment) or a general medical condition (e.g., hyperthyroidism).

Note: Hypomanic-like episodes that are clearly caused by somatic antidepressant treatment (e.g., medication, electroconvulsive therapy, light therapy) should not count toward a diagnosis of Bipolar II Disorder.

Source. American Psychiatric Association: *Diagnostic and Statistical Manual of Mental Disorders,* 4th Edition. Washington, DC, American Psychiatric Association, 1994, pp. 327, 332, 335, 338. Used with permission.

person has not been free of hypomanic or depressive symptoms for more than 2 months at a time; and that no major depressive, manic, or mixed episodes have occurred during the first 2 years of the disturbance.

• The bipolar disorder NOS category includes mood disorders with bipolar features that do not meet criteria for any specific bipolar disorder subtype. For example, this category would include patients with ultrarapid cycling, who experience rapid alternation (over days) between manic and depressive syndromes that do not meet the duration criteria for a manic, mixed, or depressive episode.

Although the Epidemiologic Catchment Area (ECA) study found that BP I disorder was more common than BP II disorder (with lifetime prevalence rates of 0.8% and 0.5%, respectively), more recent epidemiological and family studies suggest that BP II disorder may be the most common subtype of bipolar disorder in adolescents and adults (Carlson and Kashani 1988; Lewinsohn et al. 1995; Simpson et al. 1993; Wicki and Angst 1991). Some of these studies also suggest that subsyndromal forms of bipolar disorder may be more common than syndromal forms, particularly in young people. For example, in an epidemiological survey of DSM-III-R bipolar disorder in 1,709 adolescents (ages 14–18), Lewinsohn et al. (1995) found that 1% of the sample met criteria for bipolar disorder and that BP II disorder and cyclothymia were the most common bipolar subtypes. An additional 5.7% of the sample reported having experienced a distinct period of abnormally and persistently elevated, expansive, or irritable mood that never met criteria for bipolar disorder.

DSM-IV provides several specifiers to describe mood episodes and course of illness. Manic, mixed, and major depressive episodes may be specified as mild, moderate, severe without psychotic features, severe with psychotic features, in partial remission, and in full remission; with catatonic features; and with postpartum onset. Major depressive episodes also may be specified as chronic, with melancholic features, and with atypical features. Course specifiers include the following: with and without full interepisode recovery, with seasonal pattern, and with rapid cycling.

Limitations of the DSM-IV Diagnostic Criteria for Bipolar Disorder

Although the DSM-IV diagnostic criteria for bipolar disorder provide an excellent first step toward the recognition of this illness, they have several important limitations that may interfere with accurate diagnosis.

Categorical Versus Dimensional Classification

The first limitation is that DSM-IV defines bipolar disorder and its subtypes categorically. However, this illness is probably better viewed in two other ways: 1) as being on a continuum with normal mood and the depressive (and some psychotic) disorders and 2) as subtyped dimensionally according to various degrees of manic and depressive symptoms that occur cross-sectionally or simultaneously (e.g., as various pure and mixed affective states or episodes), as well as longitudinally (e.g., as BP I versus BP II versus cyclothymic disorders) (see Figures 17–1 and 17–2) (Akiskal 1995a, 1995b; Goodwin and Jamison 1990).

For example, although the DSM-IV definitions of manic, mixed, hypomanic, and major depressive episodes all specify that a certain number of symptoms must occur for a certain period of time, individuals may experience manic or mixed periods shorter than 7 days, hypomanic episodes shorter than 4 days, and depressive episodes shorter than 2 weeks, as well as protracted hypomanic and depressive states with fewer than the required number of symptoms (Akiskal 1995a; Wicki and Angst 1991). DSM-IV therefore does not recognize subthreshold, subsyndromal, or "ambulatory" forms of bipolar disorder. Similarly, because the DSM-IV definition of mixed mania requires that a full manic and full depressive syndrome occur simultaneously for at least 1 week, it does not recognize the other mixed affective states in bipolar disorder (see Figure 17–2). These include mania with mild or moderate depressive symptoms, major depression with hypomanic or mild

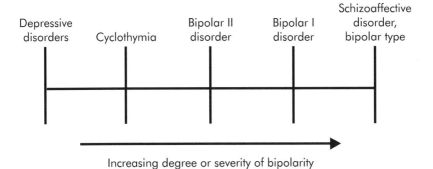

Depressive disorders — Cyclothymia — Bipolar II disorder — Bipolar I disorder — Schizoaffective disorder, bipolar type

Increasing degree or severity of bipolarity

Figure 17–1. Diagnostic dimension for mood disorders.

manic symptoms (i.e., agitated or mixed depression), hypomania with mild depressive symptoms (i.e., mixed hypomania), and mixed states briefer than 1 week (Kraepelin 1989; McElroy et al. 1992). Thus, patients with subthreshold affective symptoms may not receive a mood disorder diagnosis even if their symptoms cause distress or impairment. Patients with brief or mild manic or hypomanic symptoms alternating with prominent depressive symptoms and those with mixed affective states in which depressive symptoms predominate (e.g., mixed depression) may meet DSM-IV criteria for a depressive disorder when they in fact have bipolar disorder. This may be particularly important in diagnosing children and adolescents with incipient bipolar disorder, who are likely to present with subthreshold affective symptoms, including various mixtures of manic and depressive symptoms, before displaying full syndromal illness (Akiskal and Weller 1989; Egeland et al. 1987; Geller et al. 1994b; Lewinsohn et al. 1995).

Underrecognition of Psychosis
Another limitation of DSM-IV's criteria for bipolar disorder is that the frequency with which psychotic symptoms occur in the manic, mixed, and depressed phases of bipolar disorder is not stressed. For example, DSM-IV lists four different types of psychotic symptoms (delusions, hallucinations, disorganized speech, and grossly disorganized or catatonic behavior) as defining criteria for schizophrenia. However, it gives only grandiose delusions as a defining criterion for mania—even though mood-incongruent or bizarre delusions, hallucinations, thought disorder, and catatonic symptoms occur in mania, mixed mania, and bipolar depression (in some studies, just as frequently as in schizophrenia) (Goodwin and Jamison 1990; McElroy et al. 1996b; Pope and Lipinski 1978). This limitation may promote the continued misdiagnosis of individuals with bipolar disorder who have psychotic symptoms, especially children and adolescents, as having schizophrenia and other psychotic disorders.

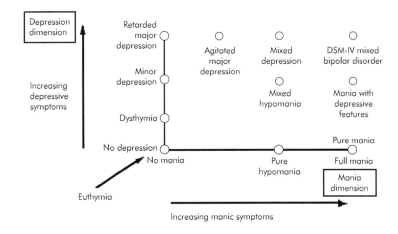

Figure 17–2. Bidimensional classification of mixed affective states.

Discussion of Antidepressant-Induced Hypomania and Mania

Unlike DSM-III-R, DSM-IV states that antidepressants can induce "manic-like mood disturbances," and it stipulates that manic, mixed, or hypomanic episodes occurring in conjunction with antidepressant treatment are to be attributed to the antidepressant (and hence to a substance-induced mood disorder) rather than to bipolar disorder. Although antidepressant-associated mania may be milder and briefer than spontaneous mania (Stoll et al. 1994a), longitudinal data suggest that a significant proportion of patients who develop manic symptoms with antidepressant treatment, especially children and adolescents, go on to develop bipolar disorder (Strober and Carlson 1982). Moreover, in a recent comparison of patients with antidepressant-associated mania and those with spontaneous mania, the two groups did not differ with respect to number of prior manic episodes (Stoll et al. 1994a). Thus, antidepressant-induced hypomania or mania may be a marker for bipolarity rather than a distinct mood disorder, particularly in younger individuals.

Age-Related Diagnostic Issues

Age-Related Phenomenological Differences

Available research (which is limited) indicates, and DSM-IV states, that the core symptoms of mania and depression are similar in persons with bipolar disorder of all ages. In other words, bipolar disorder can present in children, adolescents, and elderly persons in ways identical to those in adults—with euphoric or irritable mania, mixed mania, psychotic mania, major depression, psychotic depression, and milder mood disturbances (e.g., cyclothymia, dysthymia, and recurrent or persistent hypomania) (Carlson 1990; Carlson and Strober 1978; Coryell and Norten 1980; Fristad et al. 1992, 1995; Glasser and Rabins 1984; West et al. 1996). Hence DSM-IV's stipulation that its criteria for bipolar disorder be used for children, adolescents, and adults.

However, increasing evidence suggests that age may affect the phenomenology and course of mood disorder and that children, adolescents, and elders with bipolar disorder may present differently from similarly affected adults in several ways (Carlson 1990; Faedda et al. 1995; McElroy et al. 1997; Shulman et al. 1996; Wozniak et al. 1995). (Although developmental variations are noted in DSM-IV for major depression, dysthymia, and cyclothymia, similar accommodations have not been made for mania or hypomania.) First, affectively ill children, young adolescents, and cognitively impaired patients of all ages are often unable to articulate their affective symptoms. These symptoms may therefore go undetected or be displayed in nonspecific behavioral problems (e.g., temper outbursts or extreme hyperactivity in children, conduct problems in adolescents, and behavioral agitation in elderly persons).

Second, although core manic and depressive symptoms are similar in bipolar patients of all ages, there may be age-related differences in the severity or frequency of some specific symptoms (Carlson 1996). It has been observed that early childhood mania is more often characterized by irritability, anger, depression, mixed states, and marked affective lability than by prominent or persistent euphoria, with tantrum-like "affective storms," prolonged aggressive temper outbursts, and hyperactivity that may be more continuous than episodic. It has also been noted that childhood bipolar disorder is less likely to show clear alterations between mania and depression (Carlson 1990; Faedda et al. 1995; Weller et al. 1995; Wozniak et al. 1995). Late-childhood mania and adolescent mania have been reported to be more similar to adult mania than to prepubertal mania, with more prominent euphoria, grandiosity, pressured speech, and a more episodic course. However, compared with adult mania, adolescent mania has been described as more often associated with depressive features and psychosis, including bizarre delusions (Ballenger et al. 1982; Krasa and Tolbert 1994; McElroy et al. 1997; West et al. 1996). Also, child and adolescent bipolar disorders have been described as being frequently associated with continuous or complex rapid cycling (Geller et al. 1995). Late-life mania has been described as clinically heterogeneous and, as compared to adult mania, associated with less hyperactivity, lower sex drive, less disturbed thought processes, and lower overall severity, but more often associated with depressive features, impaired insight, "dementiform" or delirium-like symptoms, mood-incongruent (especially paranoid) delusions, and greater duration or chronicity of symptoms (Blazer and Koenig

1996; Broadhead and Jacoby 1990; Dunn and Rabins 1996; F. Post 1978; Shulman 1993; Shulman et al. 1996; Young and Falk 1989).

However, it has also been reported that adolescent mania and geriatric mania are just as likely to be mixed and associated with psychosis as is adult mania (Broadhead and Jacoby 1990; Coryell and Norten 1980). Furthermore, in a prospective comparison of the phenomenology of 40 adolescents (ages 12–18 years) and 88 adults with DSM-III-R bipolar disorder hospitalized for mania, adolescent mania was significantly more often mixed, but less often associated with psychotic features, than was adult mania (McElroy et al. 1997). To our knowledge, no single study has compared the phenomenology of mania (or depression) across the life cycle—in childhood, adolescence, adulthood, and late life. Further research into the presentation of bipolar disorder across the life span is therefore needed to definitively establish age-related phenomenological differences for mania and depression.

Prodromal or Early-Onset Bipolar Disorder

Bipolar disorder has a number of prodromal or early-onset presentations that do not include syndromal mania or hypomania (Akiskal 1995a, 1995b, 1995c; Akiskal et al. 1985; Carlson and Kashani 1988; Goodwin and Jamison 1990). These prodromes include hyperthymic, cyclothymic, and dysthymic temperaments; subsyndromal hypomanic, depressive, and mixed affective symptoms or affective instability; dysthymia, minor and major depressive episodes, and psychotic depression; anxiety disorders; episodic aggression, substance abuse, and other behavioral or conduct disturbances; and ADHD or ADHD-like symptoms. Support for such bipolar prodromes comes from the following sources:

- Retrospective reports of many adults with bipolar disorder that they experienced depressive, hypomanic, anxiety, or ADHD-like symptoms in childhood and/or adolescence before the onset of their first manic, hypomanic, or major depressive episode (Lish et al. 1994; Winokur et al. 1993)
- Findings that age at onset of bipolar disorder is earlier when defined by first symptoms or first impairment than when defined by first full manic or major depressive syndrome or first hospitalization (Egeland et al. 1987)
- Findings of low rates of early childhood mania in general and among persons with bipolar disorder (leading some to suggest that puberty might be a requirement for the onset of full mania or the biphasic occurrence of mania and depression) (Goodwin and Jamison 1990)
- Findings of significantly higher rates of depressive, hypomanic, anxiety, and ADHD symptoms and disorders (all of which overlap phe-

nomenologically with both manic and bipolar depressive symptoms), but not of mania, in the children of bipolar probands than in control children and in the childhoods of bipolar adolescents (Faedda et al. 1995; Goodwin and Jamison 1990; Grigoroiu-Serbanescu et al. 1989; Zahn-Waxler et al. 1988)

- Findings that prepubertal children with major depression (i.e., juvenile-onset major depression) and adolescents with psychotic depression are likely to display bipolar disorder on follow-up (Geller et al. 1994b; Strober et al. 1988; Strober et al. 1993). Indeed, prodromal bipolar disorder may be more common than syndromal illness in children and adolescents (Faedda et al. 1995; Lewinsohn et al. 1995)

Early onset of major depression and dysthymia may be a risk factor for subsequent bipolarity: over follow-up periods of 3–4 years, approximately 30% of prepubertal children and 20% of adolescents with depression go on to develop bipolar disorder (Akiskal 1995c; Geller et al. 1994b; Strober and Carlson 1982; Strober et al. 1993). Predictors of bipolarity among depressed children include family history of mood disorder, especially of bipolar disorder, multigenerational mood disorder, and bilineal mood disorder. Predictors of bipolarity among depressed adolescents include a depressive-symptom cluster of rapid symptom onset, psychomotor retardation, and psychosis; family history of bipolar disorder, high familial loading for mood disorder (i.e., three or more affectively ill relatives), and multigenerational mood disorder (as with children); and hypomania induced by tricyclic antidepressants (TCAs) (Strober and Carlson 1982). A greater degree of familial loading for mood disorder is associated with early onset of bipolar disorder (Strober et al. 1988). Finally, cyclothymia and BP II disorder in many instances are prodromes for BP I disorder.

Late-Life Bipolar Disorder
Epidemiological studies suggest that the prevalence of mania decreases in old age. The ECA study data, for example, found the prevalence of mania to be 1.4% in young adults and 0.1% in persons older than 65 (Weissman et al. 1988). Nonetheless, geriatric mania is an important clinical problem. Elderly patients with mania constitute at least 10% of patients treated in specialized geropsychiatry units, and they have elevated mortality compared with elderly patients with depression (Shulman 1993).

Among elderly persons, mania may occur as a recurrent episode of preexisting bipolar disorder, as the first manic episode in a preexisting major depressive disorder (sometimes referred to as latent bipolar or pseudo-unipolar disorder, or as conversion from unipolar to bipolar disorder), and as a first mood episode (Glasser and Rabins 1984; Shulman 1993; Young and Klerman 1992). Compared with elderly patients with long-standing mood disorder, elderly patients with first-episode mania are probably more likely to have an underlying organic disturbance (e.g., cerebrovascular illness) and a negative family history of mood disorder (and thus to have a mood disorder due to a general medical condition or to a substance) (Evans et al. 1995; Krauthammer and Klerman 1978; Shulman 1993; Stone 1989; Tohen et al. 1994b). It is therefore particularly important to rule out underlying organic causes of new-onset manic syndromes in older adults (Evans et al. 1995).

Psychiatric and Medical Comorbidity of Bipolar Disorder

Substantial epidemiological and clinical data show that bipolar disorder in all age groups is associated with elevated rates of most other Axis I disorders, including substance use disorders, anxiety disorders (e.g., panic disorder, obsessive-compulsive disorder, and possibly posttraumatic stress disorder), ADHD, conduct disorder (in children and adolescents), eating disorders, impulse control disorders, and possibly Tourette's disorder (Biederman et al. 1996; Goodwin and Jamison 1990; Kessler et al. 1994; Kovacs and Pollock 1995; Robins and Regier 1991; Strakowski et al. 1994; Weller et al. 1995; West et al. 1996; Winokur et al. 1993; Wozniak et al. 1995). Indeed, these data indicate that the majority of adolescents and adults with bipolar disorder have at least one other Axis I disorder. Bipolar disorder may also be associated with elevated rates of antisocial and borderline personality disorders and some medical disorders (e.g., migraine, thyroid disease) (Goodwin and Jamison 1990; Strakowski et al. 1994). Although little is known about the relationships between bipolar disorder and its comorbid psychiatric and medical disorders, this high comorbidity has diagnostic, prognostic, and treatment implications. It is therefore crucial that patients of all ages with bipolar disorder be carefully assessed for other Axis I, Axis II, and Axis III disorders and that comorbid disorders, when present, receive appropriate treatment.

General Considerations for Treatment

There are a number of general considerations for the medical treatment of bipolar disorder. A more thorough discussion of these considerations may be found in "Practice Guideline for Bipolar Disorder" (American Psychiatric Association 1994b), Goodwin and Jamison (1990), Miklowitz (1996) and Shulman et al. (1996).

Medical Evaluation

Numerous medical conditions and medications may cause affective symptoms and syndromes indistinguishable from those of bipolar disorder (Altshuler et al. 1995; Evans et al. 1995; Goodwin and Jamison 1990; Krauthammer and Klerman 1978; Strakowski et al. 1994). These include neurological disorders (e.g., head trauma, epilepsy, central nervous system [CNS] infections, multiple sclerosis, stroke, brain tumors), general medical illnesses (e.g., thyroid or adrenal disease, collagen-vascular disease, syphilis), drugs of abuse (especially cocaine, amphetamines, and anabolic steroids), corticosteroids, and dopamine agonists (e.g., bromocriptine, amantadine). (Although antidepressants are listed as substances that may cause organic manic syndromes in DSM-IV, many data suggest that these agents are better viewed as physiological triggers of latent bipolar disorder in susceptible individuals.) Persons of all ages presenting with new-onset bipolar symptoms should therefore receive a medical evaluation to rule out causes of these symptoms other than bipolar disorder. Such an evaluation should include a medical history, physical examination, and screening laboratory tests for hematological, renal, liver, and thyroid function tests. Other potential evaluations include a urine toxicology screen for drugs of abuse, a venereal disease research laboratory (VDRL) test to rule out syphilis, and a brain computed-tomography (CT) scan or magnetic resonance imaging (MRI) to rule out neurological disease—particularly if neurological abnormalities are present or family history is negative for mood disorder.

Education

As with any other lifelong illness, the successful treatment of bipolar disorder includes education and the building of a collaborative doctor-patient relationship. Patients must be educated about the following matters:

- The signs and symptoms of mania, hypomania, depression, mixed states, and psychosis
- The role of genetic factors in the etiology of bipolar disorder
- The long-term course of the illness
- Factors that may alleviate (e.g., good sleep hygiene) or exacerbate (e.g., discontinuation of mood stabilizers, sleep loss, antidepressants, and alcohol or illicit drug use) the illness
- The effect the illness may have on their interpersonal and vocational functioning
- Medical and psychological treatment options
- The potential risks of not pursuing or discontinuing treatment (e.g., suicide, psychosis, alcohol and drug abuse, promiscuity, financial ruin, and treatment refractoriness) (Maj et al. 1995; R. M. Post et al. 1992; Suppes et al. 1991)

This can be done through supportive individual psychotherapy; couple, family, or group therapy; distribution of written information and videotapes; and encouraging patient participation in self-help groups organized and run by other patients, especially the National Depressive and Manic-Depressive Association (NDMDA) and the National Alliance for the Mentally Ill (NAMI). These two organizations often provide support groups to patients and family members of a specific age or status (e.g., bipolar adolescents, parents of mentally ill children, and children with mentally ill parents).

Involvement of Others

Because bipolar disorder is often accompanied by poor insight, impaired judgment, psychosis, noncompliance with treatment, and disruption of interpersonal and vocational functioning, it is important for most patients with bipolar disorder that at least one family member (or significant other) be involved in their evaluation and treatment. The traditional dyadic patient-doctor relationship, although appropriate for some patients, must be modified for others by including family members in various ways. This is especially true for children, adolescents, young adults, and elderly patients. Interviews with family members (both at the beginning of and throughout treatment) are useful for obtaining information about past history and current progress that the patient may not provide. Moreover, family members should be educated about bipolar disorder and should be instructed to 1) encourage the patient to comply with treatment, maintain good sleep hygiene, and avoid alcohol and drugs (to minimize recurrent episodes) and 2) alert the clinician if the patient manifests symptoms and cannot notify, or refuses to notify, the clinician. Indeed, such family involvement has been shown to enhance patient compliance and reduce relapse (Goodwin and Jamison 1990; Miklowitz 1996).

The Nature of the Medical Treatment of Bipolar Disorder

The medical treatment of bipolar disorder is an empirical, sometimes complex, and lifelong process. There are no definitive means of predicting a given patient's response to a given medication. Whether a certain psychotropic will be effective for or tolerated by a certain patient can be determined only by giving that patient a therapeutic trial and observing the response. When a favorable response to an available agent occurs, the response is often incomplete. Therefore, combinations of different agents (i.e., rational polypharmacy) must often be used to obtain optimal mood stabilization. Finally, all patients with bipolar disorder, including those who have had only one episode of mania, should be considered for indefinite or lifelong medical treatment;

this recommendation includes children, adolescents, and elderly persons. Patients and their families must learn about the trial-and-effect nature of the medical treatment of bipolar disorder, the fact that multiple medications are often required for optimal response, the fact that it often takes time to find the best psychotropic regimen for a particular individual, and the recommendation that medical treatment should in most cases be lifelong. Patients and their families should also be encouraged to become active participants in this process so that compliance and outcome can be maximized.

Yet another consideration is that it is sometimes not possible to implement the best medical treatment for a given patient. Patients may refuse some but not other medications. Some patients refuse treatment altogether. In these instances, clinicians must weigh the risks of non-ideal or forced treatment, respectively, with those of no treatment. For example, it is usually safer to begin a mood stabilizer in an acutely manic patient who is refusing laboratory tests than to withhold treatment until these tests are obtained. Similarly, it is probably safer to use injectable antipsychotics in an acutely manic patient who is refusing all treatment than to not treat the patient at all.

Medical Treatment of Bipolar Disorder and Age

In contrast to the situation with adults, there are no methodologically sound, controlled studies on which to base psychopharmacological treatment recommendations for children, adolescents, and elders with bipolar disorder (American Psychiatric Association 1994b; Botteron and Geller 1995; Faedda et al. 1995; Janicak et al. 1993; Sadavoy et al. 1996). Efficacy in adults does not necessarily indicate efficacy in the very young and the very old. For example, except for one study, TCAs have not been proved superior to placebo in childhood or adolescent depression (Ambrosini et al. 1993; Kye and Ryan 1995; Papatheodorou and Kutcher 1996). Nonetheless, growing open data and clinical experience suggest that many psychotropic agents effective in adults with bipolar disorder (e.g., lithium, valproate, carbamazepine, antipsychotics, serotonin reuptake inhibitors [SRIs]) may be effective in some children, adolescents, and elders with the disorder and that the treatment of bipolar disorder in young and in elderly persons is in many ways similar to that in adults. However, because the treatment recommendations in this chapter for childhood, adolescent, and late-life bipolar disorder are based on less systematic data than are those for adults, they must be viewed as tentative until more systematic research is available.

Pharmacokinetics, Pharmacodynamics, and Age

There are important age-related changes in psychotropic drug pharmacokinetics and pharmacodynamics (Busse and Blazer 1996; Green

1995; Hardman et al. 1996; Sadavoy et al. 1996). Children and adolescents metabolize and excrete drugs very efficiently. Indeed, children and adolescents often require larger doses of psychoactive medication per unit of body weight than do adults to attain similar blood levels and therapeutic efficacy—possibly as a result of more rapid hepatic metabolism and higher glomerular filtration rates in children than in adults. With aging, however, plasma protein production decreases, volume of distribution increases, hepatic biotransformation becomes less efficient, and renal clearance (of water-soluble drugs and drug metabolites) decreases. In addition, the CNS becomes more sensitive to many psychotropics (possibly as a result of reduced neurotransmitter function). Elderly persons, therefore, are more likely than younger persons to display adverse and sometimes therapeutic effects at lower doses and serum levels of many psychotropics, including lithium, valproate, carbamazepine, antipsychotics, and many antidepressants. As bipolar patients age, modification of stable psychotropic regimens may be necessary in order to accommodate these age-related pharmacokinetic and pharmacodynamic changes.

Electroconvulsive Therapy

This chapter focuses on the psychopharmacological treatment of bipolar disorder. However, it is important that electroconvulsive therapy (ECT) always be considered a treatment option in patients of all ages (American Psychiatric Association 1994b; Bertagnoli and Borchardt 1990; Goodwin and Jamison 1990). ECT is highly effective in manic, mixed, and depressive states (with or without psychosis) and thus is truly mood stabilizing; it has a relatively rapid onset of action; it may be used safely in patients of all ages (including children, elderly patients, and pregnant women); and it may be effective and tolerated in patients resistant to or unable to tolerate mood stabilizers. Moreover, it may be used as an effective maintenance treatment.

Psychopharmacological Agents for the Treatment of Bipolar Disorder

Mood Stabilizers

Lithium
Lithium was the only drug approved by the U.S. Food and Drug Administration (FDA) for the treatment of bipolar disorder from 1974 until 1996, and it remains a primary treatment for this illness. Double-blind, placebo-controlled studies in adults have shown that lithium is effective in acute mania, in acute bipolar depression, and as a maintenance

agent in reducing recurrent manic and depressive episodes (Baldessarini et al. 1996; Davis 1976; Goodwin and Jamison 1990; Janicak et al. 1993; Price and Heninger 1994; Schou 1997; Zornberg and Pope 1993). Discontinuation of successful lithium prophylaxis in BP I disorder is associated with a nearly 100% relapse rate within 2 years (Suppes et al. 1991). Lithium also reduces affective instability between mood episodes, augments the thymoleptic properties of other mood-stabilizing and antidepressant drugs, and reduces mortality from suicide and other causes (Müller-Oerlinghausen et al. 1992; Schou 1997).

There are no adequate-size controlled studies of lithium in children, adolescents, or elderly persons with bipolar disorder. It is therefore unknown whether these patients respond to lithium as do adults with the disorder. Open data, though mixed, suggest that perhaps 60% of children, adolescents, and elders with bipolar disorder display acute antimanic, acute antidepressant, and long-term mood-stabilizing effects in response to lithium treatment (Alessi et al. 1994; Baldessarini et al. 1996; Foster 1992; Goodwin and Jamison 1990; Green 1995; Himmelhoch et al. 1980; Kafantaris 1995; Papatheodorou and Kutcher 1996; Mirchandani and Young 1993; Papatheodorou 1996; Shulman et al. 1996; Strober et al. 1990; Young 1996). However, a recent double-blind, placebo-controlled study of lithium in depressed prepubertal children with family histories of bipolar disorder found lithium no more effective than placebo (Geller et al. 1994a). Indeed, it has been suggested, but not proved, that age is associated with lithium response—that adolescents and elderly persons respond less well than adults. This variation may be due to developmental differences, higher rates of mixed features in both age groups, higher familial (i.e., genetic) loading for mood disorder in adolescents, or higher rates of complicated or secondary manic states in elderly persons (Bowden and Rhodes 1996; Evans et al. 1995; Faedda et al. 1995; Himmelhoch et al. 1980; Kafantaris 1995; Strober et al. 1988; Young and Falk 1989; Young and Klerman 1992). Conversely, it has been observed that children may respond better to lithium than adults do (Young and Falk 1989).

Onset of antimanic response to lithium usually occurs within several days to several weeks of achieving therapeutic serum levels in patients of all ages. Onset of antidepressant response is more delayed, usually occurring after several to 12 weeks of treatment. Therapeutic lithium levels for acute mania and depression typically range from 0.6 to 1.5 mEq/mL for children, adolescents, and adults but are sometimes lower for elders (i.e., 0.3 to 0.8 mEq/mL) (Alessi et al. 1994; Busse and Blazer 1996; Foster 1992; Green 1995; Kafantaris 1995; Sadavoy et al. 1996). Lower lithium levels are sometimes effective for hypomania and for augmentation of other mood stabilizers and antidepressants. Lithium levels required for prophylaxis are generally the same as or slightly lower than those required for treatment of the acute episode (Gelenberg et al. 1989). However, in adults, and possibly in younger and elderly persons, lithium clearance rates may decrease after the resolution of an acute manic episode, necessitating dosage reduction to avoid an excessive increase in serum levels (Bowden and Rhodes 1996).

Factors reported to be associated with favorable acute antimanic and/or prophylactic response to lithium are as follows:

- Response to lithium in the past
- Euphoric or pure (versus mixed) mania
- Fewer than three prior mood episodes
- Absence of rapid cycling
- Episode sequence of mania-depression-euthymia (rather than depression-mania-euthymia)
- Family history of bipolar disorder

(Gelenberg et al. 1989; Goodwin and Jamison 1990; Maj 1992; McElroy et al. 1992; O'Connell et al. 1991). Other possible predictors of favorable lithium response include less severe mania, absence of psychosis, and family history of lithium-responsive bipolar disorder.

A significant proportion of patients (20%–50%) do not respond adequately to lithium's acute or prophylactic mood-stabilizing effects (Harrow et al. 1990; Maj 1992; Price and Heninger 1994). Moreover, lithium may be a better antimanic than antidepressant agent, both acutely and prophylactically, and patients may display therapeutic tolerance after initially responding (acutely and prophylactically) to the drug (Baldessarini et al. 1996; Davis 1976; Zornberg and Pope 1993). Factors possibly associated with poor acute antimanic or prophylactic response to lithium include

- Mixed (versus pure) mania
- Formal thought disorder or mood-incongruent psychotic symptoms during mania
- Secondary or complicated mania
- Greater than three prior mood episodes
- Rapid cycling
- The episode sequence of depression-mania-euthymia (versus mania-depression-euthymia)
- Comorbid substance abuse
- Greater severity of mania
- Adolescent or geriatric presentation (as noted earlier)

(Faedda et al. 1991, 1995; Gelenberg et al. 1989; Goodwin and Jamison 1990; Maj 1992; O'Connell et al. 1991).

Factors possibly associated with lithium resistance in children and adolescents include

- Mixed states
- High familial loading for mood disorder
- Presence of an Axis I disorder before 12 years of age
- Presence of a personality disorder when euthymic

(Himmelhoch and Garfinkel 1986; Kutcher et al. 1990; Strober et al. 1988).

Factors possibly associated with lithium resistance in elders include mixed states, "dementiform" features, neurological impairment or illness (including dementia), and substance abuse (Himmelhoch et al. 1980).

Side effects, toxicity, and drug interactions. Approximately 75% of lithium-treated patients experience side effects (Goodwin and Jamison 1990; Jefferson and Greist 1994; Jefferson et al. 1987). Compliance with lithium is fairly low: 30%–50% of patients discontinue lithium against medical advice at some point during the course of their illness. Lithium has a narrow therapeutic index. Toxicity can occur with therapeutic levels (especially in elderly persons), and overdose can be fatal.

Common lithium side effects are as follows:

- Gastrointestinal distress (e.g., nausea, anorexia, diarrhea)
- Polyuria and/or polydipsia
- Cognitive complaints (e.g., cognitive dulling, impaired memory, poor concentration, confusion, and mental slowness)
- Tremor
- Sedation or lethargy
- Weight gain
- Impaired coordination
- Hair loss
- Skin complaints (onset or exacerbation of acne and folliculitis)
- Less frequently, edema

(American Psychiatric Association 1994b; Goodwin and Jamison 1990; Jefferson et al. 1987; Schou 1989).

Many of these side effects (especially cognitive dulling, impaired coordination, weight gain, and acne) are associated with noncompliance. Potentially serious side effects include the following:

- Reversible renal impairment, hypothyroidism, and goiter (which, if left untreated, may lead to delayed mental and physical development in children and adolescents and cognitive dysfunction in elders)
- Onset or exacerbation of psoriasis
- Electrocardiographic abnormalities
- Arrhythmias (primarily sinus-node)

- Pseudotumor cerebri
- Induction of confusional states (particularly in elderly patients and neurologically compromised patients)
- Teratogenicity (although recent evidence suggests that lithium is not as teratogenic as once thought [Cohen et al. 1994])

In general, lithium side effects are similar in patients of all ages. However, neurotoxicity is more common in elderly patients, and the long-term effects of lithium on growth, CNS development, and renal function in young persons are presently unknown.

Some lithium side effects (e.g., gastrointestinal distress, polyuria, polydipsia, tremor) may resolve with time or dosage reduction. Those that persist can often be managed. Persistent polyuria and/or polydipsia may be reduced by switching from divided doses to a single daily dose of lithium or by adding a diuretic (thiazide and/or potassium sparing) or a nonsteroidal anti-inflammatory agent (NSAID). Because diuretics and NSAIDs may increase serum lithium levels, lithium dosage reduction may be required. Hypothyroidism and goiter are easily treated by the addition of levothyroxine (e.g., 25–200 µg/day) or other exogenous thyroid hormone preparations. Tremor may respond to β-blockers or to the antiepileptic drug (AED) primidone. Acne can be treated with topical or systemic antibiotics and/or tretinoin (Retin-A). Cognitive dulling may improve with vitamin B_{12} or thyroid supplementation.

Lithium is not metabolized and is primarily excreted unchanged by the kidney. Thus, lithium's potential for pharmacokinetic interactions with metabolized drugs is low. However, lithium levels may be increased (and toxicity precipitated) by drugs that affect renal function, including diuretics, NSAIDs (but not aspirin or sulindac), and possibly angiotensin-converting enzyme (ACE) inhibitors. Further, lithium may potentiate tremor from valproate and antidepressants, as well as extrapyramidal symptoms (EPS) from antipsychotics.

Initiating and monitoring lithium treatment. Before lithium treatment is begun, the patient's medical history (with special reference to kidney, thyroid, dermatological, and cognitive function) should be evaluated, and baseline laboratory measures should be obtained (American Psychiatric Association 1994b; Foster 1992; Goodwin and Jamison 1990; Jefferson and Greist 1994; Jefferson et al. 1987; Schou 1989). Most authorities recommend that these include renal and thyroid function tests (serum creatinine, blood urea nitrogen [BUN], thyroxine (T_4) and thyrotropin [TSH]), a pregnancy test in females who might be pregnant, and serum electrolytes and an electrocardiogram (ECG) in patients 40 years of age or older and those with current or past cardiac disease. Other baseline measures sometimes obtained include

- Complete blood count (CBC) to establish the prelithium white blood cell count
- Urinalysis, creatinine clearance, serum electrolytes, and urine volume and osmolality (for renal function)
- Free triiodothyronine (T_3), thyroid antibodies, and a thyrotropin-releasing hormone (TRH) stimulation test (for thyroid function)
- Urine toxicology screen for surreptitious substance use

Weight should be monitored regularly in patients of all ages. Growth must be monitored in children and adolescents, and cognitive function should be monitored in elders. Renal and thyroid parameters should be retested every 1–3 months during the first 6–12 months of lithium treatment.

Lithium is usually initiated in low divided doses to minimize side effects. (Oral loading strategies with lithium may accelerate response but are generally unsuccessful because of excessive side effects.) Adolescents and young adults who are acutely manic are more likely to tolerate higher initial doses (e.g., 600–900 mg/day in divided doses) and more rapid dosage increases (e.g., 300–900 mg/day every 5–7 days). In children, elders, and patients who are hypomanic, euthymic, or depressed (rather than acutely manic), lithium should be started at lower doses (e.g., 75–600 mg/day) and titrated upward more gradually, according to response and side effects (Busse and Blazer 1996; Sadavoy et al. 1996; Weller et al. 1986). Lithium doses and levels should subsequently be adjusted to those that confer maximum acute and prophylactic efficacy and minimal side effects. To promote compliance (by enhancing convenience and/or decreasing side effects), lithium can often be administered in one daily dose (usually taken in the evening).

Authorities disagree as to how frequently lithium levels and renal and thyroid function tests should be monitored in patients on stable maintenance regimens (Schou 1997). Some advise that these parameters be determined every several (up to 6) months while patients remain on lithium, particularly in children, adolescents, and elderly patients. Others advise that the interval between regular determinations of these parameters be customized according to the patient's clinical condition, understanding of treatment guidelines and precautions, and reliability (e.g., every year in the stable adult patient). Most important is that lithium levels and renal and thyroid function tests be determined whenever clinically indicated (e.g., with breakthrough affective symptoms, side-effect changes, or development of new psychological or physical symptoms).

Valproate

Valproate, as the divalproex formulation, is the only drug other than lithium approved by the FDA for the treatment of mania (approval was given in 1996). It has been approved in the United States since 1978 for use as an AED in absence seizures, and it has been extensively used in epileptic patients of all ages. Valproate recently received FDA approval for use in migraine prophylaxis and complex partial seizures. Preliminary data (most of which are uncontrolled) suggest that valproate may also be effective in neuralgic pain syndromes, alcohol and sedative-hypnotic withdrawal, panic disorder, posttraumatic stress disorder, and dementia-related behavioral agitation (Pope and McElroy 1995).

Valproate is considered by many authorities to be a first-line mood stabilizer in patients of all ages (with the exception of children younger than 3 years because of hepatotoxicity; see below) (American Psychiatric Association 1994b; Bowden 1995, 1996; Bowden and Rhodes 1996; Papatheodorou 1996; Popper 1995). Controlled studies in adults have shown that valproate is superior to placebo and equivalent to lithium and haloperidol in acute mania: at least 50% of patients display clinically significant response (Bowden et al. 1994; McElroy et al. 1996a; Pope and McElroy 1995; Pope et al. 1991). There are no controlled studies of valproate in bipolar (or unipolar) depression, but open studies suggest that possibly 25%–30% of patients respond. Open data also suggest that valproate reduces the frequency, intensity, and duration of manic and depressive episodes in the prophylactic treatment of some bipolar patients, including those inadequately responsive to or intolerant of lithium, carbamazepine, and antipsychotics (Bowden 1996; Calabrese and Delucchi 1990; McElroy and Keck 1995; Pope and McElroy 1995). A recent open, randomized, 1½-year comparison of valpromide (the amide form of valproate) with lithium found similar prophylactic efficacy for both drugs and better tolerability with valpromide (Lambert and Venaud 1995).

As with lithium, however, valproate's acute and prophylactic antidepressant effects are less frequent and less robust than are its antimanic effects, and its acute antimanic and prophylactic mood-stabilizing effects may be incomplete or display tachyphylaxis. Valproate's antimanic effects may be augmented by other mood stabilizers (e.g., lithium, carbamazepine), typical antipsychotics, clozapine, and gabapentin (Kondo et al. 1994; McElroy et al., in press). Residual depressive symptoms may respond to the addition of antidepressants.

There are no controlled studies of valproate in children, adolescents, or elders with bipolar disorder. Open data, however, suggest that some adolescents and elders with acute mania (including those with mixed or psychotic features, rapid cycling, and lithium resistance or intolerance) may display acute antimanic and long-term mood-stabilizing effects in response to valproate (McFarland et al. 1990; Papatheodorou et al. 1995; Sadavoy et al. 1996; West et al. 1994, 1995b). A recent 2-year study of valproate versus lithium in children, adolescents, and young adults (ages 11–21) with BP I disorder found that valproate was associated with greater compliance, fewer treatment-emergent side effects, and a lower rate of relapse than was lithium (Kusumakar et al. 1996). The authors attributed the different relapse rate to better compliance with valproate. There are no published reports of the use of valproate in prepubertal bipolar disorder, but clinical experience indicates that valproate may be successfully and safely used in prepubertal patients, including children resistant to or intolerant of lithium (Bowden 1996; Popper 1995). Because valproate has been used extensively in children, adolescents, and elders with epilepsy, more is known about its adverse effects in these age groups than is known about lithium's (Dreifuss 1995; Levy et al. 1995). This experience, along with valproate's well-documented antimanic efficacy, including that in mixed mania, and generally benign side-effect profile, indicates that valproate may have advantages over lithium in young and elderly patients (Bowden and Rhodes 1996; Popper 1995).

The onset of antimanic response to valproate usually occurs within several days to 2 weeks of achieving serum levels considered therapeutic for epilepsy (50–125 or 150 mg/L) (Bowden and Rhodes 1996). However, some persons may respond to lower levels: elderly patients, hypomanic patients, and those in whom valproate is added to other partially effective mood stabilizers or antipsychotics. Substantial acute antimanic response may occur within 3 days when valproate is begun (and continued) via the oral-loading strategies of 20 or 30 mg/kg/day, which typically produce valproate levels of 80 mg/L and 100–120 mg/L, respectively, after 1 day of treatment (Keck et al. 1993; McElroy et al. 1996a). Valproate levels required for maintenance are generally the same as those required for control of acute symptoms.

Factors initially reported as associated with favorable antimanic response to valproate include mixed features, rapid cycling, neurological abnormalities (especially electroencephalographic [EEG] abnormalities), history of closed head trauma, and later age at onset of the illness (Bowden 1996; Calabrese and Delucchi 1990; Calabrese et al. 1995a; McElroy and Keck 1995; Pope and McElroy 1995; Stoll et al. 1994b). However, recent controlled data suggested that patients with mixed features or rapid cycling are just as likely to display an antimanic response to valproate as are patients with pure mania or slow cycling, but that mixed features are associated with better antimanic response to valproate than to lithium (Bowden 1995, 1996; Bowden and Rhodes 1996; Swann et al. 1997). Other possible predictors of better response to valproate than to lithium include rapid cycling, comorbid substance abuse or panic attacks, and comorbid neurological conditions such as migraine and head trauma (Brady et al. 1995; Calabrese and Delucchi 1990; McElroy and Keck 1995). Prior response to lithium or other AEDs is not associated with valproate response.

Side effects, toxicity, and drug interactions. Valproate possesses a favorable side-effect profile compared with lithium, other AEDs, and antipsychotics (Bowden 1996; Calabrese et al. 1995/1996; Dreifuss 1995; Levy et al. 1995; McElroy and Keck 1995; Pope and McElroy 1995; Tohen et al. 1995):

- It is not associated with renal, thyroid, cardiac, or extrapyramidal effects.
- It has few dermatological effects (it is generally not associated with acne, folliculitis, exacerbation of psoriasis, or allergic rash).
- It is associated with less cognitive toxicity than are other AEDs and possibly lithium.
- It is associated with a lower risk of severe blood dyscrasias and exfoliative skin reactions than is carbamazepine.

In several comparison studies in bipolar patients, valproate was better tolerated than lithium, both acutely and prophylactically (Bowden 1996; Bowden et al. 1994; Kusumakar et al. 1996; Lambert and Venaud 1995). Valproate also has a wide therapeutic index and is generally benign in overdose.

Side effects reported are listed below from the more to the less common:

- More common, dose-related side effects of valproate are gastrointestinal distress (e.g., anorexia, nausea, dyspepsia, vomiting, and diarrhea), sedation, benign hepatic transaminase elevations, tremor, hair loss, increased appetite, weight gain, and thrombocytopenia (which is reversible, usually clinically insignificant, and possibly more common in elderly patients).
- Neutropenia, coagulopathies, and impaired platelet function occur less frequently—although in one study, two-thirds of valproate-treated children with epilepsy displayed reduced factor VII complex (von Willebrand's disease, type I).
- Endocrine abnormalities (e.g., transient amenorrhea in young women, pubertal arrest, hypothyroidism, hypocortisolemia) occur rarely.
- Extremely rare, idiosyncratic, but potentially fatal adverse events include hepatic failure (which is unrelated to benign transaminase elevations), acute hemorrhagic pancreatitis, bone marrow suppression, encephalopathy with coma, and skeletal muscle weakness with respiratory failure. Valproate is also associated with a slightly elevated risk of teratogenic effects (especially neural tube defects but also craniofacial, digital, and cardiac anomalies) with first-trimester exposure.

Valproate-associated fatal hepatotoxicity is idiosyncratic and not related to valproate dosage. It usually occurs within the first 3 months of valproate treatment and is characterized by decreased alertness or lethargy, anorexia, nausea and vomiting, jaundice, hemorrhage, edema, ascites, and (in epileptic patients) increased seizures. Liver function tests, including those for hepatic transaminase levels and bilirubin levels, are often but not invariably elevated. The cause of the syndrome is unknown. However, the risk factors for the syndrome have been clearly identified. They are young age (especially less than 2 years); the use of multiple antiepileptic drugs; and the presence of developmental delay or a metabolic disorder in addition to epilepsy. With the identification of those risk factors, the rate of fatal hepatotoxicity with valproate has changed from 1/10,000 (1978–1984) to 2.5/100,000 (1985–1986) to 2.6/100,000 (1987–1993). For patients receiving valproate as their sole antiepileptic drug during the last period, the rate was 1.0/100,000. In patients older than 10 years receiving valproate monotherapy from 1978 to 1993, only 3 cases of fatal hepatotoxicity have been reported. In all 3 cases, however, the hepatotoxicity may have been due to other complicating factors. Thus, in psychiatric patients who are well over the age of 10 years and who rarely receive multiple anticonvulsants, the risk of fatal hepatotoxicity appears to be remote. However, in general, valproate should not be used for psychiatric reasons in children younger than 3 years (Papatheodorou 1996).

Pancreatitis also appears to be more frequent in young patients. It is usually reversible upon valproate discontinuation, but it can recur upon rechallenge with valproate.

Many valproate side effects (e.g., gastrointestinal distress, sedation, hepatic transaminase elevations, thrombocytopenia, hair loss, and increased appetite) are dose related and transient. Persistent gastrointestinal distress can be alleviated by dosage reduction, change of valproate preparation (e.g., use of divalproex sodium rather than sodium valproate), or by administration of a histamine$_2$ antagonist (e.g., famotidine or sulcrafate). Sedation can be reduced by administration of the entire daily valproate dosage at bedtime. Transaminase elevations and thrombocytopenia can be managed by dosage reduction or, with severe changes, by drug discontinuation. Once abnormalities resolve, valproate can usually be increased in dose or, if discontinued, restarted at a lower dose and titrated upward more gradually. Hair loss may be reduced by the addition of zinc and selenium. Tremor may respond to dosage reduction or β-blockers. Valproate-associated neural tube defects may be reduced by use of low valproate doses and folate supplementation during pregnancy.

Unlike lithium, valproate is highly protein bound and extensively metabolized and tends to inhibit hepatic metabolism. Thus, coadministration of other highly protein drugs (e.g., aspirin, phenobarbital, carbamazepine) can increase serum valproate free-fraction concentrations by displacing valproate from its binding sites and precipitate toxicity.

In addition, the levels of various metabolized drugs (e.g., TCAs, carbamazepine, phenobarbital, phenytoin, lamotrigine) may increase when they are coadministered with valproate. Conversely, valproate levels can be decreased by microsomal enzyme-inducing drugs (e.g., carbamazepine) or increased by drugs that inhibit metabolism (e.g., fluoxetine). Coadministration of valproate with lithium or antipsychotics is generally not associated with pharmacokinetic interactions, but it may produce increased tremor and sedation, respectively.

Initiating and monitoring valproate treatment. The pretreatment evaluation for valproate should include a medical evaluation (with focus on hepatic, hematological, and pancreatic function) and baseline hepatic and hematological laboratory tests. The latter should include a CBC (with differential and platelet count) and serum concentrations of lactic dehydrogenase (LDH), serum glutamic oxaloacetic transaminase (SGOT), serum glutamic pyruvic transaminase (SGPT), bilirubin, and alkaline phosphatase. Other baseline measures may include

- Bleeding time, prothrombin time (PT), and partial thromboplastin time (PTT) for patients with bleeding abnormalities
- γ-Glutamyltransferase (GGT), PT, PTT, and plasma protein level in patients with liver disease
- Renal and thyroid function tests in patients who are young or elderly or who may have renal or thyroid dysfunction
- Serum amylase in patients with pancreatic disease
- Pregnancy test in females who might be pregnant

Before valproate is begun (or, in some instances, after some degree of patient response), patients should be warned of the risk of hepatic, pancreatic, and hematological reactions, educated about the signs and symptoms of these reactions, and instructed to report them should they occur. (For children, adolescents, and cognitively impaired patients, parents or caretakers must be educated about these reactions.) Patients should also be cautioned about valproate's side effects of appetite stimulation, weight gain, and hair loss and should be considered for prophylactic zinc and selenium supplementation to reduce any hair loss experienced. Postpubertal girls and women must be warned of the drug's teratogenic effects and considered for prophylactic folate supplementation.

In acutely manic adolescents and adults, valproate may be begun via the oral-loading strategy at 20 or 30 mg/kg/day to allow therapeutic levels to be achieved on the first day of treatment, often with rapid onset of response and minimal side effects (Keck et al. 1993; McElroy et al. 1996a; West et al. 1995b). In patients who are euthymic, hypomanic, depressed, very young, or elderly, valproate should be initiated in lower, divided doses (e.g., 250–750 mg/day in adolescents and adults, and 125–250 mg/day in young children and elderly patients) to minimize gastrointestinal and neurological toxicity. Valproate loading has not been tested in children with mania (although it has been used in children with epilepsy), and it should be avoided in elderly patients because of the risk of neurotoxicity. In children or elderly patients who are unable to swallow pills, divalproex sprinkle capsules, which can be pulled apart and sprinkled on food, can be used. The valproate dose is then titrated upward (e.g., by 125–750 mg every several days) according to response and side effects, generally to a serum concentration between 50 and 125 or 150 mg/L. Occasional patients may respond best to valproate levels ranging from 150 to 200 mg/L (although side effects are more frequent with levels above 125 mg/mL). Once patients are stabilized, valproate dosage regimens can often be simplified to one daily dose, usually taken at night, to enhance convenience and compliance.

Careful clinical monitoring is probably superior to routine laboratory screening in detecting valproate-induced life-threatening hepatic, hematological, or pancreatic reactions (Pellock and Willmore 1991). However, most authorities recommend that hepatic and hematological parameters be regularly monitored in bipolar patients receiving valproate (i.e., weekly to every several months during the initiation of treatment, and, once stable, every 6–24 months while the patient is taking the drug). It has been suggested that liver function tests be monitored more frequently in children younger than 10 years (Papatheodorou 1996).

Carbamazepine
Carbamazepine has been approved by the FDA for the treatment of trigeminal neuralgia since 1968 and for temporal lobe epilepsy since 1974. It has been used extensively in epileptic patients of all ages (Levy et al. 1995). Preliminary data suggest that carbamazepine may also be effective in alcohol and sedative-hypnotic withdrawal, posttraumatic stress disorder, and episodic aggression due to a variety of disorders (e.g., dementia, borderline personality disorder, brain trauma) (R. M. Post 1995a).

Although not approved by the FDA for use in bipolar disorder, carbamazepine is generally considered to be a first-line mood stabilizer (American Psychiatric Association 1994b; R. M. Post 1995a, 1995b). Controlled studies in adults have shown that carbamazepine is superior to placebo and comparable to lithium and antipsychotics in the short-term treatment of acute mania and that approximately 50% of patients show improvement (Keck et al. 1992; McElroy and Keck 1995). Several small open and controlled trials suggest that carbamazepine may also have acute antidepressant efficacy in a small proportion of patients, including those with treatment-refractory depression (McElroy and Keck

1995; R. M. Post et al. 1986). Controlled studies (many of which have methodological limitations) suggest that carbamazepine is better than placebo and comparable to lithium in reducing recurrent mood episodes in patients with bipolar disorder over periods of 1–2 years (Baldessarini et al. 1996; Keck et al. 1992; McElroy and Keck 1995; R. M. Post 1995a). A recent 3-year controlled comparison study, however, found that lithium alone and in combination with carbamazepine was superior to carbamazepine alone in reducing the amount of time patients had manic symptoms (Denicoff et al. 1994). Lithium alone and the combination were equally effective.

As with lithium and valproate, carbamazepine's acute and prophylactic effects are possibly better for mania than for depression, are often incomplete even in responders, and may include tachyphylaxis in some patients who respond acutely or prophylactically to the drug. Carbamazepine's antimanic effects may be augmented by lithium, valproate, and antipsychotics, and its antidepressant effects may be augmented by lithium and antidepressants (McElroy and Keck 1995; Tohen et al. 1994a).

There are no controlled studies of carbamazepine in childhood, adolescent, or geriatric bipolar disorder. Open data suggest that some children, adolescents, and elders with the disorder, including patients resistant to or intolerant of lithium, may display acute antimanic and long-term mood-stabilizing responses to carbamazepine (Evans et al. 1987). However, there are also reports of the apparent induction of mania by carbamazepine in children (Levy et al. 1995; Popper 1995). Like valproate, carbamazepine has been used extensively in young and elderly patients with epilepsy, and more is known about its adverse effects in these age groups than about lithium's.

Carbamazepine's onset of acute antimanic action is comparable to that of lithium and antipsychotics: antimanic effects are usually evident within several days to 2 weeks of treatment. Carbamazepine's antidepressant effects require a longer period of time (4–6 weeks) to become apparent. In responders, therapeutic serum levels are similar to those for epilepsy, generally 4–12 or 15 mg/L with carbamazepine doses of 400–1,200 mg/day. As with lithium and valproate, however, elderly patients may respond to lower levels.

Early studies suggested that certain factors associated with poor response to lithium (more severe mania, rapid cycling, greater dysphoria during mania, and a lower incidence of familial bipolar disorder) might be associated with favorable antimanic response to carbamazepine (R. M. Post et al. 1987). Recent studies, however, have indicated that stable or decreasing episode frequencies and decreasing severity of manias correlate with favorable carbamazepine response (R. M. Post 1995b). Nonetheless, open data have suggested that carbamazepine may be more effective than lithium in patients with continuous cycling, mixed features, or psychotic symptoms (Baldessarini et al. 1996; Okuma 1993). Factors associated with favorable antidepressant response to carbamazepine in one study included more severe depression at the time of treatment, a history of more discrete episodes of depression, and a history of less chronicity (R. M. Post et al. 1986). To our knowledge, these results have not been replicated. Response to other AEDs is not predictive of carbamazepine response.

Side effects, toxicity, and drug interactions. Carbamazepine possesses a favorable side-effect profile compared with lithium, antipsychotics, and other AEDs (Levy et al. 1995; McElroy and Keck 1995; Pellock 1987; Pellock and Willmore 1991). It rarely causes extrapyramidal or renal effects; it is associated with less cognitive and neurological toxicity than are phenytoin, phenobarbital, and possibly lithium; and it is associated with less weight gain, hair loss, and tremor than is valproate.

However, one-third to one-half of patients receiving carbamazepine experience side effects, listed below:

- The most common are neurological symptoms such as diplopia, blurred vision, fatigue, nausea, vertigo, dizziness, nystagmus, and ataxia, all of which are dose-related, transient, and reversible with dosage reduction and are more common in elderly patients.
- Other side effects are transient leukopenia and thrombocytopenia (unrelated to agranulocytosis and aplastic anemia), rash, gastrointestinal complaints (e.g., constipation, diarrhea), dry mouth, hyponatremia, hepatic transaminase elevations, and, less frequently, other CNS toxicities such as mild peripheral polyneuropathies and involuntary-movement disorders.
- Rare, non–dose-related, idiosyncratic, and unpredictable but potentially fatal side effects include blood dyscrasias (e.g., agranulocytosis and aplastic anemia, occurring in 2/575,000 treated patients per year), hepatic failure, exfoliative skin reactions (e.g., Stevens-Johnson syndrome), and pancreatitis.
- Other rare side effects include systemic hypersensitivity reactions, conduction disturbances (sometimes resulting in bradycardia or Stokes-Adams syndrome), psychiatric disturbances (e.g., sporadic cases of psychosis and mania, especially in children), and (very rarely) renal effects (e.g., renal failure, hematuria, and proteinuria).
- First-trimester exposure to carbamazepine is associated with an increased risk of neural tube defects, craniofacial defects, fingertip hypoplasia, and developmental delay.

Leukopenia, thrombocytopenia, and transaminase elevations usually resolve with dosage reduction or drug discontinuation. Once abnormalities resolve, carbamazepine may be titrated upward more slowly or restarted at a lower dose. Hyponatremia is probably more common in elders, may occur after many months of treatment, and usually necessitates drug discontinuation. If rash develops, carbamazepine may be continued as long as there are no associated fever, bleeding, exfoliative skin lesions, or other signs or symptoms of hypersensitivity. Persistent rash may respond to steroids. The risk of neural tube defects with first-trimester exposure may be reduced by maintenance of low carbamazepine levels and by folate supplementation.

Carbamazepine, unlike valproate, potently induces the hepatic P450 microsomal enzyme system—inducing its own metabolism (a process called autoinduction) and the metabolism of other drugs. Coadministration of carbamazepine may therefore decrease plasma levels of antipsychotics, valproate, lamotrigine, TCAs, prednisone, theophylline, warfarin, benzodiazepines, and contraceptive pills, among others. Conversely, drugs that inhibit P450 enzymes can inhibit carbamazepine metabolism, increase carbamazepine serum levels, and precipitate toxicity. Examples are acetazolamide, the calcium-channel blockers (CCBs) diltiazem and verapamil (but not nifedipine), danazol, dextropropoxiphene, erythromycin, fluoxetine, isoniazid, and valproate.

Initiating and monitoring carbamazepine treatment. The pretreatment evaluation for carbamazepine generally includes a medical evaluation (with focus on hematological, dermatological, and hepatic disorders) and baseline hematological and hepatic function laboratory tests. The latter should include a CBC (with differential and platelet count) and serum concentrations of LDH, SGOT, SGPT, bilirubin, alkaline phosphatase, and electrolytes. Other evaluations, when indicated, include reticulocyte count, serum ferritin level, thyroid function tests, renal parameters, and a pregnancy test.

Carbamazepine is usually begun in low, divided doses (e.g., 100–400 mg/day) to minimize neurological toxicity. Acutely manic adolescents and adults generally tolerate higher initial doses and more aggressive dosage escalations than do patients who are elderly, euthymic, hypomanic, or depressed. Because correlation between response, side effects, dose, and serum level is variable, the dose is usually titrated upward (by 100 or 200 mg/day every several [up to 10] days) according to response and side effects, generally to a serum concentration between 4 and 12 or 15 mg/L. Once stabilized, carbamazepine can often be administered on a bid (and occasionally qd) schedule to enhance compliance.

Routine blood monitoring probably does not permit anticipation of blood dyscrasias, hepatic failure, or exfoliative dermatitis. Thus, for detecting these serious side effects, educating patients (or their families or guardians) about the signs and symptoms of these reactions and instructing them to report these signs and symptoms if they occur, along with careful monitoring of patient clinical status, is superior to routine laboratory screening (Pellock and Willmore 1991). Nonetheless, most authorities recommend that hematological and hepatic parameters be determined weekly to monthly during the initiation of treatment, and, once the patient is stable, every 6–24 months while the patient is taking the drug.

Calcium-Channel Blockers

A growing number of case reports, open studies, and small controlled trials suggest that various CCBs (e.g., verapamil, diltiazem, and particularly nimodipine) may have acute antimanic and long-term mood-stabilizing properties in some bipolar patients, including those with rapid cycling inadequately responsive to lithium (Dubovsky 1993; Dubovsky and Buzan 1995; Janicak et al. 1993; Pazzaglia et al. 1993). However, it has been suggested that the CCBs (especially verapamil) are most useful for manic patients who are responsive to lithium but who cannot tolerate or who refuse to take the drug (Dubovsky and Buzan 1995). Administration of CCBs (especially nimodipine) with lithium and valproate has been reported to have synergistic mood-stabilizing effects.

Many of the positive controlled trials of CCBs in acute mania, however, are methodologically flawed; one trial found verapamil no more effective than placebo, and another found verapamil less effective than lithium (Janicak et al. 1993). Methodologically sound, double-blind, placebo-controlled trials are necessary to establish definitely whether these agents have antimanic efficacy. To our knowledge, experience with CCBs in young or elderly patients with bipolar disorder is minimal.

In general, CCBs are well tolerated. Advantages of CCBs over lithium, valproate, and/or carbamazepine include less cognitive, dermatological, and hepatic toxicity and no required blood monitoring. Adverse effects of CCBs include hypotension, dizziness, headache, flushing, tachycardia, nausea, edema, constipation, coughing, rashes, somnolence, bradycardia, atrial ventricular block, and exacerbation of congestive heart failure. Cardiovascular function (blood pressure, pulse, and in patients 40 years of age or older or with heart disease, ECG) must therefore be monitored when using these agents.

CCB dose ranges reported to have antimanic effects in adults are 160–640 mg/day for verapamil, 240–360 mg/day for diltiazem, and 90–360 mg/day for nimodipine. When used to treat bipolar disorder, CCBs should be begun in low, divided doses and titrated upward according to response and side effects (including effects on cardiovascular function). Once stable, some patients may be successfully switched to once-daily dosing with long-acting forms. There have been rare reports of neurological and/or cardiac toxicity when verapamil is coadministered with lithium, carbamazepine, and antipsychotics (Dubovsky and Buzan 1995).

Antidepressants

Because the depressed phase of bipolar disorder not infrequently fails to respond to mood stabilizers, antidepressants are often necessary for the acute and maintenance treatment of bipolar depression. However, few controlled data are available regarding the use of these agents in adults with bipolar depression, and no controlled data exist for children, adolescents, and elderly patients (Kafantaris 1995; Papatheodorou and Kutcher 1996; Zornberg and Pope 1993). Moreover, most available antidepressants have been associated with the induction of mania, mixed mania, and cycle acceleration in patients of all ages (Altshuler et al. 1995; Botteron and Geller 1995; Fogelson et al. 1992; Goodwin and Jamison 1990; Zornberg and Pope 1993). Thus, antidepressants, although often necessary, may destabilize the long-term course of illness in some patients. It is currently unknown whether different antidepressants vary in their efficacy in bipolar depression or in the frequency with which they induce mania or cycle acceleration. Nonetheless, limited data suggest the following for adults:

- TCAs may be equivalent to or superior to lithium in efficacy, but they are much more likely to induce mania and cycle acceleration.
- Selective serotonin reuptake inhibitors (SSRIs) (e.g., fluoxetine, paroxetine) may be comparable or possibly superior in efficacy to TCAs (e.g., imipramine) and possibly less likely to induce mania.
- Bupropion may be comparable in efficacy to TCAs (e.g., desipramine) and possibly less likely to induce mania.
- Monoamine oxidase inhibitors (MAOIs) (e.g., tranylcypromine, phenelzine) may be superior in efficacy to TCAs (e.g., imipramine) (especially in anergic bipolar depression characterized by psychomotor retardation, hypersomnia, and hyperphagia), with similar or lower switch rates into mania (Baldessarini et al. 1995; Cohn et al. 1989; Goodwin and Jamison 1990; Himmelhoch et al. 1991; Peet 1994; Sachs et al. 1994; Stoll et al. 1994a; Zornberg and Pope 1993). Moreover, BP I or BP II depression that fails to respond to a TCA may respond to an MAOI, an SSRI, or, in our experience, the serotonin-norepinephrine reuptake inhibitor (SNRI) venlafaxine (S. Diamond, S. L. McElroy, P. E. Keck, Jr., and G. F. Kmetz, "Venlafaxine in the Treatment of Bipolar Depression," unpublished data, July 1996; Thase et al. 1992). There are also anecdotal reports of bipolar patients (particularly those with BP II disorder) displaying mood-stabilizing (i.e., antimanic as well as antidepressant) responses to SSRIs, bupropion, and nefazodone (Haykal and Akiskal 1990; Shopsin 1983; Simpson and DePaulo 1991; Worthington and Pollack 1996; Wright et al. 1985).

SSRIs, bupropion, and possibly venlafaxine and nefazodone, more so than TCAs and MAOIs, are appropriate first-line agents for bipolar depression in patients on optimized mood-stabilizer regimens in light of the following advantages they possess:

- The probable efficacy of SSRIs and bupropion in bipolar depression
- The switch rates of SSRIs and bupropion being possibly lower than those of TCAs
- Their lack of toxicity compared with TCAs and MAOIs

This may be particularly true for children and elderly patients. Double-blind, placebo-controlled trials in childhood and adolescent major depression suggest that TCAs are no more effective than placebo, although many clinicians believe they are effective (Kye and Ryan 1995; Popper 1995). In addition, desipramine has been associated with sudden death in children, and elders are particularly sensitive to the anticholinergic and cardiovascular effects of TCAs. By contrast, SSRIs are probably effective in childhood and adolescent depression, have proven efficacy in geriatric depression, and are generally better tolerated than TCAs by geriatric patients (DeVane and Sallee 1996; Popper 1995; Sadavoy et al. 1996).

MAOIs are typically reserved for patients who are inadequately responsive to SSRIs or bupropion. However, because of their fairly well-established efficacy, MAOIs are also appropriate first-line agents, especially if depression is severe or anergic.

Antidepressant doses effective in unipolar major depression, in general, are also effective in bipolar depression. However, some patients with bipolar disorder respond to subtherapeutic doses—especially patients with mild depressive symptoms and those prone to antidepressant-induced switching. Other patients, however, may require supratherapeutic doses—particularly patients with severe anergic depressions.

Typical (or Conventional) Antipsychotics

Typical antipsychotics are comparable to lithium, carbamazepine, and valproate in the early treatment of acute mania (Goodwin and Jamison 1990; Janicak et al. 1993; McElroy et al. 1996a, 1996b). These agents (e.g., chlorpromazine and haloperidol) may be superior to lithium in the initial treatment (i.e., the first week) of highly active or severely manic patients. Maintenance treatment with typical antipsychotics, including depot forms, may reduce recurrent manic symptoms and episodes. Also, antipsychotics may be effective in patients refractory to, intolerant of, or noncompliant with mood stabilizers.

However, treating bipolar disorder with typical antipsychotics is associated with several important problems:

- First, although effective acute antimanic agents, antipsychotics are less effective than lithium (and possibly other mood stabilizers) in treating core manic symptoms over longer periods (i.e., 3 weeks and longer) (Janicak et al. 1992).
- Second, typical antipsychotics may exacerbate bipolar depressive symptoms both acutely and over the long term. Thus, these agents are probably best viewed as unimodal or unidirectional antimanic agents—that is, as antimanic agents that do not possess antidepressant and hence true mood-stabilizing properties.
- Third, patients with bipolar disorder have a higher risk of developing tardive dyskinesia and possibly other extrapyramidal side effects upon exposure to typical antipsychotics than do patients with schizophrenia (Kane et al. 1992). In addition, lithium-antipsychotic combinations may be associated with increased rates of extrapyramidal and nonextrapyramidal side effects, severe psychomotor agitation (a common symptom of mania) may be a risk factor for the development of neuroleptic malignant syndrome, and antipsychotic-induced akathisia may worsen manic and mixed affective states.
- Fourth, although antipsychotics are used extensively in children with tic disorders, autism, aggressive behavior, and schizophrenia, there are no reports of the use of antipsychotics in childhood bipolar disorder (Green 1995; Richardson and Haugland 1995; Green 1995). Also, despite their extensive use in elderly patients with psychosis and dementia, there are no controlled studies of antipsychotics in geriatric mania.
- Fifth, the initial treatment of mania with an antipsychotic (alone or with a mood stabilizer), rather than with a mood stabilizer alone, obscures response to the mood stabilizer, thereby delaying determination of optimal long-term mood-stabilizer regimens. Many authorities therefore recommend that treatment of bipolar disorder with typical antipsychotics be minimized or even avoided if possible, including use during the initial treatment period of acute psychotic mania, and that benzodiazepines be used instead as adjuncts to mood stabilizers (American Psychiatric Association 1994b; Lenox et al. 1992).

Nonetheless, typical antipsychotics remain important therapeutic agents for bipolar disorder, particularly in the acute and maintenance treatment of manic patients inadequately responsive to, intolerant of, or noncompliant with mood stabilizers.

Before antipsychotics are begun, the risks and benefits of these agents must be carefully evaluated and explained to the patient (or his/her caretaker). A baseline medical evaluation should include assessment for abnormal movements—for example, with the Abnormal Involuntary Movement Scale (1976)—and, in children and adolescents, height, weight, and basic laboratory tests. When antipsychotics are used to treat bipolar disorder, conservative doses should generally be given (e.g., haloperidol 0.25–3.5 mg/day in children, 0.5–10 or 15 mg/day in older adolescents and adults, and 0.25–3.5 mg/day in elders), although higher doses are required in some patients (Green 1995; Sadavoy et al. 1996). These agents should usually be started with anticholinergic agents (rather than dopamine agonists, which may exacerbate mania) to prevent and reduce EPS. Patient response to the antipsychotic and any side effects must then be evaluated regularly in order to assess whether the agent should be reduced in dose, discontinued, continued, or replaced with another agent (i.e., a mood stabilizer).

Benzodiazepines

Available studies have not yet definitively proved that benzodiazepines possess specific antimanic, antidepressant, or long-term mood-stabilizing properties apart from their nonspecific sedative effects (American Psychiatric Association 1994b; McElroy and Keck 1995). These agents, therefore, should not be used as primary antimanic or mood-stabilizing agents. However, benzodiazepines are safe and effective adjunctive treatments for acute manic agitation, where they may be used in place of or with typical antipsychotics while waiting for the effects of primary mood-stabilizing agents to become apparent (Chouinard et al. 1993; Lenox et al. 1992). Benzodiazepines are also useful in the short-term treatment of insomnia, anxiety, and catatonia associated with either mania or depression and sometimes as adjunctive maintenance agents with mood stabilizers (particularly in patients with comorbid panic attacks or generalized anxiety). However, the safety and tolerability of these agents in young and elderly patients is not well determined. Indeed, some manic children and adolescents may display behavioral inhibition with benzodiazepines; and elders are at increased risk of cognitive impairment, other forms of neurotoxicity, and falls, particularly with long-half-life benzodiazepines (Baldessarini 1996; Papatheodorou and Kutcher 1996). In general, doses required for the adjunctive treatment of acute mania and catatonia in adolescents and adults (e.g., lorazepam 1–2 mg every 4 hours) are much higher than those useful in the treatment of anxiety and insomnia and in young and elderly patients in general (e.g., lorazepam 0.25–2 mg/day).

Atypical (or Newer) Antipsychotics

Clozapine
Substantial open data suggest that clozapine has acute antimanic and long-term mood-stabilizing effects (as well as antipsychotic properties)

in bipolar disorder (Calabrese et al. 1996; McElroy et al. 1996b; Zarate et al. 1995). These data further suggest that clozapine is effective in approximately two-thirds of manic patients refractory to standard mood stabilizers, typical antipsychotics, and ECT, including those with pure mania, mixed mania, nonpsychotic mania, psychotic mania, and rapid cycling. Indeed, the presence of manic symptoms during psychosis predicts favorable response to clozapine (Zarate et al. 1995).

Although experience with clozapine in young and elderly patients with bipolar disorder is very limited, there are reports of the successful use of clozapine in adolescents with treatment-resistant bipolar disorder and in geriatric patients with Parkinson's disease, dementia, and other neurological diseases (Kowatch et al. 1995; Sadavoy et al. 1996). Unlike typical antipsychotics, clozapine may have mild antidepressant properties. Its antimanic properties, however, are superior (Zarate et al. 1995). The onset of antimanic response to clozapine often begins within 1 week of treatment. Compared with typical antipsychotics, clozapine is also associated with significantly lower rates of EPS and tardive dyskinesia.

However, clozapine has numerous side effects, many of which are problematic for patients. These include sedation, orthostatic hypotension, appetite stimulation and weight gain, diarrhea, nighttime urinary incontinence, anticholinergic effects, seizures (especially with dosages greater than 500 mg/day), agranulocytosis, and others. Because clozapine is associated with agranulocytosis, it should be considered only after standard mood stabilizers and antipsychotics have proved inadequately effective or intolerable. Effective doses for bipolar disorder in adults are generally comparable to those for schizophrenia (e.g., 200–600 mg/day), although some patients respond to very low doses (e.g., 25–100 mg/day) and others require doses at the upper limit of the therapeutic range (e.g., 800–900 mg/day). Children and elders often respond to lower doses (e.g., 25–150 mg/day).

Clozapine should be begun in low doses (e.g., 6.25–25 mg/day) and titrated upward gradually, according to response and side effects (especially sedation and orthostatic hypotension). As with mood stabilizers and typical antipsychotics, clozapine should be started at lower doses and titrated upward more gradually in patients who are hypomanic, depressed, euthymic, very young, or elderly than in adolescents and adults who are manic. AEDs (e.g., valproate, gabapentin, or phenytoin) should generally be added for anticonvulsant prophylaxis in patients receiving clozapine at dosages of 500 mg/day or higher.

Some bipolar patients respond acutely and prophylactically to clozapine monotherapy. Others require concomitant mood stabilizers (lithium, valproate) and/or antidepressants (SSRIs, venlafaxine, TCAs) for residual or breakthrough manic, mixed, or depressive symptoms (Kondo et al. 1994). The use of clozapine in combination with valproate and some SSRIs may result in increased clozapine and norclozapine levels. The concurrent administration of clozapine and carbamazepine should be avoided—due to the blood dyscrasias associated with each drug—unless the patient clearly responds best to this regimen and is aware of the possibly increased risk of hematological toxicity. The combined use of clozapine and MAOIs should also be avoided because of potential adverse serotonergic effects.

Risperidone

Available data on the efficacy of risperidone in mania are less extensive and more mixed than are those for clozapine (McElroy et al. 1996b). Some reports suggest that risperidone has acute antimanic efficacy, especially in small dosages (e.g., 1–3 mg/day) and with mood stabilizers (Keck et al. 1995; Tohen et al. 1996). Other reports, however, suggest that risperidone may have antidepressant effects and, like other antidepressants, may induce or exacerbate manic symptoms, especially when given in higher dosages (e.g., 6–8 mg/day) and without concomitant mood stabilizers (Dwight et al. 1994; Sajatovic et al. 1996). These reports, along with the lack of double-blind, placebo-controlled data demonstrating risperidone's efficacy in acute mania, suggest that this drug should be avoided as a first-line antipsychotic in patients with mania until more is known about its thymoleptic profile. If risperidone truly has antidepressant properties, it might be particularly useful in bipolar patients with persistent psychotic depression whose manic symptoms have responded to a mood stabilizer.

Other Atypical Antipsychotics

Little is known about the thymoleptic profiles of other atypical antipsychotics. However, preliminary data on olanzapine (an atypical antipsychotic that closely resembles clozapine both structurally and pharmacologically) indicate that it may have antimanic and antidepressant properties in addition to efficacy in positive and negative symptoms in patients with schizophrenia and schizoaffective disorder (Beasley et al. 1995).

New Antiepileptic Drugs

Lamotrigine

Lamotrigine is a novel AED approved by the FDA for use as adjunctive therapy in partial seizures in patients older than 16 years (Leach and Brodie 1995; Levy et al. 1995). Lamotrigine may also be effective as monotherapy for partial seizures and as adjunctive therapy for other seizure types (e.g., intractable absence and primarily generalized seizures). It is increasingly being used in children with epilepsy.

Preliminary clinical experience suggests that lamotrigine may be effective in BP I and II depression, including patients refractory to mood stabilizers and antidepressants (Calabrese et al. 1995b; Weisler et al. 1994). Although open reports have suggested that the drug may also have acute antimanic properties, it is not yet definitely known whether the drug has bidirectional mood-stabilizing effects or whether, like other antidepressants, it induces mania or cycle acceleration. Currently our group generally reserves lamotrigine for patients with treatment-resistant BP I or II depression who are on mood-stabilizer regimens that have effectively suppressed manic symptoms.

Compared with other AEDs, mood stabilizers, and antidepressants, lamotrigine has an excellent side-effect profile (Levy et al. 1995). It is not associated with renal, hematological, or cardiac effects, has few cognitive effects, and does not require routine blood- or serum-level monitoring. Side effects include dizziness, diplopia, ataxia, headaches, blurred vision, nausea, vomiting, rash, and, less frequently, somnolence. Neurological side effects tend to occur early in treatment and resolve with time. Most instances of rash resolve with drug discontinuation and do not recur upon rechallenge, but life-threatening exfoliative skin reactions do occur. Risk factors for development of rash are greater magnitude of initial lamotrigine dose, more rapid rate of dosage escalation, and coadministration with valproate (probably due to valproate-induced inhibition of lamotrigine clearance [see below]).

Lamotrigine is moderately protein bound, extensively metabolized, and does not induce hepatic cytochrome P450 enzyme activity. Lamotrigine's metabolism is enhanced by inducers (e.g., carbamazepine) and potently inhibited by valproate.

Pretreatment evaluation for lamotrigine should include a medical evaluation with focus on hepatic and dermatological function. Patients must be warned about rash, including life-threatening exfoliative reactions.

In general, lamotrigine is started in low doses and titrated upward gradually to reduce the risk of rash and neurological side effects. It is important to note that dosing schedules vary with respect to whether the patient is also receiving a metabolic-inducing drug, no inducer, or valproate (Leach and Brodie 1995).

In patients not on inducers or valproate, lamotrigine is started at 25 mg/day in adolescents and adults and 0.5 mg/kg/day in children for 2 weeks; increased to 50 mg/day and 1 mg/kg/day, respectively, for 2 weeks; and thereafter increased to a maximum of 500 mg/day and 2–8 mg/kg/day, respectively, according to response and side effects.

In patients on inducers, lamotrigine is begun at 50 mg/day in adolescents and adults and 2 mg/kg/day in children for 2 weeks; then increased to 100 mg/day and 5 mg/kg/day, respectively, for 2 weeks; and thereafter may be increased to a maximum of 500 mg/day and 5–15 mg/kg/day, respectively.

In valproate-treated patients, lamotrigine is started at 25 mg every other day in adolescents and adults and 0.2 mg/kg every other day in children for 2 weeks; increased to 25 mg/day and 0.5 mg/kg/day, respectively, for 2 weeks; and thereafter increased to a maximum of 200 mg/day and 1–5 mg/kg/day, respectively.

Gabapentin

Gabapentin, a new AED, was released in the United States in 1993 for use as add-on therapy for refractory partial epilepsy (Levy et al. 1995). Preliminary clinical experience suggests that gabapentin may have acute antimanic and long-term mood-stabilizing properties when administered as monotherapy or as add-on therapy to lithium and/or valproate (McElroy et al., in press; Stanton et al., in press). It may also be effective in migraine and other chronic pain syndromes.

Gabapentin has an excellent side-effect and pharmacokinetic profile. It is not associated with serious renal, hepatic, gastrointestinal, hematological, cardiac, or dermatological effects; it does not require routine blood- or serum-level monitoring; it has a high therapeutic index; and it is generally safe in overdose. The most common side effects are neurological (e.g., sedation, dizziness, ataxia, and fatigue), dose related, and usually transient. Absorption of gabapentin occurs via a saturable active transport process; the drug therefore should generally be administered in divided doses. Gabapentin is not protein bound, is not metabolized (and does not induce or inhibit hepatic microsomal enzymes), is renally excreted, and thus has few pharmacokinetic interactions with other drugs (including carbamazepine and valproate). These properties make gabapentin an attractive medication for patients with bipolar disorder who are receiving multiple medications and those who are noncompliant with the required blood monitoring of standard mood stabilizers.

The pretreatment workup for gabapentin should include a medical evaluation, with focus on renal function, and a renal profile and/or urinalysis if renal impairment is suggested. In outpatients who are hypomanic, euthymic, or depressed, gabapentin should be started at lower doses (e.g., 300–900 mg/day in adolescents and adults and 100–300 mg/day in children and elders). In acutely manic patients, gabapentin may be started at higher doses (e.g., 900–1,800 mg/day). The gabapentin dose is then increased according to response and side effects. In our preliminary experience, patients may respond to a wide range of doses, from 600 to 5,200 mg/day.

Other Pharmacological Treatments

Various other somatic agents have been reported to be useful in the treatment of bipolar disorder (American Psychiatric Association 1994b;

Baldessarini et al. 1996; Goodwin and Jamison 1990). These agents include thyroid hormones, psychostimulants, older AEDs, and light therapy, among others. Open studies suggest that the thyroid hormones T_4 and T_3, sometimes in "hypermetabolic" doses and regardless of baseline thyroid status, may have mood-stabilizing effects in patients with rapid-cycling and non-rapid-cycling bipolar disorder when used adjunctively with other mood stabilizers (Bauer and Whybrow 1990; Baumgartner et al. 1994). T_3, either more than or in conjunction with T_4, may also potentiate the effects of antidepressants. Psychostimulants, usually in conjunction with TCAs, SSRIs, or MAOIs, may be helpful in treatment-resistant or geriatric bipolar depression. These agents may also be helpful in bipolar patients with comorbid ADHD who have residual ADHD symptoms despite optimal thymoleptic regimens. Various older AEDs, such as phenytoin, primidone, phenobarbital, and mephobarbital, have been reported to be effective in isolated patients with mania, including children (Hayes 1993; McElroy and Keck 1995). Light therapy has been reported to be effective in bipolar depression in adolescents and adults (Papatheodorou and Kutcher 1996). Evaluations of other drugs in acute mania, including cholinergic drugs, β-blockers, serotonergic agents (e.g., fenfluramine, methysergide, L-tryptophan), and the α_2-adrenergic antagonist clonidine, have generally been unpromising.

Psychopharmacological Treatment of Various Phases of Bipolar Disorder

Acute Mania or Hypomania

In patients of all ages, the optimal initial psychopharmacological treatment of acute mania and hypomania is a mood stabilizer. Lithium, valproate, and carbamazepine are all equally viable first-line or primary mood stabilizers in adolescents, adults, and elderly patients, as well as in first- and multiple-episode patients. Although many authorities recommend that lithium be the first-line mood stabilizer in childhood mania, growing experience indicates that valproate should also be considered a first-line agent in this age group, except in children younger than 3 years (Papatheodorou 1996; Popper 1995).

Choice of an initial mood stabilizer for a particular patient should be based on careful assessment of that patient's presenting phenomenology, past course of illness, psychiatric and medical comorbidity, family history, and response to prior treatment (if any). Examples follow:

Lithium might be considered the initial mood stabilizer in patients with euphoric mania, a family history of lithium-responsive bipolar disorder, or hepatic or hematological disease.

Valproate or carbamazepine might be chosen as the initial mood stabilizer in patients with

- Histories of lithium nontolerance, noncompliance, or refractoriness
- Mixed mania or other mixed states
- Rapid cycling (including ultrarapid or ultradian cycling)
- Neurological abnormalities or disorders
- Substance abuse
- Renal disease

Valproate might be considered before lithium and carbamazepine in patients with comorbid panic attacks, migraine, or dermatological disease (e.g., acne or psoriasis).

Once the initial mood stabilizer has been chosen, acute mania and hypomania are generally treated similarly in children, adolescents, adults, and elderly patients. In general, in adolescents and adults, the more severe the mania, the higher the initial dose and the faster the dosage titration of the mood stabilizer. In patients with hypomania and less severe mania, children, and elderly patients, the mood stabilizer should be begun at lower doses and titrated upward more slowly (i.e., via the strategy "start low, go slow"). Depending on the severity of manic symptoms, the mood stabilizer may be administered alone or with a benzodiazepine and/or an antipsychotic to promote sleep and reduce agitation. For example, hypomania might successfully respond to a mood stabilizer alone, mild to moderate mania might require a mood stabilizer in conjunction with a benzodiazepine, and severe psychotic mania might require a mood stabilizer in conjunction with high doses of a benzodiazepine and/or an antipsychotic. For the last group of patients, especially those who are suicidal, violent, or catatonic, valproate oral loading (as monotherapy or with an adjunctive benzodiazepine and/or antipsychotic) or ECT might be preferable because of the relatively rapid onset of action.

For patients of all ages, an adequate mood stabilizer trial is at least 2–3 weeks of treatment with "therapeutic" doses and/or blood levels. If the first mood stabilizer is ineffective or intolerable, another mood stabilizer should be given (e.g., valproate should be changed to lithium or carbamazepine). If the first drug is fully effective and well tolerated, however, it should be continued as maintenance treatment. If the first drug results in a partial but incomplete reduction in manic symptoms, addition of a second and sometimes a third mood stabilizer or a typical antipsychotic should be considered in patients of all ages (e.g., the addition of lithium, carbamazepine, or haloperidol to valproate). Acute mania or hypomania that has not responded to various combinations of lithium, valproate, carbamazepine, and antipsychotics may respond to addition of a CCB, another AED (e.g., gabapentin, primidone, or phenytoin), clozapine, or ECT.

Acute Mixed Mania

Mixed mania is generally treated as is pure mania in all age groups. Initial treatment is a mood stabilizer, often with an adjunctive benzodiazepine and/or antipsychotic to promote sleep and reduce anxiety and agitation. Lithium, valproate, and carbamazepine are all appropriate first-line mood stabilizers. Valproate, however, might be considered as the initial agent because it may be more effective than lithium in mixed mania (Bowden et al. 1996; Swann et al. 1997). For patients who are psychotic, suicidal, or violent—those in whom a rapid response is required—valproate oral loading or ECT may be preferable as first-line treatment.

When mixed mania is treated with mood stabilizers, there are differing patterns of response of manic and depressive symptoms in all age groups. These include

- Complete or partial response of both manic and depressive symptoms (i.e., "bidirectional" mood stabilization)
- Response of manic symptoms but persistence or exacerbation of depressive symptoms (i.e., conversion of mixed mania to pure depression)
- Less commonly, response of depressive symptoms but persistence of manic symptoms (i.e., conversion of mixed mania to pure mania)
- No response of manic or depressive symptoms

The response of both manic and depressive symptoms must therefore be followed.

As with the treatment of pure mania, lack of response or intolerable side effects with the first mood stabilizer should lead to switching to a second mood stabilizer. If the patient displays an incomplete antimanic response to the first mood stabilizer, a second mood stabilizer should be added. If manic symptoms persist, options include switching one mood stabilizer for another, adding a third mood stabilizer, and/or adding a typical antipsychotic. If various combinations of lithium, valproate, and carbamazepine (with or without standard antipsychotics) fail, addition of a CCB, another AED, clozapine, or ECT may be effective. It is important to note that, because antidepressants may induce or exacerbate mixed affective states, use of these agents should generally be avoided or minimized as long as manic symptoms persist, even if depressive symptoms are prominent.

Acute Major Depression and Dysthymia

In general, mood stabilizers should be the initial treatment for bipolar depressive symptoms, including major depressive episodes and milder (i.e., dysthymic) symptoms, in patients of all ages. Ideally, the mood stabilizer should be administered as monotherapy for at least 4–6 weeks to give it sufficient time to exert antidepressant effects. During this time, thyroid function should be normalized (and possibly maximized), and appropriate adjunctive psychosocial treatments should be used. If treatment with a mood stabilizer alone is unsuccessful, an antidepressant may be added. Another mood stabilizer may be added if the patient is prone to antidepressant-induced switches. When treating severe bipolar depression, however, initiating treatment with a mood stabilizer alone may not be feasible. In these instances, a mood stabilizer and an antidepressant may be started together. Moreover, some patients may request an antidepressant but refuse a mood stabilizer. In such patients, especially those with BP II disorder or slow cycling, antidepressant monotherapy may be begun carefully—as long as the patient understands the risk of inducing manic symptoms and agrees to stop the antidepressant and/or begin a mood stabilizer as soon as such symptoms occur.

In patients of all ages receiving mood stabilizers, postmanic or breakthrough depressions should first be managed by optimization of mood stabilizer dose and thyroid function, tapered discontinuation of antipsychotics in patients receiving such agents (because antipsychotics may be "depressogenic"), and use of psychosocial treatments. Ideally, patients should then be observed for 1 month to several months to determine whether the depression resolves spontaneously or responds to these interventions. For patients of all ages who display persistent postmanic or breakthrough depressive symptoms, an antidepressant can often be successfully added with resolution of depression but no induction of hypomania or mania, as long as manic symptoms and/or affective cycling is truly suppressed. Hypomanic symptoms occurring after the addition of an antidepressant may respond to discontinuation of the antidepressant, a reduction in antidepressant dose, an increase in mood stabilizer dose, and/or addition of a benzodiazepine or another mood stabilizer. If mania occurs, the antidepressant should be discontinued and antimanic treatments maximized—by increasing the dose of the primary mood stabilizer or by adding another mood stabilizer or an antipsychotic. If depression subsequently recurs, an antidepressant may often be successfully added to the maximized mood stabilizer regimen without mood destabilization.

As discussed earlier, few data are available in guiding antidepressant choice for bipolar depression at any age. However, antidepressants other than TCAs should generally be used as first-line agents, because of the following TCA disadvantages:

- TCAs may be less effective than SSRIs and MAOIs in adult bipolar depression.
- They may be more likely to induce switches than bupropion and SSRIs.
- They have not been shown to be superior to placebo in childhood major depression.
- They are associated with numerous side effects (including anticholinergic and arrythmogenic effects, including, for desipramine, sudden death in children).
- They are associated with higher noncompliance rates than are SSRIs.
- They are lethal in overdose.

Other antidepressants that may be used as first-line agents include SSRIs, bupropion, and possibly venlafaxine and nefazodone. If these agents are inadequately effective, MAOIs, TCAs, lamotrigine, and various strategies used for treatment-resistant unipolar depression may be considered. The last group includes

- Treatment with ultrahigh doses of MAOIs, SSRIs, or venlafaxine (e.g., tranylcypromine up to 180 mg/day, fluoxetine up to 120–200 mg/day, and venlafaxine up to 400–600 mg/day in adults)
- Augmentation with psychostimulants (e.g., D-amphetamine 5–60 mg/day)
- Augmentation with thyroid hormone (e.g., T_3, T_4, or the combination in physiological or supraphysiological doses)
- Various antidepressant combinations (e.g., an SSRI with venlafaxine, bupropion, or nefazodone)
- ECT, which should always be considered an option in all age groups

Acute Rapid (and Ultrarapid) Cycling

The treatment of acute rapid cycling in patients of all ages (like that of mania and mixed mania) first involves evaluation for possible mood-destabilizing factors, including suboptimal thyroid function, neurological illness, and use of cycle-inducing agents (e.g., antidepressants, alcohol, drugs of abuse). Thus, thyroid status should be normalized, potential cycle-inducing agents should be reduced in dose or discontinued, and the subsequent course of illness should be reevaluated.

If cycling persists, treatment with a mood stabilizer should be initiated, and response over time (preferably after at least two cycle lengths) should be carefully evaluated. Lithium, valproate, and carbamazepine may all be used as first-line agents. Valproate may be preferable, however, because it may be more effective than lithium in rapid cycling, especially in patients whose rapid cycling is accompanied by mixed states, panic attacks, or migraine headaches. Although less effective in rapid than in nonrapid cycling, lithium often has some mood-stabilizing effects in rapid-cycling patients, and it may also be used as the initial mood stabilizer—especially if manic and hypomanic episodes are pure (i.e., not associated with depressive symptoms) and are followed, rather than preceded, by depressive episodes. If hypomanic or manic symptoms and/or affective cycling persist after a therapeutic trial of the first mood stabilizer, a second and sometimes a third mood stabilizer and/or thyroid hormone can be added to or substituted for the first. For example, if valproate is partially effective, lithium, carbamazepine, a CCB, and/or gabapentin may be added. If hypomanic and manic symptoms remit but depression persists, an antidepressant may be added. Controlled data are not available regarding the administration of antidepressants to rapid cyclers (including those whose are prone to antidepressant-induced switches) once they are "covered" with mood stabilizers. However, open data suggest that antidepressants can be successfully reintroduced without reinducing cycling, if manic symptoms are suppressed and the antidepressant is administered carefully—sometimes in subtherapeutic doses or in an on-off manner (e.g., the antidepressant is taken on depressed but not on euthymic or hypomanic days).

Maintenance

Because bipolar disorder is a recurrent, lifelong, and often progressive disease, virtually all patients experiencing one manic episode, including prepubertal, adolescent, and geriatric patients, should be considered for maintenance treatment, especially if the episode is severe, there is a history of prior affective symptoms, and family history is positive for mood disorder. Patients with two or more manic episodes should receive lifetime maintenance treatment. Indeed, patients with prodromal or subsyndromal bipolar disorder might also be considered for maintenance treatment.

In general, the maintenance mood-stabilizer regimen for a particular patient consists of medications that were effective in relieving his or her acute manic symptoms. Although exceptions exist, mood-stabilizer doses and serum concentrations required for effective maintenance are similar to those required for effective treatment of acute manic, mixed, or hypomanic symptoms. However, frequent dosage adjustment and medication changes are often necessary.

Bipolar patients with a predominance of manic episodes (i.e., those with chronic or frequent manic, mixed, or rapid-cycling symptoms) should in general be maintained on single or multiple mood-stabilizer regimens (sometimes in conjunction with typical antipsychotics or clozapine), with minimal exposure to antidepressants. Bipolar patients on stable mood-stabilizer regimens that effectively prevent manic, mixed, or hypomanic symptoms, but not pure depressive symptoms (i.e., those with chronic or frequent depressive symptoms or episodes), however, may require long-term addition of an antidepressant to their mood stabilizer regimen.

Conclusion

Bipolar disorder is a lifelong illness with significant morbidity and mortality that requires lifelong medical treatment. Increased awareness of the presentation and treatment of this illness across the life span should improve the outcome of afflicted individuals.

References

Abnormal Involuntary Movement Scale (AIMS), in ECDEU Assessment Manual for Psychopharmacology, Revised. Edited by Guy W. (DHEW Publ No ADM 76-388). Rockville, MD, U.S. Department of Health, Education and Welfare, 1976

Akiskal HS: Developmental pathways to bipolarity: are juvenile-onset depressions pre-bipolar? J Am Acad Child Adolesc Psychiatry 34:754–763, 1995a

Akiskal HS: Mood disorders: clinical features, in Comprehensive Textbook of Psychiatry/VI, 6th Edition, Vol 1. Edited by Kaplan HI, Sadock BJ. Baltimore, MD, Williams & Wilkins, 1995b, pp 1123–1152

Akiskal HS: Mood disorders: introduction and overview, in Comprehensive Textbook of Psychiatry/VI, 6th Edition, Vol 1. Edited by Kaplan HI, Sadock BJ. Baltimore, MD, Williams & Wilkins, 1995c, pp 1067–1079

Akiskal HS, Weller EB: Mood disorders and suicide in children and adolescents, in Comprehensive Textbook of Psychiatry, 10th Edition, Vol 10. Edited by Kaplan HI, Sadock BJ. Baltimore, MD, Williams & Wilkins, 1989, pp 1981–1984

Akiskal HS, Downs J, Jordan P, et al: Affective disorders in referred children and younger siblings of manic-depressives: mode of onset and prospective course. Arch Gen Psychiatry 42:996–1003, 1985

Alessi N, Naylor MW, Ghaziuddin M, et al: Update on lithium carbonate therapy in children and adolescents. J Am Acad Child Adolesc Psychiatry 33:291–304, 1994

Altshuler LL, Conrad A, Hauser P, et al: Reduction of temporal lobe volume in bipolar disorder: a preliminary report of magnetic resonance imaging (letter). Arch Gen Psychiatry 48:482–483, 1991

Altshuler LL, Post RM, Leverich GS, et al: Antidepressant-induced mania and cycle acceleration: a controversy revisited. Am J Psychiatry 152:1130–1138, 1995

Ambrosini PJ, Bianchi MD, Rabinovic H, et al: Antidepressant treatment in children and adolescents, I: affective disorders. J Am Acad Child Adolesc Psychiatry 32:1–6, 1993

American Psychiatric Association: Diagnostic and Statistical Manual of Mental Disorders, 3rd Edition. Washington, DC, American Psychiatric Association, 1980

American Psychiatric Association: Diagnostic and Statistical Manual of Mental Disorders, 3rd Edition, Revised. Washington, DC, American Psychiatric Association, 1987

American Psychiatric Association: Diagnostic and Statistical Manual of Mental Disorders, 4th Edition. Washington, DC, American Psychiatric Association, 1994a

American Psychiatric Association: Practice guideline for the treatment of patients with bipolar disorder. Am J Psychiatry 151:1–36, 1994b

Baldessarini CF, Sachs GS, Stoll AL, et al: Paroxetine for bipolar depression: outcome in patients failing prior antidepressant trials. Depression 3:182–186, 1995

Baldessarini RJ, Tondo L, Suppes T, et al: Pharmacological treatment of bipolar disorder throughout the life cycle, in Mood Disorders Across the Life Span. New York, Wiley, 1996, pp 299–338

Ballenger JC, Reus VI, Post RM: The atypical clinical picture of adolescent mania. Am J Psychiatry 139:602–606, 1982

Bauer MS, Whybrow PC: Rapid cycling bipolar affective disorder, II: treatment of refractory rapid cycling with high-dose levothyroxine: a preliminary study. Arch Gen Psychiatry 47:435–440, 1990

Baumgartner A, Bauer M, Hellweg R: Treatment of intractable non-rapid cycling bipolar affective disorder with high-dose thyroxine: an open clinical trial. Neuropsychopharmacology 10:183–189, 1994

Beasley C, Tran P, Tamura G: Olanzapine versus haloperidol: results of the multi-center international trial. Paper presented at the meeting of the American College of Neuropsychopharmacology, San Juan, Puerto Rico, December 15, 1995

Bertagnoli MW, Borchardt CM: Case study: a review of ECT for children and adolescents. J Am Acad Child Adolesc Psychiatry 29:302–307, 1990

Biederman J, Faraone S, Mick E, et al: Attention-deficit hyperactivity disorder and juvenile mania: an overlooked comorbidity. J Am Acad Child Adolesc Psychiatry 35:997–1008, 1996

Blazer DG, Koenig HG: Psychiatric disorders in late life: mood disorders, in Textbook of Geriatric Psychiatry, 2nd Edition. Edited by Busse EW, Blazer DG. Washington, DC, American Psychiatric Press, 1996, pp 235–263

Botteron KN, Geller B: Pharmacologic treatment of childhood and adolescent mania. Child and Adolescent Psychiatric Clinics of North America 4:283–304, 1995

Bowden CB: Predictors of response to divalproex and lithium. J Clin Psychiatry 56 (suppl 3):25–30, 1995

Bowden CB: The efficacy of divalproex sodium and lithium in the treatment of acute mania. Directions in Psychiatry 16:i–vi, 1996

Bowden CL, Rhodes LJ: Mania in children and adolescents: recognition and treatment. Psychiatric Annals 26 [suppl]:430–434, 1996

Bowden CL, Brugger AM, Swann AC, et al: Efficacy of divalproex vs lithium and placebo in the treatment of mania. JAMA 271:918–924, 1994

Bowden CL, Janicak PG, Orsulak P, et al: Relation of serum valproate concentration to response in mania. Am J Psychiatry 153:765–770, 1996

Bowring MA, Kovacs M: Difficulties in diagnosing manic disorders among children and adolescents. J Am Acad Child Adolesc Psychiatry 31:611–614, 1992

Brady KT, Sonne S, Anton R, Ballenger JC: Valproate in the treatment of acute bipolar affective episodes complicated by substance abuse: a pilot study. J Clin Psychiatry 56:118–121, 1995

Broadhead J, Jacoby R: Mania in old age: a first prospective study. International Journal of Geriatric Psychiatry 5:215–222, 1990

Busse EW, Blazer DG (eds): Textbook of Geriatric Psychiatry, Second Edition. Washington, DC, American Psychiatric Press, 1996, pp 235–263

Calabrese JR, Delucchi GA: Spectrum of efficacy of valproate in 55 patients with rapid-cycling bipolar disorder. Am J Psychiatry 147:431–434, 1990

Calabrese JR, Bowden CB, Woyshville MJ: Lithium and anticonvulsants in the treatment of bipolar disorder, in Psychopharmacology: The Fourth Generation of Progress. Edited by Bloom FE, Kupfer DJ. New York, Raven, 1995a, pp 1099–1111

Calabrese JR, Woyshville MH, McElroy SL, et al: "Spectrum of efficacy" of lamotrigine in treatment-refractory manic depression. Paper presented at the Second International Conference on Affective Disorders, Jerusalem, Israel, September 4–8, 1995b

Calabrese JR, Goethe JW, Kayser A, et al: Adverse events in 583 valproate-treated patients. Depression 3:257–262, 1995/1996

Calabrese JR, Kimmel SE, Woyshville MJ, et al: Clozapine for treatment-refractory mania. Am J Psychiatry 153:759–764, 1996

Carlson GA: Annotation: child and adolescent mania—diagnostic considerations. J Child Psychol Psychiatry 31:331–341, 1990

Carlson GA: Clinical features and pathogenesis of child and adolescent mania, in Mood Disorders Across the Life Span. Edited by Shulman KI, Tohen M, Kutcher SP. New York, Wiley, 1996, pp 127–158

Carlson GA, Kashani JH: Manic symptoms in a non-referred adolescent population. J Affect Disord 15:219–226, 1988

Carlson GA, Strober M: Manic-depressive illness in early adolescence: a study of clinical and diagnostic characteristics in six cases. J Am Acad Child Psychiatry 17:138–153, 1978

Carlson GA, Fennig S, Bromet EJ: The confusion between bipolar disorder and schizophrenia in youth: where does it stand in the 1990s? J Am Acad Child Adolesc Psychiatry 33:453–460, 1994

Chouinard G, Annable L, Turiner L, et al: A double-blind, randomized, clinical trial of rapid tranquilization with I.M. clonazepam and I.M. haloperidol in agitated psychotic patients with manic symptoms. Can J Psychiatry 38:114–121, 1993

Cohen LS, Friedman JM, Jefferson JW, et al: A reevaluation of risk of in utero exposure to lithium. JAMA 271:146–150, 1994

Cohn JB, Collins G, Ashbrook E, et al: A comparison of fluoxetine, imipramine and placebo in patients with bipolar depressive disorder. Int Clin Psychopharmacol 4:313–322, 1989

Coryell W, Norten SG: Mania during adolescence. J Nerv Ment Dis 168:611–613, 1980

Davis JM: Overview: maintenance therapy in psychiatry, II: affective disorders. Am J Psychiatry 133:1–13, 1976

Denicoff KD, Smith-Jackson E, Disney E, et al: Outcome in bipolar patients randomized to lithium or carbamazepine prophylaxis and crossed over in year two. Paper presented at the First International Conference on Bipolar Disorder, Pittsburgh, PA, June 23, 1994

DeVane CL, Sallee FR: Serotonin selective reuptake inhibitors in child and adolescent pharmacology: a review of published experience. J Clin Psychiatry 57:55–66, 1996

Dreifuss FE: Valproic acid: toxicity, in Antiepileptic Drugs, 4th Edition. Edited by Levy RH, Mattson RH, Meldrum BS. New York, Raven, 1995, pp 641–648

Dubovsky SL: Calcium antagonists in manic-depressive illness. Neuropsychobiology 27:184–192, 1993

Dubovsky SL, Buzan R: The role of calcium channel blockers in the treatment of psychiatric disorders. CNS Drugs 4:47–57, 1995

Dunn KL, Rabins PV: Mania in old age, in Mood Disorders Across the Life Span. Edited by Shulman KI, Tohen M, Kutcher SP. New York, Wiley, 1996, pp 399–410

Dwight MM, Keck PE Jr, Stanton SP, et al: Antidepressant activity and mania associated with risperidone treatment of schizoaffective disorders. Lancet 344:554–555, 1994

Egeland JA, Blumenthal RL, Nee J, et al: Reliability and relationship of various ages of onset criteria for major affective disorder. J Affect Disord 12:159–165, 1987

Evans RW, Clay TH, Gaultheria CT: Carbamazepine in pediatric psychiatry. J Am Acad Child Adolesc Psychiatry 26:2–8, 1987

Evans DL, Byerly MJ, Greer RA: Secondary mania: diagnosis and treatment. J Clin Psychiatry 56 [suppl 3]:31–37, 1995

Faedda GL, Baldessarini RJ, Tohen M, et al: Episode sequence in bipolar disorder and response to lithium treatment. Am J Psychiatry 148:1237–1239, 1991

Faedda GL, Baldessarini RJ, Suppes T, et al: Pediatric-onset bipolar disorder: a literature review. Harvard Review of Psychiatry 3:171–195, 1995

Fogelson DL, Bystritsky A, Pasnau : Bupropion in the treatment of bipolar disorders: the same old story. J Clin Psychiatry 53:443–446, 1992

Foster JR: Use of lithium in elderly psychiatric patients: a review of the literature. Lithium 3:77–93, 1992

Fristad MA, Weller EB, Weller RA: The Mania Rating Scale: can it be used in children? a preliminary report. J Am Acad Child Adolesc Psychiatry 31:252–257, 1992

Fristad MA, Weller RA, Weller EB: The Mania Rating Scale (MRS): Further reliability and validity studies with children. Ann Clin Psychiatry 7:127–132, 1995

Gelenberg AJ, Kane JM, Keller MB, et al: Comparison of standard and low serum levels of lithium for maintenance treatment of bipolar disorder. N Engl J Med 321:1489–1493, 1989

Geller B, Cooper TB, Zimerman B, et al: Double-blind, placebo controlled study of lithium for depressed children with bipolar family histories (abstract). Neuropsychopharmacology 10 [suppl 122]:541S, 1994a

Geller B, Fox LW, Clark KA: Rate and predictors of prepubertal bipolarity during follow-up of 6- to 12-year-old depressed children. J Am Acad Child Adolesc Psychiatry 33:461–468, 1994b

Glasser M, Rabins P: Mania in the elderly. Age Ageing 13:210–213, 1984

Goodwin FK, Jamison KR: Manic-Depressive Illness. New York, Oxford University Press, 1990

Green WH: Child and Adolescent Clinical Psychopharmacology, Second Edition. Baltimore, MD, Williams & Wilkins, 1995

Grigoroiu-Serbanescu M, Christodorescu D, Jipescu I, et al: Psychopathology in children aged 10–17 of bipolar parents: psychopathology rate and correlates of severity of the psychopathology. J Affect Disord 16:167–179, 1989

Hardman JG, Limbird LE, Molinoff PB, et al: Goodman and Gilman's The Pharmacologic Basis of Therapeutics, 9th Edition. New York, McGraw-Hill, 1996

Harrow M, Goldberg JF, Grossman LS, et al: Outcome in manic disorders: a naturalistic follow-up study. Arch Gen Psychiatry 47:665–671, 1990

Hayes SG: Barbiturate anticonvulsants in refractory affective disorders. Ann Clin Psychiatry 5:35–44, 1993

Haykal RF, Akiskal HS: Bupropion as a promising approach to rapid cycling bipolar II patients. J Clin Psychiatry 51:450–455, 1990

Himmelhoch JM, Garfinkel ME: Sources of lithium resistance in mixed mania. Psychopharmacol Bull 22:613–620, 1986

Himmelhoch JM, Neil JF, May SJ, et al: Age, dementia, dyskinesias, and lithium response. Am J Psychiatry 137:941–945, 1980

Himmelhoch JM, Thase ME, Mallinger AG, et al: Tranylcypromine versus imipramine in anergic bipolar depression. Am J Psychiatry 148:910–915, 1991

Hopkins HS, Gelenberg AJ: Treatment of bipolar disorder: how far have we come? Psychopharmacol Bull 30:27–38, 1994

Janicak PG, Newman RH, Davis JM: Advances in the treatment of manic and related disorders: a reappraisal. Psychiatric Annals 22:92–103, 1992

Janicak PG, Davis JM, Preskorn SH, et al: Principles and Practice of Psychopharmacotherapy. Baltimore, MD, Williams & Wilkins, 1993

Jefferson JW, Greist JH: Lithium in psychiatry: a review. CNS Therapy 1:448–464, 1994

Jefferson JW, Greist JH, Ackerman DL, et al: Lithium Encyclopedia for Clinical Practice, 2nd Edition. Washington, DC, American Psychiatric Press, 1987

Kafantaris V: Treatment of bipolar disorder in children and adolescents. J Am Acad Child Adolesc Psychiatry 34:732–741, 1995

Kane JM, Jester DV, Barnes TRE, et al: Tardive Dyskinesia: A Task Force Report of the American Psychiatric Association. (Task Force on Tardive Dyskinesia). Washington, DC, American Psychiatric Association, 1992

Keck PE Jr, McElroy SL, Nemeroff CB: Anticonvulsants in the treatment of bipolar disorder. J Neuropsychiatry Clin Neurosci 4:395–405, 1992

Keck PE Jr, McElroy SL, Tugrul KC, et al: Valproate oral loading in treatment of acute mania. J Clin Psychiatry 54:305–308, 1993

Keck PE Jr, Wilson DR, Strakowski SM, et al: Clinical predictors of acute risperidone response in schizophrenia, schizoaffective disorder, and psychotic mood disorders. J Clin Psychiatry 56:466–470, 1995

Kessler RC, McGonagle KA, Zhao S, et al: Lifetime and 12-month prevalence of DSM-III-R psychiatric disorders in the United States: results from the National Comorbidity Survey. Arch Gen Psychiatry 51:8–19, 1994

Kondo JC, Tohen M, Castillo J, et al: Concurrent use of clozapine and valproate in affective and psychotic disorders. J Clin Psychiatry 55:255–257, 1994

Kovacs M, Pollock M: Bipolar disorder and comorbid conduct disorder in childhood and adolescence. J Am Acad Child Adolesc Psychiatry 34:715–723, 1995

Kowatch RA, Suppes T, Gilfillan SK, et al: Clozapine treatment of children and adolescents with bipolar disorder and schizophrenia: a clinical case series. Journal of Child and Adolescent Psychopharmacology 5:241–253, 1995

Kraepelin E: Manic-Depressive Insanity and Paranoia. Translated by Barclay RM. Edited by Robertson GM. Birmingham, AL, The Classics of Medicine Library, 1989

Krasa NR, Tolbert HA: Adolescent bipolar disorder: a nine-year experience. J Affect Disord 30:175–184, 1994

Krauthammer C, Klerman GL: Secondary mania: manic syndromes associated with antecedent physical illness or drugs. Arch Gen Psychiatry 30:74–79, 1978

Kusumakar V et al: Prophylaxis of early onset bipolar I disorder: a two-year follow-up study of lithium versus divalproex sodium (abstract), in Child and Adolescent Psychopharmacology News, Vol 1. Edited by Kutcher SD. New York, Guilford, 1996, p 6

Kutcher SP, Marton P, Korenblum M: Adolescent bipolar illness and personality disorder. J Am Acad Child Adolesc Psychiatry 29:355–358, 1990

Kye C, Ryan N: Pharmacologic treatment of child and adolescent depression. Child and Adolescent Clinics of North America 4:261–281, 1995

Lambert PA, Venaud G: Comparative study of valpromide versus lithium as prophylactic treatment in affective disorders. Nervure Journal de Psychiatrie 7:1–9, 1995

Leach JP, Brodie MJ: Lamotrigine: clinical use, in Antiepileptic Drugs, 4th Edition. Edited by Levy RH, Mattson RH, Meldrum BS. New York, Raven, 1995, pp 889–895

Lenox RH, Newhouse PA, Creelman WL, et al: Adjunctive treatment of manic agitation with lorazepam versus haloperidol: a double-blind study. J Clin Psychiatry 53:47–52, 1992

Lewinsohn PM, Klein DN, Seeley JR: Bipolar disorders in a community sample of older adolescents: prevalence, phenomenology, comorbidity, and course. J Am Acad Child Adolesc Psychiatry 34:454–463, 1995

Levy RH, Matson RH, Meldrum BS (eds): Antiepileptic Drugs, 4th Edition. New York, Raven, 1995

Lish JD, Dime-Meenan S, Whybrow PC, et al: The National Depressive and Manic-Depressive Association (NDMDA) survey of bipolar members. J Affect Disord 31:281–294, 1994

Maj M: Clinical prediction of response to lithium prophylaxis in bipolar patients: a critical update. Lithium 3:15–21, 1992

Maj M, Pirozzi R, Magliano L: Nonresponse to reinstituted lithium prophylaxis in previously responsive bipolar patients: prevalence and predictors. Am J Psychiatry 152:1810–1811, 1995

McElroy SL, Keck PE Jr: Antiepileptic drugs, in The American Psychiatric Press Textbook of Psychopharmacology. Edited by Schatzberg AF, Nemeroff CB. Washington, DC, American Psychiatric Press, 1995, pp 351–375

McElroy SL, Keck PE Jr, Pope HG Jr, et al: Clinical and research implications of the diagnosis of dysphoric or mixed mania or hypomania. Am J Psychiatry 149:1633–1644, 1992

McElroy SL, Keck PE, Stanton SP, et al: A randomized comparison of divalproex oral loading versus haloperidol in the initial treatment of acute psychotic mania. J Clin Psychiatry 56:142–146, 1996a

McElroy SL, Keck PE Jr, Strakowski SM: Mania, psychosis, and antipsychotics. J Clin Psychiatry 57 [suppl 3]:14–26, 1996b

McElroy SL, Soutullo CA, Keck PE, Jr, et al: Phenomenology of adolescent and adult mania in hospitalized patients with bipolar disorder. Am J Psychiatry 154:44–49, 1997

McElroy SL, Soutullo CA, Keck PE Jr, et al: A pilot trial of adjunctive gabapentin in the treatment of bipolar disorder. Ann Clin Psychiatry, in press

McFarland BH, Miller MR, Straumfjord AA: Valproate use in the older manic patient. J Clin Psychiatry 51:479–481, 1990

Miklowitz DJ: Psychotherapy in combination of drug treatment for bipolar disorder. J Clin Psychopharmacol 16 (suppl 1):56–66, 1996

Mirchandani IC, Young RD: Management of mania in the elderly: an update. Ann Clin Psychiatry 5:67–77, 1993

Müller-Oerlinghausen B, Ahrens B, Grof E, et al: The effect of long-term lithium treatment on the mortality of patients with manic-depressive and schizoaffective illness. Acta Psychiatr Scand 86:218–222, 1992

O'Connell RA, Mayo JA, Flatow L, et al: Outcome of bipolar disorder on long-term treatment with lithium. Br J Psychiatry 159:123–129, 1991

Okuma T: Effects of carbamazepine and lithium on affective disorders. Neuropsychobiol 27:138–145, 1993

Papatheodorou G: A review of valproate in acute adolescent mania. Child and Adolescent Psychopharmacology News 1:10–11,1996

Papatheodorou G, Kutcher SP: Treatment of bipolar disorder in adolescents, in Mood Disorders Across the Life Span. Edited by Shulman KI, Tohen M, Kutcher SP. New York, Wiley, 1996, pp 159–186

Papatheodorou G, Kutcher S, Katic M, et al: The efficacy and safety of divalproex sodium in the treatment of acute mania in adolescent and young adults: an open clinical trial. J Clin Psychopharmacol 15:110–116, 1995

Pazzaglia PJ, Post RM, Ketter TA, et al: Preliminary controlled trial of nimodipine in ultra-rapid cycling affective dysregulation. Psychiatry Res 49:257–272, 1993

Peet M: Induction of mania with selective serotonin re-uptake inhibitors and tricyclic antidepressants. Br J Psychiatry 164:549–550, 1994

Pellock JM: Carbamazepine side effects in children and adults. Epilepsia 28 [suppl 3]:564–570, 1987

Pellock JM, Willmore LJ: A rational guide to routine blood monitoring in patients receiving antiepileptic drugs. Neurology 41:961–964, 1991

Pope HG Jr, Lipinski JF: Diagnosis in schizophrenia and manic-depressive illness: a reassessment of the specificity of schizophrenic symptoms in the light of current research. Arch Gen Psychiatry 35:811–828, 1978

Pope HG Jr, McElroy SL: Valproate, in Comprehensive Textbook of Psychiatry/VI, 6th Edition, Vol 2. Edited by Kaplan HI, Sadock BJ. Baltimore, MD, Williams & Wilkins, 1995, pp 2112–2120

Pope HG Jr, McElroy SL, Keck PE Jr, et al: Valproate in the treatment of acute mania. Arch Gen Psychiatry 48:62–68, 1991

Popper CW: Balancing knowledge and judgement: a clinician looks at new developments in child and adolescent psychopharmacology. Pediatric Psychopharmacology II 4:483–510, 1995

Post F: The functional psychoses, in Studies in Geriatric Psychiatry. Edited by Isaacs AD, Post F. New York, Wiley, 1978, pp 77–98

Post RM: Transduction of psychosocial stress into the neurobiology of recurrent affective disorder. Am J Psychiatry 149:999–1010, 1992

Post RM: Carbamazepine, in Comprehensive Textbook of Psychiatry, 6th Edition, Vol 2. Edited by Kaplan HI, Sadock BJ. Baltimore, MD, Williams & Wilkins, 1995a, pp 1964–1972

Post RM: Mood disorders: somatic treatment, in Comprehensive Textbook of Psychiatry, 6th Edition, Vol 1. Edited by Kaplan HI, Sadock BJ. Baltimore, MD, Williams & Wilkins, 1995b, pp 1152–1177

Post RM, Uhde TW, Roy-Byrne PP, et al: Antidepressant effects of carbamazepine. Am J Psychiatry 143:29–34, 1986

Post RM, Uhde TW, Roy-Byrne PP, et al: Correlates of antimanic response to carbamaze-pine. Psychiatry Res 21:71–83, 1987

Post RM, Leverich GA, Altshuler L, et al: Lithium-discontinuation-induced refractoriness: preliminary observations. Am J Psychiatry 149:1727–1729, 1992

Price LH, Heninger GR: Lithium in the treatment of mood disorders. N Engl J Med 331:591–598, 1994

Richardson MA, Haugland G (eds): Use of Neuroleptics in Children. Washington, DC, American Psychiatric Press, 1995

Robins LN, Regier DA: Psychiatric Disorders in America: The Epidemiologic Catchment Area Study. New York, Free Press, 1991

Sachs GS, Lafer B, Stoll A, et al: A double-blind trial of bupropion versus desipramine for bipolar depression. J Clin Psychiatry 55:391–393, 1994

Sadavoy J, Lazarus LW, Jarvik LF, et al (eds): Comprehensive Review of Geriatric Psychi-atry—II, 2nd Edition. Washington, DC, American Psychiatric Press, 1996

Sajatovic M, DiGiovanni SK, Bastani B, et al: Risperidone therapy in treatment-refractory, acute bipolar and schizoaffective mania. Psychopharmacol Bull 32:55–61, 1996

Schou M: Lithium prophylaxis: myths and realities. Am J Psychiatry 146:573–576, 1989

Schou M: Forty years of lithium treatment. Arch Gen Psychiatry 54:9–13, 1997

Shopsin B: Bupropion's prophylactic efficacy in bipolar affective illness. J Clin Psychiatry 44:163–169, 1983

Shulman KI: Mania in the elderly. International Review of Psychiatry 5:445–453, 1993

Shulman KI, Tohen M, Kutcher SP (eds): Mood Disorders Across the Lifespan. New York, Wiley, 1996

Simpson SG, DePaulo JR: Fluoxetine treatment of bipolar II depression. J Clin Psycho-pharmacol 11:52–54, 1991

Simpson SG, Folstein SE, Meyers DA, et al: Bipolar II: the most common bipolar pheno-type? Am J Psychiatry 150:901–903, 1993

Stanton SP, Keck PE Jr, McElroy SL: Treatment of acute mania with gabapentin (letter). Am J Psychiatry, in press

Stoll AL, Mayer PV, Kolbrener M, et al: Antidepressant-associated mania: a controlled comparison with spontaneous mania. Am J Psychiatry 151:1642–1645, 1994a

Stoll AL, Banov M, Kilbrener M, et al: Neurologic factors predict a favorable valproate response in bipolar and schizoaffective disorders. J Clin Psychopharmacol 14:311–313, 1994b

Stone K: Mania in the elderly. Br J Psychiatry 155:220–224, 1989

Strakowski SM, McElroy SL, Keck PE Jr, et al: The co-occurrence of mania with medical and other psychiatric disorders. Int J Psychiatry Med 24:305–328, 1994

Strober M, Carlson GA: Bipolar illness in adolescents with major depression: clinical, ge-netic and psychopharmacologic predictors in a three- to four-year prospective follow up investigation. Arch Gen Psychiatry 39:549–555, 1982

Strober M, Morrell W, Burroughs J, et al: A family study of bipolar I disorder in adoles-cence: early onset of symptoms linked to increased familial loading and lithium resis-tance. J Affect Disord 15:255–268, 1988

Strober M, Morrell W, Lampert C, et al: Relapse following discontinuation of lithium maintenance therapy in adolescents with bipolar I illness: a naturalistic study. Am J Psychiatry 147:457–461, 1990

Strober M, Lampert C, Schmidt S, et al: The course of major depressive disorder in ado-lescents, I: recovery and risk of manic switching in a follow up of psychotic and non-psychotic subtypes. J Am Acad Child Adolesc Psychiatry 32:34–42, 1993

Suppes T, Baldessarini RJ, Faedda GL, et al: Risk of recurrence following discontinuation of lithium in bipolar disorder. Arch Gen Psychiatry 48:1082–1088, 1991

Swann AC, Bowden CL, Morris D, et al: Depression during mania: treatment response to lithium or divalproex. Arch Gen Psychiatry 54:37–42, 1997

Thase ME, Mallinger AG, McKnight D, et al: Treatment of imipramine-resistant recurrent depression, IV: a double-blind crossover study of tranylcypromine for anergic bipolar depression. Am J Psychiatry 149:195–198, 1992

Tohen M, Castillo J, Pope HG Jr, et al: Concomitant use of valproate and carbamazepine in bipolar and schizoaffective disorders. J Clin Psychopharmacol 14:67–70, 1994a

Tohen M, Shulman KI, Satlin A: First-episode mania in late life. Am J Psychiatry 151:130–132, 1994b

Tohen M, Castillo J, Baldessarini RJ, et al: Blood dyscrasias with carbamazepine and valproate: a pharmacoepidemiological study of 2,228 patients at risk. Am J Psychiatry 152:413–418, 1995

Tohen M, Zarate CZ, Centorrino F, et al: Risperidone in the treatment of mania. J Clin Psychiatry 57:249–253, 1996

U. S. Department of Health, Education and Welfare Medical Practice Project: A state-of-the science report for the Office of the Assistant Secretary for the U.S. Department of Health, Education and Welfare. Baltimore, MD, Policy Research, 1979

Weisler R, Risner M, Ascher J, et al: Use of lamotrigine in the treatment of bipolar disorder. American Psychiatric Association New Research Program and Abstracts, Annual Meeting, 1994, Abstract NR611, p 216

Weissman MM, Leaf PJ, Tischler GL: Affective disorders in five United States communities. Psychol Med 18:141–153, 1988

Weller EB, Weller RA, Fristad MA: Lithium dosage guide for prepubertal children: a preliminary report. J Am Acad Child Psychiatry 25:92–95, 1986

Weller EB, Weller RA, Fristad MA: Bipolar disorder in children: misdiagnosis, underdiagnosis, and future directions. J Am Acad Child Adolesc Psychiatry 34:709–714, 1995

West SA, Keck PE Jr, McElroy SL, et al: Open trial of valproate in the treatment of adolescent mania. Journal of Child and Adolescent Psychopharmacology 4:263–267, 1994

West SA, McElroy SL, Strakowski SM, et al: Attention deficit hyperactivity disorder in adolescent mania. Am J Psychiatry 152:271–273, 1995a

West SA, Keck PE Jr, McElroy SL: Oral loading doses in the valproate treatment of adolescents with mixed bipolar disorder. Journal of Child and Adolescent Psychopharmacology 5:225–231, 1995b

West SA, Strakowski SM, Sax KW, et al: Phenomenology and comorbidity of adolescents hospitalized for the treatment of acute mania. Biol Psychiatry 39:458–460, 1996

Wicki W, Angst J: The Zurich Study, 10: hypomania in a 28- to 30-year old cohort. Eur Arch Psychiatry Clin Neurosci 240:339–348, 1991

Winokur G, Clayton PJ, Reich T: Manic Depressive Illness. St. Louis, MO, CV Mosby, 1969

Winokur G, Coryell W, Endicott J, et al: Further distinctions between manic-depressive illness (bipolar disorder) and primary depressive disorder (unipolar depression). Am J Psychiatry 150:1176–1181, 1993

Worthington JJ III, Pollack MH: Treatment of dysphoric mania with nefazodone (letter). Am J Psychiatry 153:732–733, 1996

Wozniak J, Biederman J, Kiely K, et al: Mania-like symptoms suggestive of childhood-onset bipolar disorder in clinically referred children. J Am Acad Child Adolesc Psychiatry 34:867–876, 1995

Wright G, Galloway L, Kim J, et al: Bupropion in the long-term treatment of cyclic mood disorders: mood stabilizing effects. J Clin Psychiatry 46:22–25, 1985

Young RC: Treatment of geriatric mania, in Mood Disorders Across the Life Span. Edited by Shulman KI, Tohen M, Kutcher SP. New York, Wiley, 1996, pp 411–425

Young RC, Falk JR: Age, manic psychopathology and treatment response. International Journal of Geriatric Psychiatry 4:73–75, 1989

Young RC, Klerman GL: Mania in late life: focus on age at onset. Am J Psychiatry 149:867–876, 1992

Zahn-Waxler C, Mayfield A, Radke-Yarrow M, et al: A follow-up investigation of offspring of parents with bipolar disorder. Am J Psychiatry 145:506–509, 1988

Zarate CA Jr, Tohen M, Baldessarini RJ: Clozapine in severe mood disorders. J Clin Psychiatry 56:411–417, 1995

Zornberg GL, Pope HG Jr: Treatment of depression in bipolar disorder: new directions for research. J Clin Psychopharmacol 13:397–408, 1993

Chapter 18

Pharmacotherapy of Attention-Deficit/ Hyperactivity Disorder: A Life Span Perspective

Thomas Spencer, M.D., Joseph Biederman, M.D., and Timothy Wilens, M.D.

Attention-deficit/hyperactivity disorder (ADHD) is a heterogeneous disorder of unknown etiology. It is one of the major clinical and public health problems because of its associated morbidity and disability in children, adolescents, and adults. Its consequences to society are enormous in terms of financial cost, stress on families, impact on academic and vocational activities, and negative effect on self-esteem. Data from cross-sectional, retrospective, and follow-up studies indicate that children with ADHD are at risk for developing other psychiatric difficulties in childhood, adolescence, and adulthood, including antisocial behaviors, substance use disorders, and mood and anxiety symptoms and disorders.

The name and nosology of ADHD have undergone a number of changes over the last several decades. In the 1960s, in DSM-II (American Psychiatric Association 1968), motoric symptoms were stressed, and the disorder was called hyperkinetic reaction of childhood. DSM-III (American Psychiatric Association 1980) renamed the disorder as attention deficit disorder (ADD) and emphasized inattention as its core feature. In DSM-III-R (American Psychiatric Association 1987) the disorder was renamed attention-deficit/hyperactivity disorder (ADHD). Both inattention and hyperactivity were emphasized as equally important core features. The name of ADHD remained the same in DSM-IV (American Psychiatric Association 1994), but DSM-IV recognized three subtypes of ADHD, depending on which symptoms predominate: a predominantly inattentive subtype, a predominantly hyperactive-impulsive subtype, and a combined subtype.

Although the underlying neural and pathophysiological substrate of ADHD remains unknown, an emerging neuropsychological and neuroimaging literature suggests that abnormalities in frontal networks or frontostriatal dysfunction are the disorder's underlying neural substrate and that catecholamine dysregulation is its underlying pathophysiological substrate (Castellanos et al. 1994; Giedd et al. 1994; Hynd et al. 1990, 1993; Semrud-Clikeman et al. 1994; Zametkin and Rapoport 1987; Zametkin et al. 1990). Although its etiology remains unknown, data from family genetic, twin, and adoption studies, as well as segregation analysis, suggest a genetic origin for some forms of the disorder (Biederman et al. 1990a, 1992; Deutsch et al. 1990; Faraone and Biederman 1994; Faraone et al. 1992; Goodman 1989; Goodman and Stevenson 1989a, 1989b; Manshadi et al. 1983). However, other etiologies are also likely, including psychological adversity, perinatal insults, and perhaps other as yet unknown biological causes (Biederman et al. 1994; Milberger et al. 1993).

Although follow-up studies show that ADHD persists into adulthood in 10% to 60% of childhood-onset cases (Gittelman et al. 1985; Hechtman 1992; Mannuzza et al. 1991, 1993; Weiss et al. 1985), little scientific attention has been paid to the adult form of this disorder. Its high prevalence of at least 5% in childhood (Anderson et al. 1987; Bird et al. 1988), combined with the follow-up results, suggests that approximately 2% of adults may suffer from ADHD. If so, this would make ADHD a common adult psychiatric disorder that may be underidentified in adult psychiatric clinics.

In this chapter we focus on the pharmacotherapy of ADHD throughout the life cycle. However, it is important that a comprehensive treatment approach be taken when treating ADHD patients of all ages—one that attempts to address the three main areas of potential dysfunction: biological, psychosocial, and educational. Pharmacotherapy for ADHD improves attention, hyperactivity, and impulsivity, reduces abnormal behaviors at school or work, and improves the individual's family and social functioning (Gittelman-Klein 1987). Potentially useful psychotherapeutic efforts in the management of ADHD patients include behavioral and cognitive-behavioral interventions such as training in self-instruction, self-evaluation, attribution, social skills, and anger management (Hinshaw and Erhardt 1991). Because at least 30% of ADHD patients may suffer from learning disabilities that are not drug sensitive, learning-disabled ADHD patients often require additional educational support, such as tutoring, placement in special classes, and occasionally specialized schools.

Comorbidity and Attention-Deficit/ Hyperactivity Disorder

In recent years, evidence has been accumulating regarding high levels of psychiatric and cognitive (i.e., learning-disability) comorbidity between ADHD and a number of disorders, including mood and anxiety disorders and conduct disorder (Biederman et al. 1991). This high level of comorbidity has been found in culturally and regionally diverse epidemiological samples (e.g., New Zealand and Puerto Rico) (Anderson et al. 1987; Bird et al. 1988; McGee et al. 1985), clinical samples (reviewed in Biederman et al. 1991), as well as in family genetic studies (Biederman et al. 1992) indicating that ADHD is most probably a heterogeneous group of conditions rather than a single homogeneous clinical entity, with potentially different etiological and modifying risk factors and outcomes.

Conduct Disorder

Conduct disorder (CD) is the best-established comorbid condition of childhood ADHD, and it has been widely reported in epidemiological (Anderson et al. 1987; Bird et al. 1988; McGee et al. 1985), clinical (Barkley et al. 1989; Quay et al. 1987), follow-up (Gittelman et al. 1985; Loney et al. 1981a; Weiss and Hechtman 1986), and family genetic studies (Biederman et al. 1992). Consistent with childhood studies, recent studies of referred and nonreferred adults with ADHD have found high rates of childhood CD as well as adult antisocial disorders in these subjects (Biederman et al. 1990b, 1993c). The presence of CD is important to consider and identify, because it has been associated with poor prognosis (Loney et al. 1981b; McGee et al. 1984; Milich and Loney 1979) and a high risk of developing addictions (Biederman et al. 1995d; Gittelman et al. 1985).

Mood Disorders

In addition to well-documented comorbidity with CD, recent studies have also documented high rates of mood disorders in epidemiological samples of children with ADHD (Anderson et al. 1987; Bird et al. 1988; McGee et al. 1985) and clinical studies of ADHD children, adolescents, and adults (Biederman et al. 1991, 1993c; Jensen et al. 1993). Conversely, high rates of ADHD have been found in patients with mood disorders, both children and adolescents (Alessi and Magen 1988; Angold and Costello 1993; Biederman et al. 1995a; Biederman et al. 1995b; Geller et al. 1995; Wozniak et al. 1995) and adults (Alpert et al. 1996; Sachs et al. 1993). Similarly, investigators have noted high rates of anxiety in children with ADHD (Lahey et al. 1987, 1988) and high rates of ADHD in children with anxiety (Last et al. 1987). Studies have also clearly documented high levels of comorbidity with both reading and arithmetic disability in ADHD children (Biederman et al. 1991; Semrud-Clikeman et al. 1992) and, conversely, high rates of ADHD in samples of children with learning disorders (Cantwell 1985; Silver and Brunstetter 1986).

Gender and Attention-Deficit/ Hyperactivity Disorder

Although little doubt remains that ADHD affects both genders, an extraordinarily limited literature exists on ADHD in females (Gaub and Carlson, in press). This literature clearly indicates that ADHD females share with their male counterparts prototypical features of the disorder (e.g., inattention, impulsivity, hyperactivity), high rates of school failure, high comorbidity with mood and anxiety disorders and learning disabilities, and high levels of familiality (Barkley 1989; Pelham et al. 1989). However, rates of aggressive symptoms and comorbid CD are far less prevalent in females than in males. This fact perhaps accounts for the overrepresentation of males over females (up to 10:1) in clinical samples of children with ADHD (Faraone et al. 1991). The preponderance of boys over girls is much less dramatic in epidemiological and adult samples, in which the ratio of males to females approximates 2:1. The underidentification and undertreatment of females with ADHD may have substantial clinical and educational implications by depriving them of highly effective treatment programs aimed at improving impairments associated with the disorder.

Pharmacotherapy

Stimulants

Stimulants are sympathomimetic drugs structurally similar to endogenous catecholamines (e.g., dopamine and norepinephrine). The most commonly used compounds in this class include methylphenidate (Ritalin), D-amphetamine (Dexedrine), and magnesium pemoline (Cylert). These drugs are thought to act in both the central and peripheral nervous systems by preventing the reuptake of catecholamines into presynaptic nerve endings, thereby preventing catecholamine degradation by monoamine oxidase. Methylphenidate and D-amphetamine are both short-acting compounds, with an onset of action within 30–60 minutes and a usual peak clinical effect 1–3 hours after administration. Therefore, multiple daily administrations are required for a consistent daytime response. Typically, these compounds have a rapid onset of action; clinical response is evident soon after a therapeutic dose is obtained. Slow-release preparations, with a peak clinical effect between 1 and 5 hours, are available for methylphenidate and D-amphetamine and can often allow for a single dose to be administered in the morning that will last for the entire school day. Magnesium pemoline is a longer-acting compound, generally allowing for one or two daily doses. Contrary to previous indications (Conners and

Taylor 1980), a recent study has suggested that when the dose of pemoline (1–2 mg/kg) is calculated to achieve a reasonable plasma concentration (greater than 2 µg/mL), clinically measurable effects are apparent within hours (Sallee et al. 1992).

Although there are more than 150 controlled studies of stimulants, with more than 5,000 children, adolescents, and adults, the vast majority of the studies are limited to latency-age Caucasian boys treated for no longer than 2 months (Table 18–1, Figure 18–1, and Figure 18–2). These studies document the short-term efficacy and safety of stimulants in all age groups, but more clearly in latency-age children. Despite the findings on the efficacy of the stimulants, studies also have reported consistently that, on average, as many as 30% do not respond to these drugs (Barkley 1977; Gittelman 1980; Spencer et al. 1996b). Although methylphenidate is by far the most studied stimulant, the literature provides little evidence of differential response to the various available stimulants. However, some patients may respond preferentially to one or another stimulant (Elia et al. 1991).

Although the efficacy of stimulants in ADHD is most clearly documented in latency-age children, a more limited literature reveals a good response in both preschoolers and adolescents. Studies in preschoolers report improvement in structured tasks as well as in mother-child interactions (Barkley 1988; Barkley et al. 1984; Conners 1975; Mayes et al. 1994; Schleifer et al. 1975). Similarly, in adolescents, response has been reported as moderate to robust, and no abuse or tolerance has been noted (Brown RT and Sexson 1988; Coons et al. 1987; Evans and Pelham 1991; Klorman et al. 1987; Lerer and Lerer 1977; MacKay et al. 1973; Safer and Allen 1975; Varley 1983). In contrast, studies in adults with ADHD report a more variable response, ranging from 25% to 78% with an average of 54% (Gualtieri et al. 1985; Mattes et al. 1984; Spencer et al. 1995b; Wender et al. 1981; Wender et al. 1985b; Wood et al. 1976). Potential reasons for this variability in adult ADHD studies include a low average daily dose (0.6 mg/kg), diagnostic imprecision (Wood et al. 1976), differing assessment methodology, and effects of psychiatric comorbidity. The largest response in adults was reported by our group in a recent randomized, controlled study of methylphenidate in patients diagnosed with childhood-onset DSM-III-R ADHD. This investigation used standardized instruments for diagnosis; separate assessments of ADHD, depressive, and anxiety symptoms; and a robust daily dose of 1.0 mg/kg/day (Spencer et al. 1995b). This study found a markedly greater therapeutic response to methylphenidate than to placebo (78% vs. 4%), which appeared to be dose dependent. In addition, response to methylphenidate in this study was independent of gender, psychiatric comorbidity, or family history of psychiatric disorders (Figure 18–3).

The literature clearly documents a wide range of beneficial effects

Table 18–1. Psychotropics used in ADHD

Drug class	Daily dose	Daily dosage schedule	Common adverse effects
Stimulants			
dextroamphetamine	0.3–1.5 mg/kg	Twice or three times	Insomnia, decreased appetite, weight loss
methylphenidate	1.0–2.0 mg/kg	Twice or three times	Depression, psychosis (rare, with very high doses)
			Increase in heart rate and blood pressure (mild)
			Possible reduction in growth velocity with long-term use
			Withdrawal effects and rebound phenomena
magnesium pemoline	1.0–3.0 mg/kg	Once or twice	Same as other stimulants
			Abnormal liver function tests
			(Rare) liver failure
Antidepressants			
tricyclics (TCAs) (e.g., imipramine, desipramine, nortriptyline)	2.0–5.0 mg/kg (1.0–3.0 mg/kg for nortriptyline)	Once or twice	Anticholinergic (dry mouth, constipation, blurred vision)
			Weight loss
			Cardiovascular (mild increase) diastolic blood pressure and ECG conduction parameters with daily doses > 3.5 mg/kg. Treatment requires serum levels and ECG monitoring
monoamine oxidase inhibitors (MAOIs) phenelzine, tranylcypromine,	0.5–1.0 mg/kg	Twice or three times	Severe dietary restrictions (high-tyramine foods)
			Hypertensive crisis with dietetic transgression or with certain drugs
			Weight gain
selegiline	0.2–0.6 mg/kg	Twice or three times	Drowsiness
			Changes in blood pressure
			Insomnia
			Liver toxicity (remote)

	Dose	Frequency	Side effects
SSRIs			
fluoxetine	0.5–1.0 mg/kg	Once in A.M. or P.M.	Irritability
sertraline	1.5–3.0 mg/kg	Once in A.M. or P.M.	Insomnia
paroxetine	0.25–0.70 mg/kg	Once in A.M. or P.M.	GI symptoms
fluvoxamine	1.5–4.5 mg/kg	Once in A.M. or P.M.	Headaches
			Sexual dysfunction
bupropion	3–6 mg/kg	Three times	Irritability
			Insomnia
			Drug-induced seizures (in doses >6 mg/kg)
			Caution in bulimics
venlafaxine	1–3 mg/kg	Twice or three times	Similar to SSRIs
			Irritability
			Insomnia
			GI symptoms
			Headaches
			Blood pressure changes
Other drugs			
α_2 agonists			
clonidine	3–10 µg/kg	Twice or three times	Sedation (very frequent)
			Hypotension (rare)
			Dry mouth
			Confusion (with high dose)
			Depression
			Rebound hypertension
			Localized irritation with transdermal preparation

(continued)

Table 18–1. Psychotropics used in ADHD *(continued)*

Drug class	Daily dose	Daily dosage schedule	Common adverse effects
Other drugs *(continued)*			
α$_2$ agonists *(continued)*			
guanfacine	15–43 µg/kg	Once or twice	Same as clonidine (less sedation)
propranolol	2–8 mg/kg	Twice	Similar to clonidine Higher risk for bradycardia and hypotension (dose dependent) and rebound hypertension Bronchospasm (contraindicated in asthmatics) Rebound hypertension on abrupt withdrawal

Note. GI = gastrointestinal; SSRI = selective serotonin reuptake inhibitor. ECG = electrocardiographic.

A. Medication type

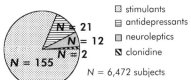

- ⊠ stimulants
- ⊟ antidepressants
- ☐ neuroleptics
- ◪ clonidine

N = 6,472 subjects

B. Age of subjects

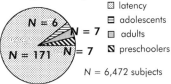

- ⊠ latency
- ⊟ adolescents
- ☐ adults
- ◪ preschoolers

N = 6,472 subjects

C. Studies of stimulants

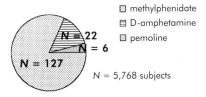

- ⊠ methylphenidate
- ⊟ D-amphetamine
- ☐ pemoline

N = 5,768 subjects

D. Studies of antidepressants

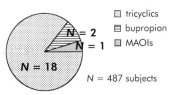

- ⊠ tricyclics
- ⊟ bupropion
- ☐ MAOIs

N = 487 subjects

Figure 18–1. Controlled studies in attention-deficit/hyperactivity disorder (all ages).
Source. Adapted from Spencer et al. (1996b).

A. Duration

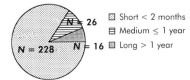

- ⊠ Short < 2 months
- ⊟ Medium ≤ 1 year
- ☐ Long > 1 year

B. Gender

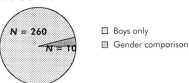

- ⊠ Boys only
- ☐ Gender comparison

C. Ethnicity

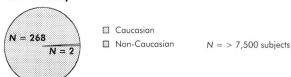

- ⊠ Caucasian
- ☐ Non-Caucasian

N = > 7,500 subjects

Figure 18–2. Medication studies in attention-deficit/hyperactivity disorder (open and controlled).
Source. Adapted from Spencer et al. (1996b).

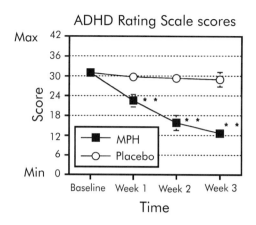

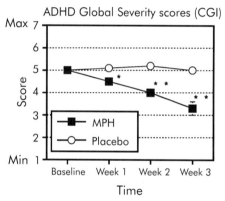

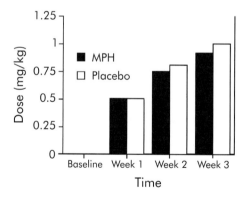

Figure 18–3. ADHD Rating Scale and ADHD Global Severity scores by week and dose.

CGI = Clinical Global Impression. MPH = methylphenidate.

*$P < .001$.**$P < .0001$.

Source. Adapted from Spencer et al. (1995b).

associated with stimulant drugs in ADHD subjects. Stimulants diminish behaviors prototypical of ADHD, including motoric overactivity, impulsivity, and inattentiveness. Stimulants can also be effective in patients with ADHD in whom hyperactivity is not a significant clinical problem (Safer and Krager 1988). In addition to improving core symptoms of ADHD, stimulants also improve associated behavioral difficulties, including on-task behavior, academic performance, and social function. These effects appear to be dose dependent and cross-situational, occurring at home, in the clinic, at school, and at work (Abikoff and Gittelman 1985; Barkley et al. 1984; Klein 1987; Rapport et al. 1986; Swanson et al. 1987; Tannock et al. 1989; Wilens and Biederman 1992). In several studies, behaviors of the child with ADHD became indistinguishable from peers without the disorder with respect to impulsivity, noncompliance, disruption, and overall hyperactivity (Whalen 1989). Observational studies have also demonstrated stimulant-enhanced social skills in school, within families, and with peers, including improved maternal-child and sibling interactions (Barkley and Cunningham 1979). Studies have also found that families of stimulant-responsive children are more amenable to psychosocial interventions (Schachar et al. 1987). Investigations of peer relationships in children with ADHD have shown that those treated with stimulants have increased abilities to perceive peer communications, self-perceptions, and situational cues. In addition, these children show improved modulation of the intensity of behavior, improved communication, greater responsiveness, and fewer negative interactions (Whalen et al. 1990). In adults with ADHD, occupational and marital dysfunction were noted to improve with stimulant treatment (Wender et al. 1985a).

These findings support the importance of treating children, adolescents, and adults with ADHD beyond school and work hours—during evenings, weekends, and vacations, should problems exist at these times. Despite beneficial effects on social skills, some interpersonal difficulties associated with ADHD could represent additional brain-based abnormal social behavior, akin to learning disabilities (Greene et al. 1996; Weintraub et al. 1981), that are not drug sensitive but may require psychosocial treatment strategies.

Numerous studies have also documented stimulant-induced improvements in children with ADHD in measures of vigilance, cognitive impulsivity, reaction time, short-term memory, and learning of verbal and nonverbal material (Barkley 1977; Klein 1987; Rapport et al. 1988). Recent studies employing a simulated classroom paradigm have shown consistent stimulant-associated improvements (Barkley 1991; DuPaul et al. 1994). It was also found that treatment with stimulants increases school-based productivity (Famularo and Fenton 1987) and improves performance in academic testing (H. Abikoff, personal communication, March 1996). However, despite these beneficial cognitive effects, it is important to be aware that children with ADHD commonly manifest additional learning disabilities that are not responsive to pharmacotherapy (Bergman et al. 1991; Faraone et al. 1993) but may respond to educational remediation.

Although short-term studies have documented rapid improvement in the core ADHD symptoms, associated functional improvement may lag behind symptom remission—a finding similar to those in other psychiatric disorders such as mood disorders and schizophrenia (Baldessarini 1996). The ultimate effectiveness of anti-ADHD medication for cognitive and academic performance, social skills, and quality of life may not be fully apparent in the existing short-term studies; hence the extent of long-term stimulant-associated functional improvement remains unknown (Schachar and Tannock 1993). In addition, there is very limited information about efficacy and safety of stimulants in females (Barkley 1989; Pelham et al. 1989) and minorities (Brown RT and Sexson 1988).

Administration and Side Effects of Stimulants

Because of their short half-life, the short-acting stimulants (methylphenidate and dextroamphetamine) should be given in divided doses throughout the day, typically 4 hours apart. The total daily dosage ranges from 0.3 mg/kg/day to 2 mg/kg/day. The starting dosage is generally 2.5–5 mg/day, given in the morning, with the dosage increased if necessary every few days by 2.5–5 mg in a divided-dose schedule. Because of the anorexogenic effects of the stimulants, it may be beneficial to administer the medication after meals. The longer–half-life agent, magnesium pemoline, is typically given once or twice daily (such as 8:00 A.M. and 2:00 P.M.), in dosages of 1–3 mg/kg/day. The typical starting dose of pemoline is 18.75 to 37.5 mg, with increments in dose of 18.75 mg every few days thereafter, until desired effects occur or side effects preclude further increments.

The relationship between dose and response remains a source of active controversy. An influential early study (Sprague and Sleator 1977) reported that higher stimulant doses were required to ameliorate behavior but that these higher doses degraded performance on cognitive tasks. Later studies, however, challenged this notion by failing to reveal evidence of cognitive impairment on standard dosages (0.3–2.0 mg/kg/day) of stimulants. Moreover, these later studies indicated that both behavior and cognitive performance improve with stimulant treatment in a dose-dependent fashion (Douglas et al. 1988; Klein 1987; Kupietz et al. 1988; Pelham et al. 1985; Rapport et al. 1987, 1989a, 1989b; Tannock et al. 1989). In addition, earlier concerns that stimulants were associated with constriction of attention or "overfocusing" have recently been refuted (Douglas et al. 1995; Solanto and Wender 1989). Furthermore, there is no evidence that improved behavior comes at the cost of "zombification": studies have shown increased prosocial behavior in those taking stimulant medication (Gittelman 1980; Whalen et al. 1990).

The most commonly reported side effects of stimulants are appetite suppression and sleep disturbances. The sleep disturbance most commonly reported is delay of sleep onset, which usually occurs when stimulants are administered in the late afternoon or early evening. Although less common, mood disturbances ranging from increased tearfulness to a full-blown, major-depression–like syndrome can be associated with stimulant treatment (Gittelman-Klein 1980). Other infrequent side effects include headaches, abdominal discomfort, increased lethargy, and fatigue. Although the cardiovascular effects of stimulants have not been fully examined, mild increases in pulse and blood pressure of unclear clinical significance have been observed (Brown RT et al. 1984). A rare stimulant-associated toxic psychosis has been observed, usually in the context of either a rapid dosage increase or very high doses. In children, this psychosis resembles a toxic phenomenon (e.g., visual hallucinosis) and is dissimilar from the stimulant-induced exacerbation of psychotic symptoms seen in schizophrenia. The development of psychotic symptoms in a child being treated with stimulants, however, requires careful evaluation to rule out the presence of a preexisting psychotic disorder. Administration of magnesium pemoline has been associated with hypersensitivity reactions involving the liver, accompanied by elevations in liver-function studies (serum glutamic oxaloacetic transaminase [SGOT] and serum glutamic pyruvic transaminase [SGPT]) after several months of treatment. Thus, baseline and repeat studies of liver function are recommended with the administration of this compound.

Other areas of controversy and concern about stimulant use include growth suppression in children (Mattes and Gittelman 1983; Safer et al. 1972), the development of tics (Lowe et al. 1982), drug abuse (Jaffe 1991), use in adolescents (Evans and Pelham 1991), and rebound (Johnston et al. 1988). Although stimulants routinely produce anorexia and weight loss, their effect on growth in height is less certain. Although initial reports suggested that there was a persistent stimulant-associated decrease in growth in height in children (Mattes and Gittelman 1983; Safer et al. 1972), other reports failed to substantiate this finding (Gross 1976; Satterfield et al. 1979). Ultimate height appears to be unaffected if treatment is discontinued in adolescence (Gittelman and Mannuzza 1988); however, there are no studies of the effects of stimulants on growth in children treated continually from childhood through adolescence and young adulthood. Moreover, the literature on stimulant-associated growth deficits does not examine the possibility that growth deficits may represent maturational delays related to ADHD itself (i.e., dysmaturity) rather than to stimulant treatment. Preliminary work from our group supports this dysmaturity hypothesis (Spencer et al. 1996a). Taken together, this evidence does not support the common practice of drug holidays in children without evidence of growth deficits. However, until more is known, it seems prudent, for children suspected of stimulant-associated growth deficits, to provide drug holidays or alternative treatments. This recommendation, however, should be carefully weighed against the risk of symptom exacerbation due to drug discontinuation.

Early reports indicated that children with personal or family histories of tic disorders were at greater risk for developing a tic disorder when exposed to stimulants (Lowe et al. 1982). However, recent work has increasingly challenged this view (Comings and Comings 1988; Gadow et al. 1992; Gadow et al. 1995). For example, in a recent short-term, controlled study of 34 children with ADHD and tics using multiple informants and direct observation, Gadow et al. reported that methylphenidate effectively suppressed ADHD symptoms, with only a weak effect on the frequency of tics (Gadow et al. 1995). Nonetheless, further studies examining larger numbers of subjects over longer periods of time are needed in order to obtain closure on this issue. Until more is known, it seems prudent to weigh risks and benefits in individual cases and to have appropriate discussion with the patient and family about the benefits and pitfalls of the use of stimulants in individuals who have both ADHD and tics.

Similar uncertainties remain about the abuse potential of stimulants in children with ADHD. Despite the concern that ADHD may increase the risk of drug abuse in adolescents and young adults (or their associates), there are no scientific data showing that stimulant-treated ADHD children abuse prescribed medication when it is appropriately administered and monitored. Moreover, recent work has shown that the most commonly abused substance in adolescents and adults with ADHD is marijuana, not stimulants (Biederman et al. 1995d).

Despite its clinical importance, interdose rebound has not been adequately examined in the literature. Poststimulant worsening of symptoms may be particularly taxing in the evening, when family life takes place. Treatment options include the use of long-acting agents, such as time-release stimulant preparations, or alternative medications, such as antidepressants.

The interactions of the stimulants with other prescription and nonprescription medications are generally mild and not a source of concern (Wilens and Biederman 1992). Whereas coadministration of sympathomimetics (i.e., pseudoephedrine) may potentiate the effects of both medications, the antihistamines may diminish the stimulant's effectiveness. Caution should be exercised when using stimulants and antidepressants of the monoamine oxidase inhibitor (MAOI) type because of the potential for hypertensive reactions with this combination.

The concomitant use of stimulants with tricyclic antidepressants (TCAs) or anticonvulsants has been associated with increases in the serum levels of both medications. Thus, when stimulants are used in combination with TCAs or anticonvulsants, the levels of these medications should be closely monitored.

Antidepressants

Tricyclic Antidepressants

Tricyclic antidepressants (TCAs) include the tertiary amines amitriptyline, imipramine, doxepin, and trimipramine and the secondary amines desipramine, nortriptyline, and protriptyline. The mechanism of action appears to be due to the blocking effects of these drugs on the reuptake of central nervous system (CNS) neurotransmitters, especially norepinephrine and serotonin. However, these agents also have variable effects on pre- and postsynaptic neurotransmitter systems, resulting in differing positive and adverse effect profiles. Unwanted side effects may emerge from activity at histaminic sites (sedation, weight gain), cholinergic sites (dry mouth, constipation), α-adrenergic sites (postural hypotension), and serotonergic sites (sexual dysfunction). In general, the secondary amines are more selective (noradrenergic) and have fewer side effects—an important consideration in sensitive populations, such as juvenile and geriatric patients.

TCAs, especially imipramine and desipramine, are the second most studied compounds in the pharmacotherapy of ADHD after the stimulants. Twenty-nine studies (18 controlled, 11 open) have evaluated TCAs in 1,016 children and adolescents and 63 adults with ADHD (Table 18–1, Figure 18–1, and Figure 18–2). Almost all these studies (93%) report at least moderate improvement. As with the stimulant studies, however, the majority of these studies included primarily latency-age children. Although most studies of TCAs and ADHD were relatively brief, lasting several weeks to several months, a few studies extended for up to 2 years. Outcomes in both short- and long-term TCA studies have been equally positive. Despite assertion to the contrary, evidence exists that improvement of ADHD symptoms can be maintained when daily doses of TCAs are titrated upward over time (Biederman et al. 1986, 1989; Gastfriend et al. 1985; Wilens et al. 1993). For example, studies using aggressive doses of TCAs reported sustained improvement for up to 1 year with desipramine (> 4 mg/kg) (Biederman et al. 1986; Gastfriend et al. 1985) and nortriptyline (2.0 mg/kg) (Wilens et al. 1993).

Thus, it could be that the apparent short-lived effects reported in previous studies of TCAs in children with ADHD could have been due to the use of relatively low (< 3 mg/kg) daily dosages.

In the largest controlled study of a TCA in children, our group reported favorable results with desipramine (DMI) in 62 clinically referred children with ADHD, most of whom had previously failed to respond to psychostimulant treatment (Biederman et al. 1989). The study was a randomized, placebo-controlled, parallel-design, 6-week clinical trial. Clinically and statistically significant differences in behavioral improvement were found for DMI over placebo, at an average daily dosage of 5 mg/kg. Specifically, 68% of DMI-treated patients were considered very much or much improved, compared with only 10% of placebo patients ($P < .001$). In a further analysis, we examined whether comorbidity of ADHD with conduct disorder, major depression, or an anxiety disorder, or a family history of ADHD, predicted response to DMI treatment (Biederman et al. 1993b). Although the presence of comorbidity increased the likelihood of a placebo response, neither comorbidity with conduct disorder, depression, or anxiety, nor a family history of ADHD yielded differential responses to DMI treatment. In addition, DMI-treated ADHD patients showed a substantial reduction in depressive symptoms compared with placebo-treated patients (Biederman et al. 1989). These data suggest that DMI may be a particularly useful treatment in children with those comorbidities and ADHD.

Our group obtained similar results in a similarly designed controlled clinical trial of DMI in 41 adults with ADHD (Wilens et al. 1996). DMI, at an average daily dosage of 150 mg (average serum level of 113 ng/mL), was statistically and clinically more effective than placebo. Sixty-eight percent of DMI-treated patients responded, compared with none of the placebo-treated patients ($P < .0001$). Moreover, at the end of the study, the average severity of ADHD symptoms was reduced below the level required to meet diagnostic criteria in patients receiving DMI. It is also important that, although the full DMI dose was achieved at week 2, clinical response improved further over the following 4 weeks, indicating a latency of response. Response was independent of dose, serum DMI level, gender, and lifetime psychiatric comorbidity with anxiety or depressive disorders.

Although controlled studies of TCAs demonstrate clear efficacy for these agents in ADHD, studies comparing TCAs and stimulants have yielded mixed results. Of the 29 TCA studies, 13 (45%) compared TCAs with stimulants. Ten studies found that TCAs were inferior ($N = 5$) (Garfinkel et al. 1983; Gittelman-Klein 1974; Greenberg et al. 1975; Rapoport et al. 1974), or equal ($N = 5$) to stimulants (Gross 1973; Huessy and Wright 1970; Kupietz and Balka 1976; Rapport et al. 1993; Yepes et al. 1977). The other three studies found that TCAs were superior to stimulants (Watter and Dreyfuss 1973; Werry 1980; Winsberg et al. 1972).

Taken together, available literature suggests that TCAs are as effective as stimulants in controlling abnormal behaviors associated with ADHD but that they may be less effective in improving cognitive impairments (Gualtieri and Evans 1988; Quinn and Rapoport 1975; Rapport et al. 1993; Werry 1980). However, more work is needed to better define the comparative cognitive effects of TCAs and stimulants in ADHD children. On the other hand, the advantages of TCAs over stimulants include a longer duration of action, the feasibility of once-daily dosing without symptom rebound or insomnia, greater flexibility in dosage, the availability of serum-level monitoring (Preskorn et al. 1983), and minimal risk of abuse or dependence (Gittelman 1980; Rapoport and Mikkelsen 1978).

Although most studies have used moderate daily dosages of TCAs (1–4 mg/kg), doses vary widely across studies, and response has been equally positive in all the dose ranges. TCA serum levels have been examined in only a few studies (Biederman et al. 1986, 1989; Donnelly et al. 1986; Gastfriend et al. 1985; Rapport et al. 1993; Wilens et al. 1993, 1994a, 1995). These studies showed high interindividual variability in serum levels, with little relationship between serum level and daily dosage or response. Nortriptyline, however, seems to have a positive association between dose and serum level (Wilens et al. 1993).

Some work suggests that children and adolescents metabolize TCAs more efficiently than do adults. Despite higher weight-corrected dosing, children often have lower plasma TCA levels than do adults (Wilens et al. 1992). For imipramine (IMI) and desipramine (DMI), an upper dose limit of 5 mg/kg has been suggested for children. However, this absolute dose limit has little clinical relevance, because children display a substantial interindividual variability in the metabolism and elimination of TCAs. Therefore, some children tolerate only low doses, whereas others may require doses greater than 5 mg/kg. TCA treatment should always be individualized in an attempt to use the lowest effective dose. High doses of IMI and DMI (up to 5 mg/kg) also have been used to treat school phobia and major depressive disorder in children (Gittelman and Klein 1971; Puig-Antich et al. 1987).

TCA treatment of children with ADHD should be initiated at 10–25 mg/day, depending on the weight of the child (approximately 1 mg/kg), and increased slowly every 4–5 days by 20%–30%. When a daily dose of 3 mg/kg (or a lower effective dose) is reached, steady-state serum levels and an electrocardiogram (ECG) should be obtained. TCA serum level monitoring is useful not only to help predict clinical response but also to determine the limits of serum TCA concentration associated with adverse cardiovascular effects. In contrast, subjective adverse effects such as dry mouth or dizziness are unrelated to drug serum levels.

Common short-term adverse effects of the TCAs include anticholinergic effects, such as dry mouth, blurred vision, and constipation. However, no known deleterious effects are associated with chronic administration of these drugs. Because the anticholinergic effects of TCAs limit salivary flow, they may promote tooth decay in some children. Regular dental care is crucial in children receiving long-term TCA treatment. Gastrointestinal symptoms, vomiting, flulike symptoms, and sleep disturbances may occur when these drugs are discontinued abruptly.

The potential benefits of TCAs in the treatment of juvenile ADHD have been clouded by rising concerns about their safety stemming from reports of sudden unexplained death in four ADHD children treated with DMI (Abramowicz 1990). The causal link between DMI and these deaths remains uncertain. A recent report estimated that the magnitude of DMI-associated risk of sudden death in children may not be much larger than the baseline risk of sudden death in this age group (Biederman et al. 1995c). Moreover, these deaths have been difficult to reconcile with the rather extensive literature evaluating cardiovascular parameters in patients of all ages who have been exposed to TCAs and with the magnitude of worldwide use of TCAs in all age groups. In most studies, TCA treatment has been associated with asymptomatic, minor, but statistically significant increases in heart rate and ECG measures of cardiac conduction times consistent with the adult literature (Biederman et al. 1993a). Because of this uncertainty, prudence mandates that until more is known, TCAs should be used as second-line treatments to stimulants for ADHD in juveniles, and only after careful weighing of the risks and benefits of treating or not treating an affected child.

Other Antidepressants

Bupropion. Bupropion hydrochloride is a novel aminoketone antidepressant related to the phenylisopropylamines but pharmacologically distinct from available antidepressants (Casat et al. 1989). Although bupropion possesses both indirect dopamine and noradrenergic agonist effects, its specific site or mechanism of action remains unknown. Bupropion has been reported to be superior to placebo in reducing ADHD symptoms in two controlled studies in children, including a four-center multisite study ($N = 72$) (Casat et al. 1987, 1989; Conners et al., in press, 1996). Bupropion also reduced ADHD symptoms in a comparison with methylphenidate ($N = 15$) (Barrickman et al. 1995). In an open study of 19 adults treated with an average of 360 mg of bupropion for 6–8 weeks, Wender and Reimherr (1990) reported a moderate to marked response in 74% of subjects and sustained improvement at 1 year in 10 subjects. The response of ADHD to bupropion appears to be rapid and sustained. Dosing of bupropion for ADHD is similar to that recommended for depression, with a suggested maximal dose of 450 mg/day, divided into three daily doses, for adults.

Bupropion is rapidly absorbed: peak plasma levels are usually achieved after 2 hours. It has an average elimination half-life of 14 hours (range = 8–24 hours). Side effects include edema, rashes, nocturia, irritability, anorexia, and insomnia. Bupropion is associated with a somewhat higher rate of drug-induced seizures (0.4%) relative to other antidepressants, particularly in daily dosages higher than 6 mg/kg. However, this risk has been linked to a previous history of seizures and eating disorders as well as to high dose. Thus, by avoiding these risk factors and by dividing the daily dose, it may be possible to keep the risk of seizures comparable to that of other antidepressants. In general, because of the limited knowledge of its use in ADHD, bupropion should be limited to patients who fail to respond or cannot tolerate more conventional treatments.

Monoamine oxidase inhibitors. The monoamine oxidase inhibitors (MAOIs) presumably exert their antidepressant effects by inhibiting the intracellular catabolic enzyme monoamine oxidase. There are two types of monoamine oxidase: MAO-A, which preferentially metabolizes norepinephrine, epinephrine, and serotonin; and MAO-B, which preferentially metabolizes phenylethylamine (PEA), an endogenous amphetamine-like substance, and N-methylhistamine. Both MAO-A and MAO-B metabolize tyramine and dopamine (Ernst 1996). Some MAOIs are selective for A or B, and some are nonselective. In addition, irreversible MAOIs (e.g., phenelzine, tranylcypromine) are more susceptible to the so-called cheese effect, whereas the reversible MAOIs (e.g., moclobemide) are less susceptible.

Preliminary studies suggest that MAOIs are effective in juvenile and adult ADHD. In a recent open study (Jankovic 1993), selegiline (L-deprenyl, a specific MAOI-B at low dose) was evaluated in 29 children with both ADHD and tics. Results showed that ADHD symptoms improved in 90% of the children, with no serious adverse effects, and with an exacerbation of tics in only 2 patients. In a 12-week double-blind crossover trial, using two MAOIs in 14 hyperactive children, Zametkin et al. (1985) reported significant and rapid reduction in ADHD symptoms with minimal adverse effects. These investigators used clorgiline (a specific MAOI-A) and tranylcypromine sulfate (a mixed MAOI-A and -B).

In open studies in adult ADHD, moderate improvements were reported in studies with pargyline and selegiline (selective MAOI-Bs) with associated adverse effects (Wender et al. 1983, 1985c). The authors reported a delayed onset of action and a post-dosing stimulant-like quality of the MAOIs on ADHD symptoms lasting up to 6 hours (Wender et al. 1983). Ernst and colleagues (Ernst 1996) reported findings in an ongoing study of selegiline in adults with familial ADHD: they found that high dose was more effective than low dose and that both were better than placebo. Although low-dose selegiline is more selective for MAOI-B, high dose produces a mixed MAOI-A and -B effect; thus the findings by Ernst and colleagues suggest that the MAOI-A effects of selegiline may be more helpful in the treatment of ADHD.

A major limitation of the use of MAOIs is the potential for hypertensive crisis (treatable with phentolamine) associated with dietetic transgressions (tyramine-containing foods—e.g., most cheeses) and drug interactions (pressor amines, most cold medicines, amphetamines). A serotonergic syndrome may occur when MAOIs are combined with predominantly serotonergic drugs (e.g., selective serotonin reuptake inhibitors [SSRIs]). Additional adverse effects include orthostatic hypotension, weight gain, drowsiness, and dizziness. There is no information on long-term adverse effects of MAOIs in children. Extrapolating from the adult literature, however, these effects may include hypomania, hallucinations, confusion, and hepatotoxicity (rare). Pediatric dose ranges have not been established. Daily doses should be carefully titrated on the basis of response and adverse effects; they range from 0.5 to 1.0 mg/kg. Although dietetic restrictions and potential drug-drug interactions complicate the use of MAOIs in this clinical population, they may nonetheless be important to consider in treatment-refractory ADHD individuals.

Selective serotonin reuptake inhibitors. Currently available SSRIs include fluoxetine, paroxetine, sertraline, and fluvoxamine. Because of their pharmacological profiles, these medications have fewer anticholinergic, sedative, cardiovascular (blood-pressure and ECG changes) and weight-affecting adverse side effects than do the TCAs. Unlike the TCAs, the SSRIs are structurally dissimilar to each other. Further, these agents vary in their pharmacokinetic and side-effect profiles. SSRIs have not been systematically evaluated in the treatment of ADHD. Although a small open study (Barrickman et al. 1991) suggested that fluoxetine may be beneficial in the treatment of children with ADHD, extensive clinical experience at our center with children, adolescents, and adults does not support the usefulness of these compounds in the treatment of core ADHD symptoms.

Suggested daily doses in pediatric patients are approximately 0.5–1.0 mg/kg. Fluoxetine and its active metabolite have a long half-life of 7–9 days. In contrast, paroxetine (dose range = 0.25–0.70 mg/kg daily), sertraline (dose range = 1.5–3.0 mg/kg daily [< 200 mg/day]), and fluvoxamine (dose range = 1.0–4.5 mg/kg [< 300 mg/day]) have moderately long half-lives: paroxetine and sertraline approximately 24 hours and fluvoxamine approximately 15 hours. Common adverse effects of SSRIs include irritability, insomnia, gastrointestinal symptoms, sexual dysfunction, and headaches. Paroxetine and sertraline have also been associated with a higher incidence of headache, sedation, dry mouth, and constipation but with less anxiety and agitation than has fluoxetine (Grimsley and Jann 1992). Antidepressants and many other psychotropics are metabolized in the liver by the cytochrome P450 system (Nemeroff et al. 1996). The coadministration of TCAs (and similar compounds) and SSRIs may result in increased levels of TCAs; great caution should therefore be exercised when using TCAs along with SSRIs.

Venlafaxine.   Venlafaxine (Effexor) is chemically unrelated to other antidepressants. It selectively blocks the reuptake of serotonin, norepinephrine, and, to a lesser extent, dopamine. Venlafaxine has been shown to be effective in adult depression and may prove to be useful in the treatment of juvenile mood disorders. Recently two open studies of venlafaxine in adults with ADHD and prominent mood symptoms reported preliminary results of moderate improvement; however, 11 of 34 adults could not tolerate adverse effects (Adler et al. 1995; Reimherr et al. 1995).

Venlafaxine has a medium half-life of approximately 5 hours (*O*-desmethylvenlafaxine approximately 11 hours). The usual dose range is 2.0–5.0 mg/kg daily in three divided doses. Venlafaxine lacks significant activity at muscarinic/cholinergic, α-adrenergic, and histaminergic sites and thus has fewer side effects (sedative, anticholinergic) than do TCAs. However, when using venlafaxine, unlike the SSRIs, there is a need to monitor for potential cardiac effects, such as diastolic hypertension.

Tomoxetine.   Because of its selective noradrenergic effects, our group evaluated the experimental antidepressant drug tomoxetine in a double-blind, placebo-controlled, 7-week crossover study of 21 adults with ADHD (Spencer et al. 1995a). Treatment with tomoxetine at an average oral dosage of 76 mg/day was well tolerated and effective. The overall response rate for ADHD symptoms was clinically and statistically higher during tomoxetine treatment than during treatment with placebo (53% versus 10.5%; $P < .05$). Tomoxetine treatment was more effective than placebo after the second week of treatment, and improvement was increasingly robust in a subsequent week. Although preliminary, these initial results are promising and warrant further research with larger samples over an extended period of time.

Other Drugs

Clonidine

Clonidine is an imidazoline derivative with α-adrenergic agonist properties that has been used primarily in the treatment of hypertension. At low doses it appears to stimulate presynaptic inhibitory autoreceptors in the CNS. Beneficial effects of clonidine in the treatment of childhood ADHD have been reported in a total of 122 patients in four studies: one open study (Hunt 1987), one retrospective review (Steingard et al. 1993), and two controlled studies (B. Gunning, "A Controlled

Trial of Clonidine in Hyperkinetic Children," unpublished thesis, Department of Child and Adolescent Psychiatry, Academic Hospital–Sophia Children's Hospital, Rotterdam, The Netherlands, 1992; Hunt et al. 1985) with daily dosages of up to 4–5 µg/kg (average dosage 0.2 mg/day). All studies reported a positive behavioral response, and 50%–70% of subjects displayed at least moderate improvement; however, beneficial effects on cognition were less clear.

Clonidine is a relatively short-acting compound with a plasma half-life ranging from approximately 5.5 hours (in children) to 8.5 hours (in adults). Daily doses should be titrated and individualized. Usual daily dosage ranges from 3 to 10 µg/kg, given generally in divided doses, twice or three times daily. Initial dose can more easily be given in the evening hours or before bedtime because of its sedation effect. The most common short-term adverse effect of clonidine is sedation; it can also produce, in some cases, hypotension, dry mouth, depression, and confusion. The potential hypotensive effects of this agent may make it problematic for use in adults. Clonidine is not known to be associated with long-term adverse effects. In hypertensive adults, abrupt withdrawal of clonidine has been associated with rebound hypertension. Thus, it requires slow tapering when discontinued. Clonidine should not be administered concomitantly with β-blockers, because adverse interactions have been reported with this combination.

Guanfacine

There is one open study ($N = 13$) of a longer-acting, more selective α_{2a} agonist, guanfacine, in children and adolescents with ADHD. Beneficial effects on hyperactive behaviors and attentional abilities were reported (Hunt et al. 1995). Side effects are similar to clonidine, although less sedation has been reported.

Propranolol

Propranolol, a nonselective β-adrenergic antagonist, blocks both β_1 and β_2 receptors. It is unclear whether the benefits obtained from propranolol are primarily due to peripheral or central effects of the drug. A small open study of propranolol for ADHD adults with temper outbursts found some improvement at dosages of up to 640 mg/day (Mattes 1986). Another report stated that β-blockers may be helpful in combination with the stimulants (Ratey et al. 1991). The drug's half-life after chronic administration is about 4 hours, and its dosage range is approximately 2–8 mg/kg/day. Propranolol can cause bradycardia and hypotension as well as increase airway resistance, and it is contraindicated in asthmatic and certain cardiac patients. No known long-term effects are associated with chronic administration of propranolol. Because abrupt cessation of this drug may be associated with rebound hypertension, gradual tapering is recommended.

Antipsychotics

Twelve controlled studies of 242 children and young adolescents have evaluated the efficacy and safety of various antipsychotics in the treatment of ADHD. Much of this literature is older and limited by diagnostic uncertainty. A review of these studies found that not more than 50% of subjects with ADHD improved on antipsychotics (Gittelman 1980). Higher daily dosages (> 90 mg, or approximately 3 mg/kg) of chlorpromazine or its equivalent were more effective than were lower doses. Although there was no evidence of antipsychotic-associated cognitive impairment in these studies, there was also no evidence of cognitive enhancement. Moreover, the spectrum of short-term (e.g., sedation, extrapyramidal and anticholinergic adverse effects) and long-term (e.g., tardive dyskinesia, tardive dystonia, hyperprolactinemia) side effects, as well as withdrawal (withdrawal dyskinesia) and idiosyncratic reactions (e.g., neuroleptic malignant syndrome), in addition to the various available alternative treatments, make the use of antipsychotics in this disorder a less desirable choice.

Lithium

One controlled, 3-month trial of lithium in the treatment of nine children with ADHD (Greenhill et al. 1973) found that ADHD children without comorbid affective disorders were unresponsive to lithium treatment.

Other Compounds

Other compounds found to be ineffective in the treatment of ADHD include antianxiety drugs, meprobamate and hydroxyzine (Cytryn et al. 1960), a sympathomimetic amine, fenfluramine (Donnelly et al. 1989), dopamine agonists (amantidine and L-dopa) (Gittelman-Klein 1987), amino acid precursors (D/L-phenylalanine and L-tyrosine) (Reimherr et al. 1987), and caffeine (Firestone et al. 1978; Garfinkel et al. 1975, 1981; Harvey and Marsh 1978).

Effect of Psychiatric Comorbidity in Pharmacotherapy

Comorbidity With Conduct Disorder and Aggression

ADHD is often accompanied by aggressive behavior and conduct disorder. Several controlled studies reported improvement in both ADHD and aggressive symptoms in ADHD subjects with comorbid aggression who were treated with stimulants (Amery et al. 1984; Barkley et al. 1989; Cunningham et al. 1991; Gadow et al. 1990; Hinshaw et al. 1989, 1992; Kaplan et al. 1990; Klorman et al. 1988, 1989, 1994; Livingston et al. 1992;

Murphy et al. 1992; Pelham et al. 1990; Pliszka 1989; Taylor et al. 1987; Whalen et al. 1987; Winsberg et al. 1972, 1974). Stimulants suppressed physical and nonphysical aggression in these children both at home and in school in a dose-dependent fashion (Gadow et al. 1990; Hinshaw et al. 1989; Murphy et al. 1992). Stimulants also reduced negative social interactions (Whalen et al. 1987) and covert antisocial behavior (stealing, destroying property, but not cheating) (Hinshaw et al. 1992). Four studies of antidepressants for ADHD children with comorbid conduct disorder also reported improvement in ADHD (Biederman et al. 1993b; Simeon et al. 1986; Wilens et al. 1993; Winsberg et al. 1972) and in aggressive symptoms in these subjects (Simeon et al. 1986; Winsberg et al. 1972).

Comorbidity With Depression and Anxiety

Little is known about the pharmacotherapy of children, adolescents, and adults with ADHD and comorbid anxiety or mood disorders. Of nine stimulant studies in ADHD children with comorbid anxiety or depression, the majority reported a diminished response to stimulants in these patients (DuPaul et al. 1994; Pliszka 1989; Swanson et al. 1978; Tannock et al. 1995; Taylor et al. 1987; Voelker et al. 1983). Because stimulants are thought to be anxiogenic and depressogenic, caution should be used in the treatment of individuals with ADHD and comorbid anxiety and mood disorders. In contrast, in the TCA studies examining the effect of medication on comorbid depressive symptoms, TCA treatment improved both ADHD and depressive symptoms (Biederman et al. 1993b; Garfinkel et al. 1983).

Despite increasing recognition of the co-occurrence of ADHD and bipolarity (West et al. 1995; Wozniak et al. 1995), nothing is known about the pharmacotherapy of the combined condition. Considering the potential for the activation of individuals with ADHD and mania with TCAs and stimulants, caution should be used in treating ADHD and mania with stimulants and antidepressants in the absence of mood stabilizers (Wozniak and Biederman 1996). Because mania can produce severe cognitive and behavioral symptoms, it is crucial first to stabilize the mood disorder in ADHD children with this comorbidity.

Comorbidity With Tic Disorders

Although stimulants have historically been contraindicated in the treatment of patients with tics and ADHD, recent literature has challenged the absolute contraindication of stimulants in patients with ADHD and tics. Methylphenidate treatment is highly effective for

ADHD behaviors, aggression, and social skill deficits in children with Tourette's syndrome or chronic tics (Comings and Comings 1984; Erenberg et al. 1985; Gadow et al. 1992, 1995; Konkol et al. 1990; Sverd et al. 1989, 1992). Although recent controlled studies, comprising 49 subjects, reported no exacerbation of tics (Gadow et al. 1995; Sverd et al. 1989, 1992), previous studies reported worsening of tics in 31% (95/306 patients, in 10 studies) of comorbid ADHD/tic patients (Caine et al. 1984; Comings and Comings 1988; Denckla et al. 1976; Erenberg 1982; Erenberg et al. 1985; Golden 1977, 1982; Konkol et al. 1990; Price et al. 1986; Shapiro and Shapiro 1981). Although many children with this comorbidity respond to stimulants without worsening of tics, until more is known, caution should be exercised in the use of stimulants in this population.

For individuals who have ADHD and tics with documented exacerbation of tics by stimulants, alternative agents should be explored. There is an emerging literature on the use of antidepressants in the treatment of children and adolescents with ADHD and tic disorders. Recent case reports and case series of the TCAs imipramine (Dillon et al. 1985), nortriptyline (Spencer et al. 1993b), and desipramine (Hoge and Biederman 1986; Riddle et al. 1988; Spencer et al. 1993a) have reported a high rate (82%) of improvement of ADHD symptoms, with no change or improvement of the tic disorder over an extended follow-up period (Spencer et al. 1993a, 1993b). In a recent controlled study, Singer et al. (1994) reported that desipramine was significantly better than both clonidine and placebo in its ability to improve ADHD symptoms associated with the full Tourette's syndrome. In this study neither desipramine nor clonidine ameliorated tic symptoms. An open study of the selective MAO-B inhibitor selegiline reported improved ADHD symptoms in 90% of children with ADHD and tics and was generally well tolerated (Jankovic 1993). Last, a small case series described precipitation ($N = 2$) or exacerbation of tics ($N = 2$) in 4 children with ADHD treated with bupropion (Spencer et al. 1993c).

In two open studies of clonidine, Steingard et al. (1993) reported a high rate (96%) of response (moderate or greater) of ADHD symptoms and improvement in tics in children with this comorbidity. However, in the controlled study mentioned above, Singer et al. (1994) reported that clonidine was not better than placebo in its ability to improve ADHD symptoms associated with the full Tourette's syndrome. Finally, there is one open study of the more selective α_{2a} agonist, guanfacine, reporting beneficial effects on phonic tics and neuropsychological measures of attention and impulsivity (the continuous performance test) in children with ADHD and tics (Chappell et al. 1995). Although clonidine and guanfacine appear effective in the combined condition for tics and excitable behavior, it remains unclear whether any cognitive improvement is associated with their use.

Comorbidity With Mental Retardation

As reviewed by Demb (1991), there is agreement among researchers that stimulants are effective for ADHD symptoms in mildly to moderately retarded children. There have been mixed findings in patients with more profound mental retardation (Aman et al. 1991; Demb 1991) and in children with pervasive developmental disorders not otherwise specified (Birmaher et al. 1988; Campbell et al. 1985; Strayhorn et al. 1988), along with concerns of increased stereotypies and constriction of attention. However, reports indicate that individual responses vary widely and that some children with moderate or profound mental retardation may improve dramatically with stimulant therapy (Demb 1991). The main predictor of response in subjects with developmental disabilities is the presence of clear ADHD symptoms (hyperactivity, impulsiveness, and inattention) as opposed to general behavioral disruption. Age, IQ, and other associated diagnoses are less predictive (Demb 1991). Considering the extraordinary importance of augmenting the functional abilities of mentally retarded individuals, clinicians should be proactive in identifying and treating ADHD in individuals with developmental disorders.

Combined Pharmacotherapy

Although in clinical practice ADHD patients commonly receive more than one psychotropic, little is known about combined pharmacotherapy in ADHD. Historically, the first reports of combined pharmacotherapy in ADHD were of antipsychotics and stimulants. Despite theoretical concern about contradictory dopaminergic mechanisms of action, there have been two controlled studies of combined neuroleptic and stimulant treatment involving 181 children (Gittelman-Klein et al. 1976; Weizman et al. 1984). In both studies the combination was superior to stimulant medication alone, although only a trend in the larger study.

In one of the few studies of its kind, Rapport et al. (1993) evaluated the separate and combined effects of methylphenidate and desipramine in 16 hospitalized children with ADHD and comorbid disorders, including major depression, dysthymia, and anxiety. These investigators found 1) that methylphenidate alone, but not desipramine, improved vigilance, 2) that both methylphenidate alone and desipramine alone improved short-term memory and visual problem solving, and 3) that the combination produced positive effects on learning of higher-order relationships. The authors speculated that performance on different cognitive measures may be modulated by separate neurotransmitter systems. Although this combined pharmacotherapy was associated with more side effects than was monotherapy, there was no evidence that the combined use of both drugs was associated with unique or serious side effects (Pataki et al. 1993).

There are several reports of the use of multiple agents in the treatment of ADHD with various comorbid disorders. For example, there is one open report of the successful use of fluoxetine with stimulants in the management of 32 patients with ADHD and depressive disorders (Gammon and Brown 1993). There are also open reports of the successful use of clonidine with stimulants for conduct disorder (D. Conners, unpublished data, October 1996) and sleep disorders (Brown and Gammon 1992; Prince et al. 1996) in ADHD children. The combined use of other agents with anti-ADHD drugs (stimulants or TCAs)—such as benzodiazepines for anxiety or lithium, valproate, or carbamazepine for mania—has not been systematically evaluated.

Although in clinical practice many ADHD patients receive multiple treatments, the literature on combined pharmacotherapy is very sparse, not permitting the development of clear therapeutic guidelines (Table 18–2). In contrast to polypharmacy, rational combined pharmacological approaches can be used for the treatment of comorbid ADHD, as augmentation strategies for patients with insufficient response to a single agent, and for the management of treatment-emergent adverse effects. Examples of the rational use of combined treatment include the use of an antidepressant plus a stimulant for ADHD and comorbid depression, the use of clonidine to ameliorate stimulant-induced insomnia, and the use of a mood stabilizer plus an anti-ADHD agent to treat ADHD comorbid with bipolar disorder (Wilens et al. 1994b).

Treatment-Refractory Patients

Despite the availability of various agents for ADHD, there appear to be a number of individuals who either do not respond to or are intolerant of the adverse effects of medications used to treat their ADHD (Table 18–2). In managing apparent medication nonresponders, several therapeutic strategies are available. If adverse psychiatric effects develop concurrent with a poor medication response, alternate treatments should be pursued. Severe psychiatric symptoms that emerge during the acute phase can be problematic, irrespective of the efficacy of the medications for ADHD. These symptoms may require reconsideration of the diagnosis of ADHD and careful reassessment of the presence of comorbid disorders. If reduction of dose or change in preparation (e.g., regular vs. slow-release stimulants) does not resolve the problem, consideration should be given to alternative treatments. Concurrent nonpharmacological interventions such as behavioral or cognitive therapies may assist with symptom reduction.

Table 18–2.   Suggested treatment algorithms for ADHD

Type of ADHD	Treatment
ADHD simplex	Stimulants clonidine (pediatric cases)/TCAs bupropion
ADHD + major depression	Stimulants + SSRIs TCAs/bupropion TCAs + stimulants
ADHD + anxiety	Stimulants + high-potency BZD Stimulants + buspirone TCAs Bupropion Stimulants + SSRIs/TCAs
ADHD + conduct disorder	clonidine (pediatric cases) clonidine (pediatric cases) + stimulants TCAs β-Blockers + stimulants
ADHD + tics	clonidine (pediatric cases) TCAs Stimulants + TCAs or clonidine Stimulants
ADHD + mania	lithium/carbamazepine/valproic acid + Stimulants/clonidine/TCAs/bupropion
ADHD + multiple comorbidities	Address each comorbidity Prioritize by severity
Tx-resistant ADHD	Assess for new or old comorbidity Consider alternative pharmacotherapies or combined approaches

Note.   ADHD = attention-deficit/hyperactivity disorder; TCA = tricyclic anti-depressant; SSRI = selective serotonin reuptake inhibitor; BZD = benzodiazepine; Tx = treatment.

Source.   Reprinted from Biederman J, Spencer T, Wilens TE, et al.: "Attention-Deficit/Hyperactivity Disorder: Pharmacotherapy," in *Treatments of Psychiatric Disorders,* 2nd Edition, Vol. 1. Edited by Gabbard G. Washington, DC, American Psychiatric Press, 1996, p. 183. Used with permission.

Clinical Guidelines

At any age, the pharmacotherapy of ADHD should be part of a treatment plan in which consideration is given to all aspects of the patient's life. The administration of medication to patients with ADHD should be undertaken as a collaborative effort with the patient and the patient's family, and the physician should guide the use and management of efficacious anti-ADHD agents. The use of medication should follow a careful evaluation of the patient, including psychiatric, social, cognitive, and vocational assessments. Careful attention should be paid to the onset of symptoms, the longitudinal history of the disorder, and differential diagnosis, including medical and neurological as well as psychosocial and educational factors contributing to the clinical presentation. Issues of comorbidity with learning disabilities and other psychiatric disorders, as well as specific academic needs, should be addressed. Patients with ongoing psychoactive substance abuse or dependence should generally not be pharmacologically treated until appropriate addiction treatments have been undertaken and the patient has maintained a drug- and alcohol-free period. Other concurrent psychiatric disorders also need to be assessed and if possible the relationship of the ADHD symptoms to these other disorders delineated.

The ADHD patient and his or her family need to be familiarized with the risks and benefits of pharmacotherapy, the availability of alternative treatments, and the likely adverse effects. Certain adverse effects can be anticipated from the known pharmacological properties of the drug (e.g., appetite change, insomnia), whereas other more infrequent effects are unexpected (idiosyncratic) and are difficult to anticipate from the properties of the drug. Short-term adverse effects can be minimized by introducing the medication at low initial doses and titrating slowly. Idiosyncratic adverse effects generally require drug discontinuation and selection of alternate treatment modalities.

Treatment should be started at the lowest possible dose, which is usually the lowest manufactured dose. Once pharmacotherapy is initiated, frequent (i.e., weekly) contact with the patient and family is necessary during the initial phase of treatment in order to carefully monitor response to the intervention and adverse effects. Evaluation of adverse effects should include both subjective reports from the patient and family (e.g., stomach aches, appetite changes) as well as appropriate evaluation of objective measurements (e.g., heart rate, blood pressure changes). Following a sufficient period of clinical stabilization (e.g., 6–12 months) it is prudent to reevaluate the need for continued psychopharmacological intervention. Withdrawal symptoms should be distinguished from the reemergence of the ADHD symptoms for which the psychotropic was prescribed. To minimize withdrawal reactions, it is important to discontinue medications gradually.

Conclusion

The available literature strongly indicates an important role for various psychopharmacological agents in the treatment of individuals with

ADHD throughout the life cycle. Pharmacological treatment leads to improvement not only of core behavioral symptoms of ADHD but also of associated impairments, including cognition, social skills, and family function. The armamentarium of anti-ADHD compounds includes not only the stimulants, but also several antidepressants and other medications such as clonidine and guanfacine. Effective pharmacological treatments for ADHD seem to share noradrenergic and dopaminergic mechanisms of action. Stimulant medications continue to be the first-line drugs of choice for uncomplicated ADHD in individuals of all ages, with TCAs and bupropion for nonresponders or patients with concurrent psychiatric disorders. There is increasing recognition that ADHD is a heterogeneous disorder with considerable and varied comorbidity. If not recognized and attended to, the combination of comorbid symptoms and ADHD may lead to high morbidity and disability, with poor long-term prognosis. Current clinical experience suggests that multiple agents may be necessary in the successful treatment of some complex ADHD patients with partial responses or psychiatric comorbidity.

References

Abikoff H, Gittelman R: Hyperactive children treated with stimulants. Arch Gen Psychiatry 42:953–961, 1985

Abramowicz M: Sudden death in children treated with a tricyclic antidepressant. The Medical Letter 32:53, 1990

Adler L, Resnick S, Kunz M, et al: Open-label trial of venlafaxine in attention deficit disorder. Paper presented at the New Clinical Drug Evaluation Unit Program, Orlando, FL, May 1995

Alessi N, Magen J: Comorbidity of other psychiatric disturbances in depressed, psychiatrically hospitalized children. Am J Psychiatry 145:1582–1584, 1988

Alpert J, Maddocks A, Nierenberg A, et al: Attention deficit hyperactivity disorder in childhood among adults with major depression. Psychiatry Res 62:213–219, 1996

Aman MG, Marks RE, Turbott SH, et al: Clinical effects of methylphenidate and thioridazine in intellectually subaverage children. J Am Acad Child Adolesc Psychiatry 30:246–256, 1991

American Psychiatric Association: Diagnostic and Statistical Manual of Mental Disorders, 2nd Edition. Washington, DC, American Psychiatric Association, 1968

American Psychiatric Association: Diagnostic and Statistical Manual of Mental Disorders, 3rd Edition. Washington, DC, American Psychiatric Association, 1980

American Psychiatric Association: Diagnostic and Statistical Manual of Mental Disorders, 3rd Edition, Revised. Washington, DC, American Psychiatric Association, 1987

American Psychiatric Association: Diagnostic and Statistical Manual of Mental Disorders, 4th Edition. Washington, DC, American Psychiatric Association, 1994

Amery B, Minichiello M, Brown G: Aggression in hyperactive boys: response to d-amphetamine. J Am Acad Child Psychiatry 23:291–294, 1984

Anderson JC, Williams S, McGee R, et al: DSM-III disorders in preadolescent children: prevalence in a large sample from the general population. Arch Gen Psychiatry 44:69–76, 1987

Angold A, Costello EJ: Depressive comorbidity in children and adolescents: empirical, theoretical, and methodological issues. Am J Psychiatry 150:1779–1791, 1993

Baldessarini RJ: Drugs and the treatment of psychiatric disorders: antimanic and antidepressant agents, in Goodman and Gilman's The Pharmacologic Basis of Therapeutics, 9th Edition. Edited by Harden W, Rudin W, Molinoff PB, et al. New York, McGraw-Hill, 1996, pp 431–459

Barkley R: Hyperactive girls and boys: Stimulant drug effects on mother-child interactions. J Child Psychol Psychiatry 30:379–390, 1989

Barkley RA: A review of stimulant drug research with hyperactive children. J Child Psychol Psychiatry 18:137–165, 1977

Barkley RA: The effects of methylphenidate on the interactions of preschool ADHD children with their mothers. J Am Acad Child Adolesc Psychiatry 27:336–341, 1988

Barkley RA: The ecological validity of laboratory and analogue assessment methods of ADHD symptoms. J Abnorm Child Psychol 19:149–178, 1991

Barkley RA, Cunningham C: The effects of methylphenidate on the mother-child interactions of hyperactive children. Arch Gen Psychiatry 36:201–208, 1979

Barkley RA, Karlsson J, Strzelecki E, et al: Effects of age and Ritalin dosage on mother-child interactions of hyperactive children. J Consult Clin Psychol 52:750–758, 1984

Barkley RA, McMurray MB, Edelbrock CS, et al: The response of aggressive and nonaggressive ADHD children to two doses of methylphenidate. J Am Acad Child Adolesc Psychiatry 28:873–881, 1989

Barrickman L, Noyes R, Kuperman S, et al: Treatment of ADHD with fluoxetine: a preliminary trial. J Am Acad Child Adolesc Psychiatry 30:762–767, 1991

Barrickman L, Perry P, Allen A, et al: Bupropion versus methylphenidate in the treatment of attention-deficit hyperactivity disorder. J Am Acad Child Adolesc Psychiatry 34:649–657, 1995

Bergman A, Winters L, Cornblatt B: Methylphenidate: effects on sustained attention, in Ritalin: Theory and Patient Management. Edited by Greenhill L, Osman B. New York, Mary Ann Liebert, 1991, pp 223–231

Biederman J, Gastfriend DR, Jellinek MS: Desipramine in the treatment of children with attention deficit disorder. J Clin Psychopharmacol 6:359–363, 1986

Biederman J, Baldessarini RJ, Wright V, et al: A double-blind placebo controlled study of desipramine in the treatment of attention deficit disorder, I: efficacy. J Am Acad Child Adolesc Psychiatry 28:777–784, 1989

Biederman J, Faraone SV, Keenan K, et al: Family-genetic and psychosocial risk factors in DSM-III attention deficit disorder. J Am Acad Child Adolesc Psychiatry 29:526–533, 1990a

Biederman J, Faraone SV, Knee D, et al: Retrospective assessment of DSM-III attention deficit disorder in non-referred individuals. J Clin Psychiatry 51:102–107, 1990b

Biederman J, Newcorn J, Sprich S: Comorbidity of attention deficit hyperactivity disorder with conduct, depressive, anxiety, and other disorders. Am J Psychiatry 148:564–577, 1991

Biederman J, Faraone SV, Keenan K, et al: Further evidence for family genetic risk factors in attention deficit hyperactivity disorder (ADHD): patterns of comorbidity in probands and relatives in psychiatrically and pediatrically referred samples. Arch Gen Psychiatry 49:728–738, 1992

Biederman J, Baldessarini R, Goldblatt A, et al: A naturalistic study of 24-hour electrocardiographic recordings and echocardiographic finding in children and adolescents treated with desipramine. J Am Acad Child Adolesc Psychiatry 32:805–813, 1993a

Biederman J, Baldessarini RJ, Wright V, et al: A double-blind placebo controlled study of desipramine in the treatment of attention deficit disorder, III: lack of impact of comorbidity and family history factors on clinical response. J Am Acad Child Adolesc Psychiatry 32:199–204, 1993b

Biederman J, Faraone SV, Spencer T, et al: Patterns of psychiatric comorbidity, cognition and psychosocial functioning in adults with attention deficit hyperactivity disorder. Am J Psychiatry 150:1792–1798, 1993c

Biederman J, Milberger S, Faraone S, et al: Family environmental risk factors for attention deficit hyperactivity disorder: a test of Rutter's indicators of adversity. Paper presented at the Scientific Proceedings of the Annual Meeting of the American Academy of Child and Adolescent Psychiatry, New York, 1994

Biederman J, Faraone S, Mick E, et al: Psychiatric comorbidity among referred juveniles with major depression: fact or artifact? J Am Acad Child Adolesc Psychiatry 34:579–590, 1995a

Biederman J, Faraone SV, Mick E, et al: High risk for attention deficit hyperactivity disorder among children of parents with childhood onset of the disorder: a pilot study. Am J Psychiatry 152:431–435, 1995b

Biederman J, Thisted R, Greenhill L, et al: Estimation of the association between desipramine and the risk for sudden death in 5- to 14-year-old children. J Clin Psychiatry 56:87–93, 1995c

Biederman J, Wilens T, Mick E, et al: Psychoactive substance use disorder in adults with attention deficit hyperactivity disorder: effects of ADHD and psychiatric comorbidity. Am J Psychiatry 152:1652–1658, 1995d

Bird HR, Canino G, Rubio-Stipec M, et al: Estimates of the prevalence of childhood maladjustment in a community survey in Puerto Rico. Arch Gen Psychiatry 45:1120–1126, 1988

Birmaher B, Quintana H, Greenhill L: Methylphenidate treatment of hyperactive autistic children. J Am Acad Child Adolesc Psychiatry 27:248–251, 1988

Brown RT, Sexson SB: A controlled trial of methylphenidate in black adolescents. Clin Pediatr 27:74–81, 1988

Brown RT, Wynne ME, Slimmer LW: Attention deficit disorder and the effect of methylphenidate on attention, behavioral, and cardiovascular functioning. J Clin Psychiatry 45:473–476, 1984

Brown TE, Gammon GD: ADHD-associated difficulties falling asleep and awakening: clonidine and methylphenidate treatments. Paper presented at the Scientific Proceedings of the Annual Meeting of the American Academy of Child and Adolescent Psychiatry, Washington, DC, October 1992

Caine E, Ludlow C, Polinsky R, et al: Provocative drug testing in Tourette's syndrome: d- and l-amphetamine and haloperidol. J Am Acad Child Adolesc Psychiatry 23:147–152, 1984

Campbell M, Green WH, Deutsch SI: Child and Adolescent Psychopharmacology, Vol 2. Beverly Hills, CA, Sage, 1985

Cantwell DP: Hyperactive children have grown up: what have we learned about what happens to them? Arch Gen Psychiatry 42:1026–1028, 1985

Casat CD, Pleasants DZ, Van Wyck Fleet J: A double-blind trial of bupropion in children with attention deficit disorder. Psychopharmacol Bull 23:120–122, 1987

Casat CD, Pleasants DZ, Schroeder DH, et al: Bupropion in children with attention deficit disorder. Psychopharmacol Bull 25:198–201, 1989

Castellanos F, Giedd J, Eckburg P, et al: Quantitative morphology of the caudate nucleus in attention deficit hyperactivity disorder. Am J Psychiatry 151:1791–1796, 1994

Chappell P, Riddle M, Scahill L, et al: Guanfacine treatment of comorbid attention-deficit hyperactivity disorder and Tourette's syndrome. J Am Acad Child Adolesc Psychiatry 34:1140–1146, 1995

Comings DE, Comings BG: Tourette's syndrome and attention deficit disorder with hyperactivity: are they genetically related? J Am Acad Child Adolesc Psychiatry 23:138–146, 1984

Comings DE, Comings BG: Tourette's syndrome and attention deficit disorder, in Tourette's Syndrome and Tic Disorders: Clinical Understanding and Treatment. Edited by Cohen DJ, Bruun RD, Leckman JF. New York, Wiley, 1988, pp 119–136

Conners C, Casat C, Gualtieri C, et al: Bupropion hydrochloride in attention deficit disorder with hyperactivity. J Am Acad Child Adolesc Psychiatry 35:1314–1321, 1996

Conners CK: Controlled trial of methylphenidate in preschool children with minimal brain dysfunction. International Journal of Mental Health 4:61–74, 1975

Conners CK, Taylor E: Pemoline, methylphenidate, and placebo in children with minimal brain dysfunction. Arch Gen Psychiatry 37:922–930, 1980

Coons HW, Klorman R, Borgstedt AD: Effects of methylphenidate on adolescents with a childhood history of ADHD, II: information processing. J Am Acad Child Adolesc Psychiatry 26:368–374, 1987

Cunningham C, Siegel L, Offord D: A dose-response analysis of the effects of methylphenidate on the peer interactions and simulated classroom performance of ADD children with and without conduct problems. J Child Psychol Psychiatry 32:439–452, 1991

Cytryn L, Gilbert A, Eisenberg L: The effectiveness of tranquilizing drugs plus supportive psychotherapy in treating behavior disorders of children: a double-blind study of eighty outpatients. Am J Orthopsychiatry 30:113–129, 1960

Demb H: Use of Ritalin in the treatment of children with mental retardation, in Ritalin: Theory and Patient Management. Edited by Greenhill L, Osman B. New York, Mary Ann Liebert, 1991, pp 155–170

Denckla MB, Bemporad JR, MacKay MC: Tics following methylphenidate administration: a report of 20 cases. JAMA 235:1349–1351, 1976

Deutsch CK, Matthysse S, Swanson JM, et al: Genetic latent structure analysis of dysmorphology in attention deficit disorder. J Am Acad Child Adolesc Psychiatry 29:189–194, 1990

Dillon DC, Salzman IJ, Schulsinger DA: The use of imipramine in Tourette's syndrome and attention deficit disorder: case report. J Clin Psychiatry 46:348–349, 1985

Donnelly M, Zametkin AJ, Rapoport JL, et al: Treatment of childhood hyperactivity with desipramine: plasma drug concentration, cardiovascular effects, plasma and urinary catecholamine levels, and clinical response. Clin Pharmacol Ther 39:72–81, 1986

Donnelly M, Rapoport JL, Potter WZ, et al: Fenfluramine and dextroamphetamine treatment of childhood hyperactivity. Arch Gen Psychiatry 46:205–212, 1989

Douglas V, Barr R, Amin K, et al: Dosage effects and individual responsivity to methylphenidate in attention deficit disorder. J Child Psychol Psychiatry 29:453–475, 1988

Douglas V, Barr R, Desilets J, et al: Do high doses of stimulants impair flexible thinking in attention-deficit hyperactivity disorder? J Am Acad Child Adolesc Psychiatry 34:877–885, 1995

DuPaul G, Barkley R, McMurray M: Response of children with ADHD to methylphenidate: interaction with internalizing symptoms. J Am Acad Child Adolesc Psychiatry 33:894–903, 1994

Elia J, Borcherding BG, Rapoport JL, et al: Methylphenidate and dextroamphetamine treatments of hyperactivity: are there true nonresponders? Psychiatry Res 36:141–155, 1991

Erenberg G: Stimulant medication in Tourette's Syndrome (letter). JAMA 248:1062, 1982

Erenberg G, Cruse RP, Rothner AD: Gilles de la Tourette's syndrome: effects of stimulant drugs. Neurology 35:1346–1348, 1985

Ernst M: MAOI treatment of Adult ADHD. Paper presented at NIMH Conference on Alternative Pharmacology of ADHD, Washington, DC, 1996

Evans SW, Pelham WE: Psychostimulant effects on academic and behavioral measures for ADHD junior high school students in a lecture format classroom. J Abnorm Child Psychol 19:537–552, 1991

Famularo R, Fenton T: The effect of methylphenidate on school grades in children with attention deficit disorder without hyperactivity: a preliminary report. J Clin Psychiatry 48:112–114, 1987

Faraone S, Biederman J: Is attention deficit hyperactivity disorder familial? Harvard Reviews in Psychiatry 1:271–287, 1994

Faraone SV, Biederman J, Keenan K, et al: A family genetic study of girls with DSM-III attention deficit disorder. Am J Psychiatry 148:112–117, 1991

Faraone S, Biederman J, Chen WJ, et al: Segregation analysis of attention deficit hyperactivity disorder: evidence for single gene transmission. Psychiatr Genet 2:257–275, 1992

Faraone SV, Biederman J, Krifcher-Lehman B, et al: Intellectual performance and school failure in children with attention deficit hyperactivity disorder and in their siblings. J Abnorm Psychol 102:616–623, 1993

Firestone P, Davey J, Goodman JT, et al: The effects of caffeine and methylphenidate on hyperactive children. J Am Acad Child Psychiatry 17:445–456, 1978

Gadow KD, Nolan EE, Sverd J, et al: Methylphenidate in aggressive-hyperactive boys, I: effects on peer aggression in public school settings. J Am Acad Child Adolesc Psychiatry 29:710–718, 1990

Gadow K, Nolan E, Sverd J: Methylphenidate in hyperactive boys with comorbid tic disorder, II: short-term behavioral effects in school settings. J Am Acad Child Adolesc Psychiatry 31:462–471, 1992

Gadow K, Sverd J, Sprafkin J, et al: Efficacy of methylphenidate for ADHD in children with tic disorder. Arch Gen Psychiatry 52:444–455, 1995

Gammon GD, Brown TE: Fluoxetine and methylphenidate in combination for treatment of attention deficit disorder and comorbid depressive disorder. Journal of Child and Adolescent Psychopharmacology 3:1–10, 1993

Garfinkel BD, Webster CD, Sloman L: Methylphenidate and caffeine in the treatment of children with minimal brain dysfunction. Am J Psychiatry 132:723–728, 1975

Garfinkel BD, Webster CD, Sloman L: Responses to methylphenidate and varied doses of caffeine in children with attention deficit disorder. Am J Psychiatry 26:395–401, 1981

Garfinkel BD, Wender PH, Sloman L, et al: Tricyclic antidepressant and methylphenidate treatment of attention deficit disorder in children. J Am Acad Child Adolesc Psychiatry 22:343–348, 1983

Gastfriend DR, Biederman J, Jellinek MS: Desipramine in the treatment of attention deficit disorder in adolescents. Psychopharmacol Bull 21:144–145, 1985

Gaub M, Carlson C: Gender differences in ADHD: a meta-analysis and critical review. J Am Acad Child Adolesc Psychiatry, in press

Geller B, Sun K, Zimmerman B, et al: Complex and rapid-cycling in bipolar children and adolescents: a preliminary study. J Affect Disord 34:259–268, 1995

Giedd JN, Castellanos FX, Casey BJ, et al: Quantitative morphology of the corpus callosum in attention deficit hyperactivity disorder. Am J Psychiatry 151:665–669, 1994

Gittelman R: Childhood disorders, in Drug Treatment of Adult and Child Psychiatric Disorders. Edited by Klein D, Quitkin F, Rifkin A, et al. Baltimore, Williams and Wilkins, 1980, pp 576–756

Gittelman R, Klein DF: Controlled imipramine treatment of school phobia. Arch Gen Psychiatry 25:204–207, 1971

Gittelman R, Mannuzza S: Hyperactive boys almost grown up, III: methylphenidate effects on ultimate height. Arch Gen Psychiatry 45:1131–1134, 1988

Gittelman R, Mannuzza S, Shenker R, et al: Hyperactive boys almost grown up, I: psychiatric status. Arch Gen Psychiatry 42:937–947, 1985

Gittelman-Klein R: Pilot clinical trial of imipramine in hyperkinetic children, in Clinical Use of Stimulant Drugs in Children. Edited by Conners C. The Hague, Netherlands, Excerpta Medica, 1974, pp 192–201

Gittelman-Klein R: Diagnosis and drug treatment of childhood disorders, in Diagnosis and Drug Treatment of Psychiatric Disorders: Adults and Children. Edited by Klein DF, Gittelman R, Quitkin F and Rifkin A. Baltimore, Williams and Wilkins, 1980, pp 576–775

Gittelman-Klein R: Pharmacotherapy of childhood hyperactivity: an update, in Psychopharmacology: The Third Generation of Progress. Edited by Meltzer HY. New York, Raven Press, 1987, pp 1215–1224

Gittelman-Klein R, Klein DF, Katz S, et al: Comparative effects of methylphenidate and thioridazine in hyperkinetic children. Arch Gen Psychiatry 33:1217–1231, 1976

Golden G: The effect of central nervous system stimulants on Tourette Syndrome. Ann Neurol 2:69–70, 1977

Golden G: Stimulant medication in Tourette's Syndrome (letter). JAMA 248:1063, 1982

Goodman R: Genetic factors in hyperactivity account for about half of the explainable variance. BMJ 298:1407–1408, 1989

Goodman R, Stevenson J: A twin study of hyperactivity, I: an examination of hyperactivity scores and categories derived from Rutter teacher and parent questionnaires. J Child Psychol Psychiatry 30:671–689, 1989a

Goodman R, Stevenson J: A twin study of hyperactivity, II: the aetiological role of genes, family relationships and perinatal adversity. J Child Psychol Psychiatry 30:691–709, 1989b

Greenberg L, Yellin A, Spring C, et al: Clinical effects of imipramine and methylphenidate in hyperactive children. International Journal of Mental Health 4:144–156, 1975

Greene R, Biederman J, Faraone S, et al: Toward a new psychometric definition of social disability in children with Attention-Deficit Hyperactivity Disorder. J Am Acad Child Adolesc Psychiatry 35:571–578, 1996

Greenhill LL, Rieder RO, Wender PH, et al: Lithium carbonate in the treatment of hyperactive children. Arch Gen Psychiatry 28:636–640, 1973

Grimsley S, Jann M: Paroxetine, sertraline, and fluvoxamine: new selective serotonin reuptake inhibitors. Clinical Pharmacy 11:930–957, 1992

Gross M: Imipramine in the treatment of minimal brain dysfunction in children. Psychosomatics 14:283–285, 1973

Gross M: Growth of hyperkinetic children taking methylphenidate, dextroamphetamine, or imipramine/desipramine. J Pediatr 58:423–431, 1976

Gualtieri CT, Evans RW: Motor performance in hyperactive children treated with imipramine. Percept Mot Skills 66:763–769, 1988

Gualtieri CT, Ondrusek MG, Finley C: Attention deficit disorders in adults. Clin Neuropharmacol 8:343–356, 1985

Harvey DHP, Marsh RW: The effects of decaffeinated coffee versus whole coffee on hyperactive children. Dev Med Child Neurol 20:81–86, 1978

Hechtman L: Long-term outcome in attention-deficit hyperactivity disorder. Psychiatr Clin North Am 1:553–565, 1992

Hinshaw S, Erhardt D: Attention-Deficit Hyperactivity Disorder in Child and Adolescent Therapy: Cognitive-Behavioral Procedures. Edited by Kendall P. New York, The Guilford Press, 1991, pp 98–128

Hinshaw S, Buhrmester D, Heller T: Anger control in response to verbal provocation: effects of stimulant medication for boys with ADHD. J Abnorm Child Psychol 17:393–407, 1989

Hinshaw S, Heller T, McHale J: Covert antisocial behavior in boys with attention-deficit hyperactivity disorder: external validation and effects of methylphenidate. J Consult Clin Psychol 60:274–281, 1992

Hoge SK, Biederman J: A case of Tourette's syndrome with symptoms of attention deficit disorder treated with desipramine. J Clin Psychiatry 47:478–479, 1986

Huessy H, Wright A: The use of imipramine in children's behavior disorders. Acta Paedopsychiatr 37:194–199, 1970

Hunt RD: Treatment effects of oral and transdermal clonidine in relation to methylphenidate: an open pilot study in ADD-H. Psychopharmacol Bull 23:111–114, 1987

Hunt RD, Minderaa RB, Cohen DJ: Clonidine benefits children with attention deficit disorder and hyperactivity: report of a double-blind placebo-crossover therapeutic trial. J Am Acad Child Psychiatry 24:617–629, 1985

Hunt R, Arnsten A, Asbell M: An open trial of guanfacine in the treatment of attention-deficit hyperactivity disorder. J Am Acad Child Adolesc Psychiatry 34:50–54, 1995

Hynd GW, Semrud-Clikeman MS, Lorys AR, et al: Brain morphology in developmental dyslexia and attention deficit/hyperactivity. Arch Neurol 47:919–926, 1990

Hynd GW, Hern KL, Novey ES, et al: Attention deficit-hyperactivity disorder and asymmetry of the caudate nucleus. J Child Neurol 8:339–347, 1993

Jaffe S: Intranasal abuse of prescribed methylphenidate by an alcohol and drug abusing adolescent with ADHD. J Am Acad Child Adolesc Psychiatry 30:773–775, 1991

Jankovic J: Deprenyl in attention deficit associated with Tourette's syndrome. Arch Neurol 50:286–288, 1993

Jensen P, Shervette R, III, Xenakis S, et al: Anxiety and depressive disorders in attention deficit disorder with hyperactivity: new findings. Am J Psychiatry 150:1203–1209, 1993

Johnston C, Pelham WE, Hoza J, et al: Psychostimulant rebound in attention deficit disordered boys. J Am Acad Child Adolesc Psychiatry 27:806–810, 1988

Kaplan SL, Busner J, Kupietz S, et al: Effects of methylphenidate on adolescents with aggressive conduct disorder and ADHD: a preliminary report. J Am Acad Child Adolesc Psychiatry 29:719–723, 1990

Klein RG: Pharmacotherapy of childhood hyperactivity: an update, in Psychopharmacology: The Third Generation of Progress. Edited by Meltzer HY. New York, Raven Press, 1987, pp 1215–1224

Klorman R, Coons HW, Borgstedt AD: Effects of methylphenidate on adolescents with a childhood history of attention deficit disorder, I: Clinical findings. J Am Acad Child Adolesc Psychiatry 26:363–367, 1987 (erratum, 26:820, 1987)

Klorman R, Brumaghim JT, Salzman LF, et al: Effects of methylphenidate on attention-deficit hyperactivity disorder with and without aggressive/noncompliant features. J Abnorm Psychol 97:413–422, 1988

Klorman R, Brumaghim JT, Salzman LF, et al: Comparative effects of methylphenidate on attention-deficit hyperactivity disorder with and without aggressive/noncompliant features. Psychopharmacol Bull 25:109–113, 1989

Klorman R, Brumaghim J, Fitzpatrick P, et al: Clinical and cognitive effects of methylphenidate on children with attention deficit disorder as a function of aggression/oppositionality and age. J Abnorm Psychol 103:206–221, 1994

Konkol R, Fischer M, Newby R: Double-blind, placebo-controlled stimulant trial in children with Tourette's syndrome and ADHD (abstract). Ann Neurol 28:424, 1990

Kupietz SS, Balka EB: Alterations in the vigilance performance of children receiving amitriptyline and methylphenidate pharmacotherapy. Psychopharmacology (Berlin) 50:29–33, 1976

Kupietz SS, Winsberg BG, Richardson E, et al: Effects of methylphenidate dosage in hyperactive reading-disabled children, I: Behavior and cognitive performance effects. J Am Acad Child Adolesc Psychiatry 27:70–77, 1988

Lahey BB, Schaughency EA, Hynd GW, et al: Attention deficit disorder with and without hyperactivity: comparison of behavioral characteristics of clinic-referred children. J Am Acad Child Adolesc Psychiatry 26:718–723, 1987

Lahey BB, Pelham WE, Schaughency EA, et al: Dimensions and types of attention deficit disorder. J Am Acad Child Adolesc Psychiatry 27:330–335, 1988

Last CG, Strauss CC, Francis G: Comorbidity among childhood anxiety disorders. J Nerv Ment Dis 175:726–730, 1987

Lerer RJ, Lerer MP: Responses of adolescents with minimal brain dysfunction to methylphenidate. Journal of Learning Disabilities 10:223–228, 1977

Livingston R, Dykman R, Ackerman P: Psychiatric comorbidity and response to two doses of methylphenidate in children with attention deficit disorder. Journal of Child and Adolescent Psychopharmacology 2:115–122, 1992

Loney J, Kramer J, Milich RS: The hyperactive child grows up: predictors of symptoms, delinquency and achievement at follow-up, in Psychosocial Aspects of Drug Treatment for Hyperactivity. Edited by Gadow KD and Loney J. Boulder, CO, Westview Press, 1981a, pp 381–416

Loney J, Whaley KMA, Ponto LB, et al: Predictors of adolescent height and weight in hyperkinetic boys treated with methylphenidate. Psychopharm Bull 17:132–4, 1981b

Lowe TL, Cohen DJ, Detlor J: Stimulant medications precipitate Tourette's syndrome. JAMA 247:1168–1169, 1982

MacKay MC, Beck L, Taylor R: Methylphenidate for adolescents with minimal brain dysfunction. New York State Journal of Medicine 73:550–554, 1973

Mannuzza S, Gittelman-Klein R, et al: Hyperactive boys almost grown up, V: replication of psychiatric status. Arch Gen Psychiatry 48:77–83, 1991

Mannuzza S, Klein RG, Bessler A, et al: Adult outcome of hyperactive boys: educational achievement, occupational rank and psychiatric status. Arch Gen Psychiatry 50:565–576, 1993

Manshadi M, Lippmann S, O'Daniel RG, et al: Alcohol abuse and attention deficit disorder. J Clin Psychiatry 44:379–380, 1983

Mattes JA: Propranolol for adults with temper outbursts and residual attention deficit disorder. J Clin Psychopharmacol 6:299–302, 1986

Mattes JA, Gittelman R: Growth of hyperactive children on maintenance regimen of methylphenidate. Arch Gen Psychiatry 40:317–321, 1983

Mattes JA, Boswell L, Oliver H: Methylphenidate effects on symptoms of attention deficit disorder in adults. Arch Gen Psychiatry 41:1059–1063, 1984

Mayes S, Crites D, Bixler E, et al: Methylphenidate and ADHD: influence of age, IQ and neurodevelopmental status. Dev Med Child Neurol 36:1099–1107, 1994

McGee R, Williams S, Silva PA: Behavioral and developmental characteristics of aggressive, hyperactive and aggressive-hyperactive boys. J Am Acad Child Psychiatry 23:270–279, 1984

McGee R, Williams S, Silva PH: Factor structure and correlates of ratings of inattention, hyperactivity, and antisocial behavior in a large sample of 9-year old children from the general population. J Consult Clin Psychol 53:480–490, 1985

Milberger S, Biederman J, Sprich-Buckminster S, et al: Are perinatal complications relevant to the manifestation of attention-deficit hyperactivity disorder? Paper presented at the Scientific Proceedings of the Annual Meeting of the American Academy of Child and Adolescent Psychiatry, San Antonio, TX, 1993

Milich R, Loney J: The role of hyperactive and aggressive symptomatology in predicting adolescent outcome among hyperactive children. J Pediatr Psychol 4:93–112, 1979

Murphy D, Pelham W, Lang A: Aggression in boys with attention deficit-hyperactivity disorder: methylphenidate effects on naturalistically observed aggression, response to provocation, and social information processing. J Abnorm Child Psychol 20:451–466, 1992

Nemeroff C, DeVane L, Pollock B: Newer antidepressants and the cytochrome P450 system. Am J Psychiatry 153:311–320, 1996

Pataki C, Carlson G, Kelly K, et al: Side effects of methylphenidate and desipramine alone and in combination in children. Am J Psychiatry 32:1065–1072, 1993

Pelham W, Greenslade K, Vodde-Hamilton M, et al: Relative efficacy of long-acting stimulants on children with attention deficit-hyperactivity disorder: a comparison of standard methylphenidate, sustained-release methylphenidate, sustained-release dextroamphetamine, and pemoline. Pediatrics 86:226–237, 1990

Pelham WE, Bender ME, Caddell J, et al: Methylphenidate and children with attention deficit disorder. Arch Gen Psychiatry 42:948–952, 1985

Pelham WE, Walker JL, Sturges J, et al: Comparative effects of methylphenidate on ADD girls and ADD boys. J Am Acad Child Adolesc Psychiatry 28:773–776, 1989

Pliszka SR: Effect of anxiety on cognition, behavior, and stimulant response in ADHD. J Am Acad Child Adolesc Psychiatry 28:882–887, 1989

Preskorn SH, Weller EB, Weller RA, et al: Plasma levels of imipramine and adverse effects in children. Am J Psychiatry 140:1332–1335, 1983

Price AR, Leckman JF, Pauls DL, et al: Gilles de la Tourette's syndrome: tics and central nervous system stimulants in twins and nontwins. Neurology 36:232–237, 1986

Prince J, Wilens T, Biederman J, et al: Clonidine for ADHD related sleep disturbances: a systematic chart review of 62 cases. J Am Acad Child Adolesc Psychiatry 35:599–605, 1996

Puig-Antich J, Perel JM, Lupatkin W, et al: Imipramine in prepubertal major depressive disorders. Arch Gen Psychiatry 44:81–89, 1987

Quay HC, Routh DK, Shapiro SK: Psychopathology of childhood: from description to validation. Annu Rev Psychol 38:491–532, 1987

Quinn PO, Rapoport JL: One-year follow-up of hyperactive boys treated with imipramine or methylphenidate. Am J Psychiatry 132:241–245, 1975

Rapoport J, Mikkelsen E: Antidepressants, in Pediatric Psychopharmacology. Edited by Werry J. New York, Brunner/Mazel, 1978, pp 208–233

Rapoport JL, Quinn P, Bradbard G, et al: Imipramine and methylphenidate treatment of hyperactive boys: A double-blind comparison. Arch Gen Psychiatry 30:789–793, 1974

Rapport MD, DuPaul GJ, Stoner G, et al: Comparing classroom and clinic measures of attention deficit disorder: differential, idiosyncratic, and dose-response effects of methylphenidate. J Consult Clin Psychol 54:334–341, 1986

Rapport MD, Jones JT, DuPaul GJ, et al: Attention deficit disorder and methylphenidate: group and single-subject analyses of dose effects on attention in clinic and classroom settings. Journal of Clinical Child Psychology 16:329–338, 1987

Rapport MD, Stoner G, DuPaul GJ, et al: Attention deficit disorder and methylphenidate: a multilevel analysis of dose-response effects on children's impulsivity across settings. J Am Acad Child Adolesc Psychiatry 27:60–69, 1988

Rapport MD, DuPaul GJ, et al: Attention deficit hyperactivity disorder and methylphenidate: the relationship between gross body weight and drug response in children. Psychopharmacol Bull 25:285–290, 1989a

Rapport MD, Quinn SO, DuPaul GJ, et al: Attention deficit disorder with hyperactivity and methylphenidate: the effects of dose and mastery level on children's learning performance. J Abnorm Child Psychol 17:669–689, 1989b

Rapport M, Carlson G, Kelly K, et al: Methylphenidate and desipramine in hospitalized children, I: separate and combined effects on cognitive function. J Am Acad Child Adolesc Psychiatry 32:333–342, 1993

Ratey J, Greenberg M, Lindem K: Combination of treatments for attention deficit disorders in adults. J Nerv Ment Dis 176:699–701, 1991

Reimherr FW, Wender PH, Wood DR, et al: An open trial of L-tyrosine in the treatment of attention deficit disorder, residual type. Am J Psychiatry 144:1071–1073, 1987

Reimherr F, Hedges D, Strong R, et al: An open-trial of venlafaxine in adult patients with attention deficit hyperactivity disorder. Paper presented at the New Clinical Drug Evaluation Unit Program, Orlando, FL, 1995

Riddle MA, Hardin MT, Cho SC, et al: Desipramine treatment of boys with attention-deficit hyperactivity disorder and tics: preliminary clinical experience. J Am Acad Child Adolesc Psychiatry 27:811–814, 1988

Sachs GS, Conklin A, Lafer B, et al: Psychopathology in children of late vs. early onset bipolar probands. Paper presented at the Proceedings of the Annual Meeting of the American Academy of Child and Adolescent Psychiatry, San Antonio, 1993

Safer DJ, Allen RP: Stimulant drug treatment of hyperactive adolescents. Diseases of the Nervous System 454–457, 1975

Safer DJ, Krager JM: A survey of medication treatment for hyperactive/inattentive students. JAMA 260:2256–2258, 1988

Safer DJ, Allen RP, Barr E: Depression of growth in hyperactive children on stimulant drugs. N Engl J Med 287:217–220, 1972

Sallee F, Stiller R, Perel J: Pharmacodynamics of pemoline in attention deficit disorder with hyperactivity. J Am Acad Child Adolesc Psychiatry 31:244–251, 1992

Satterfield JH, Cantwell DP, Schell A, et al: Growth of hyperactive children treated with methylphenidate. Arch Gen Psychiatry 36:212–217, 1979

Schachar R, Tannock R: Childhood hyperactivity and psychostimulants: A review of extended treatment studies. Journal of Child and Adolescent Psychopharmacology 3:81–97, 1993

Schachar R, Hoppe C, Schell A: Changes in family function and relationships in children who respond to methylphenidate. J Am Acad Child Adolesc Psychiatry 26:728–732, 1987

Schleifer N, Weiss G, Cohen N, et al: Hyperactivity in preschoolers and the effect of methylphenidate. Am J Orthopsychiatry 45:38–50, 1975

Semrud-Clikeman MS, Biederman J, Sprich S, et al: Comorbidity between ADHD and learning disability: a review and report in a clinically referred sample. J Am Acad Child Adolesc Psychiatry 31:439–448, 1992

Semrud-Clikeman M, Filipek P, Biederman J, et al: Attention deficit disorder: differences in the corpus callosum and shape analysis in MRI morphometric analysis. J Am Acad Child Adolesc Psychiatry 33:875–881, 1994

Shapiro AK, Shapiro E: Do stimulants provoke, cause, or exacerbate tics and Tourette syndrome? Compr Psychiatry 22:265–273, 1981

Silver LB, Brunstetter RW: Attention deficit disorder in adolescents. Hosp Community Psychiatry 37:608–613, 1986

Simeon JG, Ferguson HB, Van Wyck Fleet J: Bupropion effects in attention deficit and conduct disorders. Can J Psychiatry 31:581–585, 1986

Singer S, Brown J, Quaskey S, et al: The treatment of attention-deficit hyperactivity disorder in Tourette's syndrome: a double-blind placebo-controlled study with clonidine and desipramine. Pediatrics 95:74–81, 1994

Solanto MV, Wender EH: Does methylphenidate constrict cognitive functioning? J Am Acad Child Adolesc Psychiatry 28:897–902, 1989

Spencer T, Biederman J, Kerman K, et al: Desipramine in the treatment of children with Tic disorder or Tourette's Syndrome and attention deficit hyperactivity disorder. J Am Acad Child Adolesc Psychiatry 32:354–360, 1993a

Spencer T, Biederman J, Wilens T, et al: Nortriptyline in the treatment of children with attention deficit hyperactivity disorder and tic disorder or Tourette's syndrome. J Am Acad Child Adolesc Psychiatry 32:205–210, 1993b

Spencer TJ, Biederman J, Steingard R, et al: Bupropion exacerbates tics in children with attention deficit hyperactivity disorder and Tourette's Disorder. J Am Acad Child Adolesc Psychiatry 32:211–214, 1993c

Spencer T, Wilens TE, Biederman J: A double-blind, crossover comparison of tomoxetine and placebo in adults with ADHD. Paper presented at the Scientific Proceedings of the Annual Meeting of the American Academy of Child and Adolescent Psychiatry, New Orleans, LA, 1995a

Spencer T, Wilens TE, Biederman J, et al: A double-blind, crossover comparison of methylphenidate and placebo in adults with childhood-onset attention deficit hyperactivity. Arch Gen Psychiatry 52:434–443, 1995b

Spencer T, Biederman J, Harding M, et al: Growth deficits in ADHD children revisited: evidence for disorder-associated growth delays? J Am Acad Child Adolesc Psychiatry 1996a

Spencer TJ, Biederman J, Wilens T, et al: Pharmacotherapy of ADHD across the lifecycle: a literature review. J Am Acad Child Adolesc Psychiatry 35:409–432, 1996b

Sprague RL, Sleator EK: Methylphenidate in hyperkinetic children: differences in dose effects on learning and social behavior. Science 198:1274–1276, 1977

Steingard R, Biederman J, Spencer T, et al: Comparison of clonidine response in the treatment of attention deficit hyperactivity disorder with and without comorbid tic disorders. J Am Acad Child Adolesc Psychiatry 32:350–353, 1993

Strayhorn J, Rapp N, Donina W, et al: Randomized trial of methyphenidate for an autistic child. J Am Acad Child Adolesc Psychiatry 27:244–247, 1988

Sverd J, Gadow KD, Paolicelli LM: Methylphenidate treatment of attention-deficit hyperactibity disorder in boys with Tourette's syndrome. J Am Acad Child Adolesc Psychiatry 28:574–579, 1989

Sverd J, Gadow K, Nolan E, et al: Methylphenidate in hyperactive boys with comorbid tic disorder, I: clinic evaluations. Advances in Neurology 58:271–281, 1992

Swanson J, Kinsbourne M, Roberts W, et al: Time-response analysis of the effect of stimulant medication on the learning ability of children referred for hyperactivity. Pediatrics 61:21–24, 1978

Swanson JM, Granger D, Kliewer W: Natural social behaviors in hyperactive children: dose effects of methylphenidate. J Consult Clin Psychol 55:187–193, 1987

Tannock R, Schachar RJ, Carr RP, et al: Dose-response effects of methylphenidate on academic performance and overt behavior in hyperactive children. Pediatrics 84:648–657, 1989

Tannock R, Ickowicz A, Schachar R: Differential effects of methylphenidate on working memory in ADHD children with and without comorbid anxiety. J Am Acad Child Adolesc Psychiatry 34:886–896, 1995

Taylor E, Schachar R, Thorley G, et al: Which boys respond to stimulant medication? a controlled trial of methylphenidate in boys with disruptive behaviour. Psychol Med 17:121–143, 1987

Varley CK: Effects of methylphenidate in adolescents with attention deficit disorder. J Am Acad Child Psychiatry 22:351–354, 1983

Voelker SL, Lachar D, Gdowski LL: The personality inventory for children and response to methylphenidate: preliminary evidence for predictive validity. J Pediatr Psychol 8:161–169, 1983

Watter N, Dreyfuss FE: Modifications of hyperkinetic behavior by nortriptyline. Virginia Medical Monthly 100:123–126, 1973

Weintraub S, Mesulam MM, Kramer L: Disturbances in prosody. Acta Neurol Scand 38:742–744, 1981

Weiss G, Hechtman LT: Hyperactive Children Grown Up. New York, Guilford, 1986

Weiss G, Hechtman L, Milroy T, et al: Psychiatric status of hyperactives as adults: a controlled prospective 15-year follow-up of 63 hyperactive children. J Am Acad Child Psychiatry 24:211–220, 1985

Weizman A, Weitz R, Szekely G, et al: Combination of neuroleptic and stimulant treatment in ADHD. J Am Acad Child Psychiatry 23:295–298, 1984

Wender PH and Reimherr FW: Bupropion treatment of attention–deficit hyperactivity disorder in adults. Am J Psychiatry 147:1018–1020, 1990

Wender PH, Reimherr FW, Wood DR: Attention deficit disorder ("minimal brain dysfunction") in adults: a replication study of diagnosis and drug treatment. Arch Gen Psychiatry 38:449–456, 1981

Wender PH, Wood DR, Reimherr FW, et al: An open trial of pargyline in the treatment of attention deficit disorder, residual type. Psychiatry Res 9:329–336, 1983

Wender P, Reimherr F, Wood D, et al: A controlled study of methylphenidate in the treatment of Attention Deficit Disorder, residual type, in adults. Am J Psychiatry 142:547–552, 1985a

Wender PH, Wood DR, Reimherr FW: Pharmacological treatment of attention deficit disorder, residual type (ADDRT, "minimal brain dysfunction," "hyperactivity") in adults. Psychopharmacol Bull 21:222–232, 1985b

Werry J: Imipramine and methylphenidate in hyperactive children. J Child Psychol Psychiatry 21:27–35, 1980

West S, McElroy S, Strakowski S, et al: Attention deficit hyperactivity disorder in adolescent mania. Am J Psychiatry 152:271–274, 1995

Whalen C: Does stimulant medication improve the peer status of hyperactive children? J Consult Clin Psychol 57:545–549, 1989

Whalen C, Henker B, Swanson J, et al: Natural social behaviors in hyperactive children: dose effects of methylphenidate. J Consult Clin Psychol 55:187–193, 1987

Whalen C, Henker B, Granger D: Social judgement processes in hyperactive boys: effects of methylpheniddate and comparisons with normal peers. J Abnorm Child Psychol 18:297–316, 1990

Wilens T, Biederman J: The stimulants, in Psychiatric Clinics of North America, Vol 15. Edited by Schaffer D. Philadelphia, WB Saunders, 1992, pp 191–222

Wilens T, Prince J, Spencer T, et al: Double-blind comparison of desipramine and placebo in adults with attention deficit hyperactivity disorder: preliminary results. Paper presented at the Scientific Proceedings of the Annual Meeting of the American Academy of Child and Adolescent Psychiatry, New York, 1994a

Wilens T, Spencer T, Biederman J, et al: Combined pharmacotherapy: an emerging trend in pediatric psychopharmacology. J Am Acad Child Adolesc Psychiatry 34:110–112, 1994b

Wilens TE, Biederman J, Baldessarini RJ, et al: Developmental changes in serum concentrations of desipramine and 2-hydroxydesipramine during treatment with desipramine. J Am Acad Child Adolesc Psychiatry 31:691–698, 1992

Wilens TE, Biederman J, Geist DE, et al: Nortriptyline in the treatment of attention deficit hyperactivity disorder: a chart review of 58 cases. J Am Acad Child Adolesc Psychiatry 32:343–349, 1993

Wilens TE, Biederman JB, Mick E, et al: A systematic assessment of tricyclic antidepressants in the treatment of adult attention-deficit hyperactivity disorder. J Nerv Ment Dis 183:48–50, 1995

Wilens TE, Biederman J, Prince J, et al: Six week, double blind, placebo controlled study of desipramine for adult attention deficit hyperactivity disorder. Am J Psychiatry 153:1147–1153, 1996

Winsberg BG, Bialer I, Kupietz S, et al: Effects of imipramine and dextroamphetamine on behavior of neuropsychiatrically impaired children. Am J Psychiatry 128:1425–1431, 1972

Winsberg BG, Press M, Bialer I, et al: Dextroamphetamine and methylphenidate in the treatment of hyperactive/aggressive children. Pediatrics 53:236–241, 1974

Wood DR, Reimherr FW, Wender PH, et al: Diagnosis and treatment of minimal brain dysfunction in adults: a preliminary report. Arch Gen Psychiatry 33:1453–1460, 1976

Wozniak J, Biederman J: A pharmacological approach to the quagmire of comorbidity in juvenile mania. J Am Acad Child Adolesc Psychiatry 35:826–828, 1996

Wozniak J, Biederman J, Kiely K, et al: Mania-like symptoms suggestive of childhood onset bipolar disorder in clinically referred children. J Am Acad Child Adolesc Psychiatry 34:867–876, 1995

Yepes LE, Balka EB, Winsberg BG, et al: Amitriptyline and methylphenidate treatment of behaviorally disordered children. J Child Psychol Psychiatry 18:39–52, 1977

Zametkin A, Rapoport JL, Murphy DL, et al: Treatment of hyperactive children with monoamine oxidase inhibitors, I: clinical efficacy. Arch Gen Psychiatry 42:962–966, 1985

Zametkin AJ, Rapoport JL: Noradrenergic hypothesis of attention deficit disorder with hyperactivity: a critical review, in Psychopharmacology: The Third Generation of Progress. Edited by Meltzer HY. New York, Raven, 1987, pp 837–842

Zametkin AJ, Nordahl TE, Gross M, et al: Cerebral glucose metabolism in adults with hyperactivity of childhood onset. N Engl J Med 323:1361–1366, 1990

Chapter 19

Child and Adolescent Psychopharmacology

Scott A. West, M.D.

In this chapter, I focus on general pharmacological principles and re-cent psychopharmacological developments in psychiatric illnesses that often manifest themselves in children and adolescents and continue throughout adulthood. Some of these disorders, including bipolar dis-order, primary psychotic disorders, and attention-deficit/hyperactivity disorder, are discussed in other chapters and therefore are not ad-dressed here. This chapter provides a concise update on the current status of psychopharmacology in depressive disorders, anxiety disor-ders, eating disorders, and conduct disorder (CD)/aggression. The chapter does not include recent data in adult psychopharmacology that may have implications for the treatment of children and adolescents. Such extrapolations have inherent limitations, which are further elabo-rated on in the chapter.

It is important to emphasize that children and adolescents are de-veloping psychologically, socially, and biologically and that therefore pathological states are typically more fluid in this population than in adults. Because of this, children and adolescents should not be concep-tualized with rigid diagnostic criteria. Rather, signs and symptoms should be interpreted in the context of potentially evolving illnesses and developmental stage. Additionally, the presence of multiple psy-chiatric syndromes is common in children and adolescents (comor-bidity is approximately 50% across disorders), and an interactive effect occurs between concurrent disorders, which also has an effect on pres-entation.

When psychiatric disorders go unrecognized or untreated, they can have a profound effect on psychosocial development and can perma-nently interfere with personal identity, self-esteem, family relation-ships, peer relationships, and school and job performance. Therefore, it is imperative that psychiatric illnesses in children and adolescents are recognized early so that prompt treatment may be given. Unfortu-nately, psychopharmacological treatment in pediatric populations is not well founded, and most treatment strategies are based on anecdotal reports, small open studies, or extrapolations from controlled adult studies. This latter strategy may be especially misleading, because medications that are effective in adults may not be effective in children (e.g., tricyclic antidepressants [TCAs] in the treatment of depression), perhaps because of incomplete neuronal maturation. In addition, the substantial pharmacokinetic changes that occur throughout development must be considered when prescribing for children and adolescents, necessitating the use of higher doses of some medications (e.g., divalproex) and lower doses of others (e.g., TCAs).

Pharmacokinetics

Drug metabolism and kinetics change with physical development, and therefore the amount and frequency of dosing change as children mature into adults (Hughes and Preskorn 1994). Children have more body fat than do adults and therefore have a relatively large reservoir for psychotropic drugs, which tend to be highly lipophilic. This may be important clinically because the half-life of some medications may be prolonged in children, an effect that may affect initiating, titrating, or changing medications.

The two primary routes of drug elimination are hepatic biotransformation and renal excretion. Hepatic enzyme activity is typically fully developed by 1 year of age, allowing most medications to be readily metabolized. Prepubertal children have a much higher hepatic clearance for their body weight than do adults, and therefore, to achieve therapeutic serum concentrations and beneficial clinical results, often require larger doses or more frequent dosing of medications that are hepatically metabolized (Briant 1978). Failure to appreciate this phenomenon may result in underdosing and therefore undertreating younger patients.

As with hepatic function, renal function fully matures by 1 year of age. The glomerular filtration rate may actually be higher in children than in adolescents and adults (Popper 1985). Also, children tend to consume more fluids than do adults, adding to the rapid clearance of medications. These factors, coupled with the fact that children have more total body water and subsequently a greater volume of distribution for hydrophilic medications than do adults, means that higher doses of hydrophilic medications (such as lithium) are often required in children in order to achieve therapeutic serum concentrations (Jatlow 1987). Because drug metabolism changes with age, close monitoring is indicated with the onset of puberty so that signs of toxicity can be recognized early and medication dosages reduced as necessary. A transient decrease in drug metabolism may occur several months before the onset of puberty, which may result in sudden increases in plasma drug concentrations. The transient decrease in drug metabolism may be the result of sudden increases in circulating hormones that are competing for hepatic metabolism (Popper 1985).

Because children and adolescents are in a continual state of physical, psychological, and social development, drug toxicity may manifest itself through delayed maturation in any of these areas. This is referred to as *developmental toxicology* (Dulcan et al. 1995). These "side effects" can result in poor school performance, difficulty with peer relationships, altered family dynamics, and retarded physical growth and maturation. Therefore, being aware of this possibility in addition to monitoring specific target symptoms of the disorder being treated (and there may be considerable overlap between them) is important in providing effective long-term treatment.

Factors that influence compliance with the evaluation and treatment process in children and adolescents also tend to change with development; it is helpful to be cognizant of this tendency. For example, in prepubertal children, parental support, supervision, and structure are necessary if most children are to feel comfortable with the treatment process. Therefore, integrating parents into the treatment framework—including evaluations, psychotherapy sessions, and medication issues—is very important. Conversely, adolescents often respond more favorably to a more confidential approach, because parental involvement at this age is often interpreted as an invasion of privacy. Therefore, with adolescents it is typically more effective to minimize parental involvement, unless there are concerns about dangerousness or abuse. In short, it is helpful to remain flexible in the therapeutic approach to children and adolescents as they mature into adults.

Depression

Depression has historically been underdiagnosed in children and adolescents. Indeed, mood disorders in general have received little attention in this age group, and data on their epidemiology, phenomenology, and comorbidity are limited. The prevalence of major depression in children has been estimated at approximately 2%, affecting boys and girls equally. In adolescents, prevalence estimates are as high as 5%, and beginning in this age group females are affected twice as often as are males. Depression is also a common comorbid syndrome with other psychiatric illnesses, including ADHD, conduct disorder, anxiety disorders, substance abuse, and eating disorders.

The core symptoms of depression, according to the DSM-IV (American Psychiatric Association 1994) diagnostic criteria, are the same regardless of age, with two exceptions: in children and adolescents, but not adults, mood may be either irritable or depressed, and failure to make expected weight gain may occur instead of weight gain or loss. In addition to these two modifications, several other important caveats should be kept in mind. In prepubertal children, social withdrawal, irritability, and vague somatic complaints such as headaches and stomachaches are very common and pronounced. In adolescents, irritability, oppositional behavior, and poor school performance often become prominent. These symptoms may also be the result of comorbid conditions, whose presence can significantly influence treatment planning.

Double-blind, placebo-controlled studies evaluating the efficacy of tricyclic antidepressants (TCAs) in children and adolescents with major depression have been disappointing. Indeed, with the exception of one study that found a significant difference between imipramine and placebo (Preskorn et al. 1987), numerous studies have failed to show TCAs more effective than placebo (Hazell et al. 1995). This failure may be the result of low rates of antidepressant response rather than high rates of placebo response in this population, although that possibility remains undetermined. Clearly, some individuals respond well to TCAs, and therefore these data should not preclude the use of these agents in minors when appropriate.

Studies assessing the efficacy of selective serotonin reuptake inhibitors (SSRIs) in children and adolescents have also been tenuous, although these data are much more limited than are those for the TCAs (DeVane and Sallee 1996). One double-blind, placebo-controlled trial has been published at the time of this writing (Simeon et al. 1990a). In this study, 32 patients with depression were treated for a total of 8 weeks. In both the patients receiving fluoxetine (60 mg/day) and the patients receiving placebo, significant improvement was noted, as measured by the Hamilton Rating Scale for Depression (HAM-D), the Raskin Depression Scale, and the Covi Anxiety Scale, by the third week of treatment. However, as observed with the TCAs, there was no significant difference between treatment groups. Fluoxetine was well tolerated; headache, vomiting, insomnia, and tremor were the most frequently observed adverse effects. One other controlled trial with fluoxetine has recently been completed, and preliminary results suggest that fluoxetine was more effective than placebo (Emslie 1996).

Open trials suggest that various SSRIs may be effective in child and adolescent depression. Two open trials of fluoxetine (dosage range 5–80 mg/day), with a total of 46 patients, have reported that approximately 50% of patients improved with treatment (Boulos et al. 1992; Jain et al. 1992). One open trial with fluvoxamine has also been published; Apter et al. (1994) reported that six patients, taking daily dosages of 100–300 mg of fluvoxamine, significantly improved after 8 weeks of treatment, as measured by decreases in Beck Depression Inventory scores.

Two reports have described the effects of sertraline in children and adolescents with major depression. In the first study, McConville et al. (1996) prospectively followed 13 adolescents over a 12-week period and found that depression improved significantly in 11 patients, with marked reduction (at least 50%) in HAM-D and Montgomery-Asberg Depression Rating Scale scores. The mean dosage of sertraline was 110 mg/day, or 2 mg/kg/day. Adverse effects, which were relatively common, consisted primarily of insomnia and sedation, but they were typically manageable. One patient did become manic after 8 days of treatment with sertraline, which was subsequently discontinued. In the second report, Tierney et al. (1995) retrospectively reviewed the charts of patients 8–18 years of age treated with sertraline monotherapy and found that 11 of 17 patients improved substantially. The mean daily dosage of sertraline was 100 mg, or 1.6 mg/kg. Behavioral side effects, including mania that developed in two patients during treatment (one after 3 days, the other after 3 months), were problematic and accounted for 21% of patients' discontinuing treatment. Behavioral side effects (episodic dyscontrol, hypomania, personality change) have also been reported with fluoxetine and may be dose dependent (Riddle et al. 1990a). At this time these adverse effects should be considered a class effect, and pediatric patients on any SSRI should have dosages titrated up slowly and carefully monitored, especially if there is a family history of bipolar disorder. In that case it may be prudent to consider a mood stabilizer, such as divalproex or lithium.

In summary, data on the use of the SSRIs in children and adolescents with depression are inconsistent, and more controlled studies are needed in order to clarify the safety and efficacy of these medications in the pediatric population. However, given the favorable side-effect profile of the SSRIs, their relative safety in overdose, their lack of cardiac toxicity, and the numerous controlled trials of TCAs in children and adolescents that have failed to demonstrate this class of drugs to be more effective than placebo, it seems prudent to use the SSRIs as first-line agents in the treatment of depression. Some individuals may respond more favorably to a TCA than to an SSRI. In these patients, imipramine and desipramine should be considered, because there is a significant amount of data on the use of these agents in children and adolescents. Because four deaths have been reported thus far in patients receiving desipramine (Riddle et al. 1993), some experts (Popper 1995) have recommended using imipramine or other tricyclic medications (e.g., nortriptyline), although others (Biederman et al. 1993, 1995) have reported that desipramine is safe as long as serum concentrations remain in the therapeutic range.

As with major depression, dysthymia has been increasingly recognized in children and adolescents over the past two decades. Prevalence is estimated to be approximately 3%, and in children it is equally distributed among boys and girls. Like major depression, however, dysthymia becomes two to three times more common in females during adolescence. In this age group, irritability is a very common symptom of dysthymia; therefore, DSM-IV criteria allow for it as a criterion in lieu of depressed mood, as in major depression. It is also notable that minimum duration in children and adolescents is 1 year, according to DSM-IV—in contrast to adults, in whom symptoms must be present for 2 years before a diagnosis can be made. Diagnostic criteria are otherwise the same for children, adolescents, and adults. It should be emphasized that school performance and the development of social skills are often impaired in patients with dysthymia. These problems, when combined with pessimism and feelings of hopelessness, may lead to significant adult psychopathology if not adequately treated. Also, patients with dysthymia should be carefully monitored, because dysthymia may represent a prodrome to other psychiatric disorders (especially major depressive and bipolar disorders) in this young population (Kovacs et al. 1994).

Despite increased recognition of dysthymia in the pediatric population, there are no studies examining the efficacy of pharmacotherapy in dysthymia in children and adolescents. Indeed, only one double-blind, placebo-controlled trial in adults with dysthymia has been published; it found fluoxetine to be effective and well tolerated (Hellerstein et al. 1993). Subsequently, although the safety and efficacy of the SSRIs in dysthymic children and adolescents is unknown, if pharmacotherapy is used, it is probably prudent to use this class of medications, as with major depression.

Other types of depression, such as minor depression and brief recurrent depression, have not been studied in children and adolescents (Judd et al. 1994). This area remains a substantial one for future investigation, because depression in this age group often presents with fewer symptoms and is present for a shorter period than our current DSM-IV diagnostic criteria allow in order to make a formal diagnosis. Nevertheless, despite their brevity, such symptoms can lead to substantial functional impairment and, in adults, respond to antidepressant treatment.

Because controlled studies examining the efficacy of antidepressants in acute depression in children and adolescents have been negative, treatment guidelines for maintenance therapy have not been established. There are no long-term, controlled, systematic studies assessing the stability of remission and rates of relapse in patients who initially respond to treatment and are maintained on pharmacological regimens. However, data from open trials in acute depression, in which patients were treated for several months, suggest that it may be beneficial to continue antidepressants for an extended period once an initial response is achieved. Other clinical factors—including the degree of response, severity of depression, number of past episodes, and family history—are also important when considering maintenance treatment.

Anxiety Disorders

The characterization of anxiety disorders in children and adolescents has received a significant amount of attention. It has become well recognized that anxiety in children and adolescents often represents the early manifestation of lifelong disorders, emphasizing the need for early recognition and treatment. There has been an evolution of the nosology of anxiety disorders in this population, reflected by two significant changes in the DSM-IV. Overanxious disorder has been dropped, and most children fulfilling criteria for this disorder are now diagnosed with generalized anxiety disorder with childhood onset. Also, avoidant disorder of childhood has been deleted in favor of childhood-onset social phobia. These changes represent an attempt to maintain diagnostic integrity as illnesses evolve throughout the life span.

The pharmacotherapy of anxiety disorders in children and adolescents has also received a considerable amount of attention compared to other disorders in this age group. Indeed, there are 13 controlled trials examining the safety and efficacy of pharmacological agents in pediatric patients with various anxiety disorders, including obsessive-compulsive disorder (OCD), separation anxiety disorder, social phobia, and generalized anxiety disorder (Allen et al. 1995). Perhaps the best studied of all of these disorders is OCD, in which five controlled studies have been performed to date (DeVeaugh-Geiss et al. 1992; Flament et al. 1985; Leonard et al. 1989, 1991; Riddle et al. 1992), as well as several open trials (Apter et al. 1994; Geller et al. 1995; Riddle et al. 1990b) and case reports (Alessi and Bos 1991; Bussing and Levin 1993; Graae et al. 1992; Liebowitz et al. 1990; Simeon et al. 1990b). Clomipramine has been demonstrated to be very effective and well tolerated compared with placebo (DeVeaugh-Geiss et al. 1992; Flament et al. 1985) and desipramine (Leonard et al. 1989). Cumulatively, these studies suggest that approximately 75% of children improve substantially and that relapse occurs quickly when clomipramine is discontinued. A more recent study (Riddle et al. 1992) suggested that fluoxetine may also be effective and well tolerated in children and adolescents with OCD. This double-blind, crossover trial found that 44% of patients improved while taking fluoxetine, as measured by the Yale-Brown Obsessive-Compulsive Scale (YBOCS), compared with 27% who improved while taking placebo—a statistically insignificant difference. However, the dosage of fluoxetine was maintained at 20 mg/day, and data from open studies suggest that children and adolescents may respond more favorably to higher doses of fluoxetine (a response also commonly observed in adults).

Separation anxiety disorder is unique to children and typically manifests itself as school phobia. Five placebo-controlled studies have examined the efficacy of various medications, including imipramine (Gittelman-Klein 1971; Klein et al. 1992), clomipramine (Berney et al. 1981), clonazepam (Graae et al. 1994), alprazolam (Bernstein et al. 1990), and imipramine (Bernstein et al. 1990). Data from these studies, taken together, suggest that tricyclic antidepressants may be helpful in some patients but are disappointing overall and provide little benefit in most patients. In contrast, clonazepam appears to be slightly more beneficial: symptoms in 6 of 12 children completely remitted after 4 weeks of clonazepam, titrated as necessary up to 2 mg/day. However, side effects occurred in 10 patients and were problematic in several; they included sedation, disinhibition, and irritability.

The treatment of generalized anxiety disorder, formerly known as overanxious disorder of childhood, has received little attention. One double-blind, controlled study by Simeon et al. (1992) compared alprazolam (mean dosage 1.57 mg/day) with placebo and found no significant difference between treatment groups. Birmaher et al. (1994) examined the efficacy of fluoxetine in 21 children and adolescents in an open study. They noted substantial improvement in 17 patients as measured by the Cinical Global Impression (CGI) scale. The mean dosage of fluoxetine was 26 mg/day (range 10–60 mg/day), and it was well tolerated. These data are encouraging and need to be replicated in controlled trials.

Childhood-onset social phobia, formerly known as avoidant disorder of childhood, may involve circumscribed anxiety, such as the fear of speaking in front of a class, or a more general and persistent fear of public scrutiny. Two controlled trials have evaluated the efficacy of pharmacotherapy in this age group. The more recent study, by Black and Uhde (1994), included 15 children and adolescents with social phobia and elective mutism. This double-blind, placebo-controlled 12-week trial of fluoxetine (0.6 mg/kg/day) failed to demonstrate a substantial difference between treatments, as both groups improved. However, there was a significant difference, favoring fluoxetine, in global improvement ratings by parents. One additional controlled study using alprazolam (Simeon et al. 1992) included some patients with social phobia; the results of the study have been discussed in this chapter. More research is clearly needed assessing the safety and efficacy of pharmacotherapy in patients with social phobia so that appropriate treatment algorithms can be designed.

Although panic disorder occurs in children and adolescents and is phenomenologically similar to that observed in adults (Moreau and Weissman 1992), there are no systematic treatment data in children and adolescents. Data are limited to several case reports suggesting that imipramine, desipramine, and clonazepam may be effective in children and adolescents with panic disorder. Kutcher et al. (1992) reported preliminary findings from an ongoing double-blind study of 12 adolescents treated with clonazepam. The authors observed substantial improvement in both the intensity and frequency of panic attacks in 80% of adolescents treated with clonazepam, and it appeared to be safe and well tolerated in this population. However, controlled studies with larger numbers of patients need to be performed.

Like panic disorder, there are virtually no data on the treatment of posttraumatic stress disorder (PTSD) in children and adolescents. Despite the prevalence of sexual, physical, and emotional abuse in families today, there are no data to guide the treatment of patients who develop PTSD. Indeed, only one open-label study has been performed. This study, by Famularo et al. (1988), examined the usefulness of propranolol in 11 children with PTSD. It was found that propranolol significantly reduced the hyperarousal and autonomic symptoms of PTSD at a maximum dosage of 2.5 mg/kg/day. Overall, propranolol was well tolerated, although the dose had to be reduced in three patients as a result of intolerable side effects. Controlled data are needed to assess fully whether propranolol will be safe and effective in this population.

Eating Disorders

Anorexia and bulimia nervosa typically begin during childhood and adolescence. However, most treatment data are based on studies in young adults who have had anorexia or bulimia for a number of years before presenting for treatment. Two such studies (Trygstad 1990, Wilcox 1990) have been reported for bulimia nervosa, both of which were open trials examining the effects of fluoxetine. Trygstad (1990) followed 30 patients taking an average dosage of 60 mg/day for up to 10 months and found that bingeing and purging completely abated in 15 patients and was reduced by 75% in the remaining 15 patients. Wilcox (1990), examining 20 patients taking an average dosage of 20 mg/day, reported that only 20% of patients achieved remission of symptoms after 6 months of treatment. The difference in response rates in these two studies may be explained, at least in part, by the difference in fluoxetine dose, as it has been my experience that relatively high doses are needed to treat these disorders successfully.

As with bulimia, there are no controlled pharmacological trials in children and adolescents with anorexia nervosa. One open trial (Kaye et al. 1991) involving 31 patients (average age 20 years, range 11–40) treated with 10–80 mg/day of fluoxetine found that 10 patients responded well, 17 demonstrated some improvement, and 4 had no improvement over an average of 11 months of treatment. Two case reports (Iancu et al. 1992; Lyles et al. 1990) also suggested that fluoxetine may be beneficial, but these data need to be confirmed by controlled trials.

Disruptive-Behavior Disorders

Disruptive-behavior disorders have been some of the most challenging disorders to treat. Patients have a significant amount of comorbidity with both oppositional defiant disorder (ODD) (Iancu et al. 1992; Lyles et al. 1990) and conduct disorder (CD), including ADHD, substance abuse and dependence, bipolar disorder, depression, mental retardation, and developmental disorders (Dulcan et al. 1995). Oppositional behavior and conduct disturbances are often secondary to one of these other disorders; in that case, treatment should be focused on the primary diagnosis. Aggression is a common chief complaint in children and adolescents with disruptive behavior, and often becomes the focus of treatment in patients with a primary diagnosis of CD or ODD.

Until recently, most of the data on the treatment of disruptive behaviors were derived from open trials and case reports. Numerous medications, including β-blockers, clonidine, and neuroleptics, have been reported to be useful in some patients, although controlled trials are needed to confirm these observations. Mood stabilizers, most notably lithium and carbamazepine, have traditionally been the treatment of choice to manage symptoms of poor impulse control and aggressive behavior and have received more systematic research (Alessi et al. 1994). In a controlled study examining the efficacy of lithium, Campbell et al. (1995) compared lithium with placebo over a 6-week period in 50 children, mean age 9 years, with CD. Sixty-eight percent of patients randomized to lithium, compared with 49% of those taking placebo, were rated as moderately or markedly improved, a statistically significant difference. The mean daily dose of lithium was 1,248 mg, producing a mean serum concentration of 1.12 mEq/L. Gastrointestinal side effects were the most common group of adverse effects. This study confirmed the results of a previous study by Campbell et al. (1984). However, data from two other (as yet unpublished) double-blind and placebo-controlled trials found lithium to be no more effective than placebo (Campbell and Cueva 1995). Methodological differences may account for these discrepancies, and taken together these data suggest that lithium may be effective in some patients.

An open trial found carbamazepine to be effective in 10 hospitalized children with CD and severe aggression who were previously resistant to lithium (Kafantaris et al. 1992). However, a recent double-blind, placebo-controlled trial of carbamazepine in 22 children, ages 5 to 15 years, with CD and treatment-resistant aggressiveness and explosiveness was negative (Cueva et al. 1996). Carbamazepine dosages ranged from 400 to 800 mg/day (mean 683 mg), and serum concentrations ranged from 5 to 9 μg/mL. Treatment with carbamazepine did not differ from placebo on measures including the Overt Aggression Scale, the Global Clinical Judgments Scale, and the Children's Psychiatric Rating Scale. More research is clearly needed to further examine the efficacy of medications in general and mood stabilizers in particular in this population.

Summary

As research examining the phenomenology and comorbidity of psychiatric disorders in children and adolescents continues, more treatment studies will ensue to guide the pharmacotherapy in this population. At this time, treatment data are very limited across diagnostic groups, with a few exceptions, as noted above. Pharmacological treatment of pediatric patients is still based largely on anecdotal reports or extrapolations from adult data, which provides limited, albeit useful, guidelines. However, it is prudent to be cautious in children and adolescents, because pharmacokinetics and pharmacodynamics change with age and because daily dosage, frequency of dosing, and potential side effects may fluctuate. Nevertheless, data are beginning to accumulate that can serve as a clinically useful guide to the pharmacological management of this population.

References

Alessi N, Bos T: Buspirone augmentation of fluoxetine in a depressed child with obsessive-compulsive disorder. Am J Psychiatry 148:1605–1606, 1991

Alessi N, Naylor MW, Ghaziuddin M, et al: Update on lithium carbonate therapy in children and adolescents. J Am Acad Child Adolesc Psychiatry 33:291–304, 1994

Allen AJ, Leonard H, Swedo SE: Current knowledge of medications for the treatment of childhood anxiety disorders. J Am Acad Child Adolesc Psychiatry 34:976–986, 1995

American Psychiatric Association: Diagnostic and Statistical Manual of Mental Disorders, 4th Edition. Washington, DC, American Psychiatric Association, 1994

Apter A, Ratzoni G, King RA, et al: Fluvoxamine open-label treatment of adolescent inpatients with obsessive-compulsive disorder or depression. J Am Acad Child Adolesc Psychiatry 33:342–348, 1994

Berney T, Kolvin I, Bhate SR, et al: School phobia: a therapeutic trial with clomipramine and short-term outcome. Br J Psychiatry 138:110–118, 1981

Bernstein GA, Garfinkel BD, Borchardt CM: Comparative studies of pharmacotherapy for school refusal. J Am Acad Child Adolesc Psychiatry 29:773–781, 1990

Biederman J, Baldessarini RJ, Goldblatt A, et al: A naturalistic study of 24-hour electrocardiographic recordings and echocardiographic findings in children and adolescents treated with desipramine. J Am Acad Child Adolesc Psychiatry 32:805–813, 1993

Biederman J, Thisted RA, Greenhill LL, et al: Estimation of the association between desipramine and the risk for sudden death in 5- to 14-year-old children. J Clin Psychiatry 56:87–93, 1995

Birmaher B, Waterman GS, Ryan N, et al: Fluoxetine for childhood anxiety disorders. J Am Acad Child Adolesc Psychiatry 33:993–999, 1994

Black B, Uhde TW: Treatment of elective mutism with fluoxetine: a double-blind, placebo-controlled study. J Am Acad Child Adolesc Psychiatry 33:1000–1006, 1994

Boulos C, Kutcher S, Gardner D, et al: An open naturalistic trial of fluoxetine in adolescents and young adults with treatment-resistant major depression. Journal of Child and Adolescent Psychopharmacology 2:103–111, 1992

Briant RH: An introduction to clinical pharmacology, in Pediatric Psychopharmacology: The Use of Behavior Modifying Drugs in Children. Edited by Werry JS. New York, Brunner/Mazel, 1978, pp 3–28

Bussing R, Levin GM: Methamphetamine and fluoxetine treatment of a child with attention-deficit hyperactivity disorder and obsessive-compulsive disorder. Journal of Child and Adolescent Psychopharmacology 3:53–58, 1993

Campbell M, Cueva JE: Psychopharmacology in child and adolescent psychiatry: a review of the past seven years, II. J Am Acad Child Adolesc Psychiatry 34:126–1272, 1995

Campbell M, Small AM, Green WH, et al: Behavioral efficacy of haloperidol and lithium carbonate. Arch Gen Psychiatry 41:650–656, 1984

Campbell M, Adams PB, Small AM, et al: Lithium in hospitalized aggressive children with conduct disorder: a double-blind and placebo-controlled study. J Am Acad Child Adolesc Psychiatry 34:445–453, 1995

Cueva JE, Overall JE, Small AM, et al: Carbamazepine in aggressive children with conduct disorder: A double-blind and placebo-controlled study. J Am Acad Child Adolesc Psychiatry 35:480–490, 1996

DeVane CL, Sallee FR: Serotonin selective reuptake inhibitors in child and adolescent psychopharmacology: a review of published experience. J Clin Psychiatry 57:55-66, 1996

DeVeaugh-Geiss J, Moroz G, Biederman J, et al: Clomipramine hydrochloride in childhood and adolescent obsessive-compulsive disorder: a multicenter trial. J Am Acad Child Adolesc Psychiatry 31:45-49, 1992

Dulcan MK, Bregman JD, Weller EB, et al: Treatment of childhood and adolescent disorders, in Textbook of Psychopharmacology. Edited by Schatzberg AF, Nemeroff CB. Washington, DC, American Psychiatric Press, 1995, pp 669–706

Emslie G: The AACAP News. J Am Acad Child Adolesc Psychiatry, Jan-Feb, 1996

Famularo R, Kinscherff R, Fenton T: Propranolol treatment for childhood posttraumatic stress disorder, acute type. A pilot study. Am J Dis Child 142:1244-1247, 1988

Flament MF, Rapoport JL, Berg CG, et al: Clomipramine treatment of childhood obsessive-compulsive disorder. A double-blind controlled study. Arch Gen Psychiatry 42:977–983, 1985

Geller DA, Biederman J, Reed ED, et al: Similarities in response to fluoxetine in the treatment of children and adolescents with obsessive-compulsive disorder. J Am Acad Child Adolesc Psychiatry 34:36-44, 1995

Gittelman-Klein R, Klein DF: Controlled imipramine treatment of school phobia. Arch Gen Psychiatry 25:204–207, 1971

Graae F, Gitow A, Piacentini J, et al: Response of obsessive-compulsive disorder and trichotillomania to serotonin reuptake blockers. Am J Psychiatry 149:149–150, 1992

Graae F, Milner J, Rizzotto L, et al: Clonazepam in childhood anxiety disorders. J Am Acad Child Adolesc Psychiatry 33:372–376, 1994

Hazell P, O'Connell D, Heathcote D, et al: Efficacy of tricyclic drugs in treating child and adolescent depression: a meta-analysis. BMJ 310:897–901, 1995

Hellerstein DJ, Yanowitch P, Rossenthal J, et al: A randomized double-blind study of fluoxetine versus placebo in the treatment of dysthymia. Am J Psychiatry 150:1169–1175, 1993

Hughes CW, Preskorn SH: Pharmacokinetics in child/adolescent psychiatric disorders. Psychiatric Annals 24:76–82, 1994

Iancu I, Ratzoni G, Weitzman A, et al: More fluoxetine experience. J Am Acad Child Adolesc Psychiatry 31:755–756, 1992

Jain U, Birmaher B, Garcia M, et al: Fluoxetine in children and adolescents with mood disorders: a chart review of efficacy and adverse effects. Journal of Child and Adolescent Psychopharmacology 2:259–265, 1992

Jatlow PI: Psychotropic drug disposition during development, in Psychiatric Pharmacosciences of Children and Adolescents. Edited by Popper C. Washington, DC, American Psychiatric Press, 1987, pp 27–44

Judd LL, Rapaport MH, Paulus MP, et al: Subsyndromal symptomatic depression: a new mood disorder? J Clin Psychiatry 55(suppl):18–28, 1994

Kafantaris V, Campbell M, Padron-Gayol MV, et al: Carbamazepine in hospitalized aggressive conduct disorder children: an open pilot study. Psychopharmacol Bull 28:193–199, 1992

Kaye WH, Weltzin TE, Hsu LKG, et al: An open trial of fluoxetine in patients with anorexia nervosa. J Clin Psychiatry 52:464–471, 1991

Klein RG, Koplewicz HS, Kanner A: Imipramine treatment of children with separation anxiety disorder. J Am Acad Child Adolesc Psychiatry 31:21–28, 1992

Kovacs M, Akiskal HS, Gatsonis C, et al: Childhood-onset dysthymic disorder: clinical features and prospective naturalistic outcome. Arch Gen Psychiatry 51:365–374, 1994

Kutcher SP, Reiter S, Gardner DM, et al: The pharmacotherapy of anxiety disorders in children and adolescents. Psychiatr Clin North Am 15:41–67, 1992

Leonard HL, Swedo SE, Rapoport JL, et al: Treatment of obsessive-compulsive disorder with clomipramine and desipramine in children and adolescents: a double-blind crossover comparison. Arch Gen Psychiatry 46:1088–1092, 1989

Leonard HL, Swedo SE, Lenane MC, et al: A double-blind desipramine substitution during long-term clomipramine treatment in children and adolescents with obsessive-compulsive disorder. Arch Gen Psychiatry 48:922–927, 1991

Liebowitz MR, Hollander E, Fairbanks J, et al: Fluoxetine for adolescents with obsessive-compulsive disorder. Am J Psychiatry 147:370–371, 1990

Lyles B, Sarkis E, Kemph JP: Fluoxetine and anorexia. J Am Acad Child Adolesc Psychiatry 29:984–985, 1990

McConville BJ, Minnery KL, Sorter MT, et al: An open study of the effects of sertraline on adolescent major depression. Journal of Child and Adolescent Psychopharmacology 6:41–51, 1996

Moreau D, Weissman MM: Panic disorder in children and adolescents: a review. Am J Psychiatry 149:1306–1314, 1992

Popper CW: Child and adolescent psychopharmacology, in Psychiatry. Edited by Cavenar JO, Michaels R, Guze SB, et al. Philadelphia, PA, Lippincott, 1985

Popper CW: Balancing knowledge and judgement: a clinician looks at new developments in child and adolescent psychopharmacology. Child and Adolescent Psychiatric Clinics of North America 4:483–513, 1995

Preskorn SH, Weller E, Hughes CW, et al: Depression in prepubertal children: dexamethasone nonsuppression predicts differential response to imipramine vs. placebo. Psychopharmacol Bull 23:128–133, 1987

Riddle MA, King RA, Hardin MT, et al: Behavioral side effects of fluoxetine in children and adolescents. Journal of Child and Adolescent Psychopharmacology 1:193–198, 1990a

Riddle MA, Hardin MT, King R, et al: Fluoxetine treatment of children and adolescents with Tourette's and obsessive compulsive disorders: preliminary clinical experience. J Am Acad Child Adolesc Psychiatry 29:45–48, 1990b

Riddle MA, Scahill L, King RA, et al: Double-blind, crossover trial of fluoxetine and placebo in children and adolescents with obsessive-compulsive disorder. J Am Acad Child Adolesc Psychiatry 31:1062–1069, 1992

Riddle MA, Geller B, Ryan N: Case study: another sudden death in a child treated with desipramine. J Am Acad Child Adolesc Psychiatry 32:792–797, 1993

Simeon J, Dinicola D, Phil M, et al: Adolescent depression: a placebo-controlled fluoxetine treatment study and follow-up. Prog Neuropsychopharmacol Biol Psychiatry 14:791–795, 1990a

Simeon JG, Thatte S, Wiggins D: Treatment of adolescent obsessive-compulsive disorder with a clomipramine-fluoxetine combination. Psychopharmacol Bull 26:285–290, 1990b

Simeon JG, Ferguson HB, Knott V, et al: Clinical, cognitive, and neurophysiological effects of alprazolam in children and adolescents with overanxious and avoidant disorders. J Am Acad Child Adolesc Psychiatry 31:29–33, 1992

Tierney E, Joshi PT, Llinas JF, et al: Sertraline for major depression in children and adolescents: preliminary clinical experience. Journal of Child and Adolescent Psychopharmacology 5:13–27, 1995

Trygstad O: Drugs in the treatment of bulimia nervosa. Acta Psychiatr Scand 82 (suppl):34–37, 1990

Wilcox JA: Fluoxetine and bulimia. J Psychoactive Drugs 22:81–82, 1990

Chapter 20

Overview of Geriatric Psychopharmacology

Andrew Satlin, M.D., and Charles Wasserman, M.D.

Aging is a complex process that has physiological, psychological, and social components. These changes may render the older person more vulnerable to developing psychiatric illnesses or to having recurrences of previous disorders. Late life also is the period of greatest risk for physical disease: more than 80% of elderly patients have at least one chronic illness. These medical problems may further increase the risk of developing psychiatric illnesses and may mask or alter their presentation. Together, the changes that are age-related and those that are disease-related stress the reserves of organ function and therefore affect the metabolism, effectiveness, and side effects of the medications used to treat psychiatric conditions. An understanding of these processes that characterize growing older permits the geriatric psychiatrist to make diagnoses even when patients' presenting symptomatology does not fit typical DSM categories. Such an understanding also steers the geriatric psychiatrist's attention to medication side effects or interactions that may be the cause of the psychiatric symptoms.

At the same time, it is important to recognize that geriatric patients are not a well-defined group distinct from the population at large. Too often, psychiatric services in the hospital or outpatient clinics are divided into pediatric, adult, and geriatric programs, as if late life were no longer part of adulthood. First, of course, older people may have any of the psychiatric diseases that younger people do. Second, from a psychological perspective, aging presents developmental tasks that are equally, but not necessarily more, challenging compared to the tasks faced in younger life. From a physiological and disease perspective, elderly patients are a diverse group. Not only is the average 65-year-old vastly different from the average 85-year-old in terms of organ reserve and susceptibility to disease, but the interindividual differences among elderly persons of the same age are much greater than those among young adults of the same age. The concept of *frailty*, a useful one in geriatrics, refers to the combination of compromised reserve and function that characterizes some, but not all, elderly persons. Although frailty is associated with age, it is not age specific. An understanding of these principles enables the geriatric psychiatrist to approach patients with compassion and dignity, enhances the therapeutic alliance, prevents therapeutic nihilism, and is essential to the good practice of geriatric psychopharmacology.

The effects of age- and disease-related changes on diagnosis will be discussed in the sections on the various psychiatric syndromes. However, one important medical condition may cause many different psychiatric presentations in elderly patients and is mentioned briefly here as a paradigm of geriatric psychiatry. Delirium is often the common end point arising from a variety of losses in organ reserve coupled with the stress of medical illness or medication side effects. It may be the cause of psychosis, depression, anxiety, cognitive impairment, and sleep disturbances. Risk factors for delirium in hospitalized elderly medical patients include severity of illness, dementia, dehydration, sensory losses, metabolic and electrolyte disturbances, infections, and the use of psychotropic medications (Inouye et al. 1993).

Diagnosing delirium is the first step in determining its cause, which can then point to a simple and effective treatment for the underlying illness and its secondary psychiatric manifestations. Identification of delirium is not difficult in a patient with a fluctuating level of consciousness and other typical clinical symptoms such as autonomic dysfunction, but in elderly persons, delirium may often be more chronic, especially when it is due to the habitual use of medications with properties that are sedating or that depress the central nervous system (CNS). Sedative hypnotic medications, in particular the long-acting benzodiazepines, are commonly associated with chronic cognitive impairment (Larson et al. 1987), and anticholinergic medications may have adverse effects that are persistent and unrecognized by patients and physicians (Katz et al. 1988). Attempts to minimize inappropriate medication use and polypharmacy in elderly patients, especially in nursing homes, have included targeted physician feedback (Kroenke and Pinholt 1990), general educational programs about geriatric psychopharmacology (Avorn et al. 1992), and regulation by the federal government mandated by the Omnibus Budget Reconciliation Act (OBRA) legislation of 1987 (Shorr et al. 1994). The role of the geriatric psychiatrist in these endeavors, whether as consultant to the care of individual patients or as teacher of other physicians, is crucial.

The psychopharmacological agents used to treat elderly patients are, of course, the same as those used to treat younger patients. However, age-related changes in physiology affect the metabolism of these drugs and the brain's response to them. These changes are subsumed under the headings of *pharmacokinetic changes* and *pharmacodynamic changes*.

Pharmacokinetics usually refers to the bioavailability, distribution, metabolism, and excretion of drugs. In elderly persons, it is useful to think about pharmacokinetics more broadly: as all the steps that occur from the time that a physician writes a prescription until the drug is eliminated from the body. For some elderly patients, some prescriptions will not make it to the pharmacy—for reasons that may range from an inadequately explained rationale for the use of the medication to an inability to pay for it. Sensory deficits or cognitive impairment may make it difficult for the patient to take the medication on the prescribed schedule. Thus, many factors may interfere with adequate dosing, even before patients put the pills in their mouths.

Once the medication is swallowed, drug disposition may be affected by the degree of absorption, plasma protein binding, volume of distribution, hepatic metabolism, and renal clearance. The available evidence suggests that aging does not significantly affect the absorption of psychotropic drugs. Decreases in the amount of plasma proteins do not have a clinically meaningful effect on drug response or toxicity for most psychotropics. However, for drugs that are highly protein bound, such as valproic acid and the selective serotonin reuptake inhibitors (SSRIs), aging may be associated with increases in the relative concentration of free drug for any given dose. Changes in volume of distribution and hepatic metabolism are more important. Most psychotropic drugs are highly lipid soluble and are therefore widely distributed in fatty tissues. With aging, the proportion of the body composed of lean muscle mass decreases, whereas fatty tissue increases. As a result, the amount of drug distributed in the body for any given weight tends to increase with age. Because of this change, it takes longer for a drug to reach steady state and longer for a given percentage of the total body store of drug to be metabolized. In other words, half-life increases independently of the rate of clearance of the drug.

Decreases in hepatic biotransformation of the drug mean that clearance, too, is decreased, an occurrence that further increases half-life (Von Moltke et al. 1993). These changes have the general effect of increasing the blood level of medication for any given dose ingested, and for this reason psychopharmacological treatment of elderly patients has long been guided by the principle "Start low, go slow." However, this principle does not apply equally to all psychotropic drugs. Hepatic metabolism can be divided into two major processes: 1) microsomal enzyme oxidation and 2) glucuronide conjugation to render drugs or metabolites water soluble for renal excretion. The first process declines with age due to changes in microsomal structure and activity (Schmucker 1984), but the second does not appear to be affected by age. Thus, drugs that require hepatic oxidation for their metabolism accumulate more in elderly persons and have the potential for greater toxicity, whereas drugs that are conjugated and excreted without prior oxidation do not carry this risk. This distinction is the major reason why some benzodiazepines (e.g., lorazepam) are preferred to others (e.g., diazepam) for elderly patients.

Decreased renal clearance is clinically relevant for two types of drugs. The first includes the drugs that are water soluble and are excreted unchanged by the kidney. The only psychopharmacological agent that meets this description is lithium, which therefore must be given in lower doses to elderly patients in order to avoid toxic plasma levels and adverse cardiac and neurological effects. The other type of drug affected by renal clearance includes drugs such as the tricyclic antidepressants (TCAs), which are oxidized by the liver to water-soluble hydroxy metabolites that may retain cardiotoxic properties (Salzman et al. 1995a). Impaired renal excretion of these metabolites may lead to cardiac conduction delays, such as atrioventricular block and bundle branch block, as reflected by prolonged PR, QRS, and QT intervals on the electrocardiogram.

Pharmacodynamic changes refers to effects at the level of the interaction between drug and receptor. These changes may be relevant both in the brain and in the periphery. So far, the evidence is mixed regarding whether pharmacodynamic changes with aging have clinically significant effects on the therapeutic efficacy of psychotropic medications. That is, it is unclear whether the aging brain is more or less sensitive to the primary therapeutic actions of psychotropic drugs, and thus whether older patients respond differently to a given blood or brain level of medication. However, there is substantial evidence that pharmacodynamic effects are responsible for some of the increased side effects and toxicity seen with psychotropic medications in elderly patients. For example, diminished dopaminergic function in the brain predisposes elderly patients to more extrapyramidal side effects from neuroleptic medications. Decreased brain acetylcholine renders elderly patients more sensitive to the central effects of medications with anticholinergic properties. Older patients are therefore more prone to developing confusion, disorientation, and even delirium from TCAs and neuroleptics, especially those that are strongly anticholinergic, such as amitriptyline and thioridazine. Diminished peripheral cholinergic function with age, possibly accounting for much of the constipation and urinary hesitancy common in unmedicated older persons, is also a concern. Whereas a young adult given amitriptyline may develop constipation or delayed urination, the older adult given the same medication may become impacted or develop urinary retention.

Another factor that may affect the use of psychotropic medications in elderly patients is the presence of underlying disease states. Pathological conditions may affect the metabolism or efficacy of medications in ways that are unpredictable in the absence of research data. In particular, the effects of preexisting cardiac disease on the toxicity of most psychotropic agents are unknown. Unfortunately, drugs are often tested only in healthy adults before being approved and marketed, and frequently the numbers of elderly persons included in clinical trials are small. Thus, what are the appropriate psychotropic medications for very old, frail, or medically compromised patients remains an open question for most psychiatric disorders. In the remainder of this chapter, we review the most recent literature on the use of psychopharmacological agents in elderly patients.

Depression and Its Treatment

Depression affects nearly one million elderly Americans, coexists in at least one-third of medically ill persons, and has deleterious effects on morbidity, mortality, and functional ability. Elderly patients have the highest suicide rate of any age group, and the rate has been increasing since 1980. The estimated costs of this serious disorder are staggering, and the effect on family and caregivers is considerable. Although conceptualized as a chronic recurrent illness, risk factors are identifiable (and hence potentially modifiable), and treatment can be very successful—even when depression is comorbid with medical illnesses. Nonetheless, depression is often unrecognized, underdiagnosed, and undertreated in elderly patients.

The Epidemiologic Catchment Area (ECA) study (Weissman et al. 1991) found that the incidence of depression is actually lower in persons 65 years and older than in younger cohorts, for both 1-year (bipolar and major depression) and lifetime (bipolar, major depression, and dysthymia) estimates. However, many elderly persons with clinically significant depressive symptoms may not be diagnosed with major depression in community surveys because of the underreporting of symptoms and a tendency to attribute neurovegetative affective symptoms to medical illness. Indeed, if depressive syndromes not meeting criteria for major depression are included, the rate of clinically significant depression among elderly persons in the community is 8%–15% (Blazer 1994). In treatment settings, the rates of major depression are higher: 11% in hospitals, 5% in nonpsychiatric outpatient clinics, and 12% in long-term-care facilities. For less severe but clinically significant depression, the rates are 25% in hospitals, 10% in outpatient clinics, and 30% in long-term-care facilities. Among hospitalized patients with medical illness, depression is most prevalent in end-stage renal disease, rheumatoid arthritis, diabetes mellitus, myocardial infarction, stroke, and spinal cord injuries (Katon and Sullivan 1990). Rates of depression in late-life neurodegenerative disorders, including Parkinson's disease, Alzheimer's disease, and cortical stroke, range from 25% to 50%. As noted, suicide rates have consistently been highest among elderly persons. From 1940 to 1980 these rates declined in those 65 years and older, but from 1980 to 1992 the rates increased 36%. Elderly persons compose 12% of the population, yet they accounted for 20% of all suicides in the United States between 1980 and 1992. Men accounted for 81% of suicides among those 65 years and older. Firearms were the most common method of suicide for both men (74%) and women (31%) in this age group. A 1990 Cook County, Illinois, suicide study of 8,200 men, funded by the American Association of Retired Persons (Clark 1991), estimated that 65% had depression and 20% had alcohol problems. Although 20% had seen their primary-care physician within 24 hours and 70% within the month before suicide, only 5% had had psychiatric treatment in the prior 90 days. These figures suggest that careful screening may reduce suicide attempts and suicides (Rutz et al. 1989).

Risk factors for late-life depression include female sex, unmarried status, stressful life events, lack of a supportive social network, and concurrent medical illness (George 1994; Zisook et al. 1994). A family history of mood disorder appears to be a weaker risk factor for depression in elderly persons than it is for depression in early life. Risk factors for suicide among elders include male sex, low income, social isolation, concurrent physical illness, prior suicide attempts, alcohol abuse, and delusional affective disorder. Some of these risk factors are potentially modifiable. For example, day programs as part of support-network building, establishing regular visiting-nurse or other medical visits, and identifying and treating alcohol abuse and psychosis may reduce risk. Given that elderly persons are often reluctant to admit to depression or suicidal thoughts or to seek psychiatric care, it is important to have a high index of suspicion.

Prognosis and outcome studies have been flawed by methodological inconsistencies and a dearth of information from randomized clinical trials or controlled clinical observation in elderly patients. Given this proviso, several 1-year outcome studies found that, on the average, 50% were well, 15% had relapsed, 20% remained continuously ill, and 12% had died (Baldwin and Jolley 1986; Burvill et al. 1986; Meats et al. 1991). Factors associated with poor outcome included active physical illness, more severe depression at onset, psychosis, adverse life events, and lack of community supports. A 5-year controlled study of the efficacy of five maintenance treatment approaches in 128 midlife patients who had recovered from at least their third major depressive episode found the following cumulative probabilities of remaining well (Frank et al. 1990):

- 80% for patients receiving imipramine and interpersonal psychotherapy together and for patients receiving imipramine and medication clinic
- 40% for patients receiving interpersonal psychotherapy alone and for patients receiving interpersonal psychotherapy with placebo
- Approximately 20% for the group randomized to placebo and medication clinic

Salzman (1994) noted that the literature is an imperfect guide to the psychopharmacological treatment of depression in elderly patients, for several reasons. First, most "elderly" patients included in published clinical trials of antidepressants are between 55 and 65 years of age. Second, subjects in such studies tend to compose an atypical subset of older patients who are free from physical illness and from the medications to treat those physical illnesses. Third, most studies include only patients with moderate depression (Hamilton Rating Scale for Depression scores of 18–22, with none greater than 30; Salzman's review found only one study of delusional depressed elderly persons). Fourth, *therapeutic response* is usually defined as the percentage of decline from baseline rating-scale scores. This definition limits the clinical relevance of the findings, because many patients considered "improved" continue to have significant residual symptoms that adversely affect quality of life.

Moreover, little research has been done on the effectiveness of treatments for late-life depression. *Efficacy* is the probability of benefit from a treatment when given to a defined population under ideal conditions, whereas *effectiveness* is the performance of a treatment when given to typical patients under ordinary conditions by the average practitioner. There is also a dearth of information on the comparative efficacy of psychotherapy and medication administered separately or in combination for both acute and maintenance treatment of late-life depression. However, a randomized, double-blind, placebo-controlled comparison of four treatments (nortriptyline and medication clinic, nortriptyline with interpersonal psychotherapy, placebo and medication clinic, and placebo with interpersonal psychotherapy) in 200 patients over the age of 60 is currently in progress (Reynolds et al. 1995).

Nonetheless, some treatment guidelines can be gleaned from the literature and clinical experience. Before choosing a pharmacological intervention in the treatment of late-life depression, several factors must be considered. In cases in which substance abuse, current nonpsychotropic medications, or a general medical condition may be causing the depression, correction of these problems should be attempted first. If the depressive symptoms persist, aggressive treatment of the mood disorder should be attempted. Further, if a grief reaction persists beyond 2 months after the loss, especially if accompanied by psychotic symptoms or gross functional impairment, antidepressant treatment should be initiated. Delusional major depression often requires treatment with the combination of an antidepressant and an antipsychotic or electroconvulsive therapy (ECT), given the poor response of this disorder to monotherapy with antidepressants or antipsychotics and its malignant course.

No one antidepressant is more effective than another in treating depression, and none seems to work more rapidly than others. In addition, no studies have established preferred drug treatments for specific subtypes of depression or for specific subpopulations. Nonetheless, there are differences in the side-effect profiles of antidepressants that may guide antidepressant choice for elderly patients. An ideal antidepressant would have a rapid onset of activity, an intermediate half-life, defined therapeutic blood levels, minimal drug interactions, low toxicity associated with overdose, and no side effects. Unfortunately, no such drug exists.

The TCAs can cause orthostatic hypotension and reflex tachycardia (due to α_1 adrenergic blockade), sedation (due to histamine$_1$ [H$_1$] receptor blockade) and various anticholinergic reactions, including dry mouth, constipation, urinary retention, blurred vision, delirium, confusion, disorientation, agitation, visual hallucinations, restlessness, and memory dysfunction (due to muscarinic receptor blockade). TCA cardiotoxic effects include delayed conduction (class IA antiarrhythmic-like effect) mediated by sodium channel blockade, which contributes to the narrow therapeutic index of these drugs (Glassman and Preud'homme 1993). In addition, recent evidence from the Cardiac Arrhythmia Suppression Trial (CAST) indicates that patients with cardiac ischemia given class 1A antiarrhythmics are at increased risk for ventricular irritability and sudden death. Although this outcome has not been demonstrated with the TCAs, such findings suggest caution with the use of these agents in any elderly person with heart disease.

Many TCA side effects are more severe with the tertiary amine drugs, which should generally be avoided in the treatment of elderly patients. The secondary amines nortriptyline and desipramine are reasonable first-line TCA alternatives, starting at 10 mg/day, with increases of 10 mg every 2–4 days while monitoring blood pressure and electrocardiograms. These drugs should be titrated to plasma levels of 50–150 ng/mL and 125 ng/mL, respectively, while monitoring clinical response (Alexopoulos 1992). Other secondary-amine TCAs may be more problematic for elderly patients: protriptyline has a very long elimination half-life; maprotiline may have increased risk for grand mal seizures; and amoxapine may cause extrapyramidal side effects similar to those of the neuroleptics, presumably as a result of its blockade of dopamine$_2$ (D$_2$) receptors.

Because of their superior side-effect and safety profiles, the SSRIs have generally become the primary treatment for depression in patients of all ages. Clinical trials have documented that SSRIs are superior to placebo and comparable to TCAs in elderly patients (Dunner et al. 1992). The SSRIs have very weak H$_1$, α_1, D$_2$, and muscarinic receptor blockade effects, which accounts for their relatively low incidence of the side effects commonly seen with the TCAs (Cusack et al. 1994). Paroxetine is an exception in that its muscarinic receptor blockade is similar to that of imipramine, which may account for reports of dry mouth and constipation with its use (Boyer and Blumhardt 1992). Compared with TCAs, however, the SSRIs are more likely to cause serotonergic effects—such as gastrointestinal disturbance, anorexia, sexual dysfunction, and dose-dependent increases in anxiety. A life-threatening serotonin syndrome may occur when the SSRIs are given in combination with monoamine oxidase inhibitors (MAOIs) and possibly L-tryptophan and fenfluramine. Protein binding is 95% or greater with fluoxetine, sertraline, and paroxetine, which can result in displacement interactions (e.g., sertraline's elevating warfarin blood levels and increasing prothrombin time). Fluvoxamine has low protein-binding affinity. Other significant drug-drug interactions with SSRIs involve their differential inhibition of various cytochrome P450 isoenzymes (e.g., IID6 and IIIA4), resulting in significantly elevated blood levels of various drugs; an excellent recent review is available (Nemeroff et al. 1996). These interactions may be particularly prolonged for fluoxetine, which has the longest elimination half-life of all antidepressants—2–3 days for the parent compound and 7–15 days for its active metabolite norfluoxetine. This half-life may be further increased in elderly patients. Reasonable SSRI starting doses in elderly patients are 12.5–25 mg of sertraline; 10 mg of paroxetine; 2.5–10 mg of fluoxetine; and 25 mg of fluvoxamine.

Newer "atypical" antidepressants include trazodone, bupropion, venlafaxine, and nefazodone. Trazodone is highly sedating and has little anticholinergic activity; it can cause significant orthostatic hypotension. Trazodone is often useful for treatment of antidepressant-induced insomnia. Bupropion is a nonserotonergic, nonanticholinergic drug that at high doses may block norepinephrine and dopamine reuptake and lower the seizure threshold. Bupropion has the advantage of having been studied in elderly patients with preexisting cardiac disease, where it was found to be effective and to have minimal effects on blood pressure and no significant effects on cardiac rate, rhythm, or left ventricular function. A reasonable starting dosage for bupropion is 50 mg/day, titrating to 50 mg tid in 50-mg weekly increments.

Venlafaxine is the prototype of a new class of drugs that significantly inhibits reuptake of both norepinephrine and serotonin, with few α-adrenergic, histaminic, or muscarinic effects. Rates of seizures, cardiac conduction effects, and orthostatic hypotension are comparable to those seen with SSRIs. Hypertension appears to be a dose-related effect, which may be of greater concern in elderly patients with elevated blood pressures at baseline. Common side effects are nausea, dizziness, nervousness, and insomnia. Starting doses of 12.5–25 mg/day can be titrated to 150 mg/day in bid or tid divided doses. Nefazodone is structurally similar to trazodone, but it is also an antagonist at serotonin$_2$ (5-HT$_2$) receptors, which may account for its antianxiety effect. It inhibits the reuptake of both serotonin and norepinephrine, but more weakly than venlafaxine. Its ability to treat insomnia may make it a useful drug for the agitated, restless, and sleepless older depressive patient. Nefazodone significantly inhibits the cytochrome P450-IIIA4 isoenzyme. It is contraindicated for concomitant use with terfenadine, astemizole, and loratadine, and it should be used cautiously with triazolam and alprazolam (Nemeroff et al. 1996). As more is learned about the cardiac effects of these newer agents and about their relative efficacy compared to the SSRIs and the TCAs, they may become first-line agents for treatment of depression in elderly patients. Psychostimulants (e.g., methylphenidate, dextroamphetamine) may improve mild dysphoric, apathetic, and anergic states, especially in elderly patients with medical illnesses masking depression, and may thereby help to speed medical recovery. Despite their potential for causing tachycardia, hypertension, arrhythmia, and psychosis, elderly patients do not appear to be at greater risk for these complications than younger patients. A reasonable starting dose of methylphenidate is 2.5 mg in the morning, with titration to a maximum of 10 mg bid (in the morning and at noontime). Dextroamphetamine should be started at 2.5–5 mg once a day and increased gradually to 15 mg daily.

The MAOIs are now little used, but they remain a therapeutic choice for patients who are unresponsive to the SSRIs, the TCAs, and newer agents. Their major disadvantage in elderly patients is severe orthostatic hypotension. Hypertensive crises can be precipitated by tyramine-rich foods (e.g., aged cheese), catecholamine precursors (L-dopa, Sinemet) and drugs with indirect sympathomimetic action (phenylephrine in over-the-counter [OTC] cold preparations), as well as direct-acting sympathomimetics (epinephrine found in dental anesthetics). Other potentially fatal drug interactions include those with SSRIs and meperidine. MAOIs themselves have weak anticholinergic effects and may therefore be an alternative for elderly patients who cannot tolerate TCAs. Phenelzine can be started at 7.5 mg/day; tranylcypromine can be started at 5 mg/day. There should be at least a 14-day washout period before switching from an MAOI to a TCA or an SSRI.

Reversible and selective MAOIs of the isoenzyme A (e.g., reversible inhibitors of MAO-A [RIMAs] such as moclobemide, brofaramine, toloxatone, and cimoxatone) may prove to be well-tolerated and effective alternatives in elderly patients (Nair et al. 1995). MAO-A is partly responsible for the metabolism of the mood-regulating neurotransmitters norepinephrine and serotonin, and MAO-B metabolizes dopamine and phenylethylamine in the brain.

ECT should be considered for the following:

- For treatment of delusional depression or life-threatening depression marked by catatonia, refusal to eat or drink, or suicidality
- When antidepressants present greater risks than ECT or are ineffective
- When a rapid clinical response is needed

Efficacy in elderly patients has been established in several studies (Sackeim 1994). Although data are limited for patients older than 80 years, ECT is considered safe: associated mortality is estimated to be 1/10,000 patients, which is comparable to rates associated with anesthesia from minor surgery. Cardiovascular complications (bradycardia, tachycardia, hypertension, arrhythmia) are the most common causes of morbidity and mortality, and cerebrovascular complications are rare. Cognitive side effects include transient postictal disorientation and confusion and some degree of anterograde and retrograde amnesia, but some patients may develop prolonged delirium for several weeks. Retrograde amnesia shows gradual recovery. Although data are limited, patients with poststroke depression, depression with dementia, and depression with parkinsonism have been successfully treated with ECT (Sackeim 1994).

Mania and Its Treatment

Like depression, mania in elderly persons is a syndrome that has a number of causes. In addition to the bipolar disorders, DSM-IV (American Psychiatric Association 1994) lists "mood disorder due to a general medical condition" and "substance-induced mood disorder," which include what has been described in the literature as "secondary mania" (Krauthammer and Klerman 1978). Medical conditions that can cause mania include

- Metabolic disturbances such as vitamin B_{12} deficiency and hemodialysis
- Infections
- Cerebral disorders such as epilepsy, neoplasm, trauma, surgical lesions, cerebrovascular disease, dementia
- CNS infections such as neurosyphilis and human immunodeficiency virus (HIV)

Substances that may induce mania include

- Drug therapies such as anticholinergics, corticosteroids, L-dopa, sympathomimetics, and psychostimulants
- Alcohol
- Some illicit drugs

Recent evidence suggests that mania in elderly persons may be manifested largely in three groups of patients (Shulman et al. 1992):

- A small group who have had recurrent bipolar disorder from early life

- A group characterized by late onset of affective illness, with several episodes of depression preceding the first onset of mania, with a latency of about 10–15 years
- A group who have secondary mania associated with neurological disorders and whose mania is often their first episode of affective illness or very closely follows their first episode of depression

Positive family histories of affective illness are probably higher in those with mania than in those with depression, but lower in those with probable secondary mania than in those with primary affective illness. Further, in elderly persons, mortality is higher in those with mania than in those with depression, probably reflecting the greater preponderance of patients with underlying neurological and other medical conditions in this group. Consistent with this significant comorbidity, some studies have suggested that late-life mania tends to be more treatment resistant.

Elderly patients with mania may be treated with the same agents used to treat mania in younger patients. These include medications with both acute antimanic and long-term mood-stabilizing effects, such as lithium and the antiepileptics, and agents with predominantly acute antimanic/antipsychotic effects, such as the neuroleptics and ECT. The best treatment for any individual patient is based on that patient's clinical presentation, previous response to treatment, medical conditions, and concomitant medications. Unfortunately, there are no prospective controlled trials of lithium or of any of the anticonvulsants for either the acute or the prophylactic treatment of bipolar disorder in patients older than 65 years. Lithium and valproic acid (an antiepileptic) are both approved for use in the United States, and either may be appropriate first-line therapy. In general, longer clinical experience favors the use of lithium by most clinicians, but others prefer the use of the antiepileptics, especially when patients have

- Psychiatric histories consistent with secondary mania, rapid cycling, or mixed affective states
- A history of nonresponse or intolerable side effects to lithium
- Medical conditions that increase the risk of lithium-induced toxicity

Neuroleptics and ECT are most often used acutely and adjunctively, but they may be the sole treatment in patients unresponsive to or intolerant of any of the mood stabilizers.

Lithium has been the primary medication for the acute and prophylactic treatment of mania in elderly patients. Available evidence suggests that elderly patients both require and tolerate lower lithium levels; recommended target serum concentrations range from 0.4 to 0.7 mmol/L (Foster 1992). Higher serum levels in elderly patients compared to younger patients on the same dose are due to a reduced volume of distribution of lithium, due in turn to the relative loss of the skeletal-muscle water component, combined with reduced renal clearance of lithium. The combination of these pharmacodynamic and pharmacokinetic effects means that starting lithium doses should be low (e.g., 75–300 mg/day) and that dose increments should be smaller (e.g., 75–150 mg) and given at longer time intervals (e.g., 5–7 days) because of the increased time required to reach steady state.

Medical side effects of lithium in elderly patients are similar to those seen in younger patients, but many are more common. These include cardiac, renal, thyroid, and neurological effects. Lithium may impair sinoatrial node function and cardiac conduction, leading to bradycardia and dysrhythmias. Renal effects include reduced concentrating ability at therapeutic doses, leading to a picture of nephrogenic diabetes insipidus, and possible decreased glomerular filtration rate at toxic doses. Some reports have suggested that long-term use may be associated with tubular atrophy, glomerular sclerosis and interstitial fibrosis. Hypothyroidism may occur in 15% of patients on long-term lithium, but lithium may also be associated with a higher than expected rate of thyrotoxicosis. Hypercalcemia due to elevations in parathyroid hormone have also been reported. Neurological side effects include the following (Foster 1992):

- Cognitive impairment
- Movement disorders such as extrapyramidal syndromes, tardive dyskinesia, and oculomotor abnormalities
- Cerebellar dysfunction, manifested as ataxia, dysarthria, incoordination, intention tremor and nystagmus

In fact, neurotoxicity is often the first and most prominent sign of lithium toxicity in elderly patients, even at low therapeutic levels. Patients with underlying neurological illness or symptoms are at increased risk for neurotoxicity from lithium (Bell et al. 1993; Himmelhoch et al. 1980).

Many commonly used drugs in elderly patients can have clinically important interactions with lithium. Thiazide diuretics cause increased reabsorption of lithium in the kidney and increased lithium levels. Nonsteroidal anti-inflammatory drugs (NSAIDs), with the exception of aspirin, are also associated with higher lithium levels. Some reports suggest that elderly patients may be at increased risk for neurotoxicity, especially parkinsonism, when given lithium in combination with a neuroleptic (Ghadirian et al. 1996). Other drugs used adjunctively for the control of mania, such as carbamazepine and verapamil, have been reported to increase the risk of bradycardia (Steckler 1994) or other signs of lithium toxicity. Even low-salt diets may increase lithium levels, whereas substances that inhibit the effect of antidiuretic hormone, such as caffeine, may lower levels.

Given these potential side effects, toxicity, and interactions, the pre-treatment workup for lithium use in an elderly patient should include baseline measures of

- Cognitive function (e.g., a Mini-Mental State Examination)
- Renal function (creatinine, or creatinine clearance if the creatinine level is elevated at baseline)
- Cardiac function (ECG)
- Thyroid function (thyroxine [T4] and thyrotropin [TSH])
- Serum calcium

  as well as

- A medical and neurological examination looking for underlying conditions or medication use that may predispose to the development of lithium toxicity

Among alternatives to lithium for the treatment of mania, the antiepileptic drugs valproate and carbamazepine have received the most attention. Carbamazepine has been reported useful in one case report (Kellner and Neher 1991). The literature on valproic acid is larger (McFarland et al. 1990; Risinger et al. 1994). Two reports suggest that valproic acid may be especially useful for the treatment of mania associated with head trauma and EEG abnormalities (Pope et al. 1988; Yassa and Cvejic 1994). Both carbamazepine and valproic acid can cause hepatotoxicity, and carbamazepine is associated with blood dyscrasias, requiring regular blood monitoring with these agents, as is the case with lithium.

Anxiety and Its Treatment

In reviewing the literature on the rates of anxiety in elderly patients, the conclusions that can be drawn are similar to those described for depression. That is, large epidemiological surveys, relying on DSM criteria for diagnosis, have arrived at prevalence estimates for anxiety disorders as a group (including generalized anxiety disorder, panic disorder, phobia, obsessive-compulsive disorder, and posttraumatic stress disorder) that are lower among those older than 65 years than they are in younger persons. For example, the ECA study found 1-month prevalence rates of any anxiety disorder to be 3.6% for elderly men and 6.8% for elderly women, compared to rates of 4.7% and 9.7% for the population as a whole (Regier et al. 1990). However, surveys using scales to identify clinically significant anxiety symptoms that do not meet DSM criteria for a specific disorder have found rates of anxiety in elderly patients of 10%–20% (Himmelfarb and Murrell 1984). There also is considerable overlap between anxiety and other psychiatric disorders, particularly depression; research in elderly patients suggests that most often the anxiety is secondary to the depression (Parmelee et al. 1993). Anxiety is also a common symptom in dementia, delirium, and mania. However, alcohol abuse and dependence are not as clearly related to anxiety disorders in elderly patients as they are in younger patients (Flint 1994). Acute bereavement may be associated with anxiety, although it is not clear whether this association is independent of the effect of depression (Jacobs et al. 1990).

Anxiety frequently accompanies the chronic medical conditions that are common in elderly patients. Diseases that have the strongest association with anxiety include the following (Hocking and Koenig 1995):

- Cardiovascular illness such as angina, myocardial infarction, arrhythmias, congestive heart failure, and mitral valve prolapse
- Respiratory disorders such as chronic obstructive pulmonary disease, asthma, and pneumonia
- Endocrine disorders such as hypoglycemia, hyperthyroidism or hypothyroidism, and Cushing's disease
- Anemia or other causes of relative hypoxia

Other frequent causes of anxiety include effects of medication such as

- Stimulants (e.g., sympathomimetic decongestants, amphetamines, methylphenidate, and caffeine)
- β-Adrenergic drugs
- Thyroid replacement drugs
- Corticosteroids
- Theophylline
- Digitalis
- SSRIs
- Neuroleptic-induced akathisia
- Drug withdrawal (from sedative-hypnotics, alcohol, nicotine, caffeine, anticholinergics, and β-blockers)

Many of these medications are used chronically by elderly persons, sometimes without supervision by physicians. As a result, the anxiety caused by these medications may go unrecognized or may be attributed to other stresses or to psychiatric illness. As with depression in elderly patients, adjustment of possible offending medications or treatment of the underlying medical condition is the first line of treatment for these anxiety syndromes.

Antidepressants are the treatment of choice for anxiety associated with depression (as in agitated or anxious major depression or mixed anxiety-depression), although antianxiety agents may be useful adjuncts in the initial phases of treatment before the antidepressant achieves its therapeutic effect. Panic disorder, posttraumatic stress disorder, and obsessive-compulsive disorder should also generally be treated with antidepressants, and case reports now suggest that the SSRIs may be useful for these conditions in elderly patients (Calamari et al. 1994). For generalized anxiety disorder, or for the more prevalent anxiety syndromes associated with chronic medical conditions, the therapeutic choice is typically made between a benzodiazepine and buspirone. The benzodiazepines are highly fat soluble and thus are especially affected by the increased volume of distribution of these agents in elderly patients. Benzodiazepines that undergo oxidative hepatic metabolism have long half-lives and active metabolites, accumulate more with chronic administration, and may be associated with greater toxicity. Benzodiazepines that do not require liver biotransformation have shorter half-lives and no active metabolites. These agents, such as lorazepam and oxazepam, are therefore preferred for use in elderly persons.

Although there is some evidence that short-half-life benzodiazepines do not confer the increased risk of falls and hip fractures seen with the long-acting benzodiazepines (Ray et al. 1989), there is other evidence for a strong dose-response relationship that is independent of the type of benzodiazepine prescribed (Herings et al. 1995). These adverse events may be the result of sedation, confusion, cerebellar ataxia, or some combination of these side effects. Benzodiazepines are also associated with cognitive impairment in elderly patients (Foy et al. 1995). Hospitalized elderly patients who receive benzodiazepines are at increased risk for delirium, and patients who use them chronically may develop a dementia syndrome characterized by short-term-memory loss and impaired judgment. Benzodiazepines also depress respiration, particularly during sleep. Thus, sleep-related breathing disorders such as sleep apnea may be worsened by these medications, and elderly patients with preexisting chronic obstructive pulmonary disease may be at increased risk. Since respiratory disorders are themselves often associated with anxiety, alternative treatments, such as cognitive-behavioral therapy and improvement in respiratory function, should be attempted before turning to pharmacological management.

Buspirone is an effective anxiolytic that in open trials has had similar efficacy in older and younger patients. Studies of this drug in elderly patients with anxiety find long-term reductions in the Hamilton Anxiety Scale of more than 60%, with minimal side effects such as nausea, diarrhea, and headache (Bohm et al. 1990; Levine et al. 1988; Napoliello 1986; Singh and Beer 1988). These studies indicate that older patients require about the same doses for therapeutic efficacy as do younger patients (15–30 mg/day), consistent with the lack of effect of age on elimination half-life. Buspirone does not induce or inhibit hepatic oxidative enzymes, does not have sedative effects or effects on cognition, balance or coordination, is not addictive or associated with withdrawal effects, and does not depress respiration. In fact, one study found that respiratory function improved in four of five male patients with sleep apnea who were given 20 mg of buspirone (Mendelson et al. 1991). However, although buspirone was found to reduce anxiety symptoms in patients with chronic lung disease in one open trial (Kiev and Domantay 1988), another study found no significant effects of buspirone on anxiety scores or exercise tolerance in patients with chronic airflow obstruction (Singh et al. 1993). One drawback to the use of buspirone, compared to the benzodiazepines, is a latency of 3–4 weeks before the therapeutic effect is seen. Patients who are accustomed to the acute anxiolytic effects of benzodiazepines may tolerate this delay poorly. However, buspirone and the benzodiazepines are not cross-tolerant, and they may be combined (e.g., by continuing to prescribe a benzodiazepine while waiting for buspirone to exert its effect).

A number of other agents have been used for the treatment of anxiety, but all have significant disadvantages for elderly patients. β-Blockers may reduce the somatic symptoms of anxiety but are less effective for the psychological symptoms. Moreover, they cause hypotension and bradycardia and are relatively contraindicated in patients with congestive heart failure, diabetes, asthma, and chronic obstructive pulmonary disease. Antihistamines are sedating, but they have questionable anxiolytic efficacy as well as significant anticholinergic side effects. Neuroleptics may be preferable to the anxiolytics for patients with dementia and agitation associated with anxiety, but they carry the risk of tardive dyskinesia with long-term use and also have anticholinergic and extrapyramidal side effects.

In general, therefore, treatment of anxiety in elderly nondemented and nondepressed patients should be with either short-half-life benzodiazepines (e.g., lorazepam or oxazepam) or buspirone. Benzodiazepines are probably preferable for short-term use (e.g., less than 30 days) and for the treatment of acute anxiety due to psychosocial change or loss, especially when accompanied by sleep disorder. They also are preferable when medication is desired as needed—for example, to treat the anticipatory anxiety associated with a planned medical procedure. Buspirone is preferable to the benzodiazepines when chronic use is expected. Examples include treating generalized anxiety disorder or persistent anxiety associated with a chronic medical condition, especially in patients with respiratory disease, histories of benzodiazepine or alcohol abuse, underlying dementia (where it is desirable to avoid the cognitive toxicity of benzodiazepines), or a history of falls.

Sleep Disorders and Their Treatment

Subjective difficulty in initiating and maintaining sleep is common in elderly persons and may represent developmental changes associated with the aging of the brain mechanisms that regulate the timing and duration of sleep. Polysomnographic evidence indicates that nocturnal awakenings and stage 1 sleep (lighter sleep) increase with age, whereas sleep efficiency and slow-wave sleep (stages 3 and 4, or delta, sleep), which are subjectively associated with the refreshing function of sleep, decrease markedly with age. The multiple-sleep latency test measures the time it takes for an individual to fall asleep at different times during the day. Elderly patients have decreased latencies, suggesting that the changes occurring with age represent an inability to consolidate an adequate amount of sleep during the night rather than a decrease in the need for sleep. For this reason, a nap in the afternoon can be an effective remedy for nighttime insomnia. To avoid worsening sleep at night, the nap probably should be at a regular time and of a defined duration of not greater than an hour; patients should also adhere to regular bedtimes and rising times and should not remain in bed at night at the times when they cannot fall asleep.

Primary sleep disorders are more common in elderly persons than in younger ones. These disorders include sleep-disordered breathing, or sleep apnea, and periodic leg movements of sleep, or nocturnal myoclonus. Both have been associated with arousals at night and impaired concentration and functioning during the day. Sleep apnea and nocturnal myoclonus increase with age even in community-dwelling elderly persons without sleep complaints: sleep apnea approaches 20% of those in their 80s, and nocturnal myoclonus perhaps exceeds 90% of persons in this age group (Hoch et al. 1990). Many elderly persons with subjective complaints of drowsiness during the day may have one of these disorders.

Like anxiety and depression in elderly patients, insomnia is a symptom that increases in frequency as a result of a variety of medical and psychological conditions. Some common medical conditions (e.g., congestive heart failure with nocturnal dyspnea and chronic obstructive pulmonary disease) make it difficult for elderly persons to lie comfortably flat in bed. Other conditions cause physical sensations that interrupt sleep. Examples include pain (e.g., from arthritis, cancer, or bruxism) and nocturia (e.g., from heart disease or urinary tract disease. Psychiatric disorders associated with insomnia include

- Mood and anxiety disorders
- Pathological bereavement
- Dementia
- Delirium
- Substance abuse or withdrawal

Many medications used commonly by elderly patients interfere with sleep. These include any drugs with stimulant properties, from the SSRIs to OTC decongestants, and even the β-blockers, which can cause insomnia due to vivid dreams. Chronic use of alcohol, often started in late life in an attempt to improve sleep, can actually worsen insomnia by decreasing the amount of slow-wave sleep. Sometimes impaired hepatic metabolism results in prolonging the effects of stimulants, with the result that for some elderly persons a cup of coffee or tea at lunch may have as deleterious an effect on nighttime sleep as a cup at bedtime.

Benzodiazepines are effective hypnotics in elderly persons. Although they rapidly induce sleep, there is some evidence that they may change sleep architecture by decreasing the percentage of time spent in deep or slow-wave sleep. This change is theoretically more relevant in elderly persons, who already experience physiological decreases in slow-wave sleep. However, clinical evidence to support this contention is thus far lacking. Pharmacokinetic changes with age result in the accumulation of long-half-life benzodiazepines such as flurazepam, and therefore short-half-life drugs without active metabolites, such as temazepam, are preferable. Clinical experience suggests that these agents may lose effectiveness after daily use for a month, but elderly patients may find it particularly difficult to discontinue their use (Salzman 1990). Some clinicians suggest that discontinuation may be easier if the hypnotic is used initially only two or three times a week rather than every night. Elderly patients may also be more sensitive to the sedative effect of the benzodiazepines; therefore doses of one-quarter to one-half the usual younger adult dose should be used (e.g., 7.5 mg of temazepam; 0.125 mg of triazolam).

Because of pharmacodynamic changes, elderly patients are more susceptible to the toxic effects of the benzodiazepine sedative-hypnotics. These drugs may result in depressed mood, daytime sedation, impaired balance and coordination, and cognitive impairment. In addition, they can depress the central respiratory drive, particularly in patients with underlying asthma or chronic obstructive pulmonary disease. With the development of tolerance, rebound insomnia may occur on the first night, or sometimes the first few nights, after drug discontinuation, making it more difficult for patients to discontinue the medication.

A recent advance in the treatment of insomnia that may be of particular benefit to elderly persons is the development of the nonbenzodiazepine imidazopyridine hypnotics. The first such drug to be available in the U.S. is zolpidem. Zolpidem is believed to be relatively selective for the benzodiazepine type 1 receptor, which may account for its relative lack of muscle relaxant, anticonvulsant, and anxiolytic effects at doses adequate to achieve sedation. The half-life of zolpidem is only slightly longer in elderly patients (about 3 hours) than it is in younger patients. Initial studies in healthy geriatric patients without sleep complaints found decreases in sleep latency, increases in sleep efficiency, and subjective improvement in sleep quality, with no significant side effects, at doses ranging from 5 to 20 mg (Scharf et al. 1991). In particular, no effects on memory were found. A subsequent double-blind, placebo-controlled trial in 119 elderly psychiatric inpatients complaining of insomnia found that 10 mg/day of zolpidem improved total duration of sleep without significant daytime drowsiness or rebound upon withdrawal (Shaw et al. 1992). Preliminary data also suggest that zolpidem may not cause decreases in slow-wave sleep, but additional studies will be necessary to confirm this finding and to determine whether it has any clinical implications.

Late-Life Psychosis and Its Treatment

Psychosis may be a feature of mood disorder (unipolar or bipolar), schizophrenia, delusional disorder, dementia, and other organic mental disorders, or it may be secondary to other medical conditions, prescription medications, or substances of abuse. Any of these conditions may be present in elderly persons, but secondary psychoses are probably more common and schizophrenia less common than in younger patients. Late-life schizophrenia includes recurrences of early-onset schizophrenia and schizophrenia with a late onset; approximately 15% of all patients with schizophrenia present after age 45 (Harris and Jeste 1988). Compared to early-onset schizophrenia, the late-onset disease is more common in women than in men and has fewer negative symptoms, but it has similar positive symptoms, a similar chronic course, and a comparable response to conventional neuroleptics (Jeste et al. 1996). Neuroleptics are the primary therapy for non-mood-related psychotic disorders of any etiology, including disorders in the elderly population. In one retrospective study of 54 late-onset schizophrenic patients treated with neuroleptics, nearly half had complete remissions (defined as the absence of hallucinations, delusions, thought disorder, and catatonic behavior), and an additional 27% had a partial response (Pearlson et al. 1989). As with the use of most other psychotropic drugs in elderly patients, however, the major issues concern increased vulnerability to side effects. Because of decreased dopamine and acetylcholine function in the aging brain and peripheral organs, elderly patients are more susceptible to anticholinergic and extrapyramidal symptoms, including delirium and parkinsonism. Lower-potency neuroleptics possess more anticholinergic effects and also produce more sedation and orthostatic hypotension. With conventional neuroleptics, the traditional approach to these problems has been twofold:

- To use the lowest effective dose of medication

- To start with an intermediate-potency agent, such as perphenazine, in an attempt to avoid the extremes of either type of side effect that might be expected with a drug of low potency (e.g., chlorpromazine or thioridazine) or of high potency (e.g., haloperidol or fluphenazine)

The perphenazine starting dose should be no more than 2 mg/day. For patients who develop significant side effects even at subtherapeutic doses of an intermediate-potency drug, a switch to another agent is then warranted.

Age is a recognized risk factor for the development of tardive dyskinesia. Compared to an annual incidence of 4%–5% in younger schizophrenia patients on neuroleptics, the incidence in patients older than 45 years was found to be 26% at the end of 1 year, 52% after 2 years, and 60% after 3 years (Jeste et al. 1995). Risk factors for developing tardive dyskinesia in this study included

- The duration of prior neuroleptic use at baseline
- The cumulative amount of high-potency neuroleptics
- A history of alcohol abuse or dependence
- The presence of subtle movement disorders such as tremor at baseline

Other clinically important side effects of the neuroleptics, such as obstructive jaundice and agranulocytosis, do not appear to be more common among elderly patients. However, one recent report suggested that elderly patients with prior neuropsychiatric disorders who are prescribed high-potency neuroleptics may be at increased risk for developing neuroleptic malignant syndrome (Leipsic et al. 1995).

Recently, new antipsychotic agents combining dopaminergic and serotonergic receptor blockade have been developed, and two of these, clozapine and risperidone, have been approved for use in the United States. In younger patients, these drugs have shown promise for treatment-resistant schizophrenia (clozapine) and for the negative symptoms of schizophrenia (both drugs). They also appear to cause fewer extrapyramidal side effects than do the conventional neuroleptics, and so far, tardive dyskinesia has not been reported with their use. However, very few data are available on the use of these two drugs in elderly patients. In three small open or retrospective trials of clozapine that mostly included patients with chronic psychotic disorders, moderate to good efficacy was reported (Chengappa et al. 1995; Pitner et al. 1995; Salzman et al. 1995b). One of these studies found greater improvements in behavioral symptoms than in hallucinations and delusions (Salzman et al. 1995b). All three reports, however, noted a high incidence of side effects, especially orthostatic hypotension, lethargy, and respiratory complications. In addition, clozapine may cause agranulocytosis, and patients on this medication require weekly white blood cell counts to monitor for this adverse effect. For frail elderly patients, a starting clozapine dose of 6.25 mg/day, with a slow titration, is recommended.

Several open trials have found risperidone to be beneficial for older schizophrenic patients (Berman et al. 1996; Jeste et al. 1996; Madhusoodanan et al. 1995). In general, these studies indicate that risperidone may be effective for the negative symptoms of schizophrenia, although the time course of this response may be slower than that for positive symptoms. There are some preliminary data that risperidone may improve cognition in elderly schizophrenic patients, at least compared with haloperidol. At very low doses, risperidone lacks significant side effects, but elderly patients may develop extrapyramidal side effects, sedation, and orthostatic hypotension at considerably lower doses than may younger patients. Clinical experience suggests that risperidone be started at 0.25 mg/day in elderly patients and that the maximum daily dose should be only 2–3 mg.

Dementia and Its Treatment

Most dementia in elderly patients is caused by Alzheimer's disease, a multi-infarct state, or some combination of both. Multi-infarct disease cannot be treated, but progression of the disease may be slowed by achieving better medical control of hypertension and possibly by modifying other risk factors for vascular disease (e.g., enhancing control of diabetes, discontinuing cigarette smoking, and regularly taking low-dose aspirin).

A great deal of recent research has been directed at finding safe, effective treatments for cognitive losses due to Alzheimer's disease. Alzheimer's disease is a complex neurodegenerative disorder, marked clinically by a gradually progressive decline in memory, language, orientation, praxis, and higher cortical functions. The histopathology of Alzheimer's disease is characterized by neuronal loss, extracellular collections of abnormal proteins, known as senile plaques, and intracellular aggregations of abnormal microtubular proteins, known as neurofibrillary tangles. The cause of these pathological changes is not fully understood, and rational therapies based on these changes are not yet available. The areas of greatest neuronal loss early in the disease are the cholinergic neurons in the basal forebrain and their projections to the cortex.

Findings of reduced levels of acetylcholine in the cortex and an association between this loss and the degree of memory impairment have led to the development of drugs designed to enhance cholinergic neurotransmission. Early attempts to treat Alzheimer's disease using acetylcholine precursors such as choline or lecithin, analogous to the use of L-dopa in Parkinson's disease, were largely unsuccessful. The next step in therapeutic research based on the cholinergic hypothesis of Alzheimer's disease was the development of the cholinesterase inhibitors. Examples include the short-acting drug physostigmine and the long-acting drug tacrine, which have provided the first objectively verifiable improvements in cognitive function in Alzheimer's disease.

Tacrine has been reported to be effective in improving cognition as measured by a standardized cognitive scale in three published multicenter trials, two of which also demonstrated statistically significant improvement on a clinician's global impression of change (Davis et al. 1992; Farlow et al. 1992; Knapp et al. 1994). The results of these studies led the U.S. Food and Drug Administration (FDA) to approve tacrine for the treatment of Alzheimer's disease. However, the results of these double-blind trials and subsequent clinical experience suggest that the benefit gained from tacrine is generally modest, on the average returning the patient to the level of cognition present 6 months earlier in the course of the disease. There is no effect on the underlying progression of neurodegeneration, and patients who discontinue tacrine often experience a period of rapid deterioration that eventually leaves them where they would have been had that treatment never been tried.

Tacrine has a number of other drawbacks in clinical practice. Approximately a third of patients who reach therapeutically effective dose levels will have gastrointestinal distress. Elevations of greater than three times the upper limit of normal in liver enzymes such as serum alanine aminotransferase (ALT) are found in 25% of patients (Watkins et al. 1994). Although these changes are generally asymptomatic, they require at least temporary discontinuation of the drug. Weekly or biweekly blood tests are necessary for identifying these liver enzyme increases. Finally, because of its short half-life, tacrine must be taken four times a day, which often is difficult to arrange for an Alzheimer's disease patient whose medication use must be supervised. For these reasons, a decision to use tacrine requires a careful and detailed discussion of the risks and benefits with the patient and family. Dose increases are generally made in increments of 40 mg/day every 6 weeks, raising the dose from 10 mg qid up to 40 mg qid.

The next generation of cholinesterase inhibitors in development have more specific effects on brain cholinesterase and therefore fewer peripheral side effects. They are not associated with liver toxicity and have longer half-lives. Of these agents, donepezil hydrochloride was approved by the FDA just before the publication of this book. It has so far shown minimal side effects and no liver toxicity; it is administered in a dose of 5–10 mg once a day. Clinical trials of direct cholinergic agonists, generally somewhat specific for the M_1 muscarinic receptor, are also currently in progress.

A number of other approaches to the treatment of the cognitive symptoms of Alzheimer's disease are being tested or considered on the basis of recent clinical or laboratory findings. Neuropathological evidence for inflammatory mechanisms in the degeneration of Alzheimer's disease, together with epidemiological evidence that patients maintained on NSAIDs have lower rates of developing Alzheimer's disease, led to a trial of indomethacin in Alzheimer's disease (Rogers et al. 1993). This study found a mild protective effect compared to placebo over a 6-month period. Other treatments that are being either considered or tested include antioxidants, estrogen, MAOIs, membrane stabilizers, calcium-channel blockers, and nerve growth factors. Ergoloid mesylates, a combination of four dihydro derivatives of ergotoxine marketed under the name Hydergine, has been described as a metabolic enhancer. A recent meta-analysis of 47 trials of Hydergine found it overall more effective than placebo, but the effect was very modest, with greater effects on behavioral measures than on cognitive measures and stronger effects in a subgroup of patients with vascular dementia (Schneider and Olin 1994).

In addition to the core cognitive symptoms of Alzheimer's disease and other dementias, patients with dementia frequently develop secondary psychiatric syndromes. These include depression, psychosis, and behavioral disturbances such as agitation, restlessness, wandering, and aggressive behavior. These syndromes are often, but not consistently, responsive to the psychopharmacological agents used to treat such symptoms when they are features of primary psychiatric disorders such as major mood disorder or schizophrenia. There are few research data on the treatment of depression in dementia patients. The only double-blind trial with a placebo comparison group used imipramine and found equal improvement with both treatments (Reifler et al. 1989). Because of the anticholinergic side effects of the TCAs, it is probably preferable to use the SSRIs or other newer agents, but data from controlled trials using agents currently available in the United States are not available.

A much larger literature addresses the treatment of psychosis and behavioral disturbances in Alzheimer's disease. These problems, often unmanageable by families at home, are a common reason for the admission of Alzheimer's disease patients to nursing homes and psychiatric hospitals. Neuroleptics are effective medications for the psychotic symptoms of dementia, but these symptoms are usually less common than agitation. Most controlled studies of neuroleptics in agitated patients with dementia have important methodological limitations, including diagnostic heterogeneity, variable definitions of agitation, the use of unvalidated scales, and a lack of placebo groups. Nonetheless, a meta-analysis of the available well-designed trials concluded that neuroleptics were effective in the treatment of agitation in dementia but that the effects were small—among any theoretical sample of

100 patients, the number responsive to neuroleptics would be only 18 more than would respond to placebo (Schneider et al. 1990).

There are few direct comparisons of neuroleptics with other agents. One study found roughly equivalent effects of haloperidol, oxazepam, and diphenhydramine, but the lack of a placebo group makes interpretation of the modest efficacy difficult (Coccaro et al. 1990). Both clozapine (Oberholzer et al. 1992) and risperidone (Allen et al. 1995; Jeanblanc and Davis 1995) have been reported to be efficacious for agitation in dementia, but controlled studies are lacking. Clozapine, because of the risk of orthostatic hypotension and the need for weekly blood monitoring, is difficult to use in elderly patients with dementia unless they are in the hospital. Risperidone is preferable, because it combines the safety of the high-potency neuroleptics with a relatively low risk of extrapyramidal symptoms. However, unless risperidone doses are kept very low (probably under 1–2 mg/day), patients with dementia appear to be susceptible to parkinsonian side effects and blood pressure changes.

The mixed safety and efficacy of the neuroleptics has led to the use of a variety of other agents to treat agitation in dementia. Benzodiazepines are sometimes useful in reducing the anxiety that may lead to agitation, and short-term use, especially in patients with mild dementia, may be helpful. However, the risk of amnesia and confusion leading to greater agitation makes these drugs of doubtful use in patients with later-stage dementia. Antiepileptic drugs are beginning to receive considerable attention. In an open trial, carbamazepine reduced total Brief Psychiatric Rating Scale (BPRS) scores by 25%, and factor scores for hostility-suspiciousness and activation by 44%, in 15 inpatients with dementia who had been unresponsive to neuroleptics (Lemke 1995). Two patients had to discontinue the medication because of leukopenia and allergic reactions, but side effects were otherwise mild and well tolerated at mean daily dosages of 323 mg, with mean serum levels of 4.1 µg/mL. Valproate was useful for agitation in more than half of the patients from several case series (Lott et al. 1995; Sival et al. 1994), with minimal side effects of ataxia and sedation at doses averaging about 500 mg/day and levels slightly below 50 µg/mL. The need for blood monitoring for levels and for liver and hematological function with both of these drugs limits their ease of use in patients with dementia. Controlled trials are needed to establish the place of these agents in the treatment of dementia symptoms.

Serotonergic agents are also gaining a role in the treatment of patients with dementia. Open-label studies of buspirone have demonstrated some efficacy for agitation (Herrmann and Eryavec 1993; Sakauye et al. 1993). Buspirone has the advantage of minimal side effects, even at dosages of up to 60 mg/day, which are sometimes required for the treatment of patients with dementia. In an open trial of trazodone in 22 patients with dementia and behavioral problems, 82% of the patients had moderate or marked improvement (Houlihan et al. 1994). The most common side effect with trazodone is sedation, which may be helpful for some agitated patients with dementia. However, orthostatic hypotension also occurs frequently and may lead to falls. The SSRIs may be useful for agitation even in the absence of depression. A multicenter trial of citalopram, a very selective serotonergic agent not available in the United States, is the only double-blind, placebo-controlled trial with positive results (Nyth and Gottfries 1990). Patients showed decreases in irritability, restlessness, and depression. In an open trial, 10 patients with end-stage Alzheimer's disease who had acute behavioral changes were treated with sertraline; 6 improved, including 5 of 6 who had stopped eating (Volicer et al. 1994). In general, the SSRIs are well tolerated in patients with dementia at doses comparable to those used for the treatment of depression.

Case reports suggest possible benefit from β-blockers, lithium, selegiline, and ECT, but the indications for these medications remain unclear in the absence of well-designed trials. There is some evidence that estrogen may be useful for reducing aggressive physical behavior in men with dementia (Kyomen et al. 1991).

References

Alexopoulos GS: Treatment of depression, in Clinical Geriatric Psychopharmacology. Edited by Salzman C. Baltimore, MD, Williams & Wilkins, 1992, pp 137–174

Allen RL, Walker Z, D'Ath PJ, et al: Risperidone for psychotic and behavioural symptoms in Lewy body dementia [letter] [see comments]. Lancet 346:185, 1995

Avorn J, Soumerai SB, Everitt DE, et al: A randomized trial of a program to reduce the use of psychoactive drugs in nursing homes. N Engl J Med 327:168–173, 1992

Baldwin RC, Jolley DJ: The prognosis of depression in old age. Br J Psychiatry 149:574–583, 1986

Bell AJ, Cole A, Eccleston D, et al: Lithium neurotoxicity at normal therapeutic levels. Br J Psychiatry 162:689–692, 1993

Berman I, Merson A, Rachov-Pavlov J, et al: Risperidone in elderly schizophrenic patients: an open-label trial. American Journal of Geriatric Psychiatry 4:173–179, 1996

Blazer DG: Epidemiology of late-life depression, in Diagnosis and Treatment of Depression in Late Life: Results of the NIH Consensus Development Conference. Edited by Schneider LS, Reynolds CF, Lebowitz BD, et al. Washington, DC, American Psychiatric Press, 1994, pp 9–19

Bohm C, Robinson DS, Gammans RE, et al: Buspirone therapy in anxious elderly patients: a controlled clinical trial. J Clin Psychopharmacol 10:47S–57S, 1990

Boyer WF, Blumhardt CL: The safety profile of paroxetine. J Clin Psychiatry 53:61–66, 1992

Burvill PW, Stampfler HG, Hall WD: Does depressive illness in elderly patients have a poor prognosis? Aust N Z J Psychiatry 20:422–427, 1986

Calamari JE, Faber SD, Hitsman BL, et al: Treatment of obsessive compulsive disorder in elderly patients: a review and case example. J Behav Ther Exp Psychiatry 25:95–104, 1994

Chengappa KNR, Baker RW, Kreinbrook SB: Clozapine use in female geriatric patients with psychoses. J Geriatr Psychiatry Neurol 8:12–15, 1995

Clark DC: Suicide Among the Elderly. Chicago, IL, Center for Suicide Research and Prevention, Department of Psychiatry, Rush-Presbyterian-St. Luke's Medical Center, 1991

Coccaro EF, Kramer E, Zemishlany Z, et al: Pharmacologic treatment of noncognitive behavioral disturbances in elderly demented patients. Am J Psychiatry 147:1640–1645, 1990

Cusack B, Nelson A, Richelson E: Binding of antidepressants to human brain receptors: focus on newer generation compounds. Psychopharmacology (Berlin) 114:559–565, 1994

Davis KL, Thal LJ, Gamzu ER, et al: A double-blind, placebo-controlled multicenter study of tacrine for Alzheimer's disease. The Tacrine Collaborative Study Group. N Engl J Med 327:1253–1259, 1992

Dunner DL, Cohn JB, Walshe T, et al: Two combined, multicenter double-blind studies of paroxetine and doxepin in geriatric patients with major depression. J Clin Psychiatry 53:57–60, 1992

Farlow M, Gracon SI, Hershey LA, et al: A controlled trial of tacrine in Alzheimer's disease. (The Tacrine Study Group.) JAMA 268:2523–2529, 1992

Flint AJ: Epidemiology and comorbidity of anxiety disorders in elderly patients. Am J Psychiatry 151:640–649, 1994

Foster JR: Use of lithium in elderly psychiatric patients: a review of the literature. Lithium 3:77–93, 1992

Foy A, O'Connell D, Henry D, et al: Benzodiazepine use as a cause of cognitive impairment in elderly hospital inpatients. J Gerontol 50:M99–M106, 1995

Frank E, Kupfer DJ, Perel JM, et al: Three-year outcomes for maintenance therapies in recurrent depression. Arch Gen Psychiatry 47:1093–1099, 1990

George LK: Social factors and depression in late life, in Diagnosis and Treatment of Depression in Late Life: Results of the NIH Consensus Development Conference. Edited by Schneider LS, Reynolds CF, Lebowitz BD, et al. Washington, DC, American Psychiatric Press, 1994, pp 131–153

Ghadirian AM, Annable L, Belanger MC, et al: A cross-sectional study of parkinsonism and tardive dyskinesia in lithium-treated affective disordered patients. J Clin Psychiatry 57:22–28, 1996

Glassman AH, Preud'homme XA: Review of the cardiovascular effects of heterocyclic antidepresssants. J Clin Psychiatry 54:16–22, 1993

Harris MJ, Jeste DV: Late-onset schizophrenia: an overview. Schizophr Bull 14:39–55, 1988

Herings RM, Stricker BH, de Boer A, et al: Benzodiazepines and the risk of falling leading to femur fractures: dosage more important than elimination half-life. Arch Intern Med 155:1801–1807, 1995

Herrmann N, Eryavec G: Buspirone in the management of agitation and aggression associated with dementia. American Journal of Geriatric Psychiatry 1:249–253, 1993

Himmelfarb S, Murrell SA: The prevalence and correlates of anxiety symptoms in older adults. Journal of Psychology 116:159–167, 1984

Himmelhoch JM, Neil JF, May SJ, et al: Age, dementia, dyskinesias, and lithium response. Am J Psychiatry 137:941–945, 1980

Hoch CC, Reynolds CF, Monk TH, et al: Comparison of sleep-disordered breathing among healthy elderly in the seventh, eighth, and ninth decades of life. Sleep 13:502–511, 1990

Hocking LB, Koenig HG: Anxiety in medically ill older patients: a review and update. Int J Psychiatry Med 25:221–238, 1995

Houlihan DJ, Mulsant BH, Sweet RA, et al: A naturalistic study of trazodone in the treatment of behavioral complications of dementia. American Journal of Geriatric Psychiatry 2:78–85, 1994

Inouye SK, Viscoli CM, Horwitz RI, et al: A predictive model for delirium in hospitalized elderly medical patients based on admission characteristics. Ann Intern Med 119:474–481, 1993

Jacobs S, Hansen F, Kasl S, et al: Anxiety disorders during acute bereavement: risk and risk factors. J Clin Psychiatry 51:269–274, 1990

Jeanblanc W, Davis YB: Risperidone for treating dementia-associated aggression [letter]. Am J Psychiatry 152:1239, 1995

Jeste DV, Caligiuri MP, Paulsen JS, et al: Risk of tardive dyskinesia in older patients: a prospective longitudinal study of 266 outpatients. Arch Gen Psychiatry 52:756–765, 1995

Jeste DV, Eastham JH, Lacro JP, et al: Management of late-life psychosis. J Clin Psychiatry 57:39–45, 1996

Katon W, Sullivan MD: Depression and chronic medical illness. J Clin Psychiatry 51:3–11, 1990

Katz IR, Stoff D, Muhly C, et al: Identifying persistent adverse effects of anticholinergic drugs in elderly patients. J Geriatr Psychiatry Neurol 1:212–217, 1988

Kellner MB, Neher F: A first episode of mania after age 80. Can J Psychiatry 36:607–608, 1991

Kiev A, Domantay AG: A study of buspirone coprescribed with bronchodilators in 82 anxious ambulatory patients. J Asthma 25:281–284, 1988

Knapp MJ, Knopman DS, Solomon PR, et al: A 30-week randomized controlled trial of high-dose tacrine in patients with Alzheimer's disease. (The Tacrine Study Group.) JAMA 271:985–991, 1994

Krauthammer C, Klerman GL: Secondary mania: manic syndromes associated with antecedent physical illnesses or drugs. Arch Gen Psychiatry 35:1333–1339, 1978

Kroenke K, Pinholt EM: Reducing polypharmacy in elderly patients: a controlled trial of physician feedback. J Am Geriatr Soc 38:31–36, 1990

Kyomen HH, Nobel KW, Wei JY: The use of estrogen to decrease aggressive physical behavior in elderly men with dementia. J Am Geriatr Soc 39:1110–1112, 1991

Larson EB, Kukull WA, Buchner D, et al: Adverse drug reactions associated with global cognitive impairment in elderly persons. Ann Intern Med 107:169–173, 1987

Leipsic JS, Abraham HD, Halperin P: Neuroleptic malignant syndrome in elderly patients. J Geriatr Psychiatry Neurol 8:28–31, 1995

Lemke MR: Effect of carbamazepine on agitation in Alzheimer's inpatients refractory to neuroleptics. J Clin Psychiatry 56:354–357, 1995

Levine S, Napoliello MJ, Domantay AG: An open study of buspirone in octogenarians with anxiety. Human Psychopharmacology 4:51–53, 1988

Lott AD, McElroy SL, Keys MA: Valproate in the treatment of behavioral agitation in elderly patients with dementia. J Neuropsychiatry Clin Neurosci 7:314–9, 1995

Madhusoodanan S, Brenner R, Araujo L, et al: Efficacy of risperidone treatment for psychoses associated with schizophrenia, schizoaffective disorder, bipolar disorder, or senile dementia in 11 geriatric patients: a case series. J Clin Psychiatry 56:514–518, 1995

McFarland BH, Miller MR, Straumfjord AA: Valproate use in the older manic patient. J Clin Psychiatry 51:479–481, 1990

Meats P, Timol M, Jolley D: Prognosis of depression in elderly patients. Br J Psychiatry 159:659–663, 1991

Mendelson WB, Maczaj M, Holt J: Buspirone administration to sleep apnea patients. J Clin Psychopharmacol 11:71–72, 1991

Nair NP, Ahmed SK, Kin NM, et al: Reversible and selective inhibitors of monoamine oxidase A in the treatment of depressed elderly patients. Acta Psychiatr Scand Suppl 386:28–35, 1995

Napoliello MJ: An interim multicentre report on 677 anxious geriatric out-patients treated with buspirone. Br J Clinical Pract 40:71–73, 1986

Nemeroff CB, DeVane CL, Pollack BG: Newer antidepressants and the cytochrome P450 system. Am J Psychiatry 153:311–331, 1996

Nyth AL, Gottfries CG: The clinical efficacy of citalopram in treatment of emotional disturbances in dementia disorders. (Nordic multicentre study.) Br J Psychiatry 157:894–901, 1990

Oberholzer AF, Hendriksen C, Monsch AU, et al: Safety and effectiveness of low-dose clozapine in psychogeriatric patients: a preliminary study. Int Psychogeriatr 4:187–195, 1992

Parmelee PA, Katz IR, Lawton MP: Anxiety and its association with depression among institutionalized elderly. American Journal of Geriatric Psychiatry 1:46–58, 1993

Pearlson GD, Kreger L, Rabins PV, et al: A chart review study of late-onset and early-onset schizophrenia. Am J Psychiatry 146:1568–1574, 1989

Pitner JK, Mintzer JE, Pennypacker LC, et al: Efficacy and adverse effects of clozapine in four elderly psychotic patients. J Clin Psychiatry 56:180–185, 1995

Pope HG Jr, McElroy SL, Satlin A, et al: Head injury, bipolar disorder, and response to valproate. Compr Psychiatry 29:34–38, 1988

Ray WA, Griffin MR, Downey W: Benzodiazepines of long and short elimination half-life and the risk of hip fracture. JAMA 262:3303–3307, 1989

Regier DA, Narrow WE, Rae DS: The epidemiology of anxiety disorders: the Epidemiologic Catchment Area (ECA) experience. J Psychiatr Res 24:3–14, 1990

Reifler BV, Teri L, Raskind M, et al: A double blind trial of a tricyclic antidepressant in Alzheimer's patients with and without depression. Am J Psychiatry 146:45–49, 1989

Reynolds CF 3rd, Frank E, Perel JM, et al: Maintenance therapies for late-life recurrent major depression: research and review circa 1995. Int Psychogeriatr (suppl 7):27–39, 1995

Risinger RC, Risby ED, Risch SC: Safety and efficacy of divalproex sodium in elderly bipolar patients [letter]. J Clin Psychiatry 55:215, 1994

Rogers J, Kirby LC, Hempelman SR, et al: Clinical trial of indomethacin in Alzheimer's disease. Neurology 43:1609–1611, 1993

Rutz W, Von Knoring L, Walinder J: Frequency of suicide on Gotland after systematic postgraduate education of general practitioners. Acta Psychiatr Scand 80:151–154, 1989

Sackeim HA: Use of electroconvulsive therapy in late-life depression, in Diagnosis and Treatment of Depression in Late Life: Results of the NIH Consensus Development Conference. Edited by Schneider LS, Reynolds CF, Lebowitz BD, et al. Washington, DC, American Psychiatric Press, 1994, pp 259–277

Sakauye KM, Camp CJ, Ford PA: Effects of buspirone on agitation associated with dementia. American Journal of Geriatric Psychiatry 1:82–84, 1993

Salzman C: Anxiety in elderly patients: treatment strategies. J Clin Psychiatry 51:18–21, 1990

Salzman C: Pharmacological treatment of depression in elderly patients, in Diagnosis and Treatment of Depression in Late Life: Results of the NIH Consensus Development Conference. Edited by Schneider LS, Reynolds CF, Lebowitz BD, et al. Washington, DC, American Psychiatric Press, 1994, pp 181–244

Salzman C, Schneider LS, Alexopoulos GS: Pharmacological treatment of depression in late life, in Psychopharmacology: The Fourth Generation of Progress. Edited by Bloom FE, Kupfer DJ. New York, Raven, 1995a, pp 1471–1477

Salzman C, Vaccaro B, Lieff J, et al: Clozapine in older patients with psychosis and behavioral disruption. Am J Geriatric Psychiatry 3:26–33, 1995b

Scharf MB, Mayleben DW, Kaffeman M, et al: Dose response effects of zolpidem in normal geriatric subjects. J Clin Psychiatry 52:77–83, 1991

Schmucker DL: Drug disposition in elderly patients: a review of the critical factors. J Am Geriatr Soc 32:144–149, 1984

Schneider L, Pollack V, Lyness S: A metaanalysis of controlled trials of neuroleptic treatment in dementia. J Am Geriatr Soc 38:553–563, 1990

Schneider LS, Olin JT: Overview of clinical trials of Hydergine in dementia. Arch Neurol 51:787–98, 1994

Shaw SH, Curson H, Coquelin JP: A double-blind, comparative study of zolpidem and placebo in the treatment of insomnia in elderly psychiatric in-patients. J Int Med Res 20:150–161, 1992

Shorr RI, Fought RL, Ray WA: Changes in antipsychotic drug use in nursing homes during implementation of the OBRA-87 regulations. JAMA 271:358–362, 1994

Shulman KI, Tohen M, Satlin A, et al: Mania compared with unipolar depression in old age. Am J Psychiatry 149:341–345, 1992

Singh AN, Beer M: A dose range-finding study of buspirone in geriatric patients with symptoms of anxiety. J Clin Psychopharmacol 8:67–68, 1988

Singh NP, Despars JA, Stansbury DW, et al: Effects of buspirone on anxiety levels and exercise tolerance in patients with chronic airflow obstruction and mild anxiety. Chest 103:800–804, 1993

Sival RC, Haffmans PM, van Gent PP, et al: The effects of sodium valproate on disturbed behavior in dementia [letter]. J Am Geriatr Soc 42:906–907, 1994

Steckler TL: Lithium- and carbamazepine-associated sinus node dysfunction: nine-year experience in a psychiatric hospital. J Clin Psychopharmacol 14:336–339, 1994

Volicer L, Rheaume Y, Cyr D: Treatment of depression in advanced Alzheimer's disease using sertraline. J Geriatr Psychiatry Neurol 7:227–229, 1994

Von Moltke L, Greenblatt D, Shader RI: Clinical pharmacokinetics of antidepressants in elderly patients. Clinical Pharmacokinetics 24:141–160, 1993

Watkins PB, Zimmerman HJ, Knapp MJ, et al: Hepatotoxic effects of tacrine administration in patients with Alzheimer's disease. JAMA 271:992–998, 1994

Weissman MM, Bruce ML, Leaf PJ, et al: Affective disorders, in Psychiatric Disorders in America. Edited by Robins LN, Regier DA. New York, Free Press, 1991, pp 53–80

Yassa R, Cvejic J: Valproate in the treatment of posttraumatic bipolar disorder in a psychogeriatric patient. J Geriatr Psychiatry Neurol 7:55–57, 1994

Zisook S, Schucter SR, Sledge P: Diagnostic and treatment considerations in depression associated with late-life bereavement, in Diagnosis and Treatment of Depression in Late Life: Results of the NIH Consensus Development Conference. Edited by Schneider LS, Reynolds CF, Lebowitz BD, et al. Washington, DC, American Psychiatric Press, 1994, pp 419–435

Afterword to Section IV

Susan L. McElroy, M.D., Section Editor

I want to thank the authors for their scholarly yet practical contributions to the rapidly expanding field of psychopharmacology.

These chapters highlight several important features of this expanding area of medicine. First, the number of mental disorders amenable to psychopharmacological treatment is increasing. Second, the number of available psychopharmacological agents is increasing. Third, psychopharmacological agents effective in one mental disorder are often effective in others. Fourth, many psychiatric disorders amenable to psychopharmacological treatment are lifelong illnesses that begin early in life. Thus, the psychopharmacological treatment of these disorders should often be begun as early as possible and continued throughout the life span.

V

Psychological and Biological Assessment at the Turn of the Century

V

Psychological and Biological Assessment at the Turn of the Century

Section V

Psychological and Biological Assessment at the Turn of the Century

Foreword

John F. Clarkin, Ph.D., and John P. Docherty, M.D.,
Section Editors

There have been many reviews of psychological and neuropsychological tests and instruments (Beutler and Berren 1995; Butcher 1995; Clarkin et al. 1994; Docherty and Dewan 1995; Docherty and Streeter 1996). However, rapid developments in computer technology and profound changes in the delivery of services in psychiatry contribute to the need to take a fresh view of assessment methods and techniques.

Computer technology has fostered many advances in the standardized assessment of psychiatric patients (Butcher 1987). Such advances include computerized on-line assessment of patient diagnosis and symptoms, computerized tasks to assess the attention capacities and impulsivity of children with suspected attention-deficit/hyperactivity disorder (ADHD), and computer-scanned scoring of self-report inventories. Computer technology allows the practicing psychiatrist to provide rapid assessment of the patient in the office, and this assessment can be part of a larger computerized charting and billing system.

The transformation of the delivery of psychiatric services by managed care has created a need for rapid patient assessment and evaluation, treatments targeted to the most central problem areas, and assessment of patient satisfaction with service and symptom change. Psychiatrists in leadership roles in large systems of care need the tools to examine 1) use of treatment guidelines in the delivery of care, 2) the timely delivery of care, 3) patient outcome and satisfaction with services, and 4) the distribution of scarce treatment resources in a capitated system. The technologies to provide such assessment are also developing rapidly, and a timely review is needed.

With these developments in mind, we have organized this section around key areas of assessment in the rapidly changing treatment environment. In Chapter 21, Drs. Janicak and Winans describe the laboratory tests recommended for different subgroups of psychiatric patients. The authors address issues of economical, yet thorough and clinically appropriate laboratory testing of psychiatric patients. Chapter 22, by Drs. Mattis and Wilson, is intended to answer questions about the appropriateness of referral for specialized assessment. What symptom complexes suggest the need for neuropsychological assessment? Under what conditions can psychological testing be of use with patients whose diagnosis is not clear? In this "decade of the brain," the emphasis is on neuropsychological assessment, and not broad-band psychological assessment, and more focused assessments and interventions. In Chapter 23, Drs. Newman and Carpenter describe decision rules and criteria for selecting instruments that help clinical administrators distribute manpower in a system of care. Finally, in Chapter 24, Drs. Dewan and Carpenter address the issue of report cards and evaluation of systems of care.

References

Beutler LE, Berren MR (eds): Integrative Assessment of Adult Personality. New York, Guilford, 1995

Butcher JN (ed): Computerized Psychological Assessment: A Practitioner's Guide. New York, Basic Books, 1987

Butcher JN (ed): Clinical Personality Assessment: Practical Approaches. New York, Oxford University Press, 1995

Clarkin JF, Hurt SW, Mattis S: Psychological and neuropsychological assessment, in The American Psychiatric Press Textbook of Psychiatry, 2nd Edition. Edited by Hales RE, Yudofsky SC, Talbott JA. Washington, DC, American Psychiatric Press, 1994, pp 247–276

Docherty JP, Dewan NA: Outcomes Assessment Monograph. Washington, DC, National Association of Psychiatric Health Systems, 1995

Docherty JP, Streeter MJ: Measuring outcomes, in Outcomes Assessment in Clinical Practice. Edited by Sederer L, Dickey B. New York, Williams & Wilkins, 1996, pp 8–18

Chapter 21

The Laboratory in Clinical Psychiatry

Philip G. Janicak, M.D., and
Elizabeth A. Winans, Pharm.D.

Heightened recognition of the biological basis of many psychiatric disorders has furthered the quest for effective therapies. As a result, the need for laboratory assessments has become more frequent and, at times, clinically imperative (Anfinson and Kathol 1992; Israni and Janicak 1993; Janicak et al. 1993). Thus, in conjunction with clinical acumen, the laboratory may be utilized to 1) elucidate and quantify biological factors associated with specific psychiatric disorders, 2) serve as a guidepost for treatment selection, and 3) monitor clinical efficacy and/or toxicity of treatment.

In this chapter, we provide an overview of laboratory assessments for the psychiatric patient, as well as identify the appropriate role of therapeutic drug monitoring.

General Principles for Medical Assessment

Physical problems in the psychiatric population are often underappreciated. Further, such problems may contribute to or be the basis for psychiatric complaints. Thus, a thorough physical review is necessary to identify new or previously missed medical problems, incorrect diagnoses, or complications secondary to pharmacological treatment or substance use.

The routine ordering of a series of screening batteries is often of limited clinical utility and a waste of funds. When indicated, however, specific laboratory tests should be ordered prior to complete assessment and integration of the patient's history, mental status examination, and physical examination. Occasionally, a specific treatment such as clozapine will dictate the need for screening baseline laboratory tests and/or the ongoing utilization of laboratory data (e.g., complete blood count [CBC]). The initial clinical evaluation may then indicate the need for further medical or laboratory assessments (e.g., evidence of a substance abuse disorder or a dementia from the history and/or mental status examination).

The minimal routine laboratory workup recommended to evaluate the general physical health of a patient on admission is presented in

Table 21–1. Table 21–2 lists supplemental laboratory and diagnostic tests that should be reserved for cases in which specific clues from the history, the physical examination, and the initial laboratory screening suggest an underlying physical disorder. Finally, those laboratory tests utilized in *very* specific circumstances are listed in Table 21–3.

Laboratory Tests in Psychiatry

Laboratory abnormalities found in psychiatric disorders are often utilized as biological markers. Although these abnormalities are not specific or sensitive enough to confirm a diagnosis or identify appropriate treatment, they may be indicative of an association between a given psychiatric disorder and a particular measure that may or may not be relevant to its pathophysiology. Biological markers can be viewed as *state-dependent* and utilized as a tool to aid in the diagnosis during an exacerbation of a specific psychiatric disorder (e.g., acute depressive episode) or to monitor treatment response. Conversely, *trait-dependent* markers may be useful in identifying individuals who are susceptible to a given psychiatric disorder, even when in remission.

Neuroendocrine Tests

Endocrine disorders may present with a variety of psychiatric symptoms (e.g., mania in hyperthyroidism, depression in hypothyroidism and/or hypercortisolism, and psychosis in Cushing's syndrome), and several neuroendocrine tests are routinely used in the clinic (e.g., thyroid function tests). The limbic-hypothalamic-pituitary axis is pivotal in hormonal modulation, and endocrine changes within this system may serve as important correlates to major psychiatric disorders. These include changes in basal hormonal concentrations, as well as changes in response to a pharmacological challenge.

Dexamethasone suppression test (DST).   This procedure involves the administration of 1 mg of dexamethasone orally at 11:00 P.M. Samples for plasma concentrations of cortisol are drawn at 8:00 A.M., 4:00 P.M., and 11:00 P.M. on the following day. For outpatients, a single plasma cortisol sample should be obtained at 4:00 P.M. on the next day. In normals the administration of dexamethasone will suppress the secretion of cortisol over the next 24 hours to concentrations below 5 µg/dL. Plasma cortisol levels higher than 5 µg/dL indicate nonsuppression or a positive (abnormal) test, which indicates that there is an increased likelihood that the patient is experiencing a major depressive episode or at least that there is an affective component to the illness. Caution must be used in the interpretation of cortisol concentrations between 4 and 7 µg/dL because of variations in assay methods. In general, the DST has low

Table 21–1.   General laboratory evaluation

CBC and differential
Blood chemistries (e.g., SMAC)
Thyroid function tests (e.g., TSH, T3, T4)
Screening for syphilis (e.g., VDRL or RPR)
Urinalysis
Chest X ray

Electrocardiogram (when indicated)
Pregnancy test (in all eligible females)

Note.   CBC = complete blood count; SMAC = Sequential Multiple Analyzer
Computer; TSH = thyroid-stimulating hormone; VDRL = Venereal Disease
Research Laboratory; RPR = rapid plasma reagin.
Source.   Adapted from Janicak et al. 1993.

Table 21–2.   Supplemental assessment

Skull films; CT scan, MRI
EEG; evoked potentials
Polysomnography; nocturnal penile tumescence

Urinary toxicology screen
Blood and/or breath alcohol levels
Serum concentrations of medications
B$_{12}$ and folate levels
Heavy-metal screens
Serum ceruloplasmin

ESR
HIV testing
Antinuclear antibodies
Monospot
TB skin test

Blood cultures
Urine: porphyrins; osmolality
Stool: occult blood
Arterial blood gases
Lumbar puncture with CSF studies

Note.   CT = computed tomography; MRI = magnetic resonance imaging;
EEG = electroencephalogram; ESR = erythrocyte sedimentation rate;
HIV = human immunodeficiency virus; CSF = cerebrospinal fluid.
Source.   Adapted from Janicak et al. 1993.

Table 21–3. Specific batteries for unique clinical circumstances

Elderly psychiatric patients

CBC with differential

ESR

Serum B_{12} and folate levels

SMA-20

Liver function tests

Serological test for syphilis

Urinalysis

Lumbar puncture

Chest X ray

ECG

Skull X ray; EEG if necessary

CT scan; MRI if indicated

Suspected substance abuse

Breath and blood alcohol levels

Urine drug screen

Serum toxicological screen with gas chromatography–mass spectroscopy

Lithium

CBC with differential

Serum electrolytes

Blood urea nitrogen, serum creatinine

Thyroid function tests

ECG (if age > 45 or clinically indicated)

Urinalysis

Pregnancy test

Carbamazepine

CBC with differential

Liver function tests

Serum electrolytes

Blood urea nitrogen, serum creatinine

Pregnancy test

Divalproex sodium

CBC with differential

Liver function tests

Serum electrolytes

Pregnancy test

Clozapine

CBC with differential (as well as weekly during treatment)

Electroconvulsive therapy

CBC with differential

Blood chemistries

Chest X ray; spinal X ray (if indicated)

Urinalysis

ECG

Note. CBC = complete blood count; ESR = erythrocyte sedimentation rate; ECG = electrocardiogram; EEG = electroencephalogram; CT = computed tomography; MRI = magnetic resonance imaging.
Source. Adapted from Janicak et al. 1993.

specificity (e.g., approximately 50% false-positive rate), and it is not an adequate screening tool, because as many as 5% of healthy control subjects and approximately 19% of acutely schizophrenic patients may also demonstrate nonsuppression (Janicak et al. 1993). There are also data indicating that failure of the DST to normalize after treatment for depression might indicate a higher likelihood of relapse (Arana et al. 1985). The common causes of false positive and false negative results on the DST are listed in Table 21–4. Because of issues of sensitivity and specificity, the DST has limited application in psychiatry.

Thyroid-releasing hormone (TRH) stimulation test. This laboratory assessment is generally done on an inpatient basis. After an overnight fast, an intravenous line is placed at approximately 8:30 A.M. Baseline thyroid indices (including thyroid-stimulating hormone [TSH]) are obtained at 8:59 A.M., and immediately following, 500 µg of synthetic TRH (protirelin) is administered intravenously over 50 seconds. Plasma TSH

Table 21–4. Causes of false positive or false negative results on the dexamethasone suppression test

False positives	False negatives
Pregnancy	Addison's disease
Obesity	Hypopituitarism
Weight loss or malnutrition	Slow metabolism of dexamethasone
Alcohol abuse/withdrawal	Drugs
Infection	Exogenous corticosteroids
Trauma	Indomethacin
Diabetes mellitus	High doses of benzodiazepines
Carcinoma	High doses of cyproheptadine
Cushing's syndrome	
Anorexia nervosa	
Renal/cardiac disease	
Cerebrovascular disease	
Antipsychotic withdrawal	
Temporal lobe epilepsy	
Drugs	
Estrogens	
Narcotics	
Sedative-hypnotics	
Anticonvulsants	

Source. Adapted from Janicak et al. 1993.

samples are collected 15, 30, 60, and 90 minutes after the TRH infusion. During this period, the patient should be monitored for transient side effects, including gastrointestinal distress, genitourinary symptoms, a sensation of warmth, dry mouth, metallic taste, or tightness in the chest.

Under normal circumstances, in response to the TRH infusion, plasma TSH levels will increase by 5–15 microunits/mL. A minimal elevation in TRH concentration (generally less than 5–7 microunits/mL) is considered to be a blunted response, which may indicate a major depression. Approximately one-quarter of patients with major depression will have a blunted TRH response. When this test is used in conjunction with the DST, abnormal results in both further support the diagnosis of a major depressive episode, as well as the use of antidepressant therapy. Conversely, an "augmented" TSH response (TSH elevation > 30 microunits/mL), in conjunction with other thyroid indices, may indicate a hypothyroid state that is mimicking a depressive disorder. In this population, depressive symptoms may respond to thyroid hormone replacement.

Other neuroendocrine tests.   A variety of other neuroendocrine tests have been studied, including

- Plasma melatonin levels and urinary excretion of 6-hydroxylmelatonin, its primary metabolite, used in research as indices of noradrenergic functioning both pre- and posttreatment.
- Blunted prolactin response to serotonergic agents such as fenfluramine (Malone et al. 1996) and L-tryptophan may be secondary to a serotonergic deficiency in depression.
- Blunted growth hormone (GH) response to various stimuli may be indicative of a depressive episode. Stimuli used to assess GH response include L-dopa, 5-hydroxytryptophan, apomorphine, d-amphetamine, clonidine, growth hormone–releasing hormone (GHRH), and TRH. The GH response to clonidine is one challenge test that has been consistently replicated in the literature. This test measures the responsiveness of presynaptic α_2-adrenergic receptors, and a blunted response may be a trait marker for depression.

Biochemical Markers

After several years of research on neurotransmitters and their metabolites, researchers have identified numerous abnormalities. Unfortunately, no laboratory test has been devised to enhance diagnosis or treatment reliably and consistently. Some potentially important findings include

- An association between suicidal behavior and/or violent impulsivity and low cerebrospinal fluid (CSF) levels of the primary metabolite of serotonin, 5-hydroxyindoleacetic acid (5-HIAA) (Åsberg et al. 1976a, 1976b)

- Low urinary 3-methoxy-4-hydroxyphenylglycol (MHPG), the principal metabolite of norepinephrine, primarily in bipolar disorder, depressed phase
- Decreases in levels of plasma homovanillic acid (HVA), the primary metabolite of dopamine, which have been associated with clinical improvement of psychosis (Sharma et al. 1988)

Peripheral tissues may reflect or parallel central neuronal activity. These include receptors or high-molecular-weight complex biomolecules and enzyme systems found in platelets, lymphocytes, skin fibroblasts, and erythrocytes. Relevant findings, the clinical significance of which remains uncertain, include the following:

- Decreased platelet monoamine oxidase (MAO) in bipolar and unipolar disorders
- Increased platelet α_2-adrenergic receptors in depression
- Decreased β-adrenergic receptor binding sites on lymphocytes in affective disorders
- Significantly diminished ^{3}H-labeled imipramine binding sites in platelets from depressed or obsessive-compulsive patients
- Increased platelet serotonin2A (5-HT2A) receptors in suicidal patients independent of diagnosis (Pandey et al. 1995)

Regarding the last example, our group found that suicidal patients, regardless of diagnosis, have a significantly higher number of platelet 5-HT_{2A} receptors as compared with nonsuicidal patients or healthy control subjects. In addition, no differences in number of platelet 5-HT_{2A} receptors were noted between patients who had made suicide attempts and those with serious suicidal ideation.

Genetic Markers

Chromosomal abnormalities can be utilized to diagnose various types of mental retardation, such as Down syndrome (i.e., trisomy 21) or the fragile X syndrome (i.e., X chromosome) (Wisniewski et al. 1985). *Genetic linkage studies* attempt to establish the chromosomal locus of certain disorders (e.g., chromosome 4 in Huntington's chorea, chromosome 13 in Wilson's disease, chromosome 21 in Alzheimer's disease, X chromosome or chromosome 11 in bipolar disorder). Specific DNA sequences or *restriction fragment length polymorphisms* (RFLPs) can be used to compare the genes of patients with psychiatric disorders with those of healthy control subjects. Potential markers for candidate genes include high lithium erythrocyte/plasma ratios and high muscarinic acetylcholine receptor density in some patients with mood disorders.

Brain Imaging Techniques

While brain functional imaging has been used to study psychiatric disorders for over two decades, the data generated have not had a major impact on clinical practice (Brodie 1996). Questions that clinical psychiatrists pose and would want such technology to answer include the following:

- Can a *diagnosis* be made solely from a functional image, and can repeated scans monitor *the progress* of the disorder with or without therapy?
- Can functional imaging *localize* those areas of the brain that subserve certain symptoms (e.g., hallucinations)?
- Can functional imaging *define biochemical characteristics* of a psychiatric disorder in a reproducible, generalizable, and predictive manner?
- Can functional imaging provide a *rational basis for selecting psychopharmacotherapy,* including type of drug and dose, as well as *predict the likely outcome?*

One example is a recent report in *Nature,* in which positron-emission tomography (PET) was utilized to identify increased activity in brain areas of schizophrenic patients while they were experiencing auditory hallucinations (Silbersweig et al. 1995). Using a group (vs. individual) analysis approach, the authors found a highly significant pattern of deep activation (i.e., bilateral thalamus, left hippocampus/parahippocampal gyrus, and right ventral tegmentum). Autonomous activity in these areas is consistent with other reports and may account for the bizarre, involuntary experiences of these patients. Another example is a series of PET studies in which it has been demonstrated that there is up to 80% striatal dopamine$_2$ (D$_2$) receptor occupancy in acutely ill patients receiving antipsychotic treatment (Farde et al. 1992). More recently, Klemm and co-workers (1996) reported a similar result with a raclopride derivative ([^{123}I]benzamide) developed for single-photon emission computed tomography. The implication is that this more readily available (and less expensive) non–PET imaging procedure may be a potential tool for the clinical monitoring of patients on antipsychotics and perhaps other psychotropics.

There are several issues, however, that currently preclude the routine use of most such techniques, including that

- Many steps are required (e.g., data acquisition, tracer kinetic modeling, image processing, reconstruction and analysis).

- Analysis involves statistical techniques that may oversimplify while producing compelling visual images.
- Data may be generated in a resting (or reference) state, in response to a challenge to a putative deficiency characteristic of a clinical syndrome, or both.

Computed tomography (CT).   CT is primarily used to rule out organic lesions that might underlie and/or contribute to a psychiatric disorder. Indications for CT include the following:

- First episode after age 40 of a psychotic, mood, or personality disorder
- Abnormal motoric movements
- Delirium or dementia of unknown etiology
- Persistent catatonia
- Anorexia nervosa

Contrast is used when there are focal signs and symptoms and/or when any lesion is noted on a noncontrast scan. Some potentially relevant findings have included the following:

- Reversed cerebral asymmetry in patients with schizophrenia
- Cerebellar atrophy, third-ventricle enlargement, and high ventricle-to-brain ratios in chronic schizophrenic or bipolar patients
- A negative correlation between ventricular enlargement and response to neuroleptic treatment in chronic schizophrenic patients
- Cortical atrophy as evidenced by sulcal widening in chronic schizophrenic patients

Abnormalities have also been reported in depression, alcoholism, Alzheimer's disease, and multi-infarct dementia. In clinical practice, the CT scan is convenient, safe, relatively comfortable, less expensive than other, newer imaging techniques, and especially helpful as a diagnostic tool in patients with a history of cerebral concussion or subarachnoid hemorrhage.

Magnetic resonance imaging (MRI).   When a magnetic field is used to detect the frequencies at which chemical elements in body tissue resonate, the characteristic frequencies of various brain tissues are recorded to create an exquisitely detailed picture of brain structures. MRI has been most useful in the diagnosis of primary degenerative dementias (e.g., Alzheimer's and Pick's diseases). In addition, studies of patients with schizophrenia have demonstrated smaller frontal lobe size, ventricular enlargement (especially in the frontal horns), and temporolimbic abnormalities, including complete or partial agenesis of the corpus callosum. Advantages of MRI over CT include the following:

- Imaging in all planes
- Higher resolution
- Better differentiation of gray matter from white matter
- Better definition of lesions in demyelinating disorders
- Excellent visualization of the posterior fossa and pituitary regions
- Potential for measuring physiological variables (e.g., MRI spectroscopy)

Magnetic resonance spectroscopy (MRS).   This methodology has made it possible to measure various neurotransmitter systems in vivo, including choline-containing compounds, in the central nervous system (CNS) noninvasively and without exposure to radioactivity. For example, there have been preliminary reports of the use of MRS to evaluate choline concentrations in the subcortical nuclei of elderly depressed patients before and after treatment, as well as in younger unmedicated depressed patients (Charles et al. 1992, 1994; Renshaw et al. 1993). In the reports by Charles and co-workers (1992, 1994), there was evidence of elevated choline levels, which resolved with treatment; in the report by Renshaw and colleagues (1993), there was evidence of increased choline response in depressed patients relative to control subjects. Our group reported the first use of proton MRS in bipolar patients on lithium (Sharma et al. 1992). In comparison to healthy control subjects, these patients had basal ganglia region elevations in the choline/phosphocreatine-creatinine ratio, N-acetylaspartate/phosphocreatine-creatinine ratio, and inositol/phosphocreatine-creatinine ratio.

Regarding the impact of drug treatment, Kato and co-workers (1994) used MRS to measure lithium in the brain of manic patients and found that reduction in mania ratings did not significantly correlate with lithium serum concentrations, but that it did correlate with brain concentrations as measured by lithium MRS. Another recent report utilizing phosphorus-31 MRS found evidence for abnormal frontal lobe metabolism in unmedicated euthymic bipolar patients as compared with healthy comparison subjects (Deichin et al. 1995).

• • •

In summary, MRI and MRS provide powerful noninvasive techniques for studying both anatomic and biological activity in a variety of conditions, as well as the impact of treatment.

Positron-emission tomography (PET).   This technique provides functional images of the brain and is particularly promising in the study of neurotransmitter systems. A positron-emitting element (e.g., fluorine-18, carbon-14, carbon-11) is incorporated into a biological compound (e.g., D-glucose), which is then administered intravenously. The distribution of the compound in different regions of the brain when the patient is at rest or engaged in a specific task is then mapped. This technique can also be used to measure receptor density in a given location. Important PET scan findings include the following:

- Reduced prefrontal metabolism and increased density of D_2 receptors in schizophrenia
- Binding of antipsychotic agents to D_2 receptors, primarily in the striatum, with this binding correlating with clinical effects
- High metabolic rates in the orbital-frontal cortex and basal ganglia of OCD patients

Single-photon emission computed tomography (SPECT). This method allows the measurement of cerebral blood flow and neurotransmitter activity when certain designated brain areas are activated by having the subjects perform specific experimental tasks (e.g., cognitive challenge tests like the Wisconsin Card Sort Test). As with PET, SPECT can visualize both cortical as well as subcortical structures. Although the pictures are not as clear as those produced by PET scan, SPECT offers a much less expensive alternative to study brain activity.

Regional cerebral blood flow (rCBF) mapping techniques. These mapping techniques use radioactive probes (e.g., xenon-13) to delineate perfusion of cortical structures. Use of these techniques has generally confirmed prefrontal cortex dysfunction in schizophrenia.

. . .

Unfortunately, these complex methodologies are not typically applied uniformly across studies, making generalizability difficult. Thus, in clinical psychiatry, brain imaging offers a modest amount of information, which is chiefly useful in differential diagnosis (Israni and Janicak 1993). In research settings, however, these imaging techniques are proving to be invaluable in clarifying the relationship between neuroanatomic loci and pathophysiology.

Neurological Testing

Electroencephalogram (EEG). This technique is most useful in differentiating some neurological disorders from psychiatric syndromes and in identifying focal cortical structural lesions (Israni and Janicak 1993; Janicak et al. 1993). In some patients with episodic, paroxysmal behavioral disturbances and a presumptive diagnosis of schizophrenia, a sleep-deprived EEG with nasopharyngeal leads may help rule out a contributing or causative epileptiform disorder. An EEG may be indicated in younger patients (especially those younger than 25) presenting with a first psychotic episode, especially if there is a history of possible cerebral injury or neurological disturbance (e.g., accidents, unconsciousness, infections, seizures). Advantages of this technique include its safety, relative inexpensiveness, and freedom from discomfort. Limitations of the EEG are numerous, however, and include the following:

- An apparently normal EEG does not exclude a neurological disorder or epilepsy.
- ECT and psychotropics and a variety of other medications can affect the EEG, making interpretation difficult at times.
- Sampling error is possible because the paroxysmal electrical activity may not have occurred during the time of recording. Sleep-deprived or 24-hr ambulatory recordings might be helpful to reduce such error.

A videocamera has also been used to define the seizure type (e.g., epileptic or psychogenic) and to quantify behavior that accompanies the aberrant electrical activity.

Studies have reported various nonspecific EEG abnormalities in disorders such as schizophrenia and major mood disorders. In addition, psychiatric patients may be more sensitive to activation procedures such as sleep-deprivation, provocative stimuli (e.g., photic stimulation with flashing strobe light), and hyperventilation. No specific EEG patterns, however, can accurately aid in the diagnosis of a particular psychiatric condition.

Computed topographic mapping of the EEG (CTM/EEG). This technique, also referred to as *brain electrical activity mapping* (BEAM), involves the recording of cortical electrical activity in certain specified frequencies, which a computer then graphically visualizes in two-dimensional, color-coded maps. This procedure is chiefly used in psychopharmacological and neuropsychological research.

Polysomnography (PSG). PSG refers to sleep recordings by which various physiological parameters are simultaneously monitored (usually at nighttime). Tests that may be carried out include an EEG, electromyogram (EMG), electro-oculogram (EOG), ECG, rapid eye movement (REM), nocturnal penile tumescence (NPT), respiratory air flow, and vital signs. In a typical sleep laboratory, a 12- to 16-channel polygraph recording is made. The uses of PSG include the following:

- Investigation and diagnosis of sleep disorders, especially sleep apnea and narcolepsy
- Research in depression (e.g., REM density, latency; total sleep time)

- Drug/alcohol withdrawal studies
- Differentiation of functional from organic causes of impotence, in part, through recording NPT

Evoked potentials. Evoked potentials are electrophysiological recordings (on the order of milliseconds, as opposed to minutes as in other brain-imaging techniques such as PET) evoked from specific cortical areas (e.g., visual, auditory, somatosensory) by discrete types of sensory stimulation (e.g., flashes of light). With this technique, the clinician can differentiate between certain organic and functional disorders (e.g., visual evoked potentials [VEPs] in suspected hysterical blindness), as well as evaluate demyelinating disorders such as multiple sclerosis. Several studies have found low-amplitude, late (greater than 250 milliseconds) auditory evoked potentials in schizophrenic patients—a finding that suggests attentional and cognitive impairment (Javitt et al. 1995; McCarley et al. 1991).

Other neurological tests. An *electroretinogram* (ERG) reflects central dopaminergic function. *Abnormalities in smooth pursuit eye tracking movements* (SPEMs) may represent vulnerability markers for psychosis in general. EMG and nerve conduction studies may help in cases where myopathies or peripheral neuropathies are suspected. *Magnetoencephalography* (MEG) is a noninvasive technique that measures the weak magnetic fields generated by the electrical activity of the brain (including the deeper subcortical areas) and converts them back into electric signals, which are then recorded.

Therapeutic Drug Monitoring

The goal of pharmacotherapy for any disease state involves achievement of maximal efficacy while minimizing adverse effects. One way to achieve this goal is by monitoring plasma medication levels. Therapeutic drug monitoring (TDM) is utilized in psychiatry to monitor levels of lithium, antidepressants, and anticonvulsants on a routine basis. For other psychotropics, such as the antipsychotics (e.g., clozapine, haloperidol), TDM is utilized less routinely.

In this section, we review the theoretical basis of the blood level–clinical efficacy correlation, point out methodological problems that may confuse the interpretation of results from plasma level–clinical response studies, and integrate data from valid studies to illustrate the clinical applicability of TDM.

Theoretical Basis

The general principles that characterize the relationship between drug plasma concentrations and efficacy are as follows:

- A concentration or range exists at which maximal pharmacological response occurs.
- There is a correlation between a drug's plasma concentration and its concentration at the putative CNS site of action.
- Genetic and environmental factors alter pharmacokinetic parameters, affecting the quantity of drug that reaches receptor sites in different individuals.

Initially, at low subthreshold plasma levels, no pharmacological response will be seen. As the plasma concentration increases and reaches threshold levels, response rapidly increases. Once optimal pharmacological levels have been achieved, further elevations in plasma concentrations will usually not enhance response. Thus, a plasma level–response relationship may, when presented graphically, assume the typical sigmoidal shape, as shown by line A in Figure 21–1. In this example, higher concentrations are often associated with a greater potential for adverse events. In summary, concentrations below the response threshold produce a less-than-optimal effect or no effect, and concentrations above a putative upper end may precipitate more prominent adverse effects.

While concentrations above the upper end of the therapeutic window may be associated with toxicity, some drugs may also lose their therapeutic effects as a result of altered pharmacodynamics. The plateau in clinical effect may be seen with some drugs that have neither

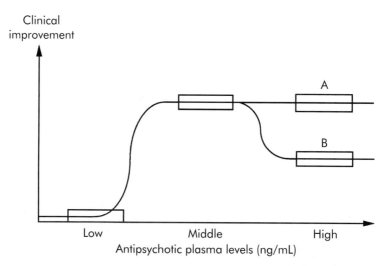

Figure 21–1. Hypothetical antipsychotic plasma level–clinical response relationship.

serious toxic effects nor loss of therapeutic action at higher concentrations. For example, data from antipsychotic plasma level studies indicate three possible outcomes that can occur at the higher concentrations:

1. No further clinical improvement (see line A in Figure 21–1)
2. Worsening because of increased adverse effects (see line B in Figure 21–1)
3. Worsening because of altered pharmcodynamics (see line B in Figure 21–1)

Drugs that produce immediate clinical effects do not require monitoring of plasma levels. For example, it is possible to observe the rapid clinical onset of pain control and adjust a narcotic's dose by monitoring the drug's effects. Conversely, with some drugs, the clinical onset of action may not occur for days to weeks after drug administration. In this scenario, if the desired plasma concentration required to produce a given effect is known, dosage regimens may be adjusted in a more timely manner to achieve the desired plasma level. Additionally, TDM is especially useful for drugs (e.g., tricyclic antidepressants) that demonstrate high interpatient variability in plasma levels on the same dose for the same diagnosis. Thus, given the large variability in plasma levels with the same dose of a psychotropic, knowledge of the potential therapeutic range for a particular agent may provide more accurate dosing guidelines as compared with empirical dosing for an individual patient.

Plasma level–clinical response studies contribute to the establishment of a minimally effective dose. Because there is a positive correlation between plasma level and response, it may be possible to estimate the average dose required to produce a desired level. Further, the time required to onset of response for many psychotropics at a given dose/plasma level is in the range of days to weeks. Thus, increasing the daily dose every few days may lead to higher-than-necessary medication doses. Although doses are frequently adjusted in response to clinical symptomatology, knowledge of the minimally effective plasma level may avoid greater-than-necessary drug exposure. Finally, TDM can be utilized to provide "fine tuning" of a dosing regimen.

Methodological Issues

The clinical applicability of results found in the plasma level–therapeutic response relationship may be confounded because of a variety of methodological problems. These problems can be grouped as relating to dosing method, assay method, patient population, and study design.

Dosing method. As noted earlier, the most insidious methodological error in serum concentration–efficacy studies is too rapid a dosage escalation when a patient is not exhibiting the expected response. Unfortunately, in this situation, a rapid escalation may obscure the lower end of the therapeutic range, because patients are not maintained on lower doses for a sufficient time to confirm a lack of response. Further, because of the lag time between initiation of drug treatment and clinical response, patients who apparently respond favorably to higher doses may have actually improved on a lower dose had they been on it for an adequate length of time.

To illustrate, consider two possible explanations for a less-than-ideal outcome. In the first scenario, lack of response may be due to a low plasma level, and dosage escalation results in a corresponding elevation in plasma level, which leads to a favorable response; but frequent dosage increases obscure the lower end of the therapeutic window. In the second scenario, lack of response may be due to treatment refractoriness despite an adequate plasma level; dosage increases result in elevations of the plasma level, but no further improvement will be achieved.

One way to avoid this confound in research trials is to utilize a fixed-dosing strategy. For example, multiple fixed doses may be utilized with patients randomly assigned regardless of baseline symptom severity to a particular dose (e.g., low, medium, or high). By using stratified fixed dosages, it is possible to investigate the lower and the upper ends of the proposed therapeutic range. Compilation of several fixed-dose studies indicating a possible therapeutic range for a given drug then allows prospective targeting of patients to plasma levels within or outside of the putative therapeutic plasma range. In this design, patients are maintained in a predetermined fixed-plasma-level range throughout the trial.

Assay method. There are two main categories of assays: chemical and biological. *Chemical assays* focus on a compound or a group of related compounds and their physiochemical characteristics in conjunction with some instrumentation. *Biological assays* are based on some biological activity of the drug (e.g., receptor blockade). In biological assays, drug concentrations are not quantified; instead, the drug's activity is transformed into a concentration equivalent. One disadvantage of biological assays is that they cannot distinguish between similarly acting compounds.

Patient population. Issues to consider regarding the patient population involve the presence of treatment-refractory patients; the impact of noncompliance, especially in outpatient treatment; and the implications of small sample sizes.

Study design. Possible biases in the design of a study include the following:

- Inadequate evaluation of clinical response, either in method of assessment or in timing of assessment
- Concurrent pharmacotherapy
- Variable time of blood sampling

Active metabolites.   Interpretation of plasma concentration–clinical response data may be clouded by the presence of active metabolites, which are produced by the majority of psychotropic medications.

Clinical Applicability

Substantial data have indicated a large interindividual variability in plasma levels achieved in patients receiving the same dose of a psychotropic medication. This finding supports the rationale for individualized monitoring of plasma drug levels to optimize therapeutic response. However, the need for large databases to establish the putative therapeutic range for each individual drug is not diminished. We believe it is imperative to examine a given plasma level in the context of the clinical picture, rather than to target slavishly to a predetermined number that falls within the proposed therapeutic range.

Therapeutic drug monitoring should be used to enhance the response to pharmacotherapy in those patients who do not respond to standard treatment approaches. Additionally, it is quite useful in other scenarios, including the following:

- When noncompliance is suspected
- For patients with a malabsorption condition
- For documenting response or lack of response to a given dose
- For minimizing the likelihood of toxicity secondary to high plasma levels
- For monitoring potential drug-drug interactions affecting steady-state concentrations or free-drug concentrations in combined therapy
- As documentation that may be utilized in potential medical-legal situations

Specific Agents

Lithium.   Traditionally within the field of psychiatry, lithium has been the medication most frequently associated with plasma level monitoring (Janicak and Davis 1987). The therapeutic window for lithium, albeit narrow, is well established. For the control of an acute manic episode, levels of 0.5 mEq/L on the low end and 1.5 mEq/L on the high end are to be targeted. As a general rule, 1.0 mEq/L is optimal for control of an acute manic episode, if tolerated by the patient. There can be large interpatient variability in terms of response and development of side effects or toxicity, however, thus necessitating close monitoring, at least initially. For healthy adults, a lithium plasma level is obtained after 4–5 half-lives (approximately 4–6 days) on a given dose before making dosage adjustments. Levels should be monitored more frequently in those individuals exhibiting unexpected responses or in those with renal impairment. Samples should be obtained 10 to 12 hours after the last lithium dose.

After resolution of an acute episode, for maintenance of the patient with bipolar disorder, lithium levels of at least 0.8 mEq/L are ideal and should be obtained every 3 to 6 months, or more frequently if clinically indicated. Additional laboratory examinations include thyroid function tests, blood urea nitrogen (BUN), serum creatinine, and an ECG when indicated.

Anticonvulsants. Currently, there is a lack of data to establish the ideal anticonvulsant serum concentrations in the treatment of psychiatric disorders, and clinicians generally employ ranges that are used for seizure control. TDM can be utilized, however, to enhance the efficacy and minimize the toxicity of anticonvulsants, to monitor compliance, and to assess and adjust for potential drug-drug interactions.

Carbamazepine levels should be monitored weekly during the initial dosage adjustment period and then every 3 months with maintenance therapy. Therapeutic plasma levels range from 4 to 15 µg/mL and must be monitored carefully after initial stabilization because of the potential for autometabolism by stimulation of the cytochrome P450 isoenzyme system. Because of potentially serious hematologic adverse effects (e.g., aplastic anemia, agranulocytosis), a CBC with a differential should be obtained at baseline, at the end of the dosage adjustment period, then monthly for 2 months, and then as indicated. More important, patients should be educated about the early warnings of hematologic disturbances, including easy bruising, malaise, sore throat, and increased temperature. The chemistry profile and serum electrolytes should be monitored at least every 12 months, in part because of the potential to develop the syndrome of inappropriate antidiuretic hormone (SIADH).

Divalproex sodium levels should be obtained weekly during initial dosage adjustments and then every 3 to 6 months for maintenance therapy. CBC with a differential, in addition to a chemistry profile, should be obtained at baseline and monitored monthly for 3 months and then at least yearly. Monitoring for signs and symptoms of hepatotoxicity such as malaise, weakness, lethargy, nausea, vomiting, and facial edema is essential, particularly during the first 6 months of treatment. The correlations between divalproex sodium dose, serum concentration, and efficacy have not been fully established; however, the therapeutic range for most psychiatric patients is thought to be between 50 and 150 µg/mL.

Antidepressants. One should consider obtaining an antidepressant plasma level for the following scenarios:

- When noncompliance is suspected
- When there is a poor response to a standard dose, possibly secondary to unexpected pharmacokinetics (e.g., slow or fast metabolizers)
- When there is poor medication tolerance, particularly at lower doses
- For patients who are more susceptible to adverse effects or toxicity, such as the elderly, children or adolescents, and the medically ill
- For patients whose therapeutic plasma level is urgently needed (e.g., severely suicidal or severely psychotic)
- For assessment of drug-drug interactions (e.g., tricyclic antidepressant augmentation with a selective serotonin reuptake inhibitor [SSRI] in refractory depression)

Some data support a correlation between plasma concentrations and response for nortriptyline, desipramine, imipramine, and amitriptyline. Studies assessing nortriptyline have found a curvilinear relationship, with desired plasma levels between 50 and 170 ng/mL. The remaining heterocyclics mentioned usually demonstrate a threshold relationship. The proposed thresholds for desipramine, imipramine, and amitriptyline are 110–160 ng/mL, 80–150 ng/mL, and above 265 ng/mL, respectively (Janicak et al. 1993).

TDM for second-generation antidepressants (e.g., SSRIs, nefazodone, venlafaxine) is usually unnecessary and not recommended, because there are no data to support a correlation between their plasma concentrations and response or toxicity. In general, these agents have a wide therapeutic range, which minimizes the need to monitor their levels.

Lastly, the pharmacokinetic parameters of specific agents also preclude the use of TDM in a rational manner. For example, clinical response to fluoxetine is often established prior to the time required to achieve a steady-state plasma concentration because of the long half-life of the drug and of its primary metabolite, norfluoxetine (1–3 days and 7–15 days, respectively). Prior to switching from this agent to a monoamine oxidase inhibitor (MAOI), however, it is necessary to obtain plasma-level data for both fluoxetine and norfluoxetine to ensure their complete elimination.

The MAOIs are generally reserved for use in refractory or atypical depression. Although there are no data to support a plasma drug concentration–response correlation, evidence suggests that response may be correlated with at least 60%–80% platelet MAO inhibition (Bresnahan et al. 1990; Stern et al. 1980).

Antipsychotics. Currently, there are no established guidelines for measuring therapeutic serum concentrations of antipsychotics. Haloperidol and fluphenazine have been the most widely studied conventional neuroleptics in terms of a serum concentration–clinical response relationship. For example, Levinson and colleagues (1995) found that fluphenazine responders showed the greatest improvement with plasma levels above 1.0 ng/mL. Marder and co-workers (1991) found that plasma levels lower than than 0.5 ng/mL were associated with significantly higher relapse rates. Finally, Dysken and colleagues (1981) reported that levels ranging from 0.2 to 2.8 ng/mL were efficacious. Therefore, fluphenazine levels between 0.5 ng/mL and 2.8 ng/mL may be the optimal range for the treatment of many psychotic disorders.

Multiple studies have addressed the relationship between serum concentrations of haloperidol and of its active metabolite (reduced haloperidol) and clinical effect. Although results have varied, the therapeutic range is thought to be between 3 and 18 ng/mL (Janicak et al. 1993). In general, levels above 18 ng/mL may be associated with an increase of side effects, without further improvement in clinical condition.

Our research group has studied three haloperidol plasma-level ranges (i.e., low, middle, and high) in the treatment of acutely psychotic patients (Janicak et al., in press). During the first 2-week treatment phase, no differences in clinical response were found among the three groups. During the second phase, nonresponders were randomly assigned to remain in their original plasma-level range or move to an alternative range. In this phase, nonresponders from the low, middle, and high groups who were reassigned to or remained in the middle group demonstrated greater improvement as compared with those patients who were not. These data indicate that 1) a low plasma level is sufficient for many patients; 2) in initial nonresponders, response may be enhanced by plasma levels averaging 10 to 12 ng/mL; and 3) higher plasma levels are unnecessary.

Clozapine.   Clozapine is unique with respect to all other antipsychotics in terms of efficacy spectrum, extrapyramidal symptom potential, and adverse effects. In the United States, mandatory weekly CBC with differential must be obtained prior to dispensing a 1-week supply of medication because of the increased risk of agranulocytosis. Weekly monitoring is performed throughout clozapine treatment and for 4 weeks after discontinuation.

Recently, investigations have begun to assess the relationship between clozapine serum concentrations and treatment response. Perry and colleagues (1991) found that response to clozapine was greater in patients whose parent compound serum concentrations were above 350 ng/mL as compared with those who had serum levels below this putative threshold. Others have found that clozapine plasma levels ≥ 450 ng/mL may be necessary to achieve an optimal response (Meltzer 1992).

Antianxiety/sedative-hypnotics. In general practice, therapeutic drug monitoring is not necessary for antianxiety and sedative-hypnotic agents because of their large therapeutic index. When cases of abuse or toxicity are suspected, monitoring of plasma concentrations may be clinically indicated. Some data have shown that a threshold plasma level of alprazolam (i.e., > 40 ng/mL) may be necessary to control symptoms of panic disorder (Shader and Greenblatt 1993).

Conclusion

The 1990s have been called the "decade of the brain." Researchers continue to use state-of-the-art techniques to search for biological correlates of psychopathology. In turn, these new findings may lead to the development of new pharmacotherapies and a more complete understanding of the pathogenesis and causation of psychiatric disorders.

The laboratory will continue to play an ever-increasing role in psychiatry as our technology and knowledge progresses. Currently, laboratory assessments are useful in the following:

- Identifying medical disorders in patients with prominent psychiatric symptomatology (e.g., cognitive, affective, or behavioral changes) or identifying medical/neurological syndromes that may present with psychiatric symptoms.
- Conducting initial and follow-up assessment for specific pharmacotherapy.
- Individualizing treatment by monitoring therapeutic drug concentrations.

It is vital for clinicians to judiciously utilize laboratory tests for a particular individual, keeping in mind the economic impact, degree of discomfort, and risk of adverse drug events. Interpretation of laboratory results must be made in conjunction with knowledge of a given method's limitations, such as specificity, sensitivity, and predictive value. Lastly, to ensure an accurate diagnosis and development of an appropriate treatment plan, laboratory data must be integrated with the patient's history, a thorough interview, and a physical examination.

References

Anfinson TJ, Kathol RG: Screening laboratory evaluation in psychiatric patients: a review. Gen Hosp Psychiatry 14:248–257, 1992

Åsberg M, Thorén P, Träskman L: "Serotonin depression"—a biochemical subgroup within the affective disorders. Science 191:478–480, 1976a

Åsberg M, Träskman L, Thorén P: 5-HIAA in the cerebrospinal fluid: a biochemical suicide predictor? Arch Gen Psychiatry 33:1193–1197, 1976b

Arana GW, Baldessarini RJ, Ornstein M: The DST for diagnosis and prognosis in psychiatry. Arch Gen Psychiatry 42:1193–1204, 1985

Bresnahan DB, Pandey GN, Janicak PG, et al: MAO inhibition and clinical response in depressed patients treated with phenelzine. J Clin Psychiatry 51:47–49, 1990

Brodie JD: Imaging for the clinical psychiatrist: facts, fantasies, and other musings (editorial). Am J Psychiatry 153:145–149, 1996

Charles HC, Lazeyras F, Boyko O, et al: Elevated choline concentrations in basal ganglia of depressed patients. Biol Psychiatry 31(5A):99A, 1992

Charles HC, Lazeyras, Krishnan KR, et al: Brain choline in depression: in vivo detection of potential pharmacodynamic effects of antidepressant therapy using hydrogen localized spectroscopy. Prog Neuropsychopharmacol Biol Psychiatry 18:1121–1127, 1994

Deichin RF, Fein G, Weiner MW: Abnormal frontal lobe phosphorus metabolism in bipolar disorder. Am J Psychiatry 152:915–918, 1995

Dysken M, Javaid J, Chang S, et al: Fluphenazine pharmacokinetics and therapeutic response. Psychopharmacology (Berl) 73:205–210, 1981

Farde L, Nordstrom AL, Wiesel FA, et al: Positron emission tomographic analysis of central D_1 and D_2 dopamine receptor occupancy in patients treated with classical neuroleptics and clozapine. Arch Gen Psychiatry 49:538–544, 1992

Israni TH, Janicak PG: Laboratory assessment in psychiatry, in Psychiatry: Diagnosis and Therapy. Edited by Flaherty J, Davis JM, Janicak PG. Norwalk, CT, Appleton & Lange, 1993, pp 30–39

Janicak PG, Davis JM: Clinical usage of lithium in mania, in Antimanics, Anticonvulsants and Other Drugs in Psychiatry. Edited by Barrows GD, Norman TR, Davies B. Amsterdam, Elsevier, 1987, pp 21–34

Janicak PG, Davis JM, Preskorn SH, et al: Principles and Practice of Psychopharmacotherapy. Baltimore, MD, Williams & Wilkins, 1993, pp 14–21

Janicak PG, Javaid JI, Sharma RP, et al: A double-blind randomized study of three haloperidol plasma levels for acute psychosis. Acta Psychiatr Scand (in press)

Javitt DC, Doneshka P, Grochowski S, et al: Impaired mismatch negativity generation reflects widespread dysfunction of working memory in schizophrenia. Arch Gen Psychiatry 52:550–558, 1995

Kato T, Inubashi T, Takahashi S: Relationship of lithium concentrations in the brain measured by lithium-7 magnetic resonance spectroscopy to treatment response in mania. J Clin Psychopharmacol 14:330–335, 1994

Klemm E, Grunwald F, Kasper S, et al: [^{123}I]-1BZM SPECT for imaging of striatal D_2 dopamine receptors in 56 schizophrenic patients taking various neuroleptics. Am J Psychiatry 153:183–190, 1996

Levinson DF, Simpson GM, Lo ES, et al: Fluphenazine plasma levels, dosage, efficacy, and side effects. Am J Psychiatry 152:765–771, 1995

Malone KM, Corbitt EM, Li S, et al: Prolactin response to fenfluramine and suicide attempt lethality in major depression. Br J Psychiatry 168:324–329, 1996

Marder SR, Midha KK, Van Putten T, et al: Plasma levels of fluphenazine in patients receiving fluphenazine decanoate: relationship to clinical response. Br J Psychiatry 158:658–665, 1991

McCarley RW, Faux SF, Shenton ME, et al: Event related potentials in schizophrenia: their biological and clinical correlates and a new model of schizophrenic pathophysiology. Schizophr Res 4:209–231, 1991

Meltzer HY: Treatment of the neuroleptic-nonresponsive schizophrenic patient. Schizophr Bull 18:515–542, 1992

Pandey GN, Pandey SC, Dwivedi Y, et al: Platelet serotonin-2A receptors: a potential biological marker for suicidal behavior. Am J Psychiatry 152:850–855, 1995

Perry P, Miller D, Arndt S, et al: Clozapine and norclozapine concentrations and clinical response in treatment-refractory schizophrenic patients. Am J Psychiatry 148:231–235, 1991

Renshaw PF, Stoll AL, Rothschild A, et al: Multiple brain LH MRS abnormalities in depressed patients suggest impaired second messenger cycling. Biol Psychiatry 33(6A):44A, 1993

Shader RI, Greenblatt DJ: Use of benzodiazepines in anxiety disorders. N Engl J Med 328:1398–1405, 1993

Sharma RP, Javaid J, Janicak PG, et al: Plasma and CSF HVA before and after pharmacological treatment. Psychiatry Res 28:91–104, 1988

Sharma RP, Venkatasubramanian PN, Barany M, et al: Proton magnetic resonance spectroscopy of the brain in schizophrenic and affective patients. Schizophr Res 8:43–49, 1992

Silbersweig DA, Stern E, Frith C, et al: A funtional neuroanatomy of hallucinations in schizophrenia. Nature 378(9):176–179, 1995

Stern SL, Rush AJ, Mendels J: Toward a rational pharmacotherapy of depression. Am J Psychiatry 137:545–552, 1980

Wisniewski KE, French JH, Fernandos S, et al: Fragile X syndrome: associated neurological abnormalities and developmental disabilities. Ann Neurol 18:665–669, 1985

Chapter 22

Psychological Assessment in a Managed Care Climate: The Neuropsychological Evaluation

Steven Mattis, Ph.D., and Barbara C. Wilson, Ph.D.

In this era of managed care, as the behavioral health system attempts to take on the full fiscal risk for such healthcare services, the role of the consultant and specialist takes on immediate fiscal import. The understanding that the managed care community will reimburse for necessary services that are provided by appropriately trained and credentialed professionals is implicit in the contract between the health service providers and the providers of managed care reimbursement plans. However, the insurers have clearly indicated that there is an emphasis on cost containment and on the cost-effectiveness of any services for which they will provide reimbursement. Psychiatrists today must make a judgment as to the probability that a referral or consultation will result in information that will be useful in the development of a treatment plan or will alter the one being entertained. The cost of such a consultation must now be carefully weighed against the benefit to be accrued in terms of accuracy of diagnosis and efficiency of treatment. It is with these considerations in mind that we consider in this chapter the clinical circumstances that favor the request for neuropsychological evaluation.

Description of a Neuropsychological Evaluation

A position paper prepared as a collaborative effort by the New York Neuropsychology Group (LeFever 1996) provides a concise description of the neuropsychological neurodiagnostic examination:

> The neuropsychological examination is one of the methods of diagnosing neurodevelopmental, neurodegenerative and acquired disorders of brain function. It is frequently a part of the overall neurodiagnostic assessment which includes other neurometric techniques such as the CT [computed tomography], MRI [magnetic resonance imaging], EEG [electroencephalogram], SPECT [single-photon emission computed tomography]. The purpose of the neuropsychological examination is to assess the clinical relationship between the brain/central nervous system (CNS) and behav-

ioral dysfunction. It is a neurodiagnostic, consultative service and NOT a mental health/psychological evaluation or psychiatric treatment service.

The Social Service Administration defines neuropsychological testing as the "administration of standardized tests that are reliable and valid with respect to assessing impairment in brain functioning." The examination is performed by a qualified neuropsychologist who has undergone specialized education and intensive training in the clinical neurosciences, including the relationship between behavioral functions and neuroanatomy, neurology, and neurophysiology. The neuropsychologist works closely with the primary or consultant physicians in assessing patient cerebral status. Neuropsychological services are designated as "medicine, diagnostic" by the federal Health Care Financing Administration (HCFA), are subsumed under "Central Nervous System Assessments" in the 1996 CTP Code Book, and have corresponding ICD diagnoses.

Neuropsychological examinations are clinically indicated and medically necessary when patients display signs and symptoms of intellectual compromise, cognitive and/or neurobehavioral dysfunction that involve, but are not restricted to[,] memory deficits, language disorders, learning disabilities, developmental disabilities, pervasive developmental disorders, impairment of organization and planning, difficulty with cognition, and perceptual abnormalities. Frequent etiologies include: head trauma, stroke, tumor, infectious disease, toxic exposure, metabolic abnormalities, autoimmune disease, genetic defects, prenatal, perinatal, neonatal complications and neurodegenerative disease. The examination entails the taking of an extensive history (including review of medical records) and the administration of a screening assessment or a comprehensive evaluation that can take many hours and requires intensive data analysis. Consultation with other medical professionals such as neurologists, neurosurgeons, pediatricians, psychiatrists, and radiologists is common. The sensitivity of the neuropsychological tests is such that they often reveal abnormality in the absence of positive findings on the CT and MRI scan. Moreover, it can identify patterns of impairment that are not determinable through other procedures, leading to appropriate treatment recommendations. . . .

Neuropsychological Assessment as a Cost-Effective Measure

There are specific areas in which neuropsychological assessment becomes a cost-saving measure. Such assessment can affect the course and efficacy of treatment by providing new information to the treating psychiatrist that is relevant to the diagnostic formulation. Further, by defining the areas of cognitive function and dysfunction, the neuropsychologist provides a baseline for decision making regarding appropriate treatment approaches and a baseline for assessment over time of efficacy of intervention. The amount of new information to be obtained from a psychological assessment and its direct relevance to treatment vary as a function of the domain of psychological function-ing to be evaluated, the treatment setting, and the reason for referral. In general, a referral for a neuropsychological evaluation is a most rele-vant referral, because it typically contains a request for the assessment of psychological domains not directly addressed in the psychiatric evaluation.

Although both psychiatry and neuropsychology deal with disorders of behavior, there is generally little overlap in the functional areas as-sessed in the psychiatric and neuropsychological evaluations. The psy-chiatric and neuropsychological evaluations do not substitute for each other; rather, they complement each other. Information obtained from the neuropsychologist may be useful in the diagnostic formulation, thereby enhancing both the probability of an appropriate prescription or proscription of specific treatment modalities and the probability of success—a most effective cost-effective outcome. For example, the documentation of a significant neurogenic language disorder rather than a hypothesized "selective mutism" would give the clinician reason for pause before recommending traditional psychotherapy, saving wear and tear on the therapist, the patient, and the managed care plan.

Neuropsychological Assessment of Adult Psychiatric Patients

In general, one assesses neurocognitive abilities in psychiatric patients for one of several reasons, among which are

- To document a specific disorder in cognition referable to a specific class of psychiatric disorders (e.g., intrusion into thought of task-irrelevant items in patients who complain of delusional or obsessive ideation, or disturbances in recall in patients with major affective disorders)
- To assist in differential diagnosis by documenting disorders in cognitive skills referable to alternative or concomitant neurogenic disorders (e.g., discriminating between a thought disorder and a language disorder or the mnemonic deficits of a depression vs. a dementia)
- To evaluate the effects of psychopharmacological intervention on neurocognitive function

Whether one is documenting specific neurocognitive deficits or is concerned about differential diagnosis, a neuropsychological assess-ment is focused on the systematic evaluation of neurocognitive func-tions. There are occasions when a brief screening battery is sufficient to answer the referral question, and in keeping with the cost-containment issue, such a screening battery should be administered when appropriate. There are other occasions when a more detailed evaluation is necessary and, in the long run, also cost-effective.

More specifically, most neuropsychological assessments of cognitive processes evaluate the presence of disorders of the following abilities: general intelligence, attention and concentration, memory and learning, perception, language, conceptualization, constructional skills, executive-motor processes, and affect. The age of the patient and the referral issue can frame the initial phase of the evaluation. The age of the patient will dictate the use of certain measures over others because of the specificity of age-related normative data. The referral issue assists in the development of initial hypotheses; a referral that had to do with neurocognitive function in a patient who had sustained a left temporal stroke and a referral of a patient for a differential diagnosis between a developmental language disorder and an autistic spectrum disorder would dictate the selection of a different set of initial measures.

Reasons for Referral

By far the most common referral in both inpatient and outpatient settings is to aid in the *differential diagnosis of early dementia versus mild delirium versus depression*. Each of the three clinical entities presents its own pattern of cognitive disorders embedded in a large number of shared cognitive deficits. The modal neuropsychological profile in *early Alzheimer s disease* demonstrates a marked memory disorder for recent events observed on both verbal and nonverbal memory tasks and on both free recall and recognition memory paradigms. Recognition memory refers to the individual's ability to recognize as familiar recently experienced stimuli from among semantically or physically similar stimuli. Delayed recall and recognition memory is especially impaired. In addition, one is likely to find a marked linguistic disorder, most typically a nominal aphasia and fluency deficits, and/or deficits on tasks requiring executive processes. Attentional processes are not markedly affected in the early stages.

The hallmark of a delirium, a *confusional state*, is exceptionally inefficient and widely fluctuating arousal and attention. With highly variable attentional processes, a mildly delirious individual will perform very unpredictably on standard tests of cognition. For example, performance on all tasks requiring sustained attention, even though the task purports to measure a different cognitive skill, will be disrupted. Given the fluctuating nature of attentional processes, performance levels often cannot be replicated for the same individual in the same session.

The major diagnostic aspects of a *clinical depression* are, of course, the cognitive, behavioral, and vegetative features. Among the cognitive findings in unipolar depression are disorders in concentration and memory, motor slowing, deficits in visuospatial or constructional skills, and tasks requiring sustained mental effort. The memory disorder with unipolar depression differs from that observed with dementia in that though free recall of recent events can be every bit as impaired as in dementia, recognition memory is quite robust. Moreover, delayed recall and recognition tend to reveal a normal "decay of trace," whereas dementia involves rapid rates of forgetting. The content of remembered material tends to be unpleasant, and, in controlled studies, depressed patients tend to remember unpleasant stimuli better than pleasant material, and at normal or near-normal levels. On vigilance or recognition memory tasks, it has been consistently observed that depressed patients, when uncertain, tend to have a very conservative response bias, saying "no" more than "yes" and being very unwilling to identify incorrectly a stimulus as a previously experienced (target) item. Dementia patients, in contrast, throw caution to the wind, tending toward a very liberal response bias; they say "yes" an inordinate number of times and thereby commit an inordinate number of errors of commission or false alarms. The examination therefore concentrates on the intensive evaluation of 1) attentional processes, 2) encoding, storage, and retrieval of new information, 3) differential processing of the hedonic tone of information, and 4) a review of linguistic, constructional, and executive processes.

The second most common referral is to aid in understanding the cognitive and affective status of an individual *post–head injury.* Traumatic brain injury consists of both diffuse axonal and multifocal impairment, the psychiatric manifestation of which will depend on 1) premorbid cognitive, psychosocial, and psychiatric status, 2) the nature and distribution of the CNS lesion, 3) the course and time since injury, and 4) the nature and extent of collateral support. The head trauma patient who comes to psychiatric attention generally presents with significant behavioral disturbance with intermittent rage and impulsivity and/or anergia and anhedonia. Although the assessment of a broad range of higher cortical functions is initially necessary for baseline evaluation and eventual assessment of the recovery course, the focus of assessment for the patient presenting with psychiatric symptomatology should be more circumscribed. The limiting factors in any systematic psychiatric intervention are not the extent of language, visuospatial, motor, or conceptual deficits, but rather the nature and magnitude of memory and executive function disorders.

Neuropsychological assessment is sensitive to changes in neurocognitive function and therefore is useful in the evaluation of the effects of psychopharmacological agents. When an appropriate set of repeatable measures are selected, it is possible to assess for effects of drug toxicity as well as for positive treatment effects. It becomes possible, therefore, to alert the treating clinician to the need for reevaluation of a prescribed medication or to provide data that support the treatment in progress. The benefits to the patient are clear in such situations; the benefits to the managed care planner lie in the possibility of a shorter treatment period, given an appropriate treatment plan, and in the diminished need for prolonged "trial and error" approaches to the prescription of psychopharmacological agents or other treatment modalities.

Approaches to Neuropsychological Assessment

In many clinical settings, the areas of higher cortical functions of interest are assessed by a formal, fixed battery of tests. Two such standardized neuropsychological batteries are the Halstead-Reitan (Boll 1981) and the Luria-Nebraska (Golden et al. 1978). In its present form, the Halstead-Reitan Neuropsychological Battery (Reed et al. 1965) consists of five tests that yield seven summary scores and a total impairment index. It includes measures of executive function, tactile perception, speech sounds perception, the Seashore rhythm test, and a finger oscillation test. A group of tests referred to as allied procedures are frequently included as part of the total examination. The entire evaluation typically takes from 4 to 6 hours, depending on the number of ancillary procedures (i.e., intelligence and academic performance) included. The reliability and validity of the tests are well established, and normative data for most comparisons of interest in clinical psychiatric populations are available.

A second widely used battery of procedures has been developed from the work of Luria (1966, 1973). Christensen (1975) was instrumental in bringing Luria's stimuli and procedures to the attention of neuropsychologists outside the former Soviet Union. Golden and his colleagues (1978) have been the primary proponents of developers of a standardized neuropsychological instrument using Christensen's published material. In its present form, the Luria-Nebraska covers the areas of motor function, rhythm (and pitch) skills, tactile and visual functions, receptive and expressive speech, writing, reading and arithmetic skills, memory, and intelligence. The complete examination consists of 269 items that yield raw scores in each area. Three additional scores for right- and left-hemisphere impairment and a pathognomonic score are computed.

Both the Halstead-Reitan and the Luria-Nebraska batteries are oriented toward an extensive evaluation of neuropsychological functioning, and in clinical practice they are typically supplemented with instruments that allow a more flexible test approach and a more intensive focus on areas of possible dysfunction. The neuropsychological areas of interest and appropriate assessment procedures are given below.

Premorbid intelligence.   A number of inferences as to the presence of neuropsychological deficits are based on observed discrepancies between present functioning and estimated premorbid abilities. Premorbid intelligence may be estimated by assessing those cognitive abilities that do not deteriorate with dementing processes. These include the *general fund of information and vocabulary,* as measured by the respective subtests of the Wechsler Adult Intelligence Scale—Revised (WAIS-R; Wechsler 1981), and *reading recognition,* as measured by the revised Wide Range Achievement Test (WRAT-3; Jastak and Wilkinson 1981) or the Nelson Adult Reading Test (Nelson 1982), which has new North American norms and with which reasonable validity has been demonstrated. It is also common to estimate premorbid intelligence on the basis of educational background. The validity of a number of different estimates of premorbid intelligence based on demographic data has been demonstrated (Karzmark et al. 1985). Premorbid intelligence may be estimated by assessing those cognitive abilities that do not rapidly deteriorate with dementing processes, such as the general fund of information and vocabulary subtests of the WAIS-R, in addition to the measures noted earlier.

General intellectual abilities.   In general, most psychological assessments include both an estimate of premorbid general intellectual abilities and some measure of present intellectual abilities in order to gauge the severity of disturbance of cognition. The most commonly used measure of general intelligence is the WAIS-R. The WAIS-R, which takes about 1 hour to administer, contains 11 subtests and offers a Verbal, Performance, and Full Scale Intelligence Quotient (IQ). Because of the length of administration, abbreviated versions of this measure are often employed, in which either only some of the subtests are used or fewer of the specific items are used and each response is weighted. Alternatively, different briefer measures, such as the Ammons Quick Test (Ammons and Ammons 1962) and the Institute of Living Scale (Shipley 1946), may be used.

Attentional disorders.   Attentional disorders are among the most common findings in psychiatric patients, since attention and concentration will be affected by both psychologically determined processes such as anxiety, depression, and personal preoccupations and neurogenic compromise of brain stem and limbic structures because of toxic-metabolic disorders, direct structural impairment, or neurophysiologically determined substrates. In adults, attentional processes are most commonly measured by the WAIS-R subtests constituting the "distractibility" triad: Digit Span, mental Arithmetic, and Digit Symbol. In addition, several variations of these procedures and other specialized procedures are commonly used. Cancellation tasks are available, in which the patient is required to cross out a given letter or design presented within rows of randomly distributed other letters or designs. An advantage of such tasks is that they can be strung together to form a lengthy continuous performance task of 10 to 15 minutes, and variation in accuracy across discrete 20-second epochs can be determined. A popular continuous performance test developed by Rosvold (Mirsky and Kornetsky 1964; Rosvold et al. 1956) has been modified and adapted for computer-assisted presentation. The advantage to this computer-assisted approach to the measure of attention lies in its flexibility and the accuracy with which stimuli can be presented and responses recorded. One can measure reaction time of each response and note fluctuations in reaction time over the duration of the task. One can systematically alter stimulus characteristics, such as stimulus duration, speed of presentation, and even size of target and duration of task.

Memory and learning disorders.   It is interesting to note that none of the subtests of the WAIS-R measure the nature and severity of memory and learning disorders that occur in patients with amnesic and dementia syndromes. In fact, in studies of classical alcoholic Korsakoff syndromes (patients with profound amnesic syndromes), care is taken to select clinical subjects whose performance on the WAIS-R are clearly within normal limits. The memory disorder of particular interest to the clinician is the one that affects "recent" memory and is generally referable to impairment of limbic system functioning. Operationally, one seeks to present the patient with a specific set of stimuli or events and then divert attention so that the stimuli cannot be rehearsed. The patient is then required to demonstrate that the target information has been encoded and stored by either reproducing the material or recognizing it among distracter items. Thus, recall of brief paragraphs or reproduction of geometric designs from memory is often used to assess mnemonic processes. Among the most commonly used standard tests of memory are the Wechsler Memory Scale—Revised (Wechsler 1987), which presents both verbal and nonverbal material as the to-be-remembered items, and the Benton Test of Visual Retention (Benton 1955), which presents only geometric designs.

Free recall of recent events has been found to be among the most sensitive of memory process. Unfortunately, in many instances, free recall has been found to be quite fragile and vulnerable to disruption because of affective arousal, depression, and motivational factors, and therefore many "false positives" may occur when one is discriminating between neurogenic and diagnostic considerations. It has been suggested that mechanisms other than free recall might be used to assess the integrity of encoding and storage processes.

Recognition memory techniques, in which the patient is asked to detect a recently presented word or design from among distracter items, have been successfully used to discriminate patients with major affective disorders from those with organic amnesias such as that associated with progressive dementia. In patients presenting with a major depression, for example, free recall might be quite consonant with that of patients with Alzheimer's disease; however, recognition memory remains intact and consonant with that of normal control subjects. It should be noted that neurological patients with focal lesions might present only a verbal or nonverbal recent memory defect, depending on the locus of lesion. It is, therefore, only in patients with bilateral or diffuse neurogenic impairment that one finds amnesic disorders in both realms. Thus, both verbal and nonverbal memory must be assessed independently, with the finding of asymmetric dysfunction strongly suggesting focal neurological impairment (Mattis et al. 1978; Squire and Shimamura 1986).

Perceptual deficits.   When care is taken to exclude significant problem-solving components from the task, and the presence of concurrent toxic-metabolic disorders is ruled out, there is little evidence for a high prevalence of perceptual deficits in a psychiatric population. However, because premorbid neuropsychological deficits may be present, related or unrelated to the presenting psychiatric problem, it is appropriate to assess the level of function in this important area. Within a psychiatric framework, this is most frequently approached by noting the integrity of perceptual processes as measured by more complex tasks given for other psychological screening purposes—for example, with above-average performance on complex constructional tasks or drawings or excellent "form level" in response to the ambiguously organized Rorschach blots. A neuropsychological approach would suggest the use of measures designed specifically for the purpose of assessing perceptual functions, such as the Benton Line Orientation Test (Benton et al. 1975), which requires the patient to match a target line at a given orientation to true vertical, with alternative lines presented at various orientations. Another such test is the Benton Face Recognition Test (Benton and Van Allen 1968), in which a photograph of a face is presented as the target and the patient is requested to detect this face from alternatives. Both of these tests have good validation as measures of the integrity of posterior cerebral, primarily nondominant hemisphere, functioning.

Auditory perception tends to be difficult to assess without hardware. However, nowadays, the fidelity available in small, portable "walkman"-type tape recorders with ear phones affords the clinician a wide range of excellent auditory stimuli. Tests such as the Goldman-Fristoe-Woodcock Test of Auditory Discrimination (Goldman et al. 1970) allow for the assessment of the efficiency of speech sound detection with and without background noise. Subtests of the Seashore Measures of

Musical Talents—Revised (Seashore et al. 1960), especially the timbre discrimination and tonal memory subtests, have been used as measures of auditory perception of nonverbal material.

The study of disorders of somatosensory perception has a long history in the field of psychophysics, and the techniques evolved from this early literature constitute a large part of the standard neuropsychological examination for peripheral and CNS disorder. Measures of pressure threshold (in which filaments of increasing caliber and stiffness, such as the Von Frey hairs, and Semmes-Ghent-Weinstein pressure esthesiometer are used), two-point discrimination, joint position sense, finger agnosia, finger order and differentiation, graphesthesia, and stereognosis are common assessment procedures for the presence of disorders of parietal lobe functioning.

Disorders of language. Among the more sensitive indices of neurogenic impairment is the presence of a language disorder. For almost all right-handed individuals and half of left-handed individuals, focal or diffuse impairment of the left hemisphere is likely to result in an aphasia (i.e., a disorder of language comprehension and/or usage). Moreover, the study of the aphasias provides some of the "hardest" evidence in the mental status examination of the presence and locus of brain impairment. There are many well-constructed tests for the assessment of aphasia. In general, all such tests are multidimensional, consisting of measures of verbal-labeling or word-finding skills, language comprehension, imitative speech, and motor-expressive speech. Many such tests also include specific measures of reading and writing. Among the most commonly used multifactorial instruments are the Multilingual Aphasia Examination (Benton and Hamsher 1976), Neurosensory Center Comprehensive Examination for Aphasia (Benton and Spreen 1969), and Boston Diagnostic Aphasia Examination (Goodglass and Kaplan 1972). Among the most widely used screening instruments for the assessment of aphasia is the Halstead-Wepman Aphasia Screening Test (Halstead and Wepman 1959).

Conceptualization disorders. The question as to whether or not the patient can assume an abstract attitude is often critical to the diagnosis and to treatment planning. This question arises most often when the differential diagnostic considerations include diffuse brain damage and, to some degree, schizophrenia. Perhaps the most direct measure of the concept of abstract or categorical thinking is the Similarities subtest of the WAIS-R, in which the patient is presented with perceptually dissimilar items and asked to determine the category to which the items both belong (e.g., "How are North and West alike?"). Proverb explanation has a long history in the psychiatric mental status exam as a task designed to measure abstract reasoning and is included among the items of the Comprehension subtest of the WAIS-R (e.g., "Shallow brooks are noisy"). However, some consider explanation of proverbs too dependent on general intellectual abilities and sociocultural factors to be a specific measure of concreteness of thought. Analogic reasoning can also be gauged with tasks such as the Conceptual Level Analogies Test (Willner 1971) for verbal reasoning and the Raven Standard Progressive Matrices (Raven 1960) for nonverbal or spatial analogic reasoning. Two measures of concept formation arising from the neuropsychological literature have recently been applied to psychiatric patients. The data to date indicate that schizophrenic patients, like patients with frontal lobe lesions, have particular difficulty with the booklet form of the Category Test (DeFilippis et al. 1979) and the Wisconsin Card Sort Test (Berg 1948; Heaton 1981).

Constructional disorders. Perhaps the quickest estimate of the integrity of the CNS can be obtained by asking the patient to draw a complex figure. Posterior sensory, central spatial, and anterior planning, monitoring, and simple motor skills must all be intact, integrated, and appropriately sequenced for this task to be successfully completed. One can alter the degree to which psychological and dynamic factors and initiative or executive planning play a role by modulating both task structure and design complexity. For example, asking the patient to draw a person or draw his or her family requires a maximum level of planning, initiative, and decision making, does not put any limit on the degree of complexity of the figures, and chooses a subject matter fraught with complex feelings and attitudes. Patients without structural impairment but with conflictual feelings about family or disordered thinking affecting planning and execution will have difficulty on such tasks. However, asking a patient to draw a clock and to set the hands to a specific time (e.g., 10 to 11:00) also requires complex planning and initiative but without the conflictual overlay. Similarly, asking the patient to copy a complex design—for example, the Rey-Osterreith figure (Rey 1941)—minimizes initiative; limits, but does not eliminate, planning; and maintains assessment of high levels of spatial constructional skills. Contrasting the patient's figure drawing to his or her clock and copy of geometric figures often allows valid inferences as to the presence and locus of CNS impairment and the degree to which affective and psychiatric factors impair otherwise intact cognitive skills. Quite often, construction tasks other than drawing, such as the Block Design and Object Assembly subtests of the WAIS-R, are used for the same assessment goals.

Disorders of executive motor skills. In general, in assessing disorders in executive motor skills, one is alert to the presence of perseveration in motor activity, thought, and affect. Perseveration of motor activity is often elicited by starting the patient on a simple repeated task and then altering one of the motor components. Thus, the patient is asked to perform a simple diadochokinetic task, such as alternating palm up–palm down, followed by another task incorporating the original task, such as palm up–palm down–fist. The shift to the next task may result in repeated performance of only two components of the task. Similarly, asking the patient to write, in script, alternating *m*'s and *n*'s will also elicit simple motor perseveration. Perseveration of thought or set is often quickly elicited by shifting task instruction. For example, in a task developed by Luria (1966) for the assessment of frontal lobe dysfunction, the patient is told, "When I raise one finger, then you raise one finger, and when I raise two fingers, you raise two fingers." After several successful completions, the patient is told, "Now when I raise one finger, you raise two fingers, and when I raise two fingers, you raise one." Patients with dorsal-lateral frontal lobe lesions have a great deal of trouble with such tasks. The Trail Making Test (Lezak 1995) is a "connect the dots" task in which the patient must first connect the dots in ascending numerical order (Trails A) and then in an alternating sequence of numbers and letters (e.g., 1 to A to 2 to B to 3 to C, etc.) (Trails B). Both the time to completion and the number of errors are noted.

Disorders in evolving or shifting more complex ideas can also be measured quite accurately. The Category Test and the Wisconsin Card Sort Test, both of which are concept formation tasks, differ in specific directions and stimuli, but both present a series of specific examples of a class of events and require the patient to derive the concept or rule of which they are an exemplar. The rule changes over time. Thus, one might observe that the patient fails to induce the first concept or perseverates the same rule well past its utility. The number of perseveration errors is among the scores obtained on both tests.

Disorders of motor skills. Disorders of simple motor skills are among the frequent concomitants of most toxic-metabolic disorders and structural lesions to both the extrapyramidal and pyramidal systems. Examination is usually exceptionally brief, and the results are quite reproducible and valid. One can measure line-quality parameters of copied geometric drawings (Mattis et al. 1975). One can, in addition, present simple fine motor coordination tasks such as the Purdue Pegboard (Costa et al. 1963) or the Grooved Pegboard. The Purdue Pegboard measures the number of slim cylinders (pegs) one can insert in a row of holes in 30 seconds. One notes the number of pegs placed with the right hand alone and the left hand alone, and the pairs of pegs placed with both hands simultaneously. The number of pegs placed simultaneously has proven to be a sensitive measure of frontal dysfunction. The Grooved Pegboard uses pegs that contain a flange on one side so that the pegs fit into a keyhole-shaped hole. The keyholes are placed in differing orientations on the board. One notes the total time to place all the pegs with each hand alone. Given the greater fine motor component to the grooved pegs, the Grooved Pegboard tends to be a more sensitive measure of tremor than the Purdue Pegboard, although one must be sensitive to the additional perceptual demands of this test.

Neuropsychological Assessment of Children

Relevance to Psychiatry

Rapoport and Ismond (1996) have pointed out that the two major influences on current diagnosis and quantitative analysis in pediatric populations have been psychopharmacology and psychiatric epidemiology. Epidemiologic studies, such as the paradigmatic Isle of Wight study, in which every child in a small island community was enrolled (Rutter et al. 1970), have contributed important findings as to the nature and course of many psychiatric disorders of childhood. Among the important findings contributed by recent epidemiologic studies are the documentation of a relatively high frequency of behavioral disorders in the pediatric population and the powerful association between a dysfunctional CNS and disordered behavior. A specific case in point is the association of learning disorders and conduct disorder. Studies of adult populations have led to an emphasis on earlier diagnosis because of the findings indicating frequent childhood or adolescent onset for many psychiatric disorders (Robins et al. 1981). On the one hand, the neuropsychological assessment can provide systematic, quantitative, and reliable assessment of psychopharmacological effects; on the other hand, it can document the presence of neurologically driven cognitive disorders such as learning disorders and communication disorders. In general, neuropsychological assessment is often more useful in the diagnostic process with children than with adults because of the relationship between cognitive function and a variety of behavioral disturbances. For example, assessment is required to make the differential diagnosis between mild mental retardation and a learning disorder.

Goals of the Neuropsychological Assessment

The pediatric neuropsychologist undertakes an evaluation of the child with goals similar to those addressed in the assessment of the adult patient:

- To provide documentation of specific patterns of cognitive dysfunction referrable to a specific class of psychiatric disorders
- To provide assistance in differential diagnosis
- To assess the impact of psychopharmacological agents or other medications on cognitive function

---

Although there is overlap in the essentials of assessment, in contrast to the neuropsychological assessment of the adult patient, the administration and interpretation of the pediatric neuropsychological assessment must be evaluated against the backdrop of normal child development. Understanding the role of maturation and development in the performance of children is crucial to the valid interpretation of assessment data and of the observed behavior of the child during the assessment. Limited attention span and motor restlessness are appropriate behaviors for a 2-year-old child; the same behaviors in a 7-year-old are considered atypical under normal circumstances. A 2-year-old is not a short 7-year-old, no more than a 12-year-old is a short adult. Although neurodevelopment and maturation underlie the elaboration and integration of cognitive functions, other variables, such as socioeconomic and sociocultural status, family structure and function, and personality characteristics, have demonstrable effects on cognitive development.

Reasons for Referral

Differential Diagnosis: Autistic Disorder, Communication Disorders, and Mental Retardation

A frequent referral issue, as well as a perennial diagnostic dilemma in the case of young children, has to do with differentiating between pervasive developmental disorders such as autism, communication disorders, and mental retardation—more specifically, between high-functioning autistic children and children with developmental language disorder, and between low-functioning autistic children and mentally retarded children. Some children may carry dual diagnoses such as autism and a communication disorder if they meet the criteria for both. Diagnosis drives treatment; in the distinction among these childhood disorders lies differentiation in therapeutic approach and, often, in prognosis.

Among the commonalities across these disorders are the paucity of expressive language, apparent deficiency in comprehension of or inattention to spoken language, limitations in social interactions, and atypical motor function. Although accurate assessment of these disorders is not always a given, there are basic questions that help to clarify the issues. Beyond the benefit to the young patient, and as with the adult patient, appropriate diagnosis and treatment offer cost benefits in the provision of appropriate intervention "the first time around" and in the possible identification of a cognitive/learning disorder rather than, or in addition to, a psychiatric disorder, in which case some, if not all, of the burden of treatment would be transferred from the managed care provider to the educational system.

History.   The importance of a detailed history has been addressed earlier in the chapter. Specificity of additional information based on the referral issue is an added consideration. In the case of this triad of clinical diagnoses, it is important to elicit as much information as possible regarding acquisition and functionality of speech and language, and descriptions of behaviors and situations that speak to social skills development. Information about play, the "work" of children, can be helpful in making inferences about "internal language" and cognitive level in the nonverbal child or the child who does not interact appropriately with others. Direct observation is best when possible, but information may be gathered from caregivers that may give some idea as to presence or absence and level of representational play, the child's ability to sustain play, and his or her willingness to allow others to join.

Behavior checklists.   The checklist is an excellent vehicle for the systematic collection of behavioral data. The Wing Autistic Disorder Interview Checklist (Wing 1996a) is used in the evaluation for autism, and the Wing Schedule of Handicaps, Behaviour and Skills (Wing 1996b) has been found useful in the assessment of children and adults with mental retardation and of those with retardation in some, but not all, aspects of development, as in autistic individuals or individuals with language disorders. Together, and in conjunction with previously gathered historical information, they provide a multidimensional picture of many areas of neurocognitive behavior.

Although more than a checklist, the Vineland Adaptive Behavior Scales (Sparrow et al. 1984), constituting a developmentally and functionally oriented structured interview, are useful in eliciting rather fine-grained information on the current level of skill acquisition and daily functional status in many of the areas of concern in this differential diagnostic evaluation.

Audiological assessment.   In instances of inadequate development of language and age-appropriate social skills, it is essential to obtain an adequate assessment of hearing. Young children with language deficits or more global developmental disorders typically are not able to be trained to respond to play audiometry; other approaches to assessment of hearing must be undertaken, including auditory evoked brain stem responses or cortical auditory evoked responses. Hearing impairment and deafness in children often go undetected for several years; children with such impairment are sometimes identified as displaying primary psychiatric disorders.

Motor functions.   The assessment of oromotor function should be undertaken in the child with a history of early feeding problems, drooling past the completion of teething, poor articulation, or inability to produce speech at an age-appropriate level. Residual primitive oromotor reflexes may contribute to speech production problems. There are children with mild, moderate, or severe developmental motor or verbal apraxia who have difficulty in producing speech or, in extreme instances, cannot produce intelligible speech beyond the one-word level, and sometimes not even that. The Screening Test for Developmental Verbal Apraxia (Blakeley 1980) includes a set of useful evaluation procedures to assist in this diagnosis. Prognosis and treatment are vastly different for these children, whose apparent psychiatric disorder may develop secondary to their compromised ability to understand spoken language and/or to communicate verbally, with the primary problem, then, being neurogenic rather than psychogenic in origin. Children in their preschool years who demonstrate significant expressive, as well as receptive, disorders are being taught sign language within a Total Communication framework. Sign language is a useful adjunct for these children and serves as an avenue of communication until aural-oral language becomes accessible (which, in most instances, it does). However, for those children with severe auditory receptive disorders and with significant oromotor deficits, sign language becomes the "bread and butter" of their communication.

In a multisite study involving children with autistic disorder, language disorder, or mental retardation, a triad of motor abnormalities— apraxia, hypotonia, and sterotypy—was found in a high percentage of autistic children in contrast to the other groups (Rapin 1996). Stereotypic motor behavior, apraxia, and hypotonia can be assessed by the neuropsychologist. Although the triad is surely not diagnostic of autism, positive motor findings in conjunction with other diagnostic criteria may heighten the probability of accurate differential diagnosis, with particular reference to the high-functioning autistic child versus the child with a communication disorder whose condition is characterized by deficits in semantic comprehension and pragmatics.

Assessment of cognitive function.   Given hearing adequate for speech and language development, assessment of cognitive function is a necessary next step. A brief and general discussion of the assessment of intelligence was given earlier in this section. A more focused assessment is required to determine whether the child is mentally retarded, demonstrates a neurocognitive profile consonant with one of the development language disorders (e.g., intact nonverbal skills in contrast to language-based measures), and/or meets the criteria for autistic disorder. Such assessment is possible if the child is at all available.

For those children who do not communicate verbally, there are standardized cognitive measures that are nonverbal in their administration and that do not require verbal responses. One such test is the Hiskey-

Nebraska Test of Learning Aptitude, which has norms for deaf and hearing children from ages 3 to 18 years and assesses a broad range of cognitive functions, ranging from form discrimination to semantic categorical skills to fine motor ability. Each subtest yields an age-equivalent score. Summary scores include an age equivalence and a Deviation IQ. The Pictorial Test of Intelligence is another visually guided measure that requires minimal auditory comprehension and a pointing, rather than verbal, response. This test extends down to the preschool years and up to age 8 years. Subtest scores and an IQ score are available. Depending on age, either the Raven Coloured Progressive Matrices (Raven 1965) or the Standard Progressive Matrices (Raven 1960, 1976) is an excellent measure of current level of visually guided cognitive function. Both require intact visual-perceptual skills and assess match-to-sample gestalt closure and analogic problem solving. Many high-functioning autistic spectrum children do well on these tests while being unable to deal with simple auditory-verbal measures.

Depending on age, the Performance Scales of either the WPPSI-R or the WISC-III are useful in determining the level of function in aspects of visuospatial, constructional, nonvocal linguistic and executive functions. The Stanford-Binet, 4th Edition, also provides a set of measures appropriate to the assessment of a broad range of verbal and nonverbal cognitive functions. If formal testing is not possible, clinical observation of behavior, with materials provided to the child in an informal situation, can be useful. Many of the cognitive functions of relevance may be observed and assessed within a neurodevelopmental, neuropsychological framework when formal testing is precluded. In instances in which the child might be cooperative enough to attempt formal assessment but is functioning at a level below that associated with 2 years of age for whatever the reason, the Bayley Scales of Infant Intelligence— Revised (Bayley 1993), normed from 1 month to 3½ years, may be administered. Although the norms are not applicable in terms of generating a Mental Development Index, item analysis provides a method of formulating a developmental profile of neurocognitve functions.

Assessment of language.   Developmental expressive language disorders are more frequently encountered than are receptive disorders, although the latter are more accessible to quantitative assessment. Expressive disorders may be quite subtle in their presentation and are typically identified on a clinical, obervational level. Language pathologists, evaluating taped language samples by comparing them with developmental criteria, are better able to provide quantitative data in relation to characteristics of expressive language such as length of utterance, grammar and morphology, and phonology. In the more subtle disorders, those of organization and formulation, several standardized subtests of the Clinical Evaluation of Language Fundamentals—

Revised (CELF-R; Semel et al. 1987) can be used to assess those aspects of language. Often, children with formulation problems can do well with these structured language stimuli, but do poorly in initiating conversational language or in responding to "wh" questions. Children who have deficiencies in expressive language are often described as shy, quiet, or not very bright. These children cannot tell mother "what happened in school today," or describe an event or retell a story just heard; they tend to have dysnomia, or word-finding problems, which may be systematically assessed by measures such as the Boston Naming Test (Kaplan et al. 1983; Kindlon and Garrison 1986), the Word Fluency subtest of the Neurosensory Center Comprehensive Examination for Aphasia (NCCEA; Gaddes and Crockett 1975a), and the word association subtests of the McCarthy Scales of Children's Abilities and the CELF-R. There are specific clusters of neurocognitive functions that serve as good indicators of an organization/formulation expressive language disorder when they are noted to be "inefficient" or deficient, relative to other cognitive skills. Preliminary data suggest that children with expressive disorders do not have difficulty in the acquisition of reading skills, but encounter problems in later grades when expressive writing demands increase (B. C. Wilson and Risucci 1988). Children with expressive language disorders are often identified as emotionally disturbed because of the paucity of spontaneous language they produce.

Children with receptive or mixed receptive-expressive disorders are at greater risk for reading disabilities (B. C. Wilson and Risucci 1988) and for the later onset of emotional or behavioral disorders. Children with developmental language disorders are, in general, overrepresented in mental health facilities (Beitchman 1985; Cantwell and Baker 1977; Cantwell et al. 1980).

The Token Test for Children (Di Simone 1978), the Test for Auditory Comprehension and Language—Revised (Carrow-Woofolk 1985), subtests of the Clinical Evaluation of Language Fundamentals (CELF; Wiig et al. 1992) and the Preschool CELF-R, and the story repetition measures, in addition to the verbal subtests of the intelligence measures, are typically sufficient to provide a profile of receptive language competence.

Attention-Deficit/Hyperactivity Disorder
Among the signal behavioral manifestations of ADHD are inattention, impulsivity, and hyperactivity. Among the key criteria that define such behavior as pathological are the observations that the behavior is inappropriate for age, occurs in more than one setting, and has an onset before 7 years of age. An accurate diagnosis is important not only in terms of immediate intervention strategies but also because some of the characteristic behaviors may herald the later occurrence of major psychiatric disorders, including schizophrenia and bipolar disorders.

Prediction, monitoring, and early intervention may offer a more positive outcome than would otherwise be possible, and certainly a more cost-effective one.

ADHD is a widely encountered diagnosis—according to some, too widely encountered. It is possible that some children are being inappropriately identified, which can lead to inappropriate therapeutic interventions. Some diagnostic evaluations may not look for the possibility of alternative or coexisting etiologies for the observed behavior. Among the possible confounders that contribute to an erroneous diagnosis of ADHD are the presence of language disorders, learning problems, agitation due to depression, sequelae of traumatic brain injury, a dysfunctional home, and physical or sexual abuse. A child's response to a dysfunctional home situation may mimic ADHD behavior because of the anxiety. Disorganized behavior, hyperactivity, and impulsivity are often the result of brain trauma. Certain medications, such as those used to treat asthma, can contribute to a picture of hyperactivity and inattention. These possible etiologic factors must be evaluated, because in each instance the orientation to treatment may differ widely.

As with any diagnostic undertaking, particularly with children, careful evaluation of the history and current status is critical. Information regarding birth and early development, medical factors, family and social information, and educational history can provide important insights as to onset, intensity, and specificity of occurrence of the behaviors in question. A psychological assessment is important to define the parameters of the behavioral and emotional concomitants; a neuropsychological assessment is necessary to rule out cognitive deficits that contribute to the observed behavior, or to define the presence of a learning disability, language disorder, or cognitive dysfunction secondary to brain injury.

In addition to obtaining behavioral rating scale data from parents and teachers, the neuropsychological assessment should include parent, teacher, and, when possible, child interviews that can provide information key to the understanding of the child's behavior. The flexibility of the interview provides maximal opportunity for addressing the issues specific to the child in question and complements the behavior rating scales that are in common use. Both the interview and behavior checklists can make important contributions to the diagnostic process.

Continuous performance tasks (CPTs) are among the complement of measures that have been used over the past several decades in the study of hyperactive children. The first computerized CPT was developed by Rosvold and colleagues (1956). Result of studies using CPT paradigms have indicated that children with ADHD tend to do more poorly on these tasks than their ADHD-free peers. A portable CPT was developed by Gordon (1983) and is being widely used in the diagnosis of ADHD. The Gordon Diagnostic System allows for the programming of a delay task, which assesses impulsivity; a vigilance task, which measures sustained attention; and a distractiblity task, which assesses sustained attention when distracting stimuli are introduced. The Test of Variables of Attention (TOVA; Greenberg 1988–1994) is another, newer CPT that can be used as part of a comprehensive ADHD evaluation. A non–language-based CPT, the TOVA serves to differentiate ADHD from learning disabilities in 80% of the cases, does not require right-left discrimination, and appears to have minimal practice effects.

In addition to the foregoing, it is important to assess levels of academic performance in reading, spelling, and arithmetic. If the child is achieving below performance levels in one or more areas as predicted by measures of cognitive function, the neuropsychologist needs to determine whether a "true" learning disability is coexisting with ADHD or whether the ADHD has contributed to the picture of underachievement. One would not expect to find systematic neurocognitive patterns reflective of a learning disabilities subtype in the ADHD child unless a learning disability was present. A typical pattern in the ADHD child without learning disabilities is one of random fluctuations on neuropsychological subtest items and evidence of dysfunction from those items that are sensitive to impulsivity and loss of focus.

Other frequently observed comorbidities in the ADHD child include behavior and emotional disorders. Frequently, these problems are the basis for the child's being brought to clinical attention. It has been estimated that between 40% and 50% of the ADHD group show signs of oppositional defiant disorder, and it is estimated that half of those children will develop a conduct disorder (Parker 1992). The prognosis for such children improves with accurate diagnosis as early on as possible, so that appropriate intervention may be provided in as timely a fashion as possible. The oppositional behavior is of more concern than the attention deficit per se and can often be addressed at home and in the school with behavioral management techniques. Psychiatric intervention may be necessary, but the best results are obtained when, drawing on the concept of ecological validity, the intervention takes place consistently and in the situations in which the target behavior occurs. Consultation provided to parents and educators in the development and implementation of an appropriate behavior management program might be more effective and cost-containing than a course of psychotherapy.

Content of the Evaluation

Similarly to the neuropsychological assessment of adults, the neuropsychological evaluation of children is structured to provide information relevant to the referral question. Portions of the evaluation are "required," and some others are "optional." History, and assessment of intellective function, typically provide the backbone of an evaluation; assessment of other aspects of neurocognitive function are called on when they are necessary to address or to clarify the issues in question.

Importance of history.   Careful history taking is always an essential part of any neuropsychlogical assessment; in the case of making a differential diagnosis among specific clinical entities, information above and beyond that obtained from the usual history may be necessary. In approaching the differential diagnosis between autism, mental retardation, and communication disorders, for example, information specific to a family history of learning disabilities, autistic traits, social skills deficits, or severe depressive or bipolar disorders becomes very important. The younger the child, the more relevant the historical information to the diagnosis. Reporting on high risk factors surrounding preganancy, birth and delivery, neonatal status, and early development often inform the diagnosis of developmental disabilities. Issues of onset of the disorder and neuropsychological findings in the preschool or school-age child need to be assessed within the framework of the functional, sociocultural, and socioeconomic status of the family. There are times when the family, rather than the child, should be identified as the "patient." It is impossible to overemphasize the importance of a detailed and focused history as a major source of data in the diagnostic evaluation of a child.

Intelligence.   The neuropsychological assessment should evaluate cognitive function in all its aspects. With children, obtaining an index of intelligence in verbal and performance areas—either with the Wechsler Preschool and Primary Scale of Intelligence—Revised (WPPSI-R; Wechsler 1989), the Wechsler Intelligence Scale for Children, 3rd Edition (WISC-III; Wechsler 1991), or the Stanford-Binet Intelligence Scale, 4th Edition (Thorndike et al. 1986)—is a good place to start, in that these measures provide an index of intelligence in verbal and performance areas. Often, a tentative pattern emerges. Assessment of some neuropsychological functions may be more relevant to one case than another, and this underscores the flexibility provided by the "process approach" in contrast to the utilization of fixed batteries. For example, it does not seem necessary to assess somatosensory functions when one is pursuing a differential diagnosis between mild mental retardation and a learning disorder, although such an assessment might be useful in the examination of a child with a high-risk birth history and abnormal development. Documentation of compromised somatosensory function and lateralizing signs may be important in explaining some of the observed behaviors, lateralization may be a useful predictor, and specific interventions might be sought as a result of this information.

Concept formation and conceptualization. These are additional important areas of inquiry for most evaluations. Concept formation and conceptualization are manifestations of higher cortical functions and are sensitive to compromised CNS function. Measures include, for example, the Absurdities subtest of the Stanford-Binet (Thorndike et al. 1986). The stimulus is visual, and the response is verbal; the task is to identify what is "funny" or "silly" about the stimulus picture. Matrix Analogies (Thorndike et al. 1986) and both the Standard Progressive Matrices (Raven 1960, 1976) and the Coloured Progressive Matrices (Raven 1965) assess concept formation and analogic reasoning. The Wisconsin Card Sort Test and the booklet form of the Category Test, mentioned earlier in the context of the neuropsychological assessment of adults, have norms that are available for the assessment of children.

Memory and learning. The evaluation of memory and learning should be pursued in most assessments. Memory and learning are critical aspects of neurocognitive function and, as with other aspects of higher cognitive function, are readily compromised by a variety of endogeneous as well as exogenous factors. There are available measures of auditory and visual sequential memory for both representational and nonrepresentational stimuli (e.g., Memory for Objects, Sentence Memory, and Bead Memory of the Stanford-Binet, 4th Edition [Thorndike et al. 1986]); visual attention span (Hiskey-Nebraska Test of Learning Aptitude [Hiskey 1966]); digit span (WISC-III); text memory (e.g., Verbal Memory II of the McCarthy Scales of Children's Abilities (McCarthy 1972); and story memory with delayed and recognition conditions (Woodcock-Johnson Psycho-Educational Battery—Revised [Woodcock and Johnson 1989–1990]). The Woodcock-Johnson Test also provides interesting measures of learning, including a list learning task, and the acquisition of a visual-verbal code, not unlike what is learned at the beginning stages of reading.

Language functions. It may not always be necessary to perform an extensive language evaluation. The cognitive measures noted above provide a good sample of receptive and expressive abilities. If, on the basis of the resulting profile, the suspicion is raised that a language disorder may be present, then a detailed examination is required. Assessment of language functions is discussed later in this section, in connection with issues of differential diagnosis.

Perceptual functions. Visual perceptual function may be assessed by a variety of instruments, based on visual discrimination (the Form Discrimination subtest of the Pictorial Test of Intelligence [French 1964]) or visuospatial function (measures such as the Block Building subtest of the Hiskey-Nebraska Test of Learning Aptitude [Hiskey 1966]). Other measures that were mentioned earlier in the context of the neuropsychological assessment of adults have children's norms as well. Aspects of auditory perception may be assesed in children with the same instruments that have been noted in the section on adult assessment. The Goldman-Fristoe-Woodcock Test of Auditory Discrimination (Goldman et al. 1970) is normed from 4 to 80 years of age. Children's norms exist for light touch and two-point perception, utilizing the Von Frey hairs, and two-point esthesiometer, respectively (J. J. Wilson et al. 1962). Children's norms are also available for assessment of stereognosis (Gaddes and Crockett 1975b; B. C. Wilson and Wilson 1967; J. J. Wilson and Wilson 1967).

Constructional praxis.   Subtests of the WPPSI-R, the WISC-III, the Stanford-Binet, the McCarthy Scales, and the Hiskey-Nebraska all provide puzzlelike tasks and block design tasks that are reliable measures of constructional abilities.

Executive functions.   The ability to plan, organize, and execute behaviors in a systematic or sequential fashion is critical to the learning process, to any rehabilitative efforts, and to academic achievement. There are a fair number of methods for the assessment of this important set of functions; the Trail Making Test (both Trails A and B) mentioned earlier has children's norms available (Reitan 1971). The Hand Positions subtest of the Kaufman Assessment Battery for Children (K-ABC; Kaufman and Kaufman 1983) assesses hand praxis but can also induce perseverative responses. The booklet form of the Category Test and the Wisconsin Card Sort Test provide information on the cognitive flexibility required for rapid shifts in set. The Coding subtest of the WISC-III and the Animal Pegs subtest of the WPPSI-R, both multimensional measures, may be viewed as indices of executive motor function.

Motor functions.   Compromised motor functions are frequently seen in association with almost every kind of developmental disability. Gross motor function is typically functional, sometimes clumsy. A brief gross motor screening is provided by subtests of the McCarthy Scales of Children's Abilities. Graphomotor function is often developmentally delayed; paper-and-pencil productions may be assessed by the Beery Developmental Test of Visual-Motor Integration (Beery 1989); the Bender Gestalt, using the Koppitz norms (Koppitz 1975); or the appropriate subtests of the WPPSI-R and the McCarthy Scales.

Fine motor function may be assessed by the Grooved Pegboard and the Purdue Pegboard (Gardner and Broman 1979), both mentioned earlier in the context of the assessment of adults. Preschool norms are available for the Purdue Pegboard (B. C. Wilson et al. 1982). Deficient abilities in motor areas put the child at risk for delay in acquiring basic skills necessary for acquisition of academic skills later in development and often lead to intense frustration unless adult intervention and facilitation are provided. Occupational therapy is frequently provided for those children who have demonstrable difficulties in these areas.

Academic achievement.   Assessment of academic skills often sheds light on the simplicity of etiology; such assessment may provide data indicating that a child with a behaviorial disorder is improperly placed in school, having lower academic or cognitive skills than is required for the work being demanded. Issues of self-esteem and heightened anxiety resulting from such a situation can contribute to a picture of attention-deficit/hyperactivity disorder (ADHD). Appropriate expectations and the provision of educational supports can positively influence the development of adequate self-esteem. Even when the problem is, in a sense, environmental rather than pathological, there is often the need for psychotherapeutic intervention. Maladaptive behaviors and expectations are sometimes difficult to unlearn without help.

· · ·

The multidimensional neuropsychological assessment outlined in this section provides an important vehicle for accurate diagnosis. As we have been indicating throughout this chapter, appropriate treatment plans flow from accurate diagnosis, and accurate diagnosis enhances the probability of better and more cost-effective outcomes.

References

Ammons RB, Ammons CH: The Quick Test (QT): provisional manual. Psychol Rep 11:111–161, 1962

Bayley N: Manual for the Bayley Scales of Infant Development, 2nd Edition. New York, Psychological Corporation, 1993

Beery KE: Developmental Test of Visual-Motor Integration. Cleveland, OH, Modern Curriculum Press, 1989

Beitchman JH: Speech and language impairment and psychiatric risk. Psychiatr Clin North Am 8:721–735, 1985

Benton AL: Visual Retention Test. New York, Psychological Corporation, 1955

Benton AL, Hamsher K: Multilingual Aphasia Examination. Iowa City, University of Iowa, 1976

Benton AL, Spreen O: Neurosensory Center Comprehensive Examination for Aphasia. Victoria, British Columbia, University of Victoria, 1969

Benton AL, Van Allen MW: Impairment in facial recognition in patients with cerebral disease. Cortex 4:344–358, 1968

Benton AL, Hannay HJ, Varney NR: Visual perception of line direction in patients with unilateral brain disease. Neurology 25:907–910, 1975

Berg EA: A simple objective test for measuring flexibility in thinking. J Gen Psychol 39:15–32, 1948

Blakeley RW: Screening Test for Developmental Apraxia of Speech. Tigard, OR, CC Publications, 1980

Boll TJ: The Halstead-Reitan Neuropsychology Battery, in Handbook of Neuropsychology. Edited by Filskov SB, Boll TJ. New York, Wiley, 1981, pp 577–607

Cantwell DP, Baker L: Psychiatric disorders in children with speech and language retardation. Arch Gen Psychiatry 34:583–591, 1977

Cantwell DP, Baker L, Mattison RE: Factors associated with the development of psychiatric disorders in children with speech and language retardation. Arch Gen Psychiatry 37:423–426, 1980

Carrow-Woofolk E: Test of Auditory Comprehension and Language—Revised. Allen, TX, DLM Teaching Resources, 1985

Christensen AL: Luria's Neuropsychological Investigation: Manual. New York, Spectrum, 1975

Costa LD, Vaughan HG, Levita E, et al: Purdue Pegboard as a predictor of the presence and laterality of cerebral lesions. Journal of Consulting Psychology 27:133–137, 1963

DeFilippis NA, McCampbell E, Rogers P: Development of a booklet form of the Category Test: normative and validity data. Journal of Clinical Neuropsychology 1:339–342, 1979

Di Simone F: The Token Test for Children. Highman, MA, Teaching Resources, 1978

French JL: The Pictorial Test of Intelligence. New York, Houghton-Mifflin, 1964

Gaddes WH, Crockett DJ: Manual for the Neurosensory Center Comprehensive Examination for Aphasia: Children's Norms. Victoria, BC, University of Victoria, 1975a

Gaddes WH, Crockett DJ: The Spreen-Benton Aphasia Test: normative data as a measure of normal language development. Brain Lang 4:257–280, 1975b

Gardner RA, Broman M: The Purdue Pegboard: normative data on 1334 school children. Journal of Clinical Child Psychology 8:156–162, 1979

Golden CJ, Hammeke TA, Purisch AD: Diagnostic validity of a standardized neuropsychological battery derived from Luria's neuropsychological tests. J Consult Clin Psychol 46:1258–1265, 1978

Goldman R, Fristoe M, Woodcock RW: Goldman-Fristoe-Woodcock Test of Auditory Discrimination. Circle Pines, MN, American Guidance Service, 1970

Goodglass H, Kaplan E: Assessment of Aphasia and Related Disorders. Philadelphia, PA, Lea & Febiger, 1972

Gordon M: The Gordon Diagnostic System. DeWitt, NY, Gordon Systems, 1983

Greenberg L: Test of Variables of Attention (TOVA). Los Alamitos, CA, Universal Attention Deficits, Inc, 1988–1994

Halstead WC, Wepman JM: The Halstead-Wepman Aphasia Screening Test. Journal of Speech and Hearing Disorders 14:9–15, 1959

Heaton RK: Manual for the Wisconsin Card Sorting Test. Odessa, FL, Psychological Assessment Resources, 1981

Hiskey MS: Hiskey-Nebraska Test of Learning Aptitude. Lincoln, NE, Union College Press, 1966

Jastak S, Wilkinson GS: The Wide Range Achievement Test—Revised. Wilmington, DE, Jastak Associates, 1981

Kaplan E, Goodglass H, Weintraub S: Boston Naming Test. Philadelphia, PA, Lea & Febiger, 1983

Karzmark P, Heaton RK, Grant I, et al: Use of demographic variables to predict full scale IQ: a replication and extension. J Clin Exp Neuropsychol 7:412–420, 1985

Kaufman AS, Kaufman NL: Kaufman Assessment Battery for Children. Circle Pines, MN, American Guidance Service, 1983

Kindlon D, Garrison W: The Boston Naming Test: norm data and cue utilization in a sample of 6- and 7-year-old children. Brain and Language 21:255–259, 1986

Koppitz EM: The Bender Gestalt Test for Young Children, Vol II. New York, Grune & Stratton, 1975

LeFever FF: President's Column, Neuropsychology Division. The Notebook 8:25–26, 1996 [Foundation of the New York State Psychological Association, Albany, NY]

Lezak MD: Neuropsychological Assessment, 3rd Edition. New York, Oxford University Press, 1995

Luria AR: Higher Cortical Functions in Man. New York, Basic Books, 1966

Luria AR: The Working Brain: An Introduction to Neuropsychology. Translated by Haigh B. New York, Basic Books, 1973

Mattis S, French JH, Rapin I: Dyslexia in children and young adults: three independent neuropsychological syndromes. Dev Med Child Neurol 17:150–163, 1975

Mattis S, Kovner R, Goldmeier E: Different patterns of mnemonic deficits in two organic amnestic syndromes. Brain and Language 6:179–191, 1978

McCarthy DA: Manual for the McCarthy Scales of Childrens' Abilities. New York, Psychological Corporation, 1972

Mirsky AF, Kornetsky C: On the dissimilar effects of drugs on the Digit Symbol Substitution and Continuous Performance Tests: a review and preliminary integration of behavioral and physiological evidence. Psychopharmacologia 5:161–177, 1964

New York State Psychological Association, Neuropsychology Division: 19__

Nelson HE: National Adult Reading Test (NART) Test Manual. Berkshire, MA, NFER-Nelson, 1982

Parker H: The ADD Hyperactivity Handbook for Schools. Plantation, FL, Impact Press, 1992

Rapin I: Neurological examination, in Preschool Children With Inadequate Communication. Edited by Rapin I. London, MacKeith Press, 1996, pp 98–122

Rapoport JL, Ismond DR: DSM-IV Training Guide for Diagnosis of Childhood Disorders. New York, Brunner/Mazel, 1996

Raven JC: Guide to the Standard Progressive Matrices. London, HK Lewis, 1960

Raven JC: Guide to Using the Raven Coloured Progressive Matrices. London, HK Lewis, 1965

Raven JC: Guide to the Standard Progressive Matrices. Oxford, UK, Oxford Psychologists Press, 1976

Reed HBC, Reitan RM, Klove H: Influence of cerebral lesions on psychological test performancess of older children. Journal of Consulting Psychology 29:247–251, 1965

Reitan R: Trail Making Test results for normal and brain-damaged children. Percept Mot Skills 33:578–581, 1971

Rey A: L'examen psychologique dans les cas d'encephalopathie traumatique. Archives de Psychologie 28(112):286–340, 1941

Robins LN, Helzer JE, Croughan J, et al: National Institute of Mental Health Diagnostic Interview Schedule: its history, characteristics, and validity. Arch Gen Psychiatry 38:381–389, 1981

Rosvold HE, Mirsky AF, Sarason I, et al: A continuous performance test of brain damage. Journal of Consulting Psychology 20:343–350, 1956

Rutter M, Tizard J, Whitmore K: Education, Health and Behaviour: Psychological and Medical Study of Childhood Development. New York, Wiley, 1970

Seashore CE, Lewis D, Saetveit DL: Seashore Measures of Musical Talents, Revised Edition. New York, Psychological Corporation, 1960

Semel E, Wiig EH, Secord W: Examiner's Manual for the Clinical Evaluation of Language Fundamentals—Revised. New York, Psychological Corporation, 1987

Shipley WC: The Institute of Living Scale. Los Angeles, Psychological Services, 1946

Sparrow SS, Balla DA, Cicchetti DV: Vineland Adaptive Behavior Scales. Circle Pines, MN, American Guidance Service, 1984

Squire LR, Shimamura AP: Characterizing amnesic patients for neurobehavioral study. Behav Neurosci 100:866–877, 1986

Thorndike RL, Hagen EP, Sattler JM: Manual for the Stanford-Binet Intelligence Scale, 4th Edition. Chicago, IL, Riverside Publishing, 1986

Wechsler D: Wechsler Adult Intelligence Scale—Revised. New York, Psychological Corporation, 1981

Wechsler D: The Wechsler Memory Scale—Revised. New York, Psychological Corporation, 1987

Wechsler D: Wechsler Preschool and Primary Scale of Intelligence—Revised. New York, Psychological Corporation, 1989

Wechsler D: Wechsler Intelligence Scale for Children, 3rd Edition. New York, Psychological Corporation, 1991

Wiig WH, Secord W, Semel E: Examiner's Manual for the Clinical Evaluation of Language Fundamentals—Preschool. New York, Psychological Corporation, 1992

Willner AE: Towards development of more sensitive clinical tests of abstraction: the Analogy Test. Proceedings of the 78th Annual Convention of the American Psychological Association 5:553–554, 1971

Wilson BC, Risucci DA: The early identification of developmental language disorders and the prediction of the acquisition of reading skills, in Preschool Prevention of Reading Failure. Edited by Masland RL, Masland MW. Parkton, MD, York Press, 1988, pp 187–203

Wilson BC, Wilson JJ: Sensory and perceptual functions in cerebral palsy, I: light pressure thresholds and two-point discrimination. J Nerv Ment Dis 145:53–60, 1967

Wilson JJ, Wilson BC: Sensory and perceptual functions in cerebral palsy, II: stereognosis. J Nerv Ment Dis 145:61–68, 1967

Wilson JJ, Wilson BC, Swinyard CA: Two-point thresholds in congenital amputees. J Comp Physiol Psychol 55:432–435, 1962

Wilson BC, Iacovello JM, Wilson JJ, et al: Purdue Pegboard performance of normal preschool children. J Clin Neuropsychol 4:19–26, 1982

Wing L: Wing Autistic Disorder Interview Checklist (WADIC), in Preschool Children With Inadequate Communication (Appendix 1). Edited by Rapin I. London, MacKeith Press, 1996a, pp 247–251

Wing L: Wing Schedule of Handicaps, Behaviour and Skills (HBS), in Preschool Children With Inadequate Communication (Appendix 5). Edited by Rapin I. London, MacKeith Press, 1996b, pp

Woodcock RW, Johnson MB: Woodcock-Johnson Psycho-Educational Battery—Revised. Allen, TX, DLM Teaching Resources, 1989–1990

Chapter 23

Guidelines for Selecting Psychological Instruments for Treatment Outcome Assessment

Frederick L. Newman, Ph.D., and Daniel Carpenter, Ph.D.

Envision what might be the situation if oncological medicine were forced to base treatment decisions on just diagnosis and cost containment rather than on clinical status and outcome:

> Mr. Smith, 90% of the tumor is now benign. Only 10% of the tumor remains malignant. Unfortunately, you have used up the 20 sessions of radiation treatment allowed under your managed care plan for this year. Please come back next year when your insurance eligibility has been renewed.

Few would argue against using health status, biological, or behavioral criteria when setting eligibility and level of care requirements for oncological medicine (or for the delivery of a baby, or for most nonelective surgery). The same logical arguments can and should be offered to support the delivery of mental health services. There are psychological assessment techniques that can be used to provide valid evidence that such criteria have been met. But how does one decide which instrument is most suitable to the circumstances?

This chapter provides guidelines that can be used by practitioners to select one or more instruments that are most suitable to the population they are serving and the treatment goals of their service(s). The guidelines can also be used to evaluate the appropriateness of an instrument(s) that is (are) currently in use or proposed. One theme of the chapter is that the guidelines must be understood within the current demands on clinical practice and the delivery of mental health services.

One contextual constraint is that of efforts to contain costs through managed care. The good news is that there are psychological assess-

This chapter was adapted, with permission, from Newman FL, Ciarlo JA: "Criteria for Selecting Psychological Instruments for Treatment Outcome Assessment," in *The Use of Psychological Testing for Treatment Planning and Outcome Assessment.* Edited by Maruish ME. Hillsdale, NJ, Lawrence Erlbaum, 1994, pp. 98–110, and from Ciarlo et al. 1986.

ment instruments available that can be usefully applied in managed care settings to determine eligibility and level of care (for reviews, see Howard et al. 1996; Newman and Tejeda 1996). Additional good news is that some behavioral health insurers now appear to understand that simple cost containment for one episode of care could lead to greater long-term expense. This is particularly true for programs serving persons with severe and persistent mental illnesses. These insurers are seeking valid procedures to address three basic questions:

- Does the individual need treatment at this time?
- What interventions are needed and by whom, and where should they be delivered?
- What outcome criteria should be applied?

Many of our research colleagues are actively involved in addressing these questions. The Internet bulletin boards serving mental health services researchers (e.g., OUTCMTEN) have active interchanges about which instruments are appropriate under what circumstances.

One problem faced by practitioners when arguing for a particular level of care is that there is little evidence in the research literature to guide decisions about the appropriate level of care (Newman and Tejeda 1996). Clinical research designs traditionally have fixed the treatment dosage level and run a horse race between experimental and control conditions or among several alternative treatments as to which achieved the best outcomes with that dosage. Yet, in practice the clinician works with the patient to achieve an agreed-on level of functioning or reduction in symptom distress, or both. There is a need to modify research strategies on mental health services effectiveness such that we can address questions such as "What type and amount of treatment will achieve a given behavioral criterion for XX% of the patients who meet the entry level of functioning?"

To be effective (and cost-effective) in the selection of an instrument or instruments by which progress can be measured, one must systematically address an additional series of questions:

- What psychological and community functioning domains do we wish to assess for this patient or this group of patients?
- What are the behaviors that we expect to have an impact on?
- What clinical or program decisions will be supported by an assessment of the person's psychological state or functional status?
- What is the most cost-effective means for performing the specified assessments?

Eleven guidelines have been offered for instrument selection. The guidelines were originally developed by a panel of experts assembled by the National Institute of Mental Health (NIMH) (Ciarlo et al. 1986)[1] and were more recently updated to consider the potential impact on managed care (Newman and Ciarlo 1994). This chapter updates those guidelines in terms of two demands on the clinical community: managed care and consumer choice. These are not, and should not be, independent. The assessment techniques used by managed care to determine eligibility, level of care, progress, and outcome can also be used as part of a delivery system "report card" to inform consumers and other purchasers of mental health services (Dewan and Carpenter, Chapter 24, in this section; see also Mulkern et al. 1995). Consumer groups are requesting that the report card go beyond that of satisfaction with the way services are provided (although that is also important), to incorporate the quality and long-term effects of the services themselves. Thus, the proper selection of psychological assessment techniques is critical to both managed care and consumer choice.

The eleven guidelines (summarized in Table 23–1) are organized under five groupings:

- Applications of measures
- Methods and procedures
- Psychometric features
- Cost considerations
- Utility considerations

It should be obvious that the guidelines are not independent of each other. Yet, each focuses on unique concerns that will help the reader consider the demands of his or her own situation, the literature, and the relationship of that guideline to the other guidelines.

This chapter does not provide a list of recommended instruments for two reasons. First, to present such a list within the context of this chapter would run counter to one of its major themes: *The selection of an instrument must be tailored to the specific circumstances of the population being served and the goals and resources of that program of services.* The second reason is that a list that would satisfy all of the possible combinations of target populations, services, and service goals would be far too long to be included here (e.g., the text by Ciarlo and coauthors [1986] was over 600 pages in length and consisted mostly of appendixes). A selection of monographs and texts in which such lists are found, as well as critiques of progress-outcome instruments for the major target populations, is provided in the appendix to this chapter.

When these references are being consulted, it is recommended that

---

[1]Members of the expert panel were A. Broskowski, J. A. Ciarlo, G. B. Cox, I. Elkins, H. H. Goldman, W. A. Hargreaves, J. Mintz, F. L. Newman, and J. W. Zinober.

Table 23–1. Guidelines for the development, selection, and/or use of progress-outcome measures

Applications of measures
  1. Relevant to target group and independent of treatment provided, although sensitive to treatment-related changes

Methods and procedures
  2. Simple, teachable methods
  3. Use of measures with objective referents
  4. Use of multiple respondents
  5. More process-identifying outcome measures

Psychometric features
  6. Psychometric strength: reliable, valid, sensitive to treatment-related change; and nonreactive

Cost considerations
  7. Low measure costs relative to its uses

Utility considerations
  8. Understanding by nonprofessional audiences
  9. Easy feedback and uncomplicated interpretation
 10. Useful in clinical services
 11. Compatibility with clinical theories and practices

once one identifies a short list of instruments that appear suitable to the population(s) one serves, one should then apply the 11 guidelines to assist in making the final selection. Or, if currently using an instrument, one should use the guidelines to contrast one or more competitors with the current instrument to determine whether use of the current instrument(s) should be continued or a switch to another instrument should be made.

Guidelines for the Development, Selection, and/or Use of Progress-Outcome Measures

Guideline 1: Relevant to Target Group

> An outcome measure or set of measures should be relevant and appropriate to the target group(s) whose treatment is being studied; that is, the most important and frequently observed symptoms, problems, goals, or other domains of change for the group(s) should be addressed by the measure(s). . . . Other factors being equal, use of a measure appropriate to a wider range of client groups is preferred. . . . Measures [should be] . . . independent of the type of treatment service provided. (Ciarlo et al. 1986, p. 26)

Common wisdom holds that treatment selection, and a person's probable response to treatment, should be based on both clinical and demographic characteristics (Beutler and Clarkin 1990). A *target group* can be described as a cluster of persons with similar clinical-demographic characteristics that are expected to have a similar response to treatment. Beutler and Clarkin (1990) have provided guidelines for treatment selection that are consistent with findings in the clinical literature. Needs assessment information from epidemiologic surveys was used by expert panels to identify target groups of persons with severe mental illness who require similar systems of services (Newman et al. 1989; Uehara et al. 1994). Another approach that has been used is a linking of the epidemiologic data with historic levels of care (Leff et al. 1994). A combination of both these approaches has also been reported (Uehara et al. 1994).

Another feature of a target group that must be considered is personal characteristics that are known to influence how the information is collected. Facets such as age, ethnicity (related to language and meaning), comorbidity with a physical illness or developmental disability, and past experiences can influence the administration of a procedure. The monographs and other texts listed in the appendix to this chapter provide a good starting point when one is attempting to identify measures that are available for a major target group. For the majority of target groups, the lists and critiques of instruments provided in these references are adequate. However, if the particular target group served by your program or practice has qualities that differ markedly from those of the overall target group, then a more detailed review of the literature cited within these references is required. The text edited by Maruish (1994) and the publication by Ciarlo and coauthors (1986) contain sections and reference lists that provide greater detail on the limits of the techniques and their potential use with other populations.

Guideline 2: Simple, Teachable Methods

As Ciarlo and co-workers (1986) pointed out, the second guideline—simple, teachable methods—was readily agreed on by all of the panelists, but the development of training manuals and methods for ensuring the quality of instrument administration had, in panelists' view, been insufficient. Since then, the development of computer-assisted administration of assessment techniques has enhanced the reliability and validity of implementation by standardizing the way in which queries are presented. The long-standing difficulty of bridging the ethnic and cultural differences between the clinician and the patient can also be helped with the use of culturally sensitive selection of an assessment technique from a computerized menu of instruments.

Even with the development of computer-assisted methods, the traditional guidelines for developing training materials and for controlling administrative quality must still be applied (see, e.g., Cronbach 1970; Nunnally and Burnstein 1994). Self-report measures (e.g., Revised Symptom Checklist–90 [SCL-90-R; Derogatis 1994], Basis-32 [Eisen et al. 1994], Beck Depression Inventory [Beck and Steer 1993]) or measures completed by a significant other (e.g., Child Behavior Checklist [Achenbach and Edelbrock 1983], completed by the parents) that have survived scrutiny and are considered to have adequate psychometric quality usually have good instructions and administration manuals. If the recommended guidelines for administration are ignored, however, there are potentially disastrous effects. For example, the instructions for most self-report instruments strongly recommend completion independent of guidance or advice from others, preferably in isolation. From our own editorial experience, this requirement has not always been adhered to adequately. It is possible that the use of computers to collect self-report information will also increase the fidelity of the data collection. This is one area in which computer-assisted applications are particularly useful. Many people are accustomed to interacting with a machine that asks them questions, sometimes of a quite personal nature (Locke et al. 1992; Navaline et al. 1994).

Measures completed by an independent clinical observer or by the treating clinician can be very useful, but often the instructions on the instrument's use, training, and quality control procedures are poorly developed. On the one hand, such measures seek to make use of the professional's trained observations; on the other hand, such scales tend to be more reactive to clinician judgment bias (Newman 1983; Patterson and Sechrest 1983). Procedures for surfacing judgment biases in a staff training format are discussed by Newman (1983) and detailed by Newman and Sorensen (1985).

Guideline 3: Use of Measures With Objective Referents

An *objective referent* is one for which concrete examples are given for each level of a measure, or at least at key points on the rating scale. A major asset of objective referents is the potential to develop reliable and usable norms for an instrument, a feature particularly critical when applied to managed care eligibility and level-of-care decisions. One of the best examples of a scale with objective referents is the Child and Adolescent Functional Assessment Scale (CAFAS; Hodges 1996; Hodges and Gust 1995). Examples of behaviors are provided at each of four levels of impairment for each of 35 categories of behavior. For example, there are five examples of behaviors at the most severe level of impairment for "Unsafe/Potentially Unsafe Behavior," two of which are "114: Dangerous behavior caused harm to household member" and "117: Sexually assaulted/abused another household member, or attempted to (e.g., sibling)."

Another approach is when multiple items within a class of behaviors are developed, and the rater is provided one referent behavior in an item and then requested to identify either:

a. The behavior's frequency (e.g., __ times in *the last 24 hours,* or in *the last week,* or in *the last 30 days*);
b. The similarity of the observed behavior to the referent behavior (e.g., *most like* to *least like* the referent behavior); or
c. The intensity of the referent behavior (e.g., from *not evident* to *mild* to *severe*)

Which approach is best suited to your situation is an empirical issue (see Guidelines 6–11).

Clinicians often proclaim the attractiveness of instruments that are individualized to the patient. The most attractive features of these instruments are 1) that the measures can be linked more directly to the consumer's own behaviors and life situation, and 2) that treatment selection, course, and outcome can be individualized to the consumer. In fact, a consistent finding in the literature is that when the patient and the clinician have agreed on the problems and goals, there is a significantly positive increase in outcome (Mintz and Kiesler 1982). Measures that are individualized to the patient include target complaints (severity of), goal-attainment scaling, problem-oriented records, and global improvement ratings.

The major argument against such measures is the issue of generalizability. Specifically, is the change in the severity of one person's complaint/problem comparable to the degree of change in another person's complaint/problem? Although the issue of generalizability plagues all measures, without objective referents, the distribution of outcomes becomes free-floating across settings or clinical groups (Cytrynbaum et al. 1979), thereby limiting the utility of the measures.

There are arguments on the other side of this issue, but mostly when data aggregation is involved. Several meta-analytic studies (e.g., Lipsey and Wilson 1993), in which effect size was standardized, have been very informative without specifically identifying the behaviors that have been modified. Howard and co-workers (1986) studied the relationship of "dosage" (i.e., number of visits) to outcome across studies in which the measure of outcome was simply whether improvement was observed. But application of data aggregation methods may be useful only for addressing research and policy questions and may not satisfy the need for a clinician or a clinical service to communicate with a patient or an insurer about an individual patient's eligibility for care.

Local conditions, including statewide funding practices or community standards of "normal functioning," will transform the distributions of any measure, with or without objective referents (Newman 1980).

Thus, studies that identify local "norms" should become standard practice for any measure used in setting funding guidelines, setting standards for treatment review, or conducting evaluation research (Newman 1980; Newman et al. 1988).

Because individualized problem identification and goal setting has beneficial outcomes, it may be possible to have the best of both worlds. This can be accomplished by using both an individualized instrument and an instrument with national norms that has objective referents. Sechrest has noted (personal communication, November 1995) that by using both individualized instruments and instruments with national norms, one can satisfy two demands. First, one can identify the individual characteristics of the patient in terms that are most useful to the local conditions. Second, one can relate these characteristics to the patient's performance on a standardized instrument. In both cases, the other guidelines that support the reliable and valid application of either assessment technique must also be applied.

Guideline 4: Use of Multiple Respondents

A number of theorists and researchers have noted that measures from the principal stakeholders (i.e., patient, therapist, significant other–collateral, research evaluator) should be obtained because each views the process and outcomes of treatment differently (Ciarlo et al. 1986; Ellsworth 1975; Lambert et al. 1983; Strupp and Hadley 1977). The importance of this guideline varies by target group and by the clinical situation involved. For example, a second informant can be helpful in the assessment of behaviors that are socially undesirable or about which someone might generally be guarded, reticent, or simply unaware. In the assessment of children, Achenbach and Edelbrock (1983) consider the parents of psychologically troubled children as primary observers, whereas teachers are considered to be secondary observers. Similar issues are being addressed in the development of assessment scales for the elderly; the adult children of the frail elderly would be considered as major stakeholders whose assessments are considered primary over self-reports (Kane and Kane 1981; Lawton and Teresi 1994; Mangen and Peterson 1984).

Several researchers have contrasted the views of the four major respondents: patient, treating clinician, significant other, and independent clinical observer. Turner and co-workers (1982) found that there is a high level of agreement across different scales originally designed specifically for use by one of the respondent groups, as evidenced through high canonical correlations across respondents (e.g., the SCL-90-R for patients, the Denver Community Mental Health Questionnaire [Ciarlo and Reihman 1977] for clinicians, and the Personal Adjustment and Role Skills Scale [Ellsworth 1975] for significant others) when instructions were modified to fit each of the respondents. High coefficients were obtained when observers described specific behaviors (where the scale had objective referents), whereas lower coefficients were obtained when observers described how another person felt (e.g., he/she felt "happy" or "sad").

The major advantages achieved by obtaining measures from multiple observers are as follows:

- Each observer's experiences result in a unique view of the patient (although Turner and co-workers' study suggests that these views can be highly similar).
- Concurrent validation of the patient's behavioral status and changes can be obtained.
- Responses are likely to be more honest if all of the respondents are aware that there are multiple respondents.
- Discrepancies between informants can enlighten the clinician to potential problem areas that can be addressed in treatment (e.g., Patient: "I am sleeping ok!" Spouse: "He paces all night long!").

A major disadvantage of using multiple sources is higher costs, particularly in terms of the time and effort of data collection and analysis. There is also the added logistical problem of attempting to collect the functional status data from multiple respondents at the same time, such that the same states are being observed. The time and effort costs are becoming more manageable with the use of computer-assisted testing and scoring procedures; however, the additional costs of hardware and software must be considered.

Guideline 5: More Process-Identifying Outcome Measures

Measure[s] that provide information regarding the means or processes by which treatments may produce positive effects are preferred to those that do not. (Ciarlo et al. 1986, p. 28)

The basic concept here is at least controversial. On one side of the issue, Orlinsky and Howard (1986) have argued that there ought to be a relationship between process and outcomes. Behavioral and cognitive-behavioral treatments involving self-management, homework assignments, and self-help group feedback often use measures with objective behavioral referents as both process and outcome measures. On the other side, Stiles and Shapiro (1995) have argued that most important interpersonal and relationship ingredients (processes) that occur during psychotherapy (and possibly other psychosocial intervention sessions as well) are not expected to correlate with outcome. Adequate empirical support for either side of the argument is still lacking, and the different perspectives appear to be based on the theoretical orientation of those involved.

It is probably best to consider this guideline in terms of measuring treatment progress or attainment of intermediate goals of the treatment plan. Progress toward these goals ought to be an integral part of the conversation between patient and clinician. Thus, a strong argument can be made that behavioral "markers" of progress or risk level should be taken regularly during the course of treatment. Examples include levels of suicidality, depression, anxiety, substance abuse, interpersonal functioning, and community functioning (Lambert 1994; Maruish 1994). These markers are not necessarily describing the actual therapeutic process. Instead, they are global indicators describing whether the person is functioning adequately to consider continuing versus altering the planned treatment. Certainly, programs serving consumers with serious and persistent illnesses should adopt a strategy of regularly collecting such "progress" measures.

Guideline 6: Psychometric Strength

> The measure used should meet minimum criteria of psychometric adequacy, including: a) reliability (test-retest, internal consistency, or interrater agreement where appropriate); b) validity (content, concurrent, and construct validity); c) demonstrated sensitivity to treatment-related change; and d) freedom from response bias and non-reactivity (insensitivity) to extraneous situational factors that may exist (including physical settings, patient expectation, staff behavior, and accountability pressures). The measure should be difficult to intentionally fake, either positively or negatively. (Ciarlo et al. 1986, p. 27)

Two issues are discussed under the topic of psychometric features. The first is obvious: It is important to use measures of high psychometric quality. The second might seem bold: The psychometric quality of the local application of an instrument is related to the quality of services.

The importance of having measures of high psychometric quality. On the surface, no one should argue to lower the standards for an instrument's psychometric qualities. Yet, the more reactive, less psychometrically rigorous global measures (e.g., global improvement ratings, global level of functioning ratings) tend to be more popular with upper-level decision-makers (e.g., program managers, legislators). Although it is possible to exert reasonable control over the application of these measures to ensure psychometric quality (Newman 1980), if such control is not enforced, then psychometric quality suffers (Green et al. 1979).

The relationship of psychometric quality of an instrument as implemented in a local program to the program's quality of care. Here, we are making a bold double-edged assertion. On the one hand, the selection and use of an instrument of poor psychometric quality could depreciate the quality of care because it is likely that the wrong information about a person would be transmitted. One the other hand, it is also possible that a service providing poor quality care can depreciate the psychometric quality of the assessment techniques. If local data collection produces low reliability and validity estimates, and evidence exists that the instrument has been demonstrated to have adequate reliability and validity in another context, then the quality and effectiveness of clinical services should be questioned.

There are three conditions that, when satisfied, lead to an increase in both the quality of care and the psychometric quality of assessment data. First, a clinical service should have clearly defined the target groups it can treat (see Guideline 1). Second, the service should have clearly defined progress and outcome goals for each target group in terms that are observable and measurable. Third, the leadership and staff of a psychological service should have identified one or more instruments whose interpretative language is useful to support clinical communication about patient status relative to service goals. When one or more instruments are selected within the context of the first two assumptions, then the instrument can support reliable and useful communication, and such support should, in turn, promote a high quality of care.

To illustrate the relationship between the quality of care and the quality of an instrument as implemented, consider the issue of psychometric reliability as it might relate to program quality. If reliability of communication (e.g., between the patient and therapist, or among two or more treatment staff) is low, then it is likely that there is inconsistent communication or understanding about the patient's psychological and functional status, the service treatment's intention, and/or the patient's progress and outcome. Inconsistent communication or understanding regarding these aspects between patient and therapist or among clinical staff would most likely result in a poor outcome (Mintz and Kiesler 1982).

How does the use of standardized measures fit into the picture of increasing the accuracy of clinical communication? There are two points to be made. First, careful selection of the progress/outcome measures must be preceded by, and based on, a clear statement of a program's purpose and goals. Second, the language describing the functional domains (i.e., factor structure) covered by the instruments represents an agreed-on vocabulary for staff to use when communicating with and about patients. If the language of communication is related to the language of the instruments, then any inconsistency in use of the instruments would reflect an inconsistency in the communication with patients and among staff when discussing patients.[2]

Another point about instrument validity in its local application should be considered. If locally established estimates of instrument validity among services or within a service deviate from established norms, the service staff's concept of "normal" needs to be studied. Classic examples of such differences are those found in estimates of community functioning between inpatient and outpatient staff (Newman et al. 1983). Kopta and co-workers (1986) found that when there were multiple frames of reference among clinicians of different theoretical orientations, there were different syntheses of the clinical material within a session and different intervention strategies and treatment plans proposed. McGovern and colleagues (1986) found that differences in attributions of problem causality and treatment-outcome responsibility were related to judgments regarding the clinicians' choices of treatment strategies. These differences in frames of reference influence (i.e., probably reduce) the estimates of concurrent validity of measures in use as well as their inter-rater reliability. However, reduced coefficients of reliability and validity are not as serious an issue as the potential negative impact on services when purpose, language, and meaning lack clarity among service staff.

A two-part recommendation should be considered. First, the leadership of a service program should implement or refine operations that satisfy the three assumptions identified earlier: 1) obtain a clear target group definition by service staff, 2) provide operational definitions of treatment goals and objectives, and 3) work toward selection of instruments whose structure and language reflect the first two assumptions. The program should also incorporate staff supervision and development procedures that will identify when and how differences in frames of reference and language meaning are occurring. Such staff development exercises can serve to document the level of measure reliability and can be conducted at relatively low costs (see Newman and Sorensen 1985). The exercises contrast staff assessments and treatment plan for the same set of patient profiles. The patient profiles could be presented via taped interviews or via written vignettes. Green and Gracely (1987) found that a two-page profile was as effective as a taped inter-

---

[2]Work with several colleagues has focused on both the methods and the results of studies that have identified factors influencing differences in clinicians' perceptions. The theoretical arguments and historical research basis for this line of work have been discussed by Newman (1983). The procedures for conducting these studies as staff development sessions have been detailed by Newman and Sorensen (1985) and Heverly and colleagues (1984). Examples of studies on factors influencing clinical assessment and treatment decisions are those by Heverly and colleagues (1984); Kopta and co-workers (1986, 1989); McGovern and co-workers 1986; and Newman and colleagues (1983, 1987, 1988).

view (and a lot less costly) in estimating inter-rater reliability. Methods for constructing such profiles and analyzing the results have been described by Newman and Sorensen (1985) and by Heverly and co-workers (1984). The data from these exercises can also be used to assess the degree to which the local use of the instruments matches the national norms.

Guideline 7: Low Measure Costs Relative to Its Uses

How much should be spent on collecting, editing, storing, processing, and analyzing progress-outcome information? The answer to this question must be considered in terms of the five important functions that the data support: screening–treatment planning, quality assurance, program evaluation, cost containment (utilization review), and revenue generation. Given these functions, a better question might be "What is the investment needed to ensure a positive return on these functions?"

There are several pressures on mental health (and physical health) services which indicate that an investment in the use of progress-assessment instruments can be cost beneficial. The first is the requirement for an initial assessment to justify entry into services and development of a treatment plan for reimbursable patients. For the seriously and persistently mentally ill, funded placement (e.g., by Medicaid in most states) in extended community services (waivered services) requires a diagnostic and functional assessment. Most third-party payers will reimburse judicious use of such activities and the affiliated resource costs if it can be shown that the testing is a cost-effective means of making screening (utilization review) decisions. Justification for continued care is also required by both public and private third-party payers. Again, the cost of the assessment can often be underwritten by the cost containment–quality assurance agreement with the third-party payer.

The second pressure is the emerging litigious culture that requires increasing levels of accountability for treatment interventions. Our own experience is that the legal profession is divided on this issue. One view says that the less hard data a service program has, the less liability it would have for its actions. The credo here appears to be "Do not put anything in writing unless required to do so by an authority that will assume responsibility." The other view says that a service program increases its liability if it does not have any hard evidence to justify its actions. There is little doubt that the former view has been the most popular view until recently. With increased legal actions by consumer groups on the "right to treatment," there is likely to be an increased need for data that can justify the types and levels of treatment provided.

A parallel force is exerted by the increased budgetary constraints by both private and public sources of revenues for mental health services. Pressures to enforce application of cost containment–utilization review guidelines appear to be far stronger than pressures for ensuring quality of care. Although the literature has indicated the efficacy of many mental health interventions, empirical literature supporting the cost effectiveness and cost benefits of these services still lags (Newman and Howard 1986; Yates and Newman 1980).

When Ciarlo assembled the panel of experts for NIMH, a cost estimate of 0.5% of an agency's total budget was considered to be a fair estimate of affordable costs for collecting and processing progress-outcome data. This total cost was to include the costs of test materials and of training personnel, as well as of collecting and processing the data. This estimate was made at a time when the public laws governing the disbursements of federal block grant funds required that 5% of the agency's budget go toward evaluations of needs and program effectiveness.

Two notable changes in service delivery have occurred since the panel of experts met. One is that the Health Care Financing Agency (HCFA) and other third-party payers now require an assessment procedure that will deflect those who do not require care or will identify the level of care required for patients applying for service. They do offer limited reimbursement for such assessment activities. The second change focuses on the use of assertive case management or continuous treatment team approaches for the seriously and persistently mentally ill or substance-abusing persons. Here, the patient tracking procedures can be part of the reimbursed overhead costs.

Assessment and patient tracking procedures are logically compatible activities. The requirement for initial and updating assessments to justify levels of care can be integrated with the patient tracking system requirement for case management or treatment team approaches. If a cost-effective technique for integrating the assessment and the patient tracking procedures is instituted, then the costs for testing become part of the costs of coordinating and providing services. It is possible that if the costs considered here were restricted to just the costs of purchasing the instrument and the capacity to process the instrument's data (and not the professionals' time), then the costs might not exceed the 0.5% estimate. Proper cost-estimation studies need to be done to provide an empirical basis to identify the appropriate levels of costs.

Guideline 8: Understanding by Nonprofessional Audiences
The scoring procedures and presentation of the results should be understandable to stakeholders at all levels: the consumer and his/her significant others, third-party payers, and administrative and legislative policy-makers at the local, state, and federal levels.

Consumer. The analysis and interpretation of the results should be understandable at the individual consumer level. Two lines of reasoning support such an assertion. First, there is an increased belief in and legal support for the consumer's right to know about the assessment's results and the associated selection of treatment and services. An understandable descriptive profile of the patient can be used in a therapeutically positive fashion. Examples for the patient or family member's consideration might include the following:

- Does the assessment score(s) indicate my need for, progress in, or success with treatment, or the need for continued treatment?
- Does a view of my assessment score(s) over time describe how I functioned in the past relative to how I am doing now?
- Does the assessment score(s) help me communicate how I feel or function to those who are trying to serve, treat, or assist me (including my family)?
- Does the assessment help me understand what I can expect in the future?

Second, there is an advantage to being able to aggregate understandable test results over groups of consumers to communicate evaluation research results to influential stakeholders (e.g., regulators, third-party payers, legislators, citizen or consumer groups). Such results include needs assessment for program and budget planning (Newman et al. 1989; Uehara et al. 1994) and evaluation of program effectiveness and/or cost effectiveness among service alternatives for policy analysis and decisions (Newman and Howard 1986; Yates and Newman 1980). Budget planners and policy decision-makers require easily understandable data. They are often reluctant to rely solely on expert opinion to interpret the data, with some even preferring to do it themselves. Examples of questions that the data should ideally be able to address include the following:

- Do the scores show whether a patient has improved in functioning to a level where he or she either requires less restrictive care or no longer requires care?
- Do the measures assess and describe the consumer's functioning in socially significant areas—for example, independent living, vocational productivity, and appropriate interpersonal and community behaviors?
- Would the measures permit comparisons of relative program effectiveness among similar programs that serve similar patients?

In summary, it is important to ensure not only that the test results are understandable to those at the front-line level (i.e., consumers, their families, and service staff) but also that the aggregate data are understandable to budget planners and policy-makers.

Guideline 9: Easy Feedback and Uncomplicated Interpretation

The discussion of Guideline 8 above is also relevant here, but here the focus is on presentation. Does the instrument and its scoring procedures provide reports that are easily interpreted? Does the report stand on its own without further explanations or training? For example, complex "look-up" tables are less desirable than a graphic display describing the characteristics of a patient or a group of patients relative to a recognizable norm. Computerized scoring and profile printouts in both narrative and graphic form are becoming more common, which is to be commended. This trend reiterates the importance of Guideline 9.

There are two important cautionary notes about the relationship between what is communicated by a report and what are the actual underlying variables captured by the scale. First, the language of the presentation should not be so "user-friendly" that it misrepresents the data. The language used to label figures and tables must be carefully developed such that the validity of the instrument's underlying constructs is not violated. Second, and related to the first caution, it should not be assumed that the language used in the report matches the language used by the patient or family members in their effort to understand and cope with their distress. For example, an elevated SCL-90 depression subscale score might not match the patient's experience of elevated depression. It is important not to allow the language of test results to mask issues that are clinically important as well as important to the patient.

Guideline 10: Useful in Clinical Services

The assessment instrument(s) used should support the clinical processes of a service with minimum interference. An important selection guideline is whether the instrument's language, scoring, and presentation of results support clinical decisions and communication. Those who need to communicate with each other include not only the clinical and service staff working with the patient but also the patient and his or her collateral-significant others. The following clinically relevant questions might be considered in discussing the instrument(s)' utility:

- Will the test results describe the likelihood that the patient needs services and be appropriately responsive to available services?
- Do the test results help in planning the array and levels of services, treatments, and intervention styles that might best meet service goals?
- Do the test results provide sufficient justification for the planned treatment to be reimbursed by third-party payers?

- Is the patient responding to treatment as planned, and if not, in what areas of functioning is he or she responding or not responding as expected?

An ideal instrument meeting this guideline would be sufficiently supportive of these processes, such that the effort required to collect and process the data would not be seen as a burden. The logic here is complementary to that of Guideline 7—that is, the measure should have low costs relative to uses in screening–treatment planning, quality assurance, cost control, and revenue generation. Here, however, the emphasis is on utilization of the measure's results. The more the instrument is seen as supporting these functions, the less expensive and interfering the instrument will be perceived by clinical staff.

Guideline 11: Compatibility With Clinical Theories and Practices

An instrument that is compatible with a variety of clinical theories and practices should have wider interest and acceptance by a broad range of clinicians and stakeholders than one based on only one concept of treatment improvement. The former would provide a base for evaluative research by allowing one to compare the relative effectiveness of different treatment approaches or strategies.

How does one evaluate the level of compatibility? A first step is to inquire as to the context in which it was developed and the samples used in developing norms. For example, if the normative sample comprised patients on inpatient units, then it would probably be too limited, because inpatient care is now seen as the most restrictive and infrequently used level of a continuum of care. The broader the initial sampling population used in the measure's development, the more generalizable the instrument. Ideally, one would want to have available norms for both clinical and nonclinical populations. For example, if an instrument is intended for a population with a chronic physical disability (e.g., wheelchair-bound), then for sampling purposes, the definition of a normally functioning population might change to persons with the chronic physical disability who function well in the community (Saunders et al. 1988).

Another indicator of measure compatibility is whether there is evidence that the use of the measure in treatment/service planning and review is consistent with the research results published in refereed journals. This is especially important when the data are used to contrast the outcomes of two or more therapeutic (or service) interventions. In reviewing this type of research, one should first review the types of patients served, the setting, and the type of diagnoses and problems treated. One should also note the differences in standard deviations among the groups in this literature. Evidence of compatibility would be indicated by similar (homogeneous) variations among the treatment groups. Homogeneity would indicate that errors of measurement (and/or individual differences and/or item difficulty) were not biased by the therapeutic intervention that was used. One note of caution needed here is that it is possible for a measure to have homogeneity of variance within and across treatment groups and to still lack equal sensitivity to the respective treatment effects. If a measure is not sensitive to treatment effects, its use as a progress- or outcome-assessment instrument is invalid. Methods for assessing these features, a topic beyond the purposes of this chapter, have been discussed by Newman (1994).

Final Comments

The 11 guidelines discussed in this chapter are designed to support the evaluation of an assessment instrument and are not presented as firm rules of conduct. Few, if any, instruments can fully meet all the guidelines. But it is expected that if the use of these guidelines provides a means of drawing together available information on an instrument, they will decrease the number of unexpected or unpleasant surprises in the adaptation and use of a measure.

The application of the 11 guidelines has its own costs. Although master's-level psychometric training is sufficient background to assemble the basic information on an instrument's ability to meet these guidelines, a full explication of the guidelines requires broader input. Some of the guidelines require clinical supervisors and managers to review clinical standards, program procedures, and policies. Other guidelines will require an interchange among clinical supervisory and fiscal management personnel in areas of inexperience. It is our contention, however, that the ultimate benefits to patients and stakeholders of applying these guidelines are well worth the costs.

References

Achenbach TM, Edelbrock CS: Manual for the Child Behavior Checklist and Revised Behavior Profile. Burlington, VT, Department of Psychology, University of Vermont, 1983

Beck AT, Steer RA: Manual for the Beck Depression Inventory. San Antonio, TX, Psychological Corporation, 1993

Beutler LE, Clarkin JF: Systematic Treatment Selection: Toward Targeted Therapeutic Interventions. New York, Brunner/Mazel, 1990

Ciarlo JA, Reihman J: The Denver Community Mental Health Questionnaire: development of a multidimensional program evaluation instrument, in Program Evaluation for Mental Health: Methods, Strategies and Participants. Edited by Coursey R, Spector G, Murrell S, et al. New York, Grune & Stratton, 1977

Ciarlo JA, Brown TR, Edwards DW, et al: Assessing Mental Health: Treatment Outcome Measurement Techniques (DHHS Publ No [ADM] 86-1301). Washington, DC, U.S. Department of Health and Human Services, 1986

Cronbach LJ: Essentials of Psychological Testing, 3rd Edition. New York, Harper & Row, 1970

Cytrynbaum S, Ginath T, Birdwell J, et al: Goal attainment scaling: a critical review. Evaluation Quarterly 3:5–40, 1979

Derogatis LR: Symptom Checklist–90—Revised (SCL-90-R) Administration, Scoring, and Procedures Manual, 3rd Edition. Minneapolis, MN, National Computer Systems, 1994

Eisen SV, Dill DL, Grob MC: Reliability and validity of a brief patient-report instrument for psychiatric outcome evaluation. Hosp Community Psychiatry 45:242–247, 1994

Ellsworth RB: Consumer feedback in measuring the effectiveness of mental health programs, in Handbook of Evaluation Research, Vol 2. Edited by Guttentag M, Struening EL. Beverly Hills, CA, Sage. 1975, pp 239–274

Green RS, Gracely EJ: Selecting a rating scale for evaluating services to the chronically mentally ill. Community Ment Health J 23:91–102, 1987

Green RS, Nguyen TD, Attkisson CC: Harnessing the reliability of outcome measures. Evaluation and Program Planning 2:137–142, 1979

Heverly MA, Fitt DX, Newman FL: Constructing case vignettes for evaluating clinical judgement. Evaluation and Program Planning 7:45–55, 1984

Hodges K: Child and Adolescent Assessment Scale (CAFAS): miniscale version. Ann Arbor, MI, Author, 1996

Hodges K, Gust J: Measures of impairment for children and adolescents. Journal of Mental Health Administration 22:403–413, 1995

Howard KI, Kopta SM, Krause MS, et al: The dose-effect relationship in psychotherapy. Am Psychol 41:159–164, 1986

Howard KI, Moras K, Brill P, et al: Evaluation of psychotherapy: efficacy, effectiveness, and patient progress. Am Psychol 51:1059–1064, 1996

Kane RA, Kane RL: Assessing the Elderly: A Practical Guide to Measurement. Lexington, MA, Lexington Books, 1981

Kopta SM, Newman FL, McGovern MP, et al: Psychotherapeutic orientations: a comparison of conceptualizations, interventions and recommendations for a treatment plan. J Consult Clin Psychol 54:369–374, 1986

Kopta SM, Newman FL, McGovern MP, et al: The relationship between years of psychotherapy experience and conceptualizations, interventions, and treatment plan costs. Professional Psychology 29:59–61, 1989

Lambert MJ: Use of psychological tests for outcome assessment, in Use of Psychological Testing for Treatment Planning and Outcome Assessment. Edited by Maruish M. Hillsdale, NJ, Lawrence Erlbaum, 1994, pp 75–97

Lambert MJ, Christensen E, DeJulio R (eds): The Assessment of Psychotherapy Outcome. New York, Wiley, 1983

Lawton MP, Teresi JA (eds): Annual Review of Gerontology and Geriatrics, Vol 14: Focus on Assessment Techniques. New York, Springer, 1994

Leff HS, Mulkern V, Lieberman M, et al: The effects of capitation on service access, adequacy, and appropriateness. Administration and Policy in Mental Health 21:141–160, 1994

Lipsey M, Wilson D: The efficacy of psychological, educational, and behavioral treatment: confirmation and meta-analyses. Am Psychol 48:1181–1209, 1993

Locke SE, Kowaloff HB, Hoff RG, et al: Computer-based interview for screening blood donors for risk of HIV transmission. JAMA 268:1301–1305, 1992

Mangen DJ, Peterson WA: Health, Program Evaluation, and Demography. Minneapolis, University of Minnesota, 1984

Maruish ME (ed): Use of Psychological Testing for Treatment Planning and Outcome Assessment. Hillsdale, NJ, Lawrence Erlbaum, 1994

McGovern MP, Newman FL, Kopta SM: Meta-theoretical assumptions and psychotherapy orientation: clinician attributions of patients' problem causality and responsibility for treatment outcome. J Consult Clin Psychol 54:476–481, 1986

Mintz J, Kiesler DJ: Individualized measure of psychotherapy outcome, in Handbook of Research Methods in Clinical Psychology. Edited by Kendall P, Butcher JN. New York, Wiley, 1982

Mulkern V, Leff HS, Green RS, et al: Section II: Performance indicators for a consumer-oriented mental health report card: literature review and analysis, in Stakeholders' Perspectives on Mental Health Performance Indicators. Edited by Mulkern V. Cambridge, MA, The Evaluation Center at the Human Services Research Institute, 1995

Navaline HA, Snider EC, Christopher JP, et al: Preparation for AIDS vaccine trials: an automated version of the Risk Assessment Battery (RAB): enhancing the assessment of risk behaviors. Aids Res Hum Retroviruses 10:281–283, 1994

Newman FL: Global scales: strengths, uses and problems of global scales as an evaluation instrument. Evaluation and Program Planning 3:257–268, 1980

Newman FL: Therapists' evaluations of psychotherapy, in The Assessment of Psychotherapy Outcome. Edited by Lambert MJ, Christensen E, DeJulio R. New York, Wiley, 1983

Newman FL: Selection of design and statistical procedures for progress and outcome assessment, in Use of Psychological Testing for Treatment Planning and Outcome Assessment. Edited by Maruish ME. Hillsdale, NJ, Lawrence Erlbaum, 1994, pp 111–134

Newman FL, Ciarlo JA: Criteria for selecting psychological instruments for treatment outcome assessment, in The Use of Psychological Testing for Treatment Planning and Outcome Assessment. Edited by Maruish ME. Hillsdale, NJ, Lawrence Erlbaum, 1994, pp 98–110

Newman FL, Howard KI: Therapeutic effort, outcome and policy. Am Psychol 41:181–187, 1986

Newman FL, Sorensen JE: Integrated Clinical and Fiscal Management in Mental Health: A Guidebook. Norwood, NJ, Ablex, 1985

Newman FL, Tejeda MJ: The need for research that is designed to support decisions in the delivery of mental health services. Am Psychol 51:1040–1049, 1996

Newman FL, Heverly MA, Rosen M, et al: Influences on internal evaluation data dependability: clinicians as a source of variance, in Developing Effective Internal Evaluation (New Directions for Program Evaluation No 20). Edited by Love AJ. San Francisco, CA, Jossey-Bass, 1983

Newman FL, Fitt D, Heverly MA: Influences of patient, service program and clinician characteristics on judgments of functioning and treatment recommendations. Evaluation and Program Planning 10:260–267, 1987

Newman FL, Kopta SM, McGovern MP, et al: Evaluating the conceptualizations and treatment plans of interns and supervisors during a psychology internship. J Consult Clin Psychol 56:659–665, 1988

Newman FL, Griffin BP, Black RW, et al: Linking level of care to level of need: assessing the need for mental health care for nursing home residents. Am Psychol 44:1315–1324, 1989

Nunnally JC, Burnstein I: Psychometric Theory, 3rd Edition. New York, McGraw-Hill, 1994

Orlinsky DE, Howard KI: Process and outcome in psychotherapy, in Handbook of Psychotherapy and Behavior Change, 3rd Edition. Edited by Garfield L, Bergin AE. New York, Wiley, 1986, pp 311–381

Patterson DR, Sechrest L: Nonreactive measures in psychotherapy outcome research. Clinical Psychology Review 3:391–416, 1983

Saunders SM, Howard KI, Newman FL: Evaluating the clinical significance of treatment effects: norms and normality. Behavioral Assessment 10:207–218, 1988

Stiles WB, Shapiro DA: Disabuse of the drug metaphor: psychotherapy process-outcome correlations. J Consult Clin Psychol 62:942–948, 1995

Strupp HH, Hadley SW: A tripartite model of mental health and therapeutic outcome. Am Psychol 32:187–196, 1977

Turner R, McGovern M, Sandrock D: A multiple perspective analysis of schizophrenic symptomatology and community functioning. Am J Community Psychol 11:593–607, 1982

Uehara E, Smukler M, Newman FL: Linking resource use to consumer level of need in a local mental health system: field test of the "LONCA" case mix method. J Consult Clin Psychol 62:695–709, 1994

Yates BT, Newman FL: Findings of cost-effectiveness and cost-benefit analyses of psychotherapy, in Psychotherapy: From Practice to Research to Policy. Edited by VandenBos G. Beverly Hills, CA, Sage, 1980, pp 163–185

APPENDIX
Monographs and Texts Containing Lists and Critiques of Instruments for Assessing Persons in the Major Target Populations

Adult: General

Ciarlo JA, Brown TR, Edwards DW, et al.: *Assessing Mental Health: Treatment Outcome Measurement Techniques* (DHHS Publ No [ADM] 86-1301). Washington, DC, U.S. Department of Health and Human Services, 1986

Docherty JP, Dewan NA: *Guide to Outcomes Management* (Monograph of the National Association of Psychiatric Health Systems). Chicago, IL, American Hospital Association Foundation Trust, 1995

Maruish M (ed): *Use of Psychological Testing for Treatment Planning and Outcome Assessment.* Hillsdale, NJ, Lawrence Erlbaum, 1994 [see Part II]

Ogles BM, Lambert MJ, Masters KS: *Assessing Outcome in Clinical Practice.* Boston, MA, Allyn & Bacon, 1996 [for outpatient clinical practice]

Sederer LI, Dickey B (eds): *Outcome Assessment in Clinical Practice.* Baltimore, MD, Williams & Wilkins, 1996

Adult: Persons With a Serious Mental Illness

Mulkern V, Leff HS, Green RS, et al: "Section II: Performance Indicators for a Consumer-Oriented Mental Health Report Card: Literature Review and Analysis, in *Stakeholders' Perspectives on Mental Health Performance Indicators.* Edited by Mulkern V. Cambridge, MA, The Evaluation Center at the Human Services Research Institute, 1995

*All the references given above as pertaining to **Adult: General** cover this subpopulation.*

Geriatric

Kane RA, Kane RL: *Assessing the Elderly: A Practical Guide to Measurement.* Lexington, MA, Lexington Books, 1981

Lawton MP, Teresi JA (eds): *Annual Review of Gerontology and Geriatrics, Vol. 14: Focus on Assessment Techniques.* New York, Springer, 1994

Mangen DJ, Peterson WA: *Health, Program Evaluation, and Demography.* Minneapolis, University of Minnesota, 1984

Children and Youth

Green RS, Newman FL: "Criteria for Selecting Instruments for Treatment Outcome Assessment." *Residential Children & Youth* (in press)

Hodges K, Gust J: "Measures of Impairment for Children and Adolescents." *Journal of Mental Health Administration* 22:403–413, 1995

LaGreco AM (ed): *Through the Eyes of the Child: Obtaining Self-Reports From Children and Adolescents.* Boston, MA, Allyn & Bacon, 1990

Maruish M (ed): *Use of Psychological Testing for Treatment Planning and Outcome Assessment.* Hillsdale, NJ, Lawrence Erlbaum, 1994 [see Part III]

Chapter 24

Performance Measurement in Healthcare Delivery Systems

Naakesh A. Dewan, M.D., and Daniel Carpenter, Ph.D.

A variety of efforts are currently under way by accreditation bodies, government agencies, and private organizations to develop and promulgate performance measures and standards in the form of "report cards" or indicator projects for medical, psychiatric, and behavioral healthcare delivery systems. Each of these efforts aims to provide "stakeholders" (i.e., patients, providers, purchasers, and anyone else who has a stake in the healthcare process) with a meaningful barometer of the quality of health care in organized systems of care. The purpose of this chapter is to compare and contrast these various approaches and to provide the reader with a general overview of this new field of systems measurement.

Background

The quest for measuring and managing clinical quality is not new (Donabedian 1966). Since the early 1900s, American medicine has led the effort to standardize and reduce the variability in both the delivery of care and the education and training of physicians providing the care. The Flexner report commissioned by the Carnegie Foundation for Advancement of Teaching was an enormous step in reforming the professional development of physicians (Flexner 1910). The efforts of Ernest Codman led to development of hospital standards and, eventually, to the Joint Commission on Accreditation of Hospitals (Roberts 1987). While associations representing hospitals and physicians were focusing on improving the quality of care, the government was developing methods to reduce the rising cost of hospital care through peer review organizations and utilization review methodologies (Institute of Medicine 1993). It was not until the American automobile industry began to suffer tremendous financial losses that government and big business were both deeply concerned about spiraling healthcare costs.

American industry began to investigate its business processes and costs utilizing total quality management techniques and started to demand lower prices and improved quality from its suppliers, including those providing healthcare services. American industry is still undergoing a "quality transformation," in which words like "reinventing" and "reengineering" are becoming part of everyday language.

American health care—and specifically American psychiatric and behavioral health care—is just beginning to transform itself (Berwick 1989; Docherty and Dewan 1995). Although it is true that the practice of medicine has always been an art grounded in fundamental scientific and ethical principles, its improvement and advances have relied on product and technological breakthroughs rather than on clinical or organizational process improvement or innovations. The cure for mental illness may lie in the basic sciences, but appropriate funding for such cure in the near future lies in the measurement and management sciences. Report cards and performance indicators in general are the first step in using evaluation and measurement to improve the accountability and functioning of a coordinated system of health care.

The steps involved in developing an evaluation system for human services have been outlined by a number of researchers (National Institute of Mental Health 1984, 1986). First, define the values and goals of the program. Then, translate the goals into measurable indicators. Finally, collect and compare the data across different programs and individuals and provide feedback to stakeholders. Despite its apparent simplicity, this process can be a tremendous burden in practice for the simple reason that *indicators* do not measure quality; *people* measure quality (Maryland Hospital Association 1993). As a result of this sociological reality, different groups will develop and implement performance measurement systems based on distinct perspective and goals. This is apparent in the current efforts to measure the performance of health plans, hospitals, and clinicians. Each initiative, however, has the potential for improving health care at a variety of levels and from different viewpoints through the appropriate use of data and statistical analysis.

The variation in language used to describe features of respective report cards reflects the diversity of approaches and viewpoints taken in their development. We have tried to use fairly consistent terminology in our discussion and will define important concepts at the outset. All report cards identify *domains* of health care, which are general categories under which the measures and indicators are grouped. A *concern* is an articulation of a value about one aspect of performance under a particular domain. A concern might also be thought of as a goal or the statement of a goal toward which a healthcare organization strives. An *indicator* is an operational definition of an organization's concern. For report cards that do not identify concerns, an indicator is an operationalization of an aspect of care grouped under a given domain. Finally, a *measure* is a specific instrument of measurement used to quantify and calculate the indicator. A measure can be an instrument with several items (e.g., a multiple-item questionnaire) or a single item (e.g., mortality rate under certain circumstances). The following section outlines the background, goals, and methodologies of the national efforts aimed at improving healthcare performance and measurement.

National Hospital-Based Efforts

The Maryland Hospital Association Quality Indicator Project was developed to measure hospital performance (Kazandjian et al. 1993). In 1985, a group of seven Maryland hospitals voluntarily initiated the testing of 10 medical and surgical inpatient indicators. This effort received a grant from the Robert Wood Johnson Foundation in 1987 and in 1994 had over 900 hospitals jointly measuring and sharing quality information data. The Maryland effort is unique in both its methodology and its philosophical approach to improving quality.

The primary mission of the Maryland project is to provide hospitals with a confidential, valid, and reliable mechanism for measuring, comparing, and improving performance. It is a research initiative, and its only customers are those actually providing care. In essence, this is a collaborative continuous quality improvement project between approximately 900 hospitals in the United States committed to supplying and sharing mutually agreed-on performance indicator data to a centralized organization. Each member receives feedback reports and participates in quarterly surveys regarding the validity, utility, and reliability of the indicator data being collected. In addition, educational seminars on topics from statistics to quality improvement techniques are provided to all participants. There has been no public release of the data, and no broad public display of the data is planned. The project and its participants have embraced the concept of continuous quality improvement, and as the public demand for accountability continues, reporting of performance data to the general public may become mandatory or even desirable to some of its members. The demand to release these data has the potential of interfering with the reliability and, eventually, the validity of the data and the process of continuous quality improvement occurring within the participants of the Maryland project.

The Maryland project focuses primarily on indicators of quality general medical care. There are 10 indicators for inpatient medical care:

1. Hospital-acquired infections
2. Surgical wound infections
3. Inpatient mortality
4. Neonatal mortality
5. Perioperative mortality
6. Cesarean sections
7. Unscheduled readmissions
8. Unscheduled admission following ambulatory procedure
9. Unscheduled returns to a special care unit
10. Unscheduled returns to the operating room

There are also five indicators for ambulatory care:

1. Unscheduled returns to the emergency department within 72 hours
2. Registered patients in the emergency department more than 6 hours
3. Emergency department cases in which discrepancy between initial and final X-ray reports required an adjustment in patient management
4. Registered patients who leave the emergency department before completion of treatment
5. Cancellation of ambulatory procedure on the day of procedure

The Maryland project began implementing a psychiatric indicator project in March of 1996. There are four indicators for psychiatric quality:

1. Unplanned departures
2. Transfers to acute medical care
3. Self-injurious behavior
4. Readmissions within 15 days

In summary, the Maryland Hospital Association Quality Indicator Project is a formative evaluation project for which providers are the key stakeholders and in which feasibility and utility of the performance measurements systems are paramount. The project needs to embrace statistical techniques such as risk adjustment and functional outcome measurement to be consistent with other efforts.

Accreditation Organizations and Performance Measurement Programs

Joint Commission on Accreditation of Healthcare Organizations

The Joint Commission on Accreditation of Hospitals was formed in 1952 as a result of a collaboration between the American College of Physicians, American Medical Association, American Hospital Association, Canadian Medical Association, and American College of Surgeons. In 1987, the Joint Commission changed its name to the Joint Commission on Accreditation of Healthcare Organizations to include all healthcare organizations because of the tremendous changes occurring in the financing and structure of healthcare delivery systems. At the same time, the Joint Commission began promoting the Indicator Management System (IMS) (Schyve 1995). This data-driven effort is designed to complement ongoing accreditation efforts and has been developed to assist hospitals in measuring and comparing outcomes and processes across a number of disease categories.

The criteria used by the Joint Commission to determine a "good" measure fall into five categories (Joint Commission on Accreditation of Healthcare Organizations [JCAHO] 1995a, 1995b):

1. The indicator must be relevant and of significant importance to patient and providers.
2. Data collection methodologies and definitions must be reliable to ensure that measurement error is minimized.
3. The indicator must be sensitive enough to discriminate between different providers and settings.
4. The data collection effort must be financially and operationally feasible.
5. The measure must have validity.

The test for validity lies in its actual utility to stakeholders and whether changes in process determined by the indicator actually change and improve performance. The IMS includes 42 indicators: 10 related to obstetrical and perioperative care, 5 to oncology care, 7 to cardiovascular care, 9 to trauma care, and 11 to medication use and infection control (Joint Commission on Accreditation of Healthcare Organizations 1996). The indicator that specifically pertains to psychiatry is the monitoring of lithium use in hospitals (JCAHO 1995a). In addition, the number of medications prescribed at discharge is another indicator that can be used to compare different patients, hospitals, and clinicians.

The attempt by the Joint Commission to develop and standardize a uniform, reliable, valid, and sensitive clinically based performance measurement system across all United States hospitals was an ambitious undertaking and a tremendous contribution to the field of quality management. The Joint Commission has decided after significant feedback and field testing that it will not mandate the use of the IMS as the standard report card for all hospitals in the country (Loeb and O'Leary 1995). Many hospitals have developed their own performance improvement system in collaboration with health services researchers. Implementing the Joint Commission's IMS would require additional expenditures and add an operational burden that hospitals cannot absorb in a managed care environment. The Joint Commission is therefore altering the IMS to make it more flexible and complete by incorporating systems developed by others.

The Joint Commission has also recently issued a request for indicators for healthcare networks (Seidenfeld et al. 1995). Clinical performance, satisfaction, and health status are the three major domains of performance outlined in the proposed network report card. In addition, seven disease categories, including substance abuse and mental health disorders, have been identified as priorities. The call for measures of enrollee, patient, provider, and purchaser satisfaction as part of this effort is unique among indicator and report card efforts. The Joint

Commission has embraced the concept that providers, payers, patients, and consumers are all important stakeholders in healthcare delivery systems. This unique philosophy will be a model for other efforts currently under way. The Joint Commission still needs to develop means to reduce the workload on provider systems and will need to set more realistic goals for the effort to succeed in a contemporary environment.

Health Plan Employer Data and Information Set

The Health Plan Employer Data and Information Set (HEDIS) was originally developed in 1989 under the auspices of The HMO Group (Corrigan and Nielsen 1993). This group, which included both staff and group model health maintenance organizations (HMOs), collaborated with four large employers (Bull HN Information Systems, Inc.; Digital Equipment Corporation; GTE; and Xerox Corporation), Towers Perrin (a benefits consulting firm), and Kaiser Permanente. The key objectives at that time were 1) to define and understand employer needs to document the "value" of a health plan, and 2) to develop performance measures that respond to those needs. HEDIS 1.0 was completed in September of 1992 and was presented to several healthcare organization and business coalitions for their use. Subsequently, The HMO Group transferred further development of HEDIS to the National Committee for Quality Assurance (NCQA), a not-for-profit organization that serves as the accreditation entity for the nation's HMOs. NCQA then assembled a variety of representatives from employers, health plans, and insurance companies, plus technical experts, to refine the performance measure developed by The HMO Group. The NCQA released HEDIS 2.0 in November 1993 (NCQA 1993), HEDIS 2.5 in January 1995 (NCQA 1995b), and a revised HEDIS 2.5 in January 1996 (NCQA 1996). Currently, HEDIS 3.0 is being developed, as well as an HEDIS for Medicaid and one for Medicare.

The original purpose of HEDIS was to help employers understand what "value" their healthcare dollar was purchasing and how to hold a health plan "accountable" for its performance. Recently, however, NCQA has included consumers of care as key stakeholders as well, but has yet to include providers as key advocates for quality. NCQA also believes that health plans are ultimately responsible for the quality of care provided to patients, and this view is currently shared by purchasers of care.

The selection of specific performance measures for HEDIS 2.0 was based on three criteria: 1) relevance to the employer community, 2) reasonable ability of health plans to develop and provide the requested data, and 3) potential impact on improving the process of care delivery. The selection criteria being utilized to develop HEDIS 3.0 are much more extensive but emphasize 1) relevance to consumers, employers, and health plans; 2) scientific validity and reliability, as well as risk adjustability; and 3) feasibility, and potential for quality improvement.

The performance measures in HEDIS 2.0/2.5 encompass the domains of quality, access and patient satisfaction, membership and utilization, finance, and descriptive information on health plan management and activities. HEDIS 3.0, which is scheduled to be released in January of 1997, is being designed to encompass the following areas (NCQA 1995a):

1. Effectiveness of care
2. Access to and availability of care
3. Satisfaction with experience of care
4. Informed healthcare choices
5. Health plan descriptive information
6. Cost of care
7. Health plan stability
8. Use of services

A comprehensive and detailed review of all the HEDIS performance measures is beyond the scope of this chapter and can be found elsewhere. It is important to note, however, that the HEDIS is a remarkable effort to measure the overall value of a healthcare delivery system. The domain of quality includes preventive measures, prenatal care, acute and chronic illness, and mental health. The selection of the items measuring quality was largely based on both academic and governmental publications (U.S. Department of Health and Human Services 1990; U.S. Preventive Services Task Force 1989; Siu et al. 1992). The item utilized to measure quality in mental health care is the percentage of patients who complete an ambulatory follow-up visit within 30 days posthospitalization for a major mood disorder. This measure was chosen because of the high prevalence of mood disorders in the United States population and the evidence in the medical literature pointing to lack of follow-up as a risk factor for relapse and increased morbidity. The other domains in HEDIS 2.0/2.5 that include mental health measures are in the membership and utilization categories. Health plans are asked to submit data on the utilization of inpatient care, including average length of stay, day/night hospital, and ambulatory services for health plan members for chemical dependency and psychiatric disorders. Readmissions within 90 days and 365 days posthospitalization for patients with major mood disorders and chemical dependency are included as well. Readmission is perhaps the only outcome measure in the HEDIS report card for mental health and will most likely remain the only outcome measure that can be agreed on by a variety of stakeholders as an important indicator of quality in psychiatric care. However, functional outcome and health status measures may be included in 1997 for medical care and potentially for psychiatric care.

In summary, the Health Plan Employer Data and Information Set is a historic effort aimed at making purchasers and patients truly rational and educated buyers of healthcare and health promotion services by providing reliable and valid information regarding the structure, process, cost, and outcome of the care provided by different health plans. The report card is still in its infancy, and variability in data collection and reporting compromises the credibility of this effort.

The Consumer Reports *Report Card*

Well before President Clinton put the term *report card* into the everyday language of healthcare researchers, *Consumer Reports* (CR) anticipated the need for some kind of performance rating for the rapidly expanding number of healthcare providers and turned to its readership for answers ("Health Care in Crisis" 1992). In a comprehensive survey of more than 20,000 readers, CR obtained consumer-based data regarding the performance of 46 HMOs across the country. For inclusion, at least 150 responses had to be received regarding a particular HMO. Consumers were asked to rate their overall level of satisfaction and their satisfaction with three specific aspects of the HMO: their primary physician, their choice of and access to a medical specialist, and the HMO administration. No data regarding behavioral health services were reported. Even the lowest rated HMOs were rated by consumers to be at least satisfactory, and 91% of the respondents were at least satisfied with their primary physician. Most (86%) were at least "satisfied" with their access to a specialist, and 79% were satisfied with the HMO administration. In the rankings, the highest-rated HMO had fewer than 5% of respondents who were "dissatisfied," whereas the lowest had more than 25% of respondents who were dissatisfied. In addition to providing satisfaction data, the survey offered information regarding the logistics of each of the plans as well.

Consumer Reports has a long-standing tradition of meeting the needs of its readers with excellent surveys and attention to the consumer's point of view. Although the 1992 CR report card was limited to 46 HMOs and is clearly not definitive as far as comparing plans in terms of outcome, it represents an early effort at providing a structure in which plans can be evaluated and consumers can make somewhat of an informed choice. A similarly helpful approach was taken by CR in its recent survey of readers regarding their satisfaction with psychotherapy ("Mental Health: Does Therapy Work?" 1995). CR is expected to publish its second survey of readers regarding HMOs in the summer of 1996.

American Managed Behavioral Healthcare Association

The American Managed Behavioral Healthcare Association (AMBHA) was founded in 1994 and represents most of the managed mental healthcare companies in the United States. Soon after its formation,

AMBHA formed the Quality Improvement and Clinical Services Committee (referred to here as the Committee) to oversee the development of a report card structure by which adherence to high standards of mental health care on the part of the member organizations could be shown. The Committee identified two phases of work, which might be loosely described as *development* and *implementation*. Data on the development phase have been published, but data on the implementation of the report card developed in phase I are not yet available.

The development of the AMBHA report card involved the definition of results or levels of performance that the committee felt characterized an efficient and effective healthcare program. The Committee's first report was published in August 1995 and described those standards of performance as the Performance-Based Measures for Managed Behavioral Healthcare Programs, Version 1.0 (PERMS 1.0). PERMS 1.0 is meant to be the first step toward the development of a report card for the members of AMBHA. The report identifies three principles on which the selection of performance indicators was based: meaningfulness, measurability, and manageability.

1. *Meaningful.* The performance indicators had to be comprehensive in their assessment of quality of care across the wide range of clinical services and enrolled populations. The indicators also had to be amenable to risk adjustment.
2. *Measurable.* The performance indicators had to be consistent with accepted standards of measurement of the quality of care.
3. *Manageable.* The performance indicators had to be realistically obtainable in the context of the member organizations.

To avoid large amounts of missing data on measures that might be difficult for some of its members to obtain, the Committee recommended measures that were readily available to the member organizations.

With these principles as guidelines, the Committee then identified performance measures in three domains: access to care, consumer satisfaction, and quality of care.

Access to Care
Making access to services as easy as possible for healthcare consumers is widely agreed to be central to any report card on healthcare services. The PERMS indicators of access to care have to do with the percentage of enrolled persons who utilize the wide range of services offered by the system and with the concrete details of contacting the system by telephone and obtaining services. The indicators involve the demographics, clinical characteristics, and types of services used by its enrollees; utilization of services by the severely mentally ill; and telecommunication issues or ease of telephone access to the plan.

Consumer Satisfaction

The PERMS indicators of consumer satisfaction involve enrollees being asked how satisfied they are with services in five main areas: access to services; the intake worker; clinical care, which involves ratings of their therapist's competence and whether they would refer a friend to the clinic; outcome; and global satisfaction. In addition to explicitly describing its indicators, the AMBHA report requires minimum standards for accepting survey data as representative of the enrollees of a program. The standards describe methodological features such as a minimum response rate of 79%; a minimum number of responses of 500; requirements for the reporting of raw, as well as percentage, data; the manner in which the sample is chosen; and the timing of sampling relative to the utilization of services.

Quality of Care

The indicators for the quality of care are divided into three categories: effectiveness, efficiency, and appropriateness.

Effectiveness.   The concept of the *effectiveness* of healthcare services essentially refers to whether the treatments being given or the services being offered by a system of care are effective in addressing the problems and concerns of its enrollees. The PERMS offers indicators of effectiveness in the treatment of major depressive disorder (MDD) and substance abuse. For MDD, the indicator is the number of patients who receive outpatient follow-up within 30 days of an inpatient admission. For substance abuse, the indicator is the percentage of patients treated with a first detoxification service who need another detoxification service within 90 days of the first.

Efficiency.   The *efficiency* of health care is the extent to which services are provided in such a way that good outcome is maximized while resource utilization is minimized. The quality of a program can be judged in terms of the way it meets these sometimes competing goals. The PERMS offers indicators of efficiency for mental health in general and for substance abuse in particular. The efficiency indicator for mental health is the distribution of patients in each of four categories based on the follow-up contact after a hospitalization: no follow-up, follow-up contact, follow-up contact plus readmission to an inpatient unit, or readmission only. The efficiency indicator for substance abuse is similar to that for mental health and is defined as the distribution of patients in four categories based on the follow-up after an inpatient detoxification.

Appropriateness.   The *appropriateness* of care is defined by PERMS as the extent to which enrollees receive an accepted standard of care. PERMS offers three indicators of the appropriateness of care divided by target populations: patients with schizophrenia, children age 12 years and younger, and individuals with an adjustment disorder. For patients with schizophrenia, the indicator of appropriateness is meant to assess the availability of medication management services and is based on the number of brief contacts with a psychiatrist in a year's time. The standard is that such patients should receive at least four medication management visits with a psychiatrist in a year. The appropriateness indicator for children age 12 years and younger is based on the standard that if a child in this age range receives any services under the plan, at least one collateral family visit should also be held. The appropriateness indicator for adults with adjustment disorder is based on the number of persons with that diagnosis who are seen for 10 visits or fewer in a calendar year.

$$\cdot \;\; \cdot \;\; \cdot$$

The AMBHA report card represents a major leap forward in terms of having involved the cooperation of members who are, in many cases, competing with each other in the very aggressive market of managed psychiatric health care. The report card is described by its authors as a first-generation effort and includes several self-critical comments on its limitations and on potential areas of future work. This acknowledgment of its limitations is commendable and bespeaks a commitment to the development of a report card that enhances the quality of care delivered by the member organizations. In general, the limitations of the AMBHA report card involve a lack of consistency with existing literature on report card development, outcomes assessment, and consumer satisfaction. The scope of the report card is narrow, with the report card offering assessment of only two disorders (MDD and substance abuse), making the assessment of an entire system of care difficult. The Committee had limited consultation with academic centers and experts regarding measurement technology and the measurement sciences as they have been applied to the behavioral health field.

Perhaps the aspect of the AMBHA report card of most concern so far is the lack of attention to research regarding utilization of behavioral healthcare services for special populations. For example, how well the provider handles linguistic issues is not included in the indicators. Non-English-speaking individuals are not included in the sampling of survey respondents, and race is not one of the blocking variables when penetration of services is evaluated.

In summary, the AMBHA report card represents a remarkable effort by a brand-new industry to come to a consensus regarding standards of care and performance reporting. In its report card effort so far, AMBHA has faced revolutionary changes in the way behavioral health care is delivered, with relatively little guidance from established standards of assessment and quality. It is certain that AMBHA will begin to involve consumers and special-needs populations. The fact that the development of this report card was initiated by the very industry that it will ultimately scrutinize bodes well in terms of its prospects for implementation.

Mental Health Statistic Improvement Program

In response to President Clinton's proposed 1993 Health Security Act (HSA) and in anticipation of ensuing changes in the healthcare industry, the Mental Health Statistic Improvement Program (MHSIP) of the Center for Mental Health Services formed a task force to make recommendations regarding the composition of and methodology for developing a mental health report card that would be comparable to report cards in other areas of health care. Membership of the task force was quite broad, including consumers; officials from local, state, and federal governments; and health services researchers. It was planned that once a national healthcare system was in place, the federal government would require providers to report their performance using a standard report card structure. In such a system, the MHSIP recommendation would have been central in establishing the report card structure and the accompanying performance standards. Even though a national healthcare system is very unlikely as of this writing, the recommendations of the MHSIP task force should be considered required study for any system developing a report card.

The MHSIP Report Card Task Force identifies itself as being committed to helping develop a report card from the mental healthcare consumer's point of view. Consumers have been included at every step in the process, and performance indicators have been reviewed in terms of their ability to inform the consumer about his or her healthcare options. The task force also has identified the additional priorities of being research based, inclusive of issues associated with serious mental illness, inclusive of outcomes assessment, and conscious of cost and administrative burden. The MHSIP effort is extremely ambitious in terms of the broad range of issues and concerns that it sought to address.

The task force has conceptualized its work in three phases. The first two have been completed, and some documentation has been published. Phase I, chaired by John A. Hornik, Ph.D., included a thorough review of the literature on existing report cards in general and on mental health report cards specifically (Center for Mental Health Services 1994). Phase II, chaired by Vijay Ganju, Ph.D., involved a more thorough and specific review of indicators and measures that the earlier work of the task force had identified as candidates for inclusion in the mental health report card (Center for Mental Health Services 1995). Although the final Phase II report has not been published, preliminary reports are available (e.g., Center for Mental Health Services 1995;

Mulkern et al. 1995; Sherman and Kaufman 1995). Phase III is expected to involve pilot testing of the specific measures identified in Phase II. The present discussion includes material currently available.

The structure of the MHSIP Report Card Task Force report is based on the basic domains that were identified by President Clinton's HSA as crucial in the evaluation of general healthcare delivery systems. These domains are access, appropriateness, outcomes, health promotion, and prevention. Consumer satisfaction concerns were subsumed under the other domains. In each domain, a list of concerns is identified that represent value statements about the performance of a health plan or delivery system. For each identified concern, one to four indicators are given as gauges of progress toward addressing the concern. The complete list of Phase II concerns, including a sample indicator for each concern, is presented in Table 24–1 by the respective domains.

One of the strengths of the MHSIP report card is that it identifies specific instruments and sources of data for its indicators. Each of the measures is critiqued in terms of its psychometric characteristics and ability to cover the indicator being assessed. Consistent with other report cards, the sources of information for the measures include consumer self-report, financial data, enrollment/encounter data, medications prescribed, and data from the doctor's examination. The consumer self-report data are obtained by a 44-item survey that was pilot-tested with good success in patients with serious mental illnesses. In addition, a brief inventory tapping symptom distress and three items assessing level of functioning are also given. Clinicians are given brief measures for different situations, including a functioning scale for children and adolescents, a measure of involuntary movement for adults with serious mental illnesses, and rating scales for drug and alcohol use. The consumer and clinician measures are given in the task force report and their origins are specified. The report also specifies precise definitions of the measures associated with claims, enrollment, and expenditures.

To summarize: the MHSIP Report Card Task Force reports represent a more thorough review of existing report cards and literature on performance indicators than that provided by other report cards under development. Twenty-nine report cards in various stages of development were reviewed, including all of those in the current chapter except for the *Consumer Reports* survey. The reports associated with Phase I and II of the development of the MHSIP report card are excellent handbooks for anyone devising or evaluating an outcomes assessment system in general or a mental health report card in particular. Adopting its structure will allow a behavioral healthcare delivery system to merge its continuous quality improvement goals with large-scale services delivery research goals. For example, the consumer self-report questions regarding missed work days provide an elegant basis on which to build

Table 24–1. Mental Health Statistic Improvement Program (MHSIP) Report Card Phase II Task Force domains and concerns with sample indicators

Domain	Concern	Sample indicator
Access	Entry into MH services is quick, easy, and convenient.	Average length of time from the first face-to-face meeting with a mental health professional.
	A full range of MH service options is available.	Average resources expended on mental health services.
	Enrollees have access to a primary care MH provider who meets their needs in terms of ethnicity, language, culture, age, and disability.	Proportion of enrollees who report not seeking services because of perceptions of incompatibility related to ethnicity, language, culture, and age.
	The out-of-pocket costs to enrollees do not discourage the use of necessary MH services.	Proportion of enrollees who report cost as an obstacle to service utilization.
Appropriateness	Persons using MH services do so voluntarily and in collaboration with service providers. The use of involuntary MH interventions is minimized.	The proportion of service recipients who report active participation in decisions regarding their services plans.
	The plan offers services that promote the process of recovery.	Average resources expended on services that promote recovery.
	Persons using MH services have meaningful involvement in program policy, planning, evaluation, quality assurance, and service delivery.	The proportion of enrollees who are consumers and/or family members and serve on planning and development groups and/or paid staff positions in the Plan.

Service recipients receive information to enable them to make informed choices about services.	The proportion of service recipients reporting that they had received adequate information to make choices.
Services are delivered, where possible, in accordance with known and accepted best-practiced guidelines.	The percentage of service recipients whose services follow specific accepted best-practice guidelines.

Outcome

Physical health

MH service recipients have equal access to effective general health care relative to general population.	The percentage of people with mental illness who are connected to primary care.
Service recipients experience minimal adverse iatrogenic effects.	Average level of involuntary movements resulting from the use of psychotropic medications for specified service recipient groups.

Psychological health

Level of psychological distress from symptoms is minimized.	The percentage of persons receiving MH services who report a decreased level of psychological distress.
Service recipients experience an increased sense of personhood.	The percentage of service recipients who experience an increased sense of self-respect and dignity.

Level of independence

Enrollees experience minimal impairment from use of substances.	Average reduction in impairment in service recipients with substance abuse problems.
Recipients experience minimal interference with productive activity such as work, school, or volunteer activities as a result of alcohol, drugs, and/or mental disorders.	Average change on self-report of the extent to which alcohol, drugs, or mental problems interfere with performance of productive activity.

(continued)

Table 24–1. Mental Health Statistic Improvement Program (MHSIP) Report Card Phase II Task Force domains and concerns with sample indicators (*continued*)

Domain	Concern	Sample indicator
Outcome *Level of independence* (continued)	Enrollees function in community settings with optimal independence from formal service systems.	Percentage of adults with severe psychiatric disabilities living in residences that they themselves *own or lease.*
	Service recipients experience increased independent functioning.	Percentage of service recipients experiencing increased level of functioning on a given scale.
	Recipients take an active role in managing their own illness.	Proportion of service recipients doing self-help services.
	Persons experiencing an episode of acute psychiatric illness receive care that reduces the likelihood of recurrence within a short period of time.	The percentage of readmissions that are within 30 days of discharge.
	Services result in positive change in problems as defined by consumers.	The percentage of MH service users reporting that the services received resulted in positive change in the problems for which they sought help.
Social relationships	Service recipients experience increased natural supports and social integration.	Proportion of adults experiencing increased activities with family, friends, neighbors, or social groups.
Environment	Service recipients live in situations of their choice.	None specified.

Prevention

Environment

Enrollees are provided information that helps lower the risk of mental and/or substance use disorders.

Expenditures on dissemination of preventive information per enrollee.

Populations at risk are provided interventions designed to reduce risk of developing mental disorders.

Proportion of enrollees participating in selected or indicated preventive interventions.

Family support and skill training is provided.

Proportion of parents (of children at high risk) receiving skill training and parenting education.

Note. MH = mental health.
Source. Center for Mental Health Services 1995.

studies of the cost-offset associated with more appropriate use of care. The eventual product could be expected to be a report card structure that is implemented nationwide and that would lead to a series of national performance standards for providers of mental health services based on the report card. The MHSIP effort is one of the few report cards based on the consumer perspective and provides an excellent framework by which to understand the issues involved in developing a mental healthcare report card.

Conclusions

Behavioral healthcare is undergoing massive change. Report cards are being finalized as this chapter is being published. The final MHSIP Report Card Phase II Task Force report will have been made available and will have a much more definite report card structure, *Consumer Reports* will have published its second survey on HMOs, and AMBHA will probably have implemented their report card in some sites. A summary of the relative differences between the three major national report card effects is provided in Table 24–2. It is clear that changes will occur in an ongoing way for the next several years as report card developers respond to their critics and to the challenges involved in implementing systemwide change.

One challenge is that the report card structure must be seamlessly woven into the day-to-day administration of the delivery system. Nelson and colleagues (1995) have written about the distinction between a *report card*, which is a static document summarizing the performance of a system over a specified period of time (usually a year), and an *instrument panel*, which is an assembly of performance indicators that provides data on a real-time basis to the administrators of a system. A report card for a delivery system, as described above, is analogous to reports given to students each semester by the teacher. An instrument panel for a delivery system is analogous to the instrument panel of an aircraft, which provides the pilot with various indicators of the plane's performance at every moment of the flight so that corrective action can be taken if problems arise. The instrument panel for a psychiatric hospital might include the average length of stay for current patients or the follow-up medication compliance of recently discharged patients. The latter indicator might ideally be used to gauge whether efforts to improve medication compliance have been effective. Successful report cards will essentially be instrument panels with a fixed-time frame of reference. The system administrators will be able to start each day with an analysis of the report card for the previous day, week, or month. This will help fund the report cards as a necessary part of the clinical and administrative operation and pull us toward the model of a healthcare delivery

Table 24–2. Comparison of report cards in regard to mental health issues

	HEDIS 2.5	AMBHA	MHSIP[a]
Access and utilization	4 Indicators; 12 items	8 Indicators; 17 items	11 Indicators; 15 items
Satisfaction	1 Indicator; 1 item	5 Indicators; 6 items	Satisfaction indicators are measured as satisfaction with performance on the other domains (e.g., satisfaction with access)
Outcome	2 Indicators; 4 items	None	18 Indicators; 91 items
Prevention	None	None	4 Indicators; 5 items
Quality of care and appropriateness	1 Indicator; 1 item	7 Indicators; 7 items	8 Indicators; 19 items
Financial performance	2 Indicators; 16 items	None	Financial performance indicators are measured as expenditures on the other domains (e.g., expenditures on prevention education)
Source(s) of data	Administrative data; telecommunications data; medical records; consumer self-report	Administrative data; telecommunications data; medical records; consumer self-report	Administrative data; consumer self-report; plan expenditures; enrollment/encounter data; examination by physician; medical records

(continued)

Table 24–2. Comparison of report cards in regard to mental health issues *(continued)*

	HEDIS 2.5	AMBHA	MHSIP[a]
Additional concepts included as measures	None	None	Staff Composition vis-à-vis inclusion of consumers in decision and policy making Percentage of primary care physicians who receive continuing education on mental health and substance abuse Patient self-report of lost productivity because of mental health problems

Note. HEDIS 2.5 = Health Plan Employer Data and Information Set, Version 2.5; AMBHA = American Managed Behavioral Healthcare Association; MHSIP = Mental Health Statistic Improvement Program.
[a]Some MHSIP indicators are based on a single measure that has many individual items, but these are counted as one measure. For example, the SF-36 has 36 items but is tallied above as one measure.

system in which quality improvement and clinical care are based on ongoing services utilization and treatment effectiveness data.

Another problem that developers of report cards will have to face is the extent to which consumers will have access to the data or even the reports themselves. Although large companies and state governments will hopefully include the report cards of bidding providers in their decision as to which plans they should offer their employees, the way in which employers will pass along the report card information to the employees is not at all clear. This is an issue of transferring the data published in the report card to the consumers who ultimately use the services. Such consumers are much more likely to read something like the *Consumer Reports* article and avoid the lowest ranked plans than they are to read through several volumes of report card data that are kept on file in the human resources office of their employer. New ways of communicating information to consumers must be developed. The advances in information technology, quality management, and organizational metrics in the form of report cards on instrument panels will parallel the advances in the neurosciences as psychiatry heads into the 21st century. These advances may provide the answers to mental health as its parity with physical health is sought.

References

Berwick DM: Continuous quality improvement as a ideal in health care. N Engl J Med 320:53–56, 1989

Center for Mental Health Services, MHSIP Mental Health Report Card Phase I Task Force: Progress Report. Cambridge, MA, Center for Mental Health Services, 1994

Center for Mental Health Services, MHSIP Mental Health Report Card Phase II Task Force: Draft Final Report. Cambridge, MA, Center for Mental Health Services, 1995

Corrigan JM, Nielsen DM: Toward the development of uniform reporting standards for managed care organizations: The Health Plan Employer Data and Information Set (Version 2.0). Jt Comm J Qual Improv 19:566–575, 1993

Docherty JP, Dewan NA: Guide to Outcomes Management. Washington, DC, National Association of Psychiatric Health Systems, 1995

Donabedian A: Evaluating the quality of medical care. Milbank Q 44:166–206, 1966

Flexner A: Medical Education in the United States and Canada: Report to the Carnegie Foundation for Advancement of Teaching. New York, Marymount Press, 1910

Health care in crisis: are HMOs the answer? Consumer Reports 57(8):519–531, 1992

Institute of Medicine: Access to Health Care in America. Edited by Millman M. Washington, DC, National Academy Press, 1993

Joint Commission on Accreditation of Healthcare Organizations: Indicator Measurement System, Medication Use Indicator Information Form (Draft). Oakbrook Terrace, IL, JCAHO, 1995a

Joint Commission on Accreditation of Healthcare Organizations: Request for Indicators on Healthcare Networks. Oakbrook Terrace, IL, JCAHO, 1995b

Joint Commission on Accreditation of Healthcare Organizations: IM System General Information. Oakbrook Terrace, IL, JCAHO, 1996

Kazandjian VA, Lauthers J, Cernak CM, et al: Relating outcome to processes of care: the Maryland Hospital Association's Quality Indicator Project. Jt Comm J Qual Improv 19:530–538, 1993

Loeb JM, O'Leary DS: A call for collaboration in performance measurement. JAMA 273:1405, 1995

Maryland Hospital Association: Target: Quality. Lutherville, MD, MHA, 1993

Mental health: does therapy work? Consumer Reports 60(11):734–739, 1995

Mulkern V, Leff HS, Green RS, et al: Section II: Performance indicators for a consumer-oriented mental health report card: literature review and analysis, in Stakeholders Perspectives on Mental Health Performance Indicators. Edited by Mulkern V. Cambridge, MA, The Evaluation Center at the Human Services Research Institute, 1995

National Committee for Quality Assurance: Health Plan Employer Data and Information Set, Version 2.0. Washington, DC, NCQA, 1993

National Committee for Quality Assurance: Call for HEDIS 3.0 Measures. Washington, DC, NCQA, December 1995a

National Committee for Quality Assurance: Health Plan Employer Data and Information Set, Version 2.5. Washington, DC, NCQA, 1995b

National Committee for Quality Assurance: Health Plan Employer Data and Information Set, Version 2.5 (Revised). Washington, DC, NCQA, 1996

National Institute of Mental Health: Program Performance Measurement: Demands, Technology, and Dangers (Ser BN No 5; DHHS Publ No [ADM] 84-1357). Edited by Windle C. Washington, DC, U.S. Department of Health and Human Services, 1984

National Institute of Mental Health: Mental Health Program Performance Measurement (Ser BN No 7; DHHS Publ No [ADM] 86-1441). Edited by Windle C, Jacobs JH, Sherman PS. Washington, DC, U.S. Department of Health and Human Services, 1986

Nelson EC, Batalden PB, Plume SK, et al: Report cards or instrument panels: who needs what. Jt Comm J Qual Improv 21:155–165, 1995

Roberts J, Coale J, Redman R: A history of the Joint Commission on Accreditation of Hospitals. JAMA 258:936–940, 1987

Schyve PM: Models for relating performance measurement and accreditation. International Journal of Health Planning and Management 10:231–241, 1995

Seidenfeld J, Hanold LS, Loeb JM: Requests for indicators. JAMA 273:691, 1995

Sherman PS, Kaufman C: A Compilation of the Literature on What Consumers Want From Mental Health Services. Cambridge, MA, Human Services Research Institute, 1995

Siu A, McGlynn E, Beers M: Choosing quality-of-care measures based on the expected impact of improvement quality care for the major causes of mortality and morbidity (JR-03). Santa Monica, CA, Rand Corporation, 1992

U.S. Department of Health and Human Services: Healthy People 2000: National Health Promotion and Disease Prevention Objectives (DHHS Publ No 91-50213). Washington, DC, U.S. Department of Health and Human Services, 1990

U.S. Preventive Services Task Force: Guide to Clinical Preventive Services: An Assessment of the Effectiveness of 169 Interventions. Baltimore, MD, Williams & Wilkins, 1989

Afterword to Section V

John F. Clarkin, Ph.D., and John P. Docherty, M.D.,
Section Editors

This section on assessment should be viewed in the larger context in which psychiatry and the healthcare system are operating today. First, we are in an era of quantification. Second, automation is providing the capacity for rapid communication, including telecommunications. Third, there is a strong demand for accountability. Physicians no longer operate as independent practitioners, but are accountable to their patients and the healthcare system. The demand for accountability was an outgrowth of the difficulties in the healthcare system. At the heart of the difficulties was the lack of a rational cost-containment system, problems of patient access to services, and a nonrational distribution of resources.

Historically, the fields of psychiatry and psychology have developed instruments to implement a laboratory assessment of the patient, which in turn informs clinical practice and the care of the patient. At present, we are beginning to examine the healthcare system as a whole, using our capacity for quantification, autometrics, and telecommunications. Of course, there are risks in focusing on the healthcare system as a whole, because when such a perspective is adopted, the individual could potentially be treated as simply an entity rather than as a human being in need. On the other hand, there are benefits to this approach, and, when used correctly, such an approach should not ignore the individual. This process makes judgments more open, so that they can be challenged and examined; leads to more equitable distribution of resources; enables one to define procedures of care that are teachable; and provides for systems of care that can improve themselves on an ongoing basis.

Why is the field heading toward a solution that emphasizes assessment of the entire healthcare delivery system? First, such assessment is now feasible. Computerization, for instance, enables the rapid assessment of large numbers of patients. Second, this approach is based upon science and a scientific value system and can lead to more efficient use of services and the betterment of the individual patients.

It is in this context that assessment instruments are useful tools. Assessment instruments can yield quantifiable data on the individual that can be compared with large samples for meaning and interpretation.

Test instruments are public in their methodology and results. Thus, the results are open to inspection by others, and the method for obtaining the results is clear and verifiable. The tests and their results are tools that can be used in a decision-making process. The test results do not by themselves determine or necessarily indicate a course of action. However, they are information that can be used by clinical and systems decision-makers to further the treatment of the individual patient, guide the distribution of care across a sample of patients, or measure the relative quality of care of a particular delivery system.

Tests and their results are, therefore, one step away from treatment guidelines. Treatment guidelines are agreed-on models of care that have been arrived at by polling groups of experts. One could see how the content of Chapter 21, laboratory tests for psychiatric patients, could be turned into treatment guidelines by a panel of experts. The determination of when to refer a psychiatric patient for specialized neuropsychiatric care, as discussed in Chapter 22, could likewise form the basis for clinical guidelines on referral for assessment.

The rapid changes in the healthcare system and the concomitant changes in assessment of patients reflected in this section have many implications, including ones for psychiatric education and the larger healthcare system that relates to psychiatry. The education of psychiatrists should include the resident's relating to a system of care in which resources are limited, having access to feedback from patients to help inform the shape and trajectory of the treatment itself, and having the quality of his or her performance monitored. In the larger picture, primary care physicians will need enhanced assessment tools. Efficient, automated assessment tools for depression, for example, will enable primary care doctors to carry out efficiently and with quality what they have been asked by the system to do.

VI

*Computers, the Patient,
and the Psychiatrist*

VI

Computers, the Patient, and the Psychiatrist

Contents

Section VI

Computers, the Patient, and the Psychiatrist

Foreword

Zebulon Taintor, M.D.

Computers are not new to the mental health field. It has been 40 years since Dr. Stanley Yolles, then director of the National Institute of Mental Health (NIMH), touring the exhibit area of the 1956 World Psychiatric Association World Congress in Madrid, found people of various nationalities carrying psychiatric histories that were produced by filling out checklists in various languages. His enthusiasm led to what stood for years as the largest NIMH grant ever to Dr. Eugene Laska and the New York State Research Foundation for Mental Hygiene for the Multi-State Information System (MSIS). The Missouri Mental Standard System of Psychiatry (SSOP) was developed by George Ulett and James Hedlund, while Bernard Gluek had developed a system for the Institute of Living that was widely appreciated. The systems had many similarities (e.g., mental status examinations) and some special virtues, such as the Missouri system's actuarial predictions of risk of suicide, elopement, and so forth. All of these systems were meant to be of immediate help to the clinician, but were more appreciated by administrators, researchers, and statisticians. None is in much use today, although the MSIS survived until Internal Revenue Service (IRS) regulations about not-for-profit foundations abolished it on the basis of its potential earnings. Other systems were developed over the years and met a similar fate.

It is easy to trace developments from the first few articles published in 1958 through 1978, a total of 1,399 included in a superb annotated bibliography by Hedlund et al. (1981). Hedlund's group at the Missouri Institute of Psychiatry continued to disseminate bibliographies regularly, and their categories for classifying articles provide a convenient way of tracing developments to understand how we have gotten to the present condition of having no broadly used software in mental health practice. In general, applications that could be put easily into digital form prospered, especially if development funds were available, and few people were displaced by the new use of computers. Growth was guaranteed if whatever the computer did became indispensable to the operation of the enterprise, as happened almost always with business applications and rarely with clinical programs.

In the field of psychiatry, computer technology has aided the following business and clinical applications:

- *Administration.*   Business necessities have driven many developments in computer technology. Growth in using computers in the field of psychiatry has been fueled by the easy adaptation of concepts and software from other areas of medicine and business, which contributes to critical mass development and purchasing. Development funding is plentiful, and managers see their administrative power increases with their store of facts.
- *Alcohol abuse programs.*   Computer technology in alcohol abuse programs is relatively undeveloped, despite the recurring finding that patients are more honest in detailing their drinking behavior to a computer than to a live interviewer.
- *Patient assessment.*   Patient assessment was the largest category in the original Hedlund et al. (1981) bibliography, accounting for one third of the publications reviewed.
- *Artificial intelligence.*   Decision making by computer has never justified the hopes or fears of those who took it seriously. Instead, arguments against seeing computer processing as similar to the workings of the human mind have mounted (e.g., Mender 1994).
- *Behavior therapy.*   Desensitization programs have progressed, with virtual reality now being used for acrophobia, fear of flying, and translating cognitive misperceptions into something closer to the reality that others experience, but there has not been widespread use.
- *Biofeedback.*   Despite many reports on the efficacy of alpha training and other forms of biofeedback, there has not been widespread use.
- *Computer-aided instruction.*   Computer-aided instruction has become widespread, largely because there have been development funds and because of its efficiency. Computers can be available all the time, offer multimedia responses to students, and use programs that link to other topics matching the students' responses or link to the literature, and the programs are updated more easily than textbooks. Generally, teachers have not felt threatened by new technology and tend to worry about being criticized for not using it.
- *Case register.*   Case registers were more prominent when they were stand-alone applications. They seem to be casualties of the substitution of a managed care approach for a public health approach that accompanied community mental health centers (CMHCs). However, there are some prominent databases, such as the schizophrenia registry for Suffolk County, New York, operated by the State University of New York at Stony Brook. In the Scandinavian countries, computers have been used with great effect to automate their many

careful registries, bringing data to bear on important questions. For example, Finland maintains registries of both patients with violence and schizophrenia and patients receiving clozapine that are now being combined to determine if there is an effect of clozapine on violence. The case registry challenge is not in hardware and software, because all that is needed is a good database management system, but in the challenge of maintaining data entry.

- *Community mental health.* Community mental health systems have risen and fallen with CMHCs, most of the survivors of which are currently attempting some sort of transition to managed care. Business applications have had some longevity, and there have been a few clinically oriented information systems, but none have achieved notable market share or distinction.

- *Computer-generated text.* Although computer-generated text is discussed in greater detail in Chapter 26 of this volume, by Warren et al., it is clear that enthusiasm for computer-generated output from checklists has waned, paradoxically, as ability to generate it flexibly has grown. Clinicians want to generate their own text, not deal with what comes out of a machine.

- *Computed tomography.* There has been enormous growth in computed tomography as images, such as sound, have been digitized. It is now possible to manipulate images in many ways, incorporate them into text, and reproduce them easily. Similar progress has been made in the related fields of magnetic resonance imaging, more recently high-speed magnetic resonance imaging, positron-emission tomography, and single photon emission computed tomography.

- *Diagnosis.* Although computerized diagnosis is discussed in Chapter 25, this is less of a hardware and software problem than an inability to obtain enough input to really help the clinician. Software tends to depend on recognizing key words.

- *Drug abuse programs.* Patients tend, as noted in the discussion of alcohol abuse programs, to be more truthful in reporting to computers the amount and frequency of substances they use than when they are faced by a human interviewer, despite having generally more sociopathy than people with alcoholism. Management programs have been developed to satisfy regulatory requirements.

- *Education.* There has been considerable use of databases for measuring outcome in general education, especially standardized test scores, but relatively little has been done to measure the efficacy of professional psychiatric education, although the work that has been done is encouraging.

- *Electroencephalography.* Electroencephalography also has been digitalized, enabling actuarial comparisons with large databases and probability statements about possible abnormalities. John et al. (1988) has linked these to probable diagnoses. However, computerized electroencephalograms have not progressed into widespread clinical use.

- *Evoked potentials.* Another digitalized area, with many applications, is evoked potentials (e.g., P300, mismatched negativity). Little has progressed into general clinical practice.
- *Laboratory computer (psychiatry).* General laboratory tests are highly automated and are communicated quickly by computer. Computerized databases enable the retrieval and comparison of results.
- *Natural language.* This category distinguishes text from alphanumerically coded responses (e.g., the word *yes* instead of a coding convention in which entering the number 1 in a certain spot means "yes"). Word processing programs have come into widespread use and have powerful word-searching and -replacing capabilities. Statistical summaries are not yet widely available.
- *Medical records.* As discussed in Chapter 25 by Taintor, Schwartz, and Miller, the medical record can be paperless, easily transmitted, and reconfigured and large sections can be automated, but this is not yet widely done.
- *Modeling mental processes.* This category is similar to artificial intelligence, except that it takes a piecemeal approach to modeling mental processes and has been incrementally more successful. Work has progressed on using computers to simulate neural networks, but this has not had a clinical application.
- *Minnesota Multiphasic Personality Inventory.* This test was highly automated; use is stable or slightly reduced.
- *Management information systems.* Management information systems were highly developed for billing, scheduling, recording services, tracking staff time not spent in direct patient contact, and so forth. They require modification and adaptation to new hardware and software drivers. As discussed in Chapter 25 by Taintor, Schwartz, and Miller, health maintenance organizations have added a new dimension of comparing as much data as possible to practice norms.
- *Modeling and simulation.* Related to modeling and simulation is the recent explosive growth of virtual reality programs.
- *Mental status.* Computerized mental status findings have become a routine application, resulting in an increased number of mental status examinations.
- *Mental retardation and developmental disabilities.* Cognitive rehabilitation programs developed for patients with mental retardation and developmental disabilities have been used in general psychiatry. Many programs have been developed for patients with head injuries. There has been some abuse by staff who leave patients alone with computers when they still need help.

- *Modeling psychopathology.* Model patients were produced by computers to simulate interaction with clinicians and caught the attention of the field of psychiatry when computerized models began interacting with each other, but more development did not occur. Increased interest by clinicians in simulating evaluations may stimulate new developments.
- *Modeling social processes.* Although there was some initial interest in providing software for sociograms, not much work has been done in this area, although new sociotherapeutic interests, such as Galanter's (1993) network therapy for substance abuse, may lead to more work. Consistent with psychiatry's interests and developments in genetics, a considerable number of software programs have been developed to create family trees, trace relatives, and diagram genetic traits and therefore have contributed to psychiatry's genetic investigations.
- *Peer review.* Computers have been used not only for peer review but also for quality assurance. Algorithms enable exceptional instances of patient care to be selected for review based on very large samples that could not possibly be reviewed manually. In this situation, computers work well as an adjunct to the human effort. A prime example is the *PHARMAKON* system in New York State that keeps track of all orders for all medications written in the Office of Mental Health's 21 adult and 7 child psychiatric facilities. With input from any interested psychiatrist, an expert committee sets the guidelines for review of drug interactions, polypharmacy, high and low dosage, and so forth. Exceptions generated from the orders are printed at each facility and reviewed by a drug-monitoring committee. This system is remarkable in its assumption that exceptions are to be expected in the population being treated because admission into an Office of Mental Health hospital generally involves a failure to respond to conventional treatment. Reviews are collegial and supportive. The principal problem with the system has been the enormous size of the databases, which has been handled only by CD-ROMs and frequent archiving.
- *Problem-oriented medical record.* Once popular because of the inadequacies of the diagnostic system, the problem-oriented medical record has become less popular with the advent of DSM-III and subsequent versions. The problem with the problem-oriented record was the lack of an agreed-on list of problems. Some facilities limited choices to a few, whereas others had many (e.g., Butler Hospital, Providence, Rhode Island, offered about 10,000 choices). The result was a tower-of-Babel phenomenon that prevented agreement on a path of development or a critical mass of software.
- *Prediction.* Both logical and actuarial predictions have flourished but have occasionally foundered on legal issues. The high accuracy

of actuarial predictions in the Missouri system led to the output being suppressed because of inability to resolve the problem of how to handle high-risk patients. Logical prediction has been less successful. A major success for psychiatry in resisting the imposition of diagnosis-related groups (DRGs) was the use of large databases to show that psychiatric diagnosis did not predict the utilization of resources.

- *Program evaluation.* Myriad program evaluation applications have been developed. These applications attempt to answer the usual managerial questions. A decade ago, the emphasis was on measuring and evaluating process; now the emphasis has shifted to outcome. This shift will be much more demanding of databases and continuity of care, although it may be subject to criticism for being too short term. Emphasis on long-term outcome is cost-effective and part of the shift to the longitudinal dimension of natural history in diagnosis in which psychiatry has been increasingly involved since publication of DSM-III in 1980. Such work will require large information systems similar to case registers, albeit probably organized by managed care plans rather than community.
- *Psychological testing.* Virtually every test that has any base of acceptance has had some computerization (e.g., scoring, reliability, validity, derivation of norms, usefulness of each item).
- *Psychophysiology.* Physiological data have lent themselves to digitalization, so abundant material is ready for linking with psychological data, but this linking has occurred infrequently outside the experimental laboratory.
- *Psychotherapy.* Programs can help clinicians in treating depression, obsessive-compulsive disorder, excessive smoking, and other disorders. Even larger is the pool of self-help programs, which patients are encouraged to use to treat themselves.
- *Research.* Computers have become virtually indispensable for research, holding databases and offering all sorts of statistical programs; so many, in fact, that mistaken choices of which tests to apply are not infrequent.
- *Screening and history.* Many screening and history applications exist, and use is increasingly widespread.
- *Treatment.* Again, many treatment applications exist, some of which are mentioned in Chapter 25.
- *Utilization review.* As with peer review, the mere existence of data in a computer lends itself to the derivation of tests that can be run to ensure completeness, timeliness, and accuracy. Norms are derived easily, and deviations from those norms can be flagged and assessed easily.

Although developments in all of the above mentioned areas have been important over the past 16 years, many new areas aided by computer technology have emerged. The foremost technology is the Internet, the subject of Chapter 26 in this volume, by Warren et al. Developments in managed care have provided quite different content for the chapters in this section than would have been included 3 years ago. Software development has mushroomed, and some programs deserve special mention. The common denominator is the patient using the computer.

- *Self-help.* All sorts of programs have been sold to the general public, including many on how to curb undesirable habits, diagnose and alleviate one's problems, and acquire skills useful in surmounting some of life's obstacles or in gaining the competitive edge.
- *Cognitive rehabilitation.* Computers have been used in the developmental disabilities field for years because they can reward nicely with colored pictures, hopeful messages, and pleasant sounds. They never lose patience and are not critical unless programmed to be so. How much can be accomplished in using computers to treat patients with head injuries is somewhat controversial. In psychiatry, at least four programs have been developed. The need for staff supervision remains high; one cannot simply leave patients alone with computers (see Chapter 25 for a more detailed description).
- *Professional associations.* Using computers to support professional associations—ranging from simple files of members, mailing labels, letters, and dues billing to complicated databases on membership and member activities (often sought by the government, as gathering data directly requires permission from the Office of Management and Budget), member lobbying by fax, fax broadcasting, electronic mail, home pages on the Internet, chat groups, and desktop and electronic publishing—has had a broad range of effects. There are many more associations than before, by a variety of measures. Associations that use computing power well have acquired a voice out of proportion to their membership and resources. The American Psychiatric Association has been slow to use computer technology, having started only in 1994 regular presentation of software at annual meetings (but having had no continuing medical education [CME] courses on how to use computers since 1993), but is increasing its computer proficiency.

Despite these many developments, the use of computers has not met the predictions of Dr. Howard Rome (1967):

Psychiatry is now on the threshold of a fourth quantum advance. Automation of information-processing will achieve what never has been available heretofore—a valid database for psychiatry's assumptions, treatments, logistics, and at the same time it offers a potential solution for psychiatrist's administrative complexities. Moreover, automation techniques will breach psychiatry's most isolating barrier: its idiosyncratic system of communication which poses an almost impenetrable cognitive screen within psychiatry as well as among psychiatry's communications with other sectors of the scientific and medical community. (p. 37)

Hedlund (1987) quoted Rome's remarks as part of a review of trends in 1985 and noted that the promise had not been filled. Some trends Hedlund noted then are still prevalent now, namely, 1) clinically oriented, general mental health information systems have given way to more narrowly defined, special purpose management information systems; 2) computerizing hospital psychiatric records continues to be an elusive reality; and 3) the most frequently cited need for an automated clinical record involves quality assurance. He was correct about the microcomputers of the time not being able to handle more than a few clinical applications, but now they can. He correctly doubted that psychological testing had entered a golden age. Although he noted that computerized clinical interviews had continued to proliferate, that patient acceptance of automated testing and interviewing was well documented, and that computer diagnosis in mental health was well established in principle if not in practice—implying that great strides were to be made in this area—patients rarely encountered a computer. Hedlund and Greist urged proceeding vigorously with the tools at hand, but only a few have done so. There finally is a society of psychiatrists interested in using computers, but its membership numbers only 150.

Some of the reasons for clinician nonacceptance of computer technology are the same reasons Hedlund cited for information systems' failure, including lack of top-level agency support, lack of adequate funding, difficulties transferring research projects to clinical settings, piggybacking clinical onto statistical reporting systems, "softness" of mental health data, ambiguity of mental health goals and criteria, lack of an overall guiding conceptual framework for systems, lack of a standard clinical language and an inability to gain wide acceptance for standard or highly structured clinical forms, complex data and distribution systems that have been unable to ensure either timely or reliable information return, duplicate (manual and computerized) clinical reporting systems, distrust of mental health clinicians for information that has been obtained or processed "impersonally," resistance related to issues of privacy and confidentiality, and lack of clinical commitment to making computer technology work for mental health needs. Psychiatrists may be more concerned with arguments such as computers have subtle, malignant influences (Mowshowitz 1976) or the human mind does not lend itself to computer modeling (Mender 1994; Penrose 1994). These reasons persist while Hedlund's more technical reasons are less true.

Despite the great numbers of practitioners who use computers for necessities such as billing patients, most psychiatrists preserve "medicine's responsibility for the personal and intuitively sensitive provision of care" (Rome 1968). They should continue to do so.

These arguments have little to do with the rapid spread of computers as communications tools. Large numbers of students are taking courses in which computers are studied not for computer theory but for enhancing content (Chartrand 1995), and the Rand Corporation argues that electronic mail can be the new foundation of democracy (Bickson 1995). Relatively simple concepts can be translated into relatively simple computer applications quickly, for example, programming a patient information system into *Paradox for Windows*. There are now adequate input devices for high-volume entry from a wide variety of clinical settings. Computer-generated reports, as described in Chapter 25, need no longer be stereotyped, and data for special needs need not be inaccessible. Technical improvements in data retrieval make it clear that the problem is more likely related to human factors. In short, computers have changed, being more accessible, flexible, and in greater use than ever before. There are personal data assistants. The cost of a computer, with no bottom price in sight (Francis and Ouellette 1996), in present dollars is the same as the cost of an IBM Selectric typewriter in the days when having one was considered de rigueur, and the computer can do many of the things the typist did. Although computers have changed rapidly, human beings have changed slowly. The following chapters review recent developments that may be an update for some and a way of easing changes for others.

References

American Psychiatric Association: Diagnostic and Statistical Manual of Mental Disorders, 3rd Edition. Washington, DC, American Psychiatric Association, 1980

Bickson T, et al: Universal Access to E-Mail: Feasibility and Social Implications. Los Angeles, CA, Rand Corporation, 1995

Chartrand S: Computer theory as social science. The New York Times, December 5, 1995, pp D1, D5

Francis B, Ouellette T: PC prices remain in free fall. Computerworld, May 13, 1996, p 10

Galanter M: Network Therapy for Alcohol and Drug Abuse: A New Approach to Practice. New York, Basic, 1993

Hedlund JL: Mental health computing in the 1980s, in Research in Mental Health Computer Applications: Directions for the Future (DHHS Publ No ADM-87-1468). National Institute of Mental Health Series DN No 8. Edited by Greist JH, Carroll JA, Erdman HP, et al. Washington, DC, U.S. Government Printing Office, 1987, pp 7–38

Hedlund JL, Vieweg BW, Wood JB, et al: Computers in Mental Health: A Review and Annotated Bibliography (DHHS Publ No ADM-81-1090). National Institute of Mental Health, Series FN No 7. Washington, DC, U.S. Government Printing Office, 1981

John ER, Prichep L, Fridman J, et al: Neurometrics: computer-assisted differential diagnosis of brain disorders. Science 293:162–169, 1988

Mender D: The Myth of Neuropsychiatry. New York, Plenum, 1994

Mowshowitz A: The Conquest of Will: Information Processing in Human Affairs. Reading, MA, Addison-Wesley, 1976

Penrose R: The Emperor's New Mind. New York, Oxford University Press, 1994

Rome HP: Prospects for a PSI-NET: the fourth quantum advance in psychiatry. Compr Psychiatry 8:450–454, 1967

Rome HP: Human factors and technical difficulties in the application of computers to psychiatry, in Computers and Electronic Devices in Psychiatry. Edited by Kline NS, Laska EM. New York, Grune & Stratton, 1968, pp 37–44

Chapter 25

Computers and Patient Care

Zebulon Taintor, M.D., Marc Schwartz, M.D., and Marvin Miller, M.D.

In this chapter we review 1) the scope and location of an information system a clinician might use, 2) the relationship between computerized data and paper records, 3) the use of computers in an office, 4) the use of computers according to the flow of work with patients, and 5) the special considerations about dealing with managed care organizations. The references cited in this chapter are drawn entirely from non-Internet sources. Chapter 26 offers practitioners more details on using the Internet, with references drawn only from the Internet.

Lag of Software Development Behind Hardware Marketing

One of the most difficult things about information systems is getting information about them. These days, advertisers promise that almost anything can be done with a personal computer. One major manufacturer asks whether it has changed your life yet, implying that all you need is a personal computer. In this chapter, we describe what psychiatrists and patients can do sitting at a computer without using Internet connections. However, many clinicians will use personal computers that are somehow connected to some other machine in a network. Hardware is improving rapidly, but connections and software lag, and the connections required may be complicated:

> The PC you just bought will have to be replaced before your controller has depreciated it. Windows 95 has been out for nearly a year and you're still using DOS. . . . In the past, a single comprehensive system was the goal. But today, obtaining a single comprehensive system from one company is a myth. You cannot expect a single system to be the best of everything. (Rowland 1996, p. 72)

Hardware has become more complicated, with mobile devices, distributed (client-server) processing, and the continuance of mainframe (large) computers, and the specialized mobile devices have developed a market niche (Brekka 1995). Portable computers have been useful in a primary-care clerkship (Maulitz et al. 1996). The MMX chip is the first that brings laptop development close to that of desktop units (Campanelli 1997). Resisting the temptation to wax enthusiastic about hardware, we focus on software for mental health. Operating systems and connectivity software will vary. Caveat emptor: The reader interested in specific software mentioned within this chapter must investigate it further before purchasing it for a particular computer.

Scope and Location of Information Systems

The software we use has many sources: 1) in-house systems developers, 2) commercial software developers hoping to sell to healthcare systems or individuals, 3) general medical systems, and 4) colleagues in the mental health professions. Each source has its advantages and disadvantages, but the immediate consequences vary, including availability, costs (initial and upgrade), location and participation requirements, appropriateness, and adaptability. For example, a facility may very much want to use a general laboratory or pharmacy system developed in the general medical sector but may find that it is difficult to develop and bring in-house a record that includes an assessment, mental status, treatment plan, or progress notes. We point out these differences where especially relevant, but we again caution that these factors must be explored.

General Medical Systems

One can try a general information system. There is no shortage of vendors or products. The March 1, 1996, issue of *Health Management Technology* lists more than 750 companies, with a similar number occupying about 100 pages of the December 1996 issue of *Healthcare Informatics*. The Spring 1996 issue (Vol. 14, No. 1) of *Computertalk* constitutes a directory of medical computer systems. *Healthcare Informatics* lists the top 75 general medical information systems annually in its July issue. In 1993, revenue varied from $469.6 to $0.67 million from the 1st to the 75th.

Applications typically include patient care. financials, radiology, laboratory, pharmacy, materials management, surgery scheduling, managed care, clinic system, physician office, critical care, consulting outsourcing, claims administration, and miscellaneous other modules. A typical advertisement by Integrated Medical System (IMS) for *Medacom*, directed at helping physicians to cope with managed care, adds to the usual clinical and fiscal packages by offering an electronic bulletin board that posts

> critical information such as policies and procedures, guidelines and newsletters . . . custom electronic forms—fulfil two-way provider communication needs for internal departments; Automated report distribution—

delivers reports such as claim submission summaries, claim expense reports and referral log summaries, E-Mail capabilities—provide electronic communications with and among providers . . . Links to Others—full integration and information exchange with hospitals, labs, home care, employers . . . (Integrated Medical Systems 1996, p. 5)

The systems directed at managed care emphasize interactivity, outcomes, and patient satisfaction as attractions for everyone (Campbell 1996), but the attraction that may be most appealing to managed care organizations is the ease with which various computer analyses and simulations can be applied to the data to answer questions about how to reduce costs and to foresee the consequences of various payment strategies (Cave 1995). Since computer applications come from many sources, they often are incompatible, and additional software or operational reorganization is needed to put them together (Morrissey 1993).

Despite the fact that the cost benefit of data integration is hard to prove, integration of clinical and financial data is proceeding from its preliminary stages, as seen in the Healthcare Financial Management Association's survey of 17 systems (5 of which are medical school–based) thought most likely to have achieved such integration, to be able to comment on its costs (Morrissey 1996a). Few of these systems have much that is specific to psychiatry. Review of recent conference programs (e.g., Second Annual Conference on the Computerized Record, November 1993, in Chicago, organized by Temple University; Health Care Information Technology Solutions Conference, April 1994, in Washington, D.C.) shows that the systems are all institutionally based but not related to psychiatry. The trend has continued to the present. For example, there were 100 delegates at the European Information Systems Conference in August 1996, but only one who could be said to represent mental health, and there were no presentations related to mental health (Rigby 1996).

General medical computer-based patient records typically are assessed according to the following criteria: operating system (MS-DOS, Windows, Unix, etc.), platform (hardware requirements), access (hours/day, security, backup, view modifiability by customer, etc.), clinical resources (direct entry by clinicians, rationale for decisions, relationship with decision support, etc.), and patient case management (at point of care, automation of scheduling, assessments, progress notes, treatment planning, ordering, care protocols, scheduling outcomes data, outcomes variances, results reporting, clinical alerts, workload management, patient severity/acuity). Links to fiscal and other systems are assumed, although integrating (rather than just linking) automated systems remains a challenge and lags behind system integration in the 301 largest integrated healthcare delivery systems being tracked (Work 1996). Of the 40 systems rated in the July 1996 issue of *Health Management*

Technology (Braly 1996), none has become well known for its mental health applications. The Computer-Based Patient Record Institute in Schaumberg, Illinois, is collaborating with other health information organizations and the Los Alamos National Laboratory to offer a nonproprietary master-patient index that can be downloaded from its web site ("CPRI Offering Non-Proprietary MPI Application," *Health Care Technology* 1996). Those wishing to keep up with general medical information systems are now able to visit trade shows and download demonstration packages and work with them via the Internet ("Visit Virtual Trade Shows," *Health Systems Technology* 1996).

Although general medical systems may not include much for the psychiatrist, they should be followed for three reasons: 1) intake, assessment, treatment, and outcome measure templates may be applied to psychiatry whether they fit or not, 2) technology developed for such systems may carry psychiatric traffic, and 3) confidentiality of both general medical data and psychiatric data may be an issue at several levels and in several ways. For example, the brochure for ACCESS HealthNet (1996)—a firm that started with satellite transmission of laboratory data and has moved on to managed care and provider site communications—states that with one key stroke, information can be sent to payers and providers, and "everyone knows what is going on within minutes."

Psychiatry is unlikely to be immune as the medical record itself changes as a result of information technology. The paperless record is an endpoint on a continuum that may include combinations of electronically stored data, papers, voice and other sound, pictures, video clips and other images, and so forth. Frisse and co-workers (1994) suggest including databases, patient-centered (and -generated) sections that turn the present "diary-monologue" into a forward-looking planning entity that has not been available heretofore. The electronic medical record (EMR) is different from the computer-based patient record (CPR) in that the EMR is "an electronic, machine-readable version of much of the patient data typically found in today's PPR [paper-based patient record]," whereas the CPR "is a representation of all of the data found in the PPR in a coded and structured, machine readable form." This requires agreement on and support for a clinical data dictionary, standardized vocabulary, terminology standard, nosology and coding structure, standard codes, messaging standard, document and diagnostic imaging, clinical documentation, clinical decision support, management analysis, access to remote databases, feedback, and dictation support. The clinician does not have to produce all of the above; much is generated automatically from computerized systems. A 1996 list of vendors numbers 45 (Andrew and Dick 1996).

Responding to the Institute of Medicine's recommendation that there be support for a CPR in place by 2000 (saving $40–$80 billion ["New Momentum for Electronic Patient Record," *New York Times*

1993]), Furfaros and colleagues (1996) surveyed 360 acute hospitals for progress on the six steps to be taken to achieve that goal, finding that only 9% had succeeded in computerizing all of the functions required for step one. The 1996 Healthcare Information and Management Systems Society survey of 1,200 chief information officers and their peers in similar titles found expenditures increasing, with 35% indicating that physician offices were the highest department priority for the coming year, but with only 29% making a substantial investment in hardware and software for a CPR.

Although the Internet is the subject of the next chapter, the technological changes related it (e.g., Intranets, using the technology in-house) may alter the record and how practices and facilities operate (Wheeler 1997). Frisse (1996a) argues that use of Intranets promotes academic activity and that academic centers are lagging.

It may be of interest to note that healthcare organizations have not yet particularly distinguished themselves in their own information processing. Only one (Cigna) not related to pharmaceuticals made the annual ranking of the 100 corporations regarded as world leaders in information processing (CIO [Chief Information Officer] 1996). Moreover, psychiatrists are not alone in not wishing to computerize practices. A survey of 484 physicians and group practices found that 77% have not taken steps to computerize patient records and that only 8% of those that had done so used the systems for clinical purposes ("Clinical Systems Do Not Enamor Group Physician Practices," *Healthcare Informatics* 1996).

More data on general medical systems can be obtained from journals such as *MD Computing* (Springer-Verlag, 175 Fifth Avenue, New York, NY 10010), which is mostly on institutional systems (also covered in *HealthCare Informatics* [see list in September 1996 special section], *Managed Healthcare News, Modern Healthcare,* and, to some extent, *Health Management Technology,* all of which are free), and *Physicians and Computers* (free from 810 S. Waukegan Road, Suite 200, Lake Forest, IL 60045); from evaluations of software (e.g., Medical Society of New York County survey, discussed later in this chapter); and (caveat emptor!) from vendor listings such as Medical Software (1-800-444-4570). The American Hospital Association offers a guide for physician involvement in hospital systems (Bria and Rydell 1992). One can join the American Medical Informatics Association (AMIA), but at its 1996 meeting there was only one session dealing with mental health (AMIA 1996).

Psychiatric Systems

For years, the National Institute of Mental Health (NIMH) served as the rallying point for mental health computing and the development of data definitions and standards. The initial hope of being able to offer one information system from which aggregate data could easily be retrieved that had led to the Multi-State Information System had given way to a recognition that computer hardware and software were becoming too diverse to expect a consensus on their use. The NIMH, therefore, started the Mental Health Statistics Improvement Program in 1976. In addition to publications on computers, costs, quality assurance, and technical support, the project has focused on design and content issues (Patton and Leginski 1983), uniform data definitions (Leginski 1989), and general concerns such as usefulness, confidentiality, and, more recently, consumer involvement.

Different task forces have developed different indicators for different sorts of programs (public, private, child, etc.) in five basic areas. In addition, they have suggested a number of items for a minimum and for additional auxiliary data sets (given as minimum-auxiliary) for providers (0–25), patients (29–28), human resources (23–25), the event (service provided) (10–10), and finance (15–9). This approach allows process evaluations of treatment with performance indicators for appropriateness, adequacy, efficiency, and effectiveness (Kamis-Gould and Waizer 1991).

The main consumers of NIMH support—a function now ably carried out by the Substance Abuse and Mental Health Services Administration (SAMHSA), particularly the Center for Mental Health Services (CMHS)—have been in the public sector, especially state governments and agencies, epidemiologists, and administrators. As commercial systems have become available, the NIMH/CMHS properly has refrained from comparing or endorsing any of them, instead offering minimum data sets and performance criteria against which individual systems can be judged. At the hospital/community mental health center level, there has been a proliferation of systems. Facilities have learned from each other what usefully can be put onto computers (e.g., fund raising) (Klynstra 1991) and clinical information used in formulating treatment plans and linked to continuous quality improvement (White and Wingfield 1991). Hospitals have been able to choose from inventories of software available (Rowland and Rowland 1991).

The individual practitioner wanting to use some systems in the office has been able to obtain information from books, such as those by Schwartz (1984), Lieff (1987), and others; occasional articles in general medical journals; and computer columns in particular journals (e.g., *Hospital and Community Psychiatry* [now *Psychiatric Services*] since 1982 or *Academic Psychiatry* since 1996). They have also been able to follow developments through publications such as *Computers in Psychiatry/Psychology* (edited by one of us [MS] from 1975 to 1988) and *Computers in Human Services* (Richard Schoech, editor, 1985–1992), and through newsletters such as that of the Psychiatric Society for Informatics (c/o Marvin Miller, M.D., 1315 W. 10th Street, Indianapolis, IN 46202) or

Michael Zarr's *Psychiatrists and Computers* (subscribe from Dr. Zarr at 1455 Kings Pointe Road, Grand Blanc, MI 48439). *Behavioral Health Management,* a free publication from MEDQUEST (P.O. Box 20179, Cleveland, OH 44120), has occasional articles on psychiatric information systems.

There are proprietary sheets such as Mental Health Connections (Mental Health Connections, Inc., 21 Blossom Street, Lexington, MA 02173, 1-800-788-4743, mhc@mhc.com www.mhc.com) that are free, offer some news, and offer software such as *Generic Questionnaire Driver; Easy Psychiatric Record Keeper,* a program that includes perfectly worded DSM-IV diagnoses, with all new modifiers properly placed, and prints prescriptions; and *Civer-Psych,* a multifunction (intake/assessment, diagnosis, treatment planning, patient monitoring, billing/claims processing) practice helper (Civerex Systems, 48 Lakeshore Road, Suite 1, Pointe Claire, Quebec, Canada H9S 4H4, 514-630-1005, Fax: 514-630-1456, civerex@civerex.com). Mental Health Connections will send a disc containing about 100 programs for psychiatrists. (Mental Health Connections also offers *Quick-Doc, Anxiety Expert* [psychopharmacology], *Clozapine Expert, OCD Expert, PDR Library on CD-ROM,* and *AskRx Plus.*)

Information on computer systems in psychiatry can be obtained at conferences and meetings. Some conferences are specific to psychiatry, such as "Behavioral Informatics Tomorrow," sponsored by the Institute for Behavioral Healthcare, which held its first annual conference in February 1994 in Orlando and met in San Francisco in September 1996. There are presentations at psychiatry meetings. The Information Systems Committee of the American Psychiatric Association (APA) has offered an update on developments as its component workshop since 1989 and has been cooperating in software demonstrations as part of the media track of the program since 1994. The media track also deals with basic computing and how to get started, replacing courses of such types that were offered occasionally at the APA annual meetings in the 1980s. APA's other meeting, of the Institute on Psychiatric Services, has followed a similar track since 1994, thanks to Ian Alger. The Psychiatric Services Institute's 1996 meeting included presentations on treatment of agoraphobia, fear of flying, cognitive therapy, cognitive rehabilitation, and so forth. Psychiatric subspecialty groups generally include presentations on software and uses of computers relevant to the work of the group (e.g., American Association of Directors of Psychiatry Residency Training on how to keep logs, which residents are required to keep on the patients they treat). Psychiatrists can join the Psychiatric Society for Informatics (PSI), which has had a separate all-day meeting in conjunction with the APA meeting since 1995 (having, in effect, met separately since 1990 in conferences organized by its president, Marvin Miller, whose book *Computer Applications in Mental Health* [Miller 1992] is recommended by the other coauthors of this chapter). At the 1996 meeting there were presentations on global technology, telepsychiatry, multimedia for psychiatric education, office systems, clinical databases, managing information, and business process re-engineering, in addition to general discussions about developments in the field. Software can be obtained free or for a nominal charge (Shareware) from colleagues as described in Chapter 26 on the Internet.

Computer system exhibits are to be found at most psychiatric meetings, but these have tended to be either from commercial firms interested in profits or from idealistic psychiatrists who have developed programs they and others have found useful and who have started commercial ventures. Examples of the latter are *Decisionbase*, by Philip Long, and *The Treatment Planner*, by James Kennedy. Applications are difficult to judge on the basis of the exhibit, which often leaves unanswered questions of how users can get together to compare notes on how they use the system, whether the system will still be in business next year, availability and cost of upgrades, and so forth.

There is a need for software reviews, such as those published in the Southern California Psychiatric Society newsletter by Freedman (1996). He has developed a comprehensive set of criteria (ease of use, interface, documentation, customer support, security, patient symptom assessment, clinician progress notes, treatment planner, medication tracker/prescription writer, laboratory monitor, treatment monitor, patient demographics, insurance information, billing package, clinical accounting package, clinical calendar, M.D. professional information, electronic claims submission, networkability, cost). He evaluated *CBS, PM/2, Shrink, Touched, SOS,* and *PBS3,* producing overall scores by which to rank the software. Touched ranked the highest, with 2.5 stars, while four systems had only 1.5 stars. The next versions reviewed might reverse the standings. Zarr has provided software reviews for the *American Journal of Psychotherapy* since 1989, and he and others have written for the *Psychiatric Times* since 1991.

Other disciplines have banded together around uses of computers in human services. The School of Social Work at Rutgers University has organized conferences on human service information technology applications (HUSITA), incorporating the national nursing computer conference. (HUSITA conference information is available from School of Social Work, 536 George Street, Rm. 206, New Brunswick, NJ 08903.)

Computerized Record Versus Paper Record

Several problems and benefits must be considered in using computerized records. Problems to be considered involve

- Data entry
- Data maintenance
- Data retrieval
- Time expenditure on learning applications, struggling with hardware and software, or implementing ill-conceived projects that take a long time to go nowhere
- Keeping up with hardware and software changes and upgrades

These difficulties should not be minimized. Recently, it was disclosed that the Internal Revenue Service wants to start over again after spending $4 *billion* on computer systems (Johnston 1997).

The benefits of using computerized records are

- Data from other sources can be entered easily.
- The record can be reconfigured to suit a variety of purposes.
- Multimedia applications are available.
- The record can be part of the forward thrust in patient care. Two randomized double-blind studies showed that physicians were better able to predict their patients' future symptom changes and laboratory test results from outpatient visits to an arthritis clinic when a computerized record was added to the paper record (Whiting-O'Keefe et al. 1985). The result was fewer tests and some cost savings, achieved largely through the flexibility of the computerized record in presenting data to clinicians.
- Data are more readily available.
- Word-processing applications enable related documents to be produced from the record, and multiple copies of any document can be produced easily, reducing the risk of loss.
- Patients' progress can be assessed easily.
- Links to other data for decision support can be automatic.
- Expert knowledge–base links can be automatic.
- Templates can be used to ensure that documentation requirements are met for quality assurance and to reduce the risk of malpractice.
- Paperwork can be reduced. Paperwork abounds almost everywhere psychiatrists work. The public sector, apart from billing and reimbursement, often generates repetitive forms. The New York State Office of Mental Health (OMH) found that in 1984 its physicians spent an average of about one-third of their time each week filling out forms (107 of them) to comply with regulations for federal and state governments; OMH facilities and local planning, monitoring, and administration; community agencies; and patient care (New York State Office of Mental Health: "Reducing the Paperwork on Professional Staff in OMH Facilities." Unpublished manuscript, October 1984). However, a large amount of paperwork generally exists 13 years later, the state not having implemented recommended

changes (J. M. Tien, M. F. Cahn, J. A. McClure: "An Information Systems Assessment of the New York State Department of Mental Hygiene," December 1984).

- Literature access and review are more efficient.
- Quality assurance can be done by applying guidelines to all (not just a sample of) records and selecting those for closer scrutiny automatically.
- Billing can be automated, with an automated form sometimes being the only form payers will accept.
- Databases can be used for research without having to find cases or enter data manually.
- Programs can be used for predicting patient outcome, for therapies, for treatment planning, and for simulations and models.

Powsner (1997) describes how some of the advantages can be obtained for $2,420. However, more complicated systems of the sort a group may need in order to deal with managed care will cost more and require expertise in many areas. Systems will become obsolete and require replacement. Dunbrack (1996) estimates that annual costs for the practice management market will reach $1 billion by 1999. The health information systems market value reached $19 billion in 1996 (Schneider 1996). There will be a higher initial cost and perhaps some subsequent savings as the federal standards to be developed as a requirement of the Health Insurance Portability and Accountability Act (PL 104-91, August 21, 1996) are implemented. These standards for electronic exchange of administrative and financial data must be developed by February 20, 1998, and cover health claims or equivalent encounter information, health claims attachments, enrollment and disenrollment in a health plan, eligibility for a health plan, healthcare payment and remittance advice, health plan premium payments, first report of injury, health claim status, and referral certification and authorization. Additional standards must be developed for unique identifiers, code sets, security and privacy, and electronic signatures (Hammond 1997). The development of such standards is overdue and will promote integration. Similar standards are needed in psychiatry for the data elements that psychiatrists use frequently.

Use of Computers in an Office

All of us dream of being able to avoid having to use keyboards and instead say whatever we want into the computer and to have it do whatever we want. About 30 programs that provide aids to dictation are currently being advertised. Automatic speech recognition (ASR) can help with dictation. Part of this chapter was produced using

DragonDictate (Dragon Systems, 320 Nevada Street, Newton, MA 02160). This program, *Powersecretary* (Articulate Systems), and *VoiceOATH* (Kurzweil Applied Intelligence, Waltham, MA, 1-800-380-1234) require a brief pause between words, but have been stable enough to have a user base broad enough to be described in the scientific literature (C. Gardner et al. 1996). Other applications claim to accommodate normal rate and rhythm of speech (*SpeechWriter for Mental Health*) or to recognize the written word (*ScriptWriter XL*) (available from CMHC Systems, 570 Metro Place North, Dublin, OH 43017, 1-880-97VOICE), and IBM offers a system (*VoiceType 3.0 for Windows 95* [can be obtained from IBM, Somers, NY, 1-800-825-5263]) that links words. Most of these products have been reviewed recently (Morrey et al. 1996).

Systems Issues and Use of Computers According to Work Flow

The discussion in this subsection generally follows the recommendations of *The Perfect Chart User's Manual* (Schwartz 1995) in listing data elements to be put in notes. In *The Perfect Chart,* most of the notes are generated easily through macros in WordPerfect. A macro comprises lines of text or program instruction that can be generated from a few keystrokes. For example, one can turn on the macro by pressing a key or two together (in WordPerfect 5.1, Alt-F10) and then, say, type one's initials and produce one's name, title, address, telephone number, and so forth. *The Perfect Chart* is a large and growing collection of macros that cover most aspects of patient care. Anyone can develop a system of macros, given the time and expertise.

In *The Perfect Chart,* one is prompted to enter information in the following areas:

First contact. Patient name, date, address, telephone number(s), and complaint(s) will start a file.

Intake. Data elements include patient demographics, referral source demographics, fee and insurance information, payment responsibility, emergency information, information about pharmacy, family and significant others, patient problems, and treatment goals. Computer-assisted interviews (that function "more like a person than a computer" [Naditch 1994]) can be linked to managed care concerns, such as eventual outcomes. One such application has been developed for substance abuse (Kane et al. 1994). *First Visit Solutions* (RingTrue, Inc., 3425 Martin Road, Mosinee, WI 54455) is perhaps best mentioned here, although it aspires to be a complete system.

History. The user is prompted to call for past history (previous treatment), psychiatric medications being taken (present and past), history of emotional disorder in blood relatives, psychotropic medications taken by other members of the family, the patient's feeling about taking medication, and other items.

Family and significant others. Basic data are entered on each person who matters to the patient, with the information updatable as more knowledge is gained.

Problems and treatment goals. An extensive list of problems, goals, objectives, and intervention is offered. Being just words, these can be edited for each patient. Other systems are in code, which cannot be edited. *Documentor* (LANSTAR, 315 E. Eisenhower Parkway, Ste. 310, Ann Arbor, MI 48108, 1-800-822-0888, Fax: 313-663-6363) uses the Actus 4th Dimension relational database and includes appointment book, patient profile, symptom profiles, diagnoses and codes, prescription writer, and a few other features.

Diagnostic templates. *The Perfect Chart* has ways of linking words and marshaling the history but does not make diagnostic suggestions. Foremost among programs that do so is *DTREE,* which is currently available from Multi-Health Systems, Inc. (908 Niagara Falls Boulevard, North Tonawanda, NY 14120, 800-456-3003, Fax: 416-424-1736), or privately (First et al. 1988). Computers also offer new ways of looking at data—for example, the bar graphs of Behavioral MAPS (Master Assessment and Progress Scale) offered by Goknar and Kemal (1989). A short interview can be very efficient for screening and obtaining an overview of a patient's lifetime psychiatric status (see Bucholz et al. 1996).

Mental status. Although there are many different mental status outlines, *The Perfect Chart* outline, together with the Health Care Financing Administration (HCFA) guidelines, yields the following: appearance and behavior, orientation (recorded by day, time, day of week, date, season, type of place, name of place, person) and memory, speech, affect, thinking, attitude toward interviewer, intelligence and how it is estimated, general information, abstractions, calculations (and actual test used), insight, and judgment.

Psychological and assessment information. Psychological testing has been extensively automated and in this form is well accepted by patients, even those with severe illnesses. Numerous studies have shown generally good equivalence between old (usually paper-and-pencil) and computerized versions. Some patients are computer phobic; one study found that these patients had higher Beck Depression

Inventory scores (Beck 1967). Several studies have shown that patients are more willing to divulge sensitive information about substance abuse to a computer than to a human interviewer (e.g., Lucas et al. 1977). Computers enable precise measurement of response time. The shortest response latencies are noted in random responding, followed by faking good responses, honest responses, and, lastly, faking bad responses (Holden and Fekken 1988). It is estimated that more than 500 computerized tests are available (see catalogs from, e.g., Multi-Health Systems, Inc., and The Psychological Corporation [c/o Harcourt, Brace and Co., 555 Academic Court, San Antonio, TX 78204-2498]). Miller and Tharp (1996) describe how a psychiatrist can construct a custom interview. Although scoring of tests is easily done by computer, interpretive statement quality may vary widely, since it is a function of whoever wrote the software. The results of reliability and validity studies should be published in the professional literature and a bibliography reviewed by a clinician before a specific test is used in practice. Some tests enjoy wide popularity among the public and some clinicians even without evidence of concurrent or predictive validity. However, some tests have been shown to correlate well with other measures. The computerized Continuance Performance Test has been significantly correlated with teacher ratings of school performance, subtests of the Wechsler Intelligence Scale for Children—Revised that relate to attention, and some scales from the Conners Parent and Teacher Rating Scales (Seidel and Joschko 1991).

There has been some decline in the use of tests that provide narrative interpretations. Some tests, such as the Minnesota Multiphasic Personality Inventory (MMPI), have been around so long as to have some items interpreted quite differently from how they were interpreted when the test first was developed. In managed care, long testing sessions with psychologists may require preauthorization (Schlosser 1995), so new forms are being developed that are shorter and "managed care friendly" (Bindler and Shapiro 1995; Ficken 1995; Werthman 1995). On the other hand, a long session with a computer may require no preauthorization. Testing costs may be as low as $1 per hour if amortized over the life of the computer, and costs are further lowered by scoring being done automatically and available immediately for the clinician. Thus, clinicians with computers tend to perform more tests and do a broader evaluation of the patient (Flowers et al. 1993). Multi-Health Systems bundles *SHRINK 6.0* and other applications for assessment and diagnostic information. Kobak (1996) has recently reviewed computer-administered symptom rating scales.

Laboratory and electroencephalogram (EEG) data. The digitalization of EEG data has resulted in several machines being developed that have personal computers as their main hardware. These can be used by individual practitioners, or EEG recordings taken in an office can be transmitted over ordinary telephone lines to be read elsewhere. Output usually includes a brain map and a comparison with other brain maps. These machines have been useful in drug trials (Itil and Itil 1995; Itil et al. 1996), as well as in usual clinical practice (Tele-Map EEG Services [HZI Research Center, 150 White Plains Road, Tarrytown, NY 10591, 914-631-3315, Fax: 914-631-8815]). Not only can they provide conventional analog EEGs to be read in the traditional way, but they can remove artifacts, scan signals for various patterns, and so forth (NEUROSCAN, 1035 Sterling Road, Ste. 103, Herndon, VA 22070-3806, 703-787-7575, Fax: 703-787-0297) and provide probability data that the EEG is consistent with various psychiatric diagnoses (John et al. 1988).

Diagnostic conclusions. DSM-IV (American Psychiatric Association 1994) is available on disk from American Psychiatric Press, Inc. Two excellent DSM-III-R (American Psychiatric Association 1987) interview packages have been updated for DSM-IV: the Diagnostic Interview Schedule (Robins and Helzer 1994) and the Structured Clinical Interview for DSM-IV (Spitzer et al. 1995; software available from Multi-Health Systems). These are available as stand-alone programs or as part of *Decisionbase* (Suite 1206, 750 West Broadway, Vancouver, British Columbia, Canada V5Z 1J2, Tel: 604-876-2254), a monumental program developed by Philip Long (since 1983) that also includes a computerized history, psychiatric textbook, graphed progress chart, statistics, tutorials, text retrieval, word processor, and so forth.

Somewhere in this chapter it should be observed that no one believes that computers will replace, rather than help, psychiatrists, least of all in making diagnoses. Computers are useful for marshaling data, checking against guidelines, and so forth. More than 15 years ago, it was observed that computers do not do as well as humans in situations where they have all of the data (e.g., chess), and there is no way of putting in all of the data a good clinician uses to make a diagnosis (Taintor 1980)

Treatment planning. James Kennedy's *The Psychiatric Assistant* is recommended. (*The Psychiatric Assistant* can be obtained by calling 1-800-535-5680 [in Louisiana: 504-748-8183].) Built around treatment planning as described in his book (Kennedy 1992), this software includes diagnosis, psychiatric databases, medication reviews, information tracking, a variety of clinical scales such as the NOSIE (Nurse's Observation Scale for Inpatient Evaluation), and so forth. It uses the DayFlo Tracker, a text-oriented relational database management system. Another program, the *Computer-Assisted Service Plan* (available since 1994 from PSP Information Group, Inc., 1700 Broadway, Ste. 800, Oakland, CA 94612, 1-800-304-8322), is a stand-alone package that runs with Windows 3.0+, an outgrowth of client tracking and billing programs currently used by more than 5,000 clinics and programs. Another program, *Quick-Doc* (Mental Health Connections), offers quality assurance and treatment plans on a single computer. Willie Kai Yee's *Problem-Knowledge Coupler System* (available from Dr. Yee at 21 Tricor Avenue, New Paltz, NY 12561, 914-255-0660) feeds several sources into decision making. Another program, *TxPlan* (available from Earley Corporation, 407 West Ponce de Leon Aveune, Decatur, GA 30030, in a 1995 version) generates a nice-looking treatment plan.

Prescriptions.   Several pharmacy data programs are available: *Anxiety Expert* (psychopharmacology), *Clozapine Expert, OCD Expert, PDR Library on CD-ROM*, and *AskRx Plus* (Mental Health Connections). One may be linked to a large-scale system. The field is growing and consolidating (DePietro et al. 1995). Systems such as *PHARMAKON* in New York State offer guidelines for dosage, polypharmacy, and drug interactions (see foreword to this section). Patient medication leaflets are available on disk from several sources (e.g., Mental Health Connections) and can be tailored to specific patients (done by *The Perfect Chart*), including *Ask Advice* and *MedCoach*.

Psychotherapy.   Documentation of treatment is most important and is available in *The Perfect Chart*. There are many computer-assisted therapy programs, including *Assertiveness Training, Help-Assert, Help-Esteem, Help-Stress, Help-Think, Overcoming Depression, Personal Problem-Solving Guide*, and *Stress Management* (Mental Health Connections); Greist's pioneering work using touch telephones as simple computer terminals to treat depression (Dean Foundation 1996); and a program for adult development (Gould 1992). The *Therapeutic Learning Program* (Gould 1994) is an adjunct to help patients and therapists learn a brief, problem-solving approach, but does not substitute for the specifics of therapy. Programs generally do not distinguish between those that are to be used in conjunction with a psychiatrist, with some one else, or by a person alone in a self-help mode. Greist and Marks compared the efficacy of a psychiatrist, a nurse, an interactive computer program, and reading Marks's book in relieving symptoms of anxiety. They found that the computer program did well for some patients. Generally, however, computer-assisted therapy is thought to work better with human reinforcement and, often, vice versa. Patients left alone with computers usually do not do much with them. Colby (1995) has reported on a computer program using cognitive therapy to treat depression.

Virtual reality will be a useful adjunct in psychotherapy, especially desensitization for phobias and guided imagery. The American Psychiatric Association cooperated in part ("Virtual Reality and Mental Health") of the conference "Medicine Meets Virtual Reality" in 1996.

Cognitive rehabilitation.   There have been reports of home-grown programs that have improved memory and spatial relationships ("Tireless Tutor" *Business Week* 1985). One program is *Shift Notes,* developed by Alice Medalia and associates (available from The Information Exchange, Inc., 20 Squadron Blvd., New City, NY 10956). Software for the treatment of attention-deficit disorder is available (BrainTrain, 727 Twin Ridge Lane, Richmond, VA 23235; Psychiatric Information and Education Systems, 2129 Belcourt Avenue, Nashville, TN 37212; Universal Attention Disorders, Inc., 4281 Katella Avenue, Ste. 215, Los Alamitos, CA 90720). Computer-assisted cognitive rehabilitation is an impressive part of the rehabilitation mall at Middletown Psychiatric Center (Bopp et al. 1996), where assessment instruments such as the Wisconsin Card Sort Test are practiced in such a way that they have the potential to become the remediation instruments.

Rehabilitation.   Some programs, such as *Employee Appraiser* and *Psyber Dx* (Mental Health Connections), are geared toward assessing people in work situations,

Billing.   Mandatory electronic claims submission is increasing. Benefits claimed include reduced paperwork, lower mailing costs, reduced administrative costs, no electronic exclusions, improved cash flow with rapid payment (often by electronic funds transfer), easy monitoring of claims, and so forth. But physicians resist. Courtroom battles did not delay scheduling for mandatory electronic submission starting October 1, 1996, for the five Blue Cross and Blue Shield plans in New York State (MSSNY 1996), although individual practitioners may seek exemptions. A useful source is the January 1993 report "Electronic Commerce in U.S. Health Care: Input Research Report" (from Input, Mountain View, CA), which discusses medical claims processing, payment, procurement, and utilization review. The report addresses how to eliminate intermediaries and how to re-engineer practices and offers some product comparisons and cost-benefit analyses.

As long as one is dealing with intermediaries, the key is coding. One has to know how which service will be handled by which provider. Reimbursements sometimes can be improved with coding (Heckler 1996). Workshops to improve coding and claims submission typically are held in large cities (e.g., Kathy Dunphy's popular Medicare workshops in New York City). One program that can assist at the coding level is *Medicode* (Medicode Systems, Inc., 5225 Wiley Post Way, Ste. 500, Salt Lake City, UT 84116-2889, Tel: 1-800-999-4600). But one can get a system to do bills (among other things). Jerome Blumenthal, a psychiatrist, developed a system for himself years ago that has acquired enough of a critical mass of users to keep up with necessary changes (Jerome Blumenthal, M.D., 4100 Old Vestal Road, Binghamton, NY

13903, Tel: 607-770-0081). A typical system of interest is *Billing Practice Management Software (PM/2)* (Available from Practice Management Software, 285 Engle Street, Englewood, NJ 07631, 1-800-874-2159). It provides bills and statements in various formats, insurance claim preparation, electronic claim submission via clearinghouse to all third-party payers, open item or balance-forward posting of items, treatment plan writer, progress notes, accounting reports, mailing labels, face sheets, and other forms. Compulink (Compulink Business Systems, Inc., 31300 Via Colinas, Ste. 104, Westlake Village, CA 91362, Tel: 1-800-456-4522) offers the *Psych Advantage* package, which generates information for billing, scheduling, patient records, and prescriptions. This package also features a word processor and accommodates multiple users at multiple sites. Compulink is an interesting company because it initially made its fortune selling its software to run on Everex computers, which are no longer made; this illustrates the difficulty of selling software linked to particular hardware. *CaseWatch* (Watchung Software Group, Inc., 1090 King Georges Post Road, Ste. 708, Edison, NJ 08837, 201-417-0200, Fax: 201-417-1968) uses the PICK operating system, a powerful database management system that is "platform independent," in that it runs on a variety of hardware systems, inadvertently illustrating the problems of going from code to words by advertising it "includes an *English-like* [italics added] report generator for easy production of ad hoc reports." Custom Businessware, Inc. (22 Brevoort Rd., Chappaqua, NY 10514), is a recent arrival, emphasizing billing software. *Medical Claims Assistance* (127 South Broadway, Yack, NY 10960) is a general medical billing system.

Quality assurance. Available in the United States are such programs as *Quick-Doc* (quality assurance and treatment plans on a single computer), *Psyber Net,* and *Psyber Com* (prediction of length of stay) (Mental Health Connections). The European Psychiatric Association is trying to define outcome (I. Marks, comment at World Psychiatric Association Information Systems Symposium, Madrid, August 24, 1996). *CORM* (Clinical Outcome and Resource Monitoring) is a program developed to automate what Isaac Marks has been doing since 1979 at the Maudsley to check outcome of patients treated by his staff. (*CORM* is available from Qualcare Ltd., 9/10 Chiltern House, Leys Rd., Brockmoor, Brierly Hill, DY5 3UT United Kingdom.) Also available from the same private source is *HoNOS-COM:V4,* a computer information system for efficient delivery of Britain's *Health of the Nation*–type scales for mental health, a measure used throughout Britain by the Department of Health as part of the routine assessment of mentally ill patients (Marks 1996).

Patient uses. Patients have many uses for their records. Automated records are readily available to them in printed form, in whole or part.

For some years, we (Taintor et al. 1993) have routinely given our patients at Manhattan Psychiatric Center copies of what the psychiatrists write about them and find this improves communication.

Learning and support.   It is estimated that there are more than 1,000 electronic discussion groups, which are wide-ranging and mostly organized by diagnosis. They cover new treatments, emotional concerns, pain relief, and all aspects of physician care (Lamberg 1996). Psychiatrists should welcome patient participation in these groups as additional sources of information and support, part of the process that can help the person objectify and get distance from the illness, bearing in mind such problems as confidentiality, hidden commerciality, junk mail exposure, and inadequacy compared with face-to-face communication.

Self-help.   *IT'S YOUR CALL* is an expert system for sending and receiving voice-mail messages from smoking cessation experts. Experts found that of 800 unscreened smokers, almost two-thirds quit temporarily; the 1-year quit rate of those who called five times or more was approximately equal to that in most face-to-face counseling programs. There is no need to schedule sessions or to be concerned about being judged. Computer-assisted programs also help people lose weight and manage other behaviors (Petersen 1993). There is a recent comprehensive guide to general medical self-help (Ferguson 1996).

In addition to using the Internet, patients can use other customized educational resources. For example, one health maintenance organization (HMO) offered a worker a 10% premium reduction to become a certified "health partner" with her employer and to distribute and attempt to implement with her family the data and recommendations in a prevention news service customized for her and her family. The news service reminds them about clinical preventive services falling due, makes appointments, helps with multimedia educational projects, and so forth (Harris and Crawford 1996).

Special Considerations in Dealing With Managed Care Organizations

As we examine the topic of dealing with managed care organizations in greater detail, it is important to note the different types of managed care organizations and their transiency. The rapid growth of managed care concerns and their move to provide coverage for more and more Americans (about 108 million by October 1995 [Manderscheid and Henderson 1995]) have surprised many people, including both the traditional fee-for-service insurance industry and the traditional not-for-profit HMOs such as Kaiser-Permanente. Fee-for-service insurance companies, by buying managed care firms, have contributed to the notion that many of these firms are basically businesses guided by the profit motive—for example, the sale of U.S. Healthcare to Aetna for $8.9 billion (of which almost a billion went to U.S. Healthcare's founder) ("Aetna Completes U.S. Healthcare Deal" *Modern Healthcare* 1996). For-profit Cigna's 1995 revenues of $15.6 billion surpassed Kaiser-Permanente's not-for-profit revenues of $12.3 billion (*Modern Healthcare* 1996).

The idea of profit is related to the transiency and multiplication of insurance entities and to the United States' unique position (as a result of wage freezes in World War II, which made attractive fringe-benefit packages the means for recruiting good workers) of having health coverage so dependent on employer payments. It is paradoxical to start an insurance plan focusing only on young, healthy people and their usually limited and equally young families. As an insurance plan matures, it inevitably accumulates older people, retired workers, and larger families of dependents, some of whom are likely to be chronically ill. Companies offer "open enrollment" for switching insurance plans, which adds to the transiency of such plans, since workers will switch to any plan that offers the same coverage at lower rates. Such a plan is always the youngest plan, because it has not accumulated costly users of its benefits.

The result has been a proliferation of insurance companies, peaking at about 1,600. New corporate entities are born in an effort to select a healthy population, leaving behind the high users in plans that are increasingly deficit-ridden. Thus, we see not-for-profit firms, such as Blue Cross and Blue Shield, setting up for-profit entities, such as Greenspring. Adding to the chaos is each firm's drive not to pay the first dollar of benefits, which tends to penalize the customer who has gotten into several plans to guarantee coverage. He may have the coverage, but he also has the inconvenience of the firms fighting over who will pay first by refusing to pay at all. Firms have refined this art by using different claim forms that often serve as a method to deny benefits.

The consequences of this multiplicity of claim forms and insurance companies have been disastrous for information systems. Firms are rarely interested in having anything other than fiscal data used for getting rates or for reimbursement from companies. This situation has complicated health systems research. Although the United States has led in developing computer hardware and software, other countries offer superior databases for health services research because they have fewer, more stable payers for health care. The lack of comparability data, unfortunately, will leave unanswered the major question of whether new firms can seem (at least financially) to be doing things better as a result of utilization review or because of their clientele. Nothing much should be expected from utilization review in the public sector or Medicare, both of which also have many factors cooperating to reduce comparability and often lack accurate data or good data retrieval software.

The information age must be distinguished from the age of managed care. It is clear that most managed care firms regard information systems as key to their survival and profitability. However, the information system–based drive to track and reduce costs is occurring throughout the economy. New software is credited with making it possible finally to reduce legal bills (Geer 1997). Managed care competition will reduce administrative costs, which had become bloated in the American pay-any-fee-for-service environment that existed in some places before managed care. Fee-for-service in Canada historically has featured lean administrative structures, and specialists in Ontario recently successfully struck to keep administrative costs to 2.2%. Although some firms initially reaped (and, some say, concealed) profits by charging large (say, 30%) administrative costs, overheads are negotiated and typically are 11%–12% for new plans. Profits made by reducing administrative costs are universally applauded, while those resulting from reducing medical care expenditures are increasingly unpopular. There are many ways informatics can drive managed care; decentralization and distributed processing constitute one likely direction.

Meanwhile, software supposedly specific to managed care is being marketed. Borch (1996) provides a useful overview and a list of more than 60 vendors.

Confidentiality Concerns as Promoters of Physician Control

Not only are some organizations perceived as just out for profits, but fears of outright criminality have been strengthened by one report of the Mafia's allegedly siphoning money from group healthcare programs serving a million patients. Confidentiality issues were raised as investigators "warned that the medical industry was a potential treasure trove for mobsters who could use sensitive and personal information gleaned from group-care programs to blackmail and exploit patients and health-care providers" (Raab 1996, A1).

There are many candidates for running managed care organizations, and it is expected that those interested in profit will soon pocket it and be gone from the scene, leaving systems that now cover the majority of Americans. However, the focus on outcomes and continuity as medical goals is having the effect of forcing continuity onto the corporations that have been practicing discontinuity. The resulting consolidations consist largely of profiteers selling to others who believe they can make a go of it by staying in the business for the long term. Not surprisingly, many of the latter are already committed to the field by having chosen medical careers. Thus, we see more physician-owned healthcare organizations The well-heeled physician who did not have to worry about costs is now less well heeled as physician income has dropped ("Physician Incomes Drop" *New York Times* 1996), but in a group that is keeping careful track of costs and having to use information systems to do it. Various organizations are vying to lead the professionals with whom they have a relationship. The American Hospital Association wants to be the national leader in representing provider-based integrated delivery systems and "the single most influential national organization" for hospitals and hospital systems (*Modern Healthcare* 1996). Whoever is running them, managed care companies see information systems as the key to their future; they having emerged as the first priority in research for the agenda of the 1996 National Managed Health Care Congress. Physician-owned and managed firms emerged as the second priority (ahead of quality), which may reflect the next generation of ownership (Campbell 1996).

With the proliferation of managed care organizations, there are, of course, efforts to sell computer systems that supposedly have special competence for dealing with managed care. Data systems such as those offered at the Disease Management Congress (September 16–19, 1996, Washington, D.C.) are designed "to gather, classify and interpret the data that is necessary to determine whether disease management efforts are cost- and quality effective, and to identify areas in the process that can be continuously improved." This conference included one session with a psychiatrist on psychosocial issues in asthma management. (For more information, contact National Managed Health Care Congress, 70 Blanchard St., Ste. 4000, Burlington, MA 01803, 617-270-6000, Fax: 617-270-6004.) Systems can be developed or repackaged to report on or otherwise emphasize quality (Edlin 1996). The Medical Society of New York County Committee on Office Computer Systems has been surveying medical office systems and noting features claimed to be of special help dealing with managed care, such as deductible copays, fee schedules, patient eligibility, receipts, referral authorizations, and withholds. (One of us [ZT] co-chairs the committee. The survey is available [$50 for nonmembers] from the Medical Society of New York County, 26 East 25th Street, 11th floor, New York, NY 10016.)

So far, psychiatric specialty concerns about confidentiality have not become a focus in managed care didactics. The APA series on managed care mentions computer systems only in response to questions. Books on managed care do not mention automation, computers, or documentation, with the exception of Zieman's (1995) discussion of how to design an information system. Yet the APA books offer language that can easily be incorporated into macros about patients in documentation submitted to managed care companies for approval of patient care (e.g., the patient impairment definitions and individual psychotherapy interventions in Goodman et al. 1992, Appendixes A and B, respectively; and the forms and protocols in Wyatt 1994). But the real issue will be whether anyone can guarantee integrity and security at the level one would expect from a physician, the sort of behavior Robert Newman showed in going to jail rather than show police photos of patients enrolled in his methadone clinic.

Confidentiality is much more of a concern now than 20 years ago, when it could be argued that there were no recorded breaches of confidentiality in a psychiatric information system (Laska and Bank 1976). Reasons that security concerns should mount now include

- More data are collected on each person in a system. Increasing detail means more data of potential interest to more people.
- Data are collected on more persons and are retrieved by more people, many of whom leave systems on when they should be turned off, post passwords on the wall near the computer, or act otherwise carelessly.
- Making systems user-friendly involves making data more accessible. Managed care organizations generally want to have all data online.
- Communications systems are more easily tapped. If a computer is left on and connected to a telephone line, the chances are good something can be gotten out of it by someone with enough skill, time, expertise, and motivation.

Okstein (1996) offers suggestions for physicians trying to reduce these risks:

- Control access.
- Deter unauthorized access.
- Limit access by user type and only to certain parts.
- Prevent unauthorized copying.
- Prevent chart tampering, and physically protect the chart.
- Have an overall security plan.

Computers do add risks, such as the current American Medical Association (AMA) study of health data clearinghouses that collect information on patients' conditions from insurance companies and then sell it back to insurers trying to determine if applicants have unreported preexisting conditions. Unauthorized access can lead to embarrassment, job loss, and a breakdown in doctor-patient trust. Federal legislation, introduced by Senator Robert Bennett, is pending and controversial, since it seems to do more to aid the formation industry than to protect confidentiality (*American Medical News* 1996). In the "1996 Computer Crime and Security Survey" ("Industry Watch" *Health*

Management Technology 1996), 41% of information systems surveyed had had their security compromised by detecting unauthorized access. Of these, 50% were traced to current employees, but many were also traced to remote dial-in sources and Internet connections, and 36.8% of site attacks in medical institutions were the result of altering data in an unauthorized manner. A child rapist got little girls' telephone numbers from a hospital information system and made obscene calls to them, using a password that should have been canceled. Yet half the hospitals surveyed reported it takes longer than a day to cancel a password. Just a partial list of security concerns involves pages of questions to be answered (Brandt 1995). Frisse (1996b) is concerned that recent requirements for Medicare and other reimbursement may require too much data to leave the physician's office and that questions asked on the Internet must be protected. With all this going on, patients are likely to seek small, physician-controlled firms that protect confidentiality.

Different Comparisons Made Possible by Different Kinds of Data

Populations and Treatment Norms

The first version of the Health Plan Employer Data and Information Set (HEDIS), developed by the National Committee for Quality Assurance (NCQA), was released in 1993 (see Chapter 24 in Section V, Volume 16 of the *Review of Psychiatry*). The NCQA is important in and of itself, since it represents a major alternative to the Joint Commission on the Accreditation of Healthcare Organizations (JCAHO). Its approach is to be less concerned with looking at the process of care as JCAHO has done and, instead, to focus on outcomes. The HEDIS is a set of integrated performance measures according to which plans can specify, calculate, and report performance information. For example, childhood immunization data from a healthcare plan can be compared with data for all children in the area and with the plan's own performance. HealthPartners reported increasing the percentage of children immunized against childhood diseases from 54% to 89% over 4 years.

Healthcare plans are having to adapt to HEDIS after having developed their own ways of reporting. Currently, HEDIS is used by 330 healthcare plans, with more plans adopting it as it becomes a standard report card to businesses and consumers.

Although HEDIS will be the industry standard, it has many blank areas—including mental health—that it is trying to fill in rapidly. The next version has been released in draft form and will go into effect in January 1997. It expands the original 60 items to 75, moving from the areas of prevention and immunization to heart disease, asthma, and diabetes, with a second tier of measures in the testing stage for evaluating certain outpatient, follow-up, and diagnostic track records.

Reports are expected to be generated from patient care and management data: "Figure out how to use the information systems to improve care, and the rest all follows from this" (Morrissey 1996b, p. 2).

Managed care organizations can be expected to single out for review a provider whose work falls more than two standard deviations outside the HEDIS or other norms. Cigna has announced this publicly (Medical Society of New York County, *Managed Care Forum*, February 28, 1996). In the example above, 4 years ago, the pediatrician whose patient immunization rate was below 40% would be looked at; now the expectation would be 76%. The pediatrician would be expected to anticipate immunization needs, schedule appointments, and provide educational materials, all of which are tasks made easier with the help of computers.

Public sector plans can be evaluated under the expanded HEDIS, including Medicaid managed care and Medicare HMOs. A draft Medicaid HEDIS has been developed and reviewed for mental health indicators by the CMHS (Robinson et al. 1996) and placed in context with other report cards.

Although, so far, data relevant to mental health and psychiatry are limited, the amount of data released for analysis (Colorado Health Data Commission 1992; National Committee for Quality Assurance 1993; Pennsylvania Healthcare Cost Containment Council 1991) is staggering to anyone used to the sparse tidbits available during an era when many are concerned about reputation, confidentiality, and due process. In data released to the public, individual patients supposedly are protected by being kept anonymous, because the system wants aggregate data that can be compared with other aggregate data in a test of means, modes, and standard deviations. But even with aggregate data, the identity of some localities and practitioners and information about socioeconomic status inevitably will be revealed (Brook et al. 1996). However, within a plan, increasingly detailed data on individual treatment will be entered to ascertain how the result compares with norms. Thus, Keatley and colleagues (1995) describe both an outcome report comparing treatments and another comparing patients: ". . . you can compare patient M.G's treatment to the 'norm' who received Protocol II. It is apparent that the patient's outcome was excellent, with improvement across all areas and a cost that was $577 less than predicted . . ."

The notion that quality and outcome will turn on data systems is axiomatic in the managed care literature, despite data entry and other limitations, so we can expect that a lot of data will be accumulated. The data so entered may well hang around and be retrievable. Morrissey (1996b) describes ways of limiting access but reports that this is often neglected in planning and maintaining systems. The prospectus for *Behavioral Informatics Tomorrow* (March 1997) offers help in designing information systems to meet "emerging . . . confidentiality guidelines": "Improve quality and reduce costs through computer-assisted outcomes management, clinical intervention and decision support systems. . . . Enhance patient and provider access to essential treatment information through online services. . . . Integrate your delivery system with applications that connect all levels of care and facilitate electronic communications with other organizations."

A Community Health Information System (CHIN) is also in the cards. "CHIN" was one of the buzz words of 1995 (Rushing et al. 1995), and some states, such as Massachusetts, are trying to build CHINs from the ground up by ensuring that information systems of various providers are mutually compatible (Morrissey 1996c). Wisconsin has been most advanced in CHIN building. A limited data set has been implemented in Alberta (McDougall et al. 1995). CHINs will eventually be linked to create a national healthcare information infrastructure (Vijay 1994). According to one report, "The CHIN movement will engulf nearly every healthcare provider, payor, third party administrator and patient in America" ("CHINs" *Infocare* 1994). The American Hospital Association has published a guide to developing CHINs (Wakerly and First Consulting Group Authors 1994).

HMOs and Behavioral Health Care
In an effort to get nine million federal employees to choose their health plans on the basis of quality as well as price, the *Federal Employee Health Benefit Guide* issued in November 1996 included NCQA ratings of some of the 388 plans that compete for employee premiums during the open enrollment period. The NCQA has accredited 243 of the more than 600 HMOs in the United States, but only 102 fully (for 3 years). Other accreditation data, such as those of the JCAHO, are likely to be included in future guides; consumer satisfaction data were included in 1995 (J. Gardner 1996).

Strategies for Dealing With Managed Care

Groups of Practitioners
Munoz (1996) has offered a step-by-step list of maneuvers that some managed care firms have carried out to hold on to as many dollars as possible (Table 25–1). It is useful as a worst-case scenario to show how computers and information systems can be used both for attack and for defense.

Regarding Munoz's recommendations to form clinical groups and develop regional and national groups, little can be accomplished without following one in particular: Clinicians must understand, use, and control information systems. In this respect, the Substance Abuse and Mental Health Administration's Center for Mental Health Services offers a great deal of technical assistance for practitioners and consumers through its dozens of publications. The CMHS has also marshaled the

Table 25–1.   Contracting tactics of managed care firms

Attack (set limits on)	Defense (use data to show)
Pretreatment	
Benefits	Costs of lack of treatment
Coverage	Costs of episodic treatment versus continuity
Providers	One is as good as any other provider
During treatment	
Concurrent review	One's own, better concurrent review[a]
Discharge plan	Why the patient is not ready to go
Case management	One is managing the case better
Prepayment	
Appropriate care	Why the care was better than "appropriate"
Pattern analysis	What is wrong with the pattern analysis
Procedure review	What any reasonable person would consider
Billing process	How slowly payment comes
Postpayment	
Billing audits	Charges were justified
Record review	The patient's record
Denial of claims	Claims were justified
"Fraud" detection	There is no fraud; repeated witch-hunts are harassment
Provider profile	Statistics require that some data be outside standard deviations; the particular patient, defined in one's own rich database, was more ill and his or her case was more complicated than defined by the sparse descriptors available in the firm's data set
Report cards	One's report is good (recalculate if necessary)
Costs	Costs are competitive
Quality	One's own set of defensible measures
Services	Have been duly rendered and compare in type and frequency
Outcomes	Objective measures show what progress has been made
Patient satisfaction	Subjective measures also have been obtained (bear in mind Marks's (1996) observation that satisfaction and outcome may differ, which is as much the payer's problem as anyone else's)

[a]Concurrent review, currently done by asking questions about the patient and record, will increasingly be done through real-time availability of an electronic record.
Source.   Adapted from Munoz 1996.

data that were used to argue for more coverage for mental health in healthcare reform and the recent press for parity. Such data are bound to be useful in dealing with managed care providers. Among the many publications, several stand out as particularly useful in dealing with information systems and managed care. One should start with *Managed Behavioral Healthcare: History, Models, Key Issues, and Future Course* (Freeman and Trabin 1995). Of general interest are a summary of federally supported managed care activities, mostly evaluations and innovations (Center for Mental Health Services 1995); the *MHSIP Consumer-Oriented Mental Health Report Card*, which is currently being field-tested and is consumer-oriented, but also research-based, cost-conscious, and value-based, including outcomes and concerns related to serious mental illness (Center for Mental Health Services 1996); and *First Quarterly Report: Public Sector Moves Managed Care to Forefront of Behavioral Health Services* (The Policy Resource Center 1996), which shows the methodology and rapid progress of public-sector managed behavioral care, noting what data are collected and how they are used.

Academic departments have a chance to develop systems for their own needs (Fuller et al. 1995) and to compete favorably for business, but must be able to make the productivity argument. Psychiatry can learn from what medical colleagues have done (Lewis 1996). Wong and Abendroth (1996) argue that "providers recognize data as a strategic asset." The need to band together could lead to bypassing the struggle to look at individual office-based systems and consider an integrated data network, such as that offered by InStream (300 Unicorn Park Drive, Woburn, MA 01801).

As physicians develop their own managed care groups and contract with patients and employers, eliminating the HMO or BHCO in the middle, they will need managed care software, which includes, in addition to all that has gone before, the following: contract management and billing for the hospital(s) (patient management, billing, decision support); contract management and billing support for physician practices (benefits, coverage, and copayments); accurate billing according to managed care contracts; accurate accounts receivable and collection); and, if there is a physician-hospital organization (PHO), membership/enrollment, benefit and plan management, authorizations and referrals, provider management and relations, capitation management, claims processing, utilization review, and provider profiling (Ribka 1996).

Individual Strategies

The first task is to become computer literate. Frisse (1994) provides a useful overview. One way is to use the computer for one's own education, an activity promoted by some medical schools (Dev 1994) and some psychiatry residencies (Burt et al. 1996). Other medical schools are lagging and still at the stage of curriculum development (Koschmann 1995). Information technology is seen as a plus in recruiting and being hired (Colucci 1996).

The individual practitioner taking on any sort of managed care organizational (MCO) decision in the processes listed in Table 25–1 should understand that the initial determination may have been produced automatically. By June 1996, it was possible to list 46 companies providing clinical and financial decision-support tools (HOTLIST 1996), and larger information systems doubtlessly have built in such modules. Software specifically directed at outcomes is offered by Health Outcomes, Inc. (4558 4th Avenue NE, Seattle, WA 98105). Psychiatrists must understand the internal rules by which the software is programmed and work to ensure that key variables are handled well.

Office systems of the sort described in this chapter can provide data on patient benefits and coverage. Getting provider data to MCOs can be tedious and may be required in different forms. A psychiatrist must keep credentialing data in a computer to retrieve them easily and put them into whatever format is required. Issues during treatment are best handled by having more documentation than does the MCO. *The Perfect Chart* or any other program that uses words rather than code is likely to have the advantage here, as will the individual practitioner, who will always know patients in the practice better than does the MCO, which must have some data on all the patients in all the practices with which it deals. Words, rather than codes, document exactly what is done and why. If, for example, the argument is over who is managing the case better, the first objective is to have more data on the case, the second is to have more on the management, and the third is to show why the outcome so far is the best that can be expected.

In summary, information systems can be used to deal with managed care, but by having more, not less, data and documentation.

References

ACCESS HealthNet (brochure). Westlake Village, CA, ACCESS HealthNet, 1996

Aetna completes U.S. Healthcare deal. Modern Healthcare 26(30)(July 22):11, 1996

American Medical News, July 8/15, 1996, p 36

American Medical Informatics Association (AMIA): Beyond the Superhighway: Exploiting the Internet With Medical Informatics. Bethesda, MD, American Medical Informatics Association, 1996

American Psychiatric Association: Diagnostic and Statistical Manual of Mental Disorders, 3rd Edition, Revised. Washington, DC, American Psychiatric Association, 1987

American Psychiatric Association: Diagnostic and Statistical Manual of Mental Disorders, 4th Edition. Washington, DC, American Psychiatric Association, 1994

Andrew W, Dick R: On the road to the CPR: where are we now? Healthcare Informatics 13(5):48–88, 1996

Beck AT: Depression: Clinical, Experimental and Theoretical Aspects. New York, Harper & Row, 1967

Bindler P, Shapiro R: Psychological testing in brief psychotherapy. Behavioral Health Management 15(5):18–20, 1995

Bopp JH, Ribble DJ, Cassidy JJ, et al: Re-engineering the state hospital to promote rehabilitation and recovery. Psychiatr Serv 47:697–698, 701, 1996

Borch K: Companies define managed care software. Health Management Technology 17(5):58–66, 1996

Braly D: HOTLIST: computer-based patient records/electronic medical records. Health Management Technology 17(8):40–44, 1996

Brandt M: How safe is your system? Healthcare Informatics 12(10):24–32, 1995

Brekka T: Select mobile computers tailored to healthcare environment. Health Management Technology 16(13):48–50, 1995

Bria WF, Rydell RL: The Physician-Computer Connection. Chicago, IL, American Hospital Publishing, 1992

Brook RH, Kamberg CJ, McGlynn EA: Health system reform and quality. JAMA 276:476–480, 1996

Bucholz KK, Marlon SL, Shayka JJ, et al: A short computer interview for obtaining psychiatric diagnoses. Psychiatr Serv 47:293–297, 1996

Burt T, Ishak WW, Taintor Z, et al: Psychiatry residents use of Internet resources. Presentation at the annual meeting of the American Psychiatric Association, New York, May 1996

Campanelli M: Multimedia to the Max. Mobile Computing and Communications 8(2):52–63, 1997

Campbell GR: Info systems, outcomes and interactivity are all the rage at NMHCC 1996. Managed Health Care 6(5):40–44, 1996

Cave DG: The marketbasket approach to cost control in capitated plans. Managed Health Care 6(5):46–60, 1995

Center for Mental Health Services: Managed Care Activities (Publ No MC96-58). Rockville, MD, Center for Mental Health Services, Substance Abuse and Mental Health Services Administration, 1995

Center for Mental Health Services: The MHSIP Consumer-Oriented Mental Health Report Card. Rockville, MD, Center for Mental Health Services, Substance Abuse and Mental Health Services Administration, 1996

CHINs—their value defined, their building described in AHA book. Infocare [Supplement to Healthcare Informatics], September 1994, p 4

CIO (Chief Information Officer), August 1996 (Special Issue)

Clinical systems do not enamor group physician practices. Healthcare Informatics 13(9):§§8–24, 1996

Colorado Health Data Commission: Colorado Hospital Outcomes: Mortality, Length of Stay and Charges for Cardiovascular and Other Diseases. Clinical Data Project. Denver, Colorado Health Data Commission, 1992

Colby KM: Clinical computing: a computer program using cognitive therapy to treat depressed patients. Psychiatr Serv 46:1223–1226, 1995

Colucci MP: Information technology: the new edge in recruiting. Health Systems Review 29(3):16–17, 1996

CPRI offering non-proprietary MPI application free to users. Health Care Technology 17(8):38, 1996

DePietro S, Tocco M, Tramontozzi A: Pharmacy systems: keeping pace. Healthcare Informatics, 1995, pp 29–44

Dev P: Consortia to support computer-aided medical education. Acad Med 69:719–721, 1994

Dunbrack L: Practice-management market to reach $1 billion by 1999. Health Management Technology 17(7):31–34, 1996

Edlin ML: Refine your health plan's value with quality reporting. Health Management Technology 17(8):17–19, 1996

Ferguson T: Health Online: How to Go Online to Find Health Information, Support Forums, and Self-Help Communities in Cyberspace. Reading, MA, Addison-Wesley, 1996

Ficken J: New directions for psychological testing. Behavioral Health Management 15(5):12–14, 1995

First MB, Williams JB, Spitzer RL: Concise Guide to Using DTREE: The Electronic DSM-III-R. Toronto, MultiHealth Systems, 1988

Flowers JV, Booraem CD, Schwartz B: Impact of computerized rapid assessment instruments on counselors and client outcome. Computers in Human Services 10:9–18, 1993

Freedman J: Review of office systems. Presentation at the Psychiatric Society for Informatics, New York, May 1996

Freeman MA, Trabin T: Managed Behavioral Healthcare: History, Models, Key Issues, and Future Course (Publ No MC95-44). Rockville, MD, Center for Mental Health Services, Substance Abuse and Mental Health Services Administration, 1995

Frisse ME: Acquiring information management skills. Acad Med 69:803–806, 1994

Frisse ME: The commerce of ideas: Internets and Intranets. Acad Med 71:749–753, 1996a

Frisse ME: What is the Internet learning about you while you are learning about the Internet? Acad Med 71:1064–1067, 1996b

Frisse ME, Schnase JL, Metcalfe ES: Models for patient records. Acad Med 69:546–550, 1994

Fuller S, Braude R, Florance V, et al: Managing information in the academic medical center: building an integrated information environment. Acad Med 70:887–891, 1995

Furfaros CJ, Muchoney KK, Anania-Firouzan PA: CPR by the year 2000—a myth? Healthcare Informatics 13(5):45–47, 1996

Gardner C, Bower J, Rogers: Speech Technology 1(3):18–21, 1996

Gardner J: Federal workers to get HMO data. Modern Healthcare 26(November 11):33, 1996

Geer CT: Haggle no more. Forbes 159(2):96, 1997

Goknar M, Kemal M: Behavioral M.A.P.S. Oak Park, IL, 1989 [810-968-3887, Fax: 810-968-2886]

Goodman M, Brown J, Dietz P: Managing Managed Care. Washington, DC, American Psychiatric Press, 1992

Gould R: Adult development and brief computer-assisted therapy in mental health and managed care, in Managed Mental Health Care. Edited by Feldman J, Fitzpatrick RJ. Washington, DC, American Psychiatric Press, 1992 [Describes the Treatment Learning Program (TLP). Dr. Gould was writing as CEO, Interactive Health Systems.]

Gould R: The computer as "co-therapist." Behavioral Health Management 14(1):11–13, 1994

Hammond WE: '96 Health Insurance and Portability Act. Healthcare Informatics 14(1):50, 1997

Harris LM, Crawford CM: Electronic umbilical cords bring healthcare back home. Healthcare Forum Journal 39(1):26–31, 1996

Heckler C: Improving reimbursement with coding. Healthcare Informatics 13(9):104–106, 1996

Holden RR, Fekken GC: Using reaction time to detect faking on a computerized inventory of psychopathology. Paper presented at the Canadian Psychological Association Annual Convention, Montreal, Quebec, Canada, 1988

HOTLIST: Clinical and Financial Decision-Support Software. Health Management Technology 17(7):46–50, 1996

Industry Watch: 1996 Computer Crime and Security Survey. Health Management Technology 17(8):10, 1996

Integrated Medical Systems: Advertisement for Medacom. Managed Health Care 6(5):5, 1996

Itil TM, Itil KZ: Quantitative EEG brain mapping in psychotropic drug development, drug treatment section, and monitoring. American Journal of Therapeutics 2:367–369, 1995

Itil TM, Eralp E, Tsambis E, et al: Central nervous system effects of Ginkgo biloba, a plant extract. American Journal of Therapeutics 3:63–73, 1996

John ER, Prichep LS, Fridman J, et al: Neurometrics: computer-assisted differential diagnosis of brain disorders. Science 293:162–169, 1988

Johnston DG: IRS admits lag in computerization; urges contracting. New York Times, January 31, 1997, A1

Kamis-Gould E, Waizer J: National data standards for mental health management and performance indicators. The Psychiatric Hospital 23(1):23–28, 1991

Kane RL, Bartlett J, Potthoff S: Integrating outcomes information into managed care for substance abuse. Behavioral Healthcare Tomorrow 3(3):57–61, 1994

Keatley MA, Lemmon J, Miller T, et al: Using "normative data" for outcomes comparisons. Behavioral Health Management 15(3):20–21, 1995

Kennedy J: Fundamentals of Psychiatric Treatment Planning. Washington, DC, American Psychiatric Press, 1992

Kirkby KC: Clinical computing: computer-assisted treatment of phobias. Psychiatr Serv 47:139–140, 1996

Klynstra JH: Information systems management under pressure. The Psychiatric Hospital 23(1):13–17, 1991

Kobak KA: Computer-administered psychiatric rating scales. Psychiatr Serv 47:367–370, 1996

Koschmann T: Medical education and computer literacy: learning about, through, and with computers. Acad Med 70:818–821, 1995

Lamberg L: Patients go ONLINE for support. American Medical News, April 1, 1996, pp 10–13

Laska E, Bank R (eds): Safeguarding Psychiatric Privacy. New York, Wiley, 1976

Leginski WA: Data standards for mental health decision support systems (DHHS Publ No [ADM]-89-1589). Rockville, MD, National Institute of Mental Health, 1989

Lieff J: Computer Applications in Psychiatry. Washington, DC, American Psychiatric Press, 1987

Lewis JE: Improving productivity: the ongoing experience of an academic department of medicine. Acad Med 71:317–328, 1996

Lucas RW, Mullin PJ, Luna CBX, et al: Psychiatrists and a computer as interrogators of patients with alcohol-related illness: a comparison. Br J Psychiatry 131:160–167, 1977

Manderscheid RW, Henderson MJ: Federal and state legislative program directions for managed care: implications for case management [pamphlet]. Rockville, MD, Center for Mental Health Services, Substance Abuse and Mental Health Services Administration, October 1995

Marks I: CORM: a computer-assisted quality assurance system. Psychiatr Serv 47:811–812, 1996.

Maulitz RC, Ohles JA, Schnuth RL, et al: The CyberDoc Project: using portable computing to enhance a community-based primary care clerkship. Acad Med 71:1325–1328, 1996

McDougall GM, Adair-Bischoff CE, Grant E: Development of an integrated clinical database system for a regional mental healthservice. Psychiatr Serv 46:826–828, 1995

Miller M (ed): Computer Applications in Mental Health. Binghamton, NY, Haworth, 1992

Miller M, Tharp M: How to create your own computerized questionnaires, in Mental Health Computing. Edited by Miller M, Hammond KW, Hile MG. New York, Springer-Verlag, 1996, pp 115–124

Modern Healthcare 26(30)(July 22):2, 3, 16, 1996

Morrey B, Ginchereau B, Welch J: Put words in your mouth. Infoworld 18(40):66–79, 1996

Morrissey J: Integrating the incompatible. Modern Healthcare 23:39–42, 1993

Morrissey J: Cost benefit of integration hard to prove. Modern Healthcare, July 1, 1996a, p 38

Morrissey J: HEDIS to expand performance. Modern Healtchcare 26(30)(July 22):2–3, 1996b

Morrissey J: Mass plan seeks to build regional link from the ground up. Modern Healthcare 26(1)(January 1):52–53, 1996c

MSSNY: News of New York, August 1996, p 3

Munoz R: Hispanic patients and managed care. Presentation at the World Psychiatric Association, Madrid, August 26, 1996

Naditch MP: Shifting to a new paradigm to measure outcomes. Behavioral Healthcare Tomorrow 3(3):51–55, 1994

National Committee for Quality Assurance (NCQA): Report Card Pilot Project (NCQA Technical Report). Washington, DC, National Committee on Quality Assurance, 1993

New momentum for electronic patient record. New York Times, May 9, 1993, A1

Okstein CJ: Security of medical records deserves close scrutiny. American Medical News, July 8/15, 1996, p 17

Patton RE, Leginski WA: The design and content of a National Mental Health Statistics System (DHHS Publ No [ADM]-83-1095). Rockville, MD, National Institute of Mental Health, 1983

Pennsylvania Healthcare Cost Containment Council: A Consumer Guide to Coronary Artery Bypass Graft Surgery: Pennsylvania's Declaration of Health Care Information. Harrisburg, Pennsylvania Health Care Cost Containment Council, 1991

Petersen C: How well am I? Let me check with my computer. Managed Healthcare News, 1993, pp 25–26

Physician incomes drop for the first time. New York Times, September 3, 1996, A1

The Policy Resource Center and the George Washington University, Center for Health Policy Research: First Quarterly Report: Public Sector Moves Managed Care to Forefront of Behavioral Health Services. Rockville, MD, Center for Mental Health Services, Substance Abuse and Mental Health Services Administration, 1996

Powsner S: Medical informatics and the quality of professional life. Psychiatr Serv 48(1):27–28, 1997

Raab S: New Jersey officials say Mafia infiltrated health-care industry. New York Times, August 21, 1996, A1

Ribka JP: Strategic planning for managed care information systems. Health Management Technology 17(12):30–33, 1996

Rigby A: Information systems in psychiatry. Presentation at the World Psychiatric Association Symposium, Madrid, August 24, 1996

Robins LH, Helzer J: Diagnostic Interview Schedule. The C-DIS Group, Ottawa Civic Hospital, 737 Parkdale Avenue, Ottawa, Ontario, Canada K1Y 4E9 [Tel: 613-761-4746]

Robinson G, et al: Mental Health Measures in Medicaid HEDIS (Publ No MC96-57). Rockville, MD, Center for Mental Health Services, Substance Abuse and Mental Health Services Administration, 1996

Rowland DL: Facility-wide networks are now a necessity. Contemporary Long-Term Care 19(8):72, 1996

Rowland HS, Rowland BL: Hospital Software Source Book. Rockville, MD, Aspen Publications, 1991

Rushing, Singer C, Anderson G: Buzzwords, acquisitions shaping healthcare I/T. Health Management Technology 16(13):20–29, 1995

Schlosser B: Psychological testing: past and future. Behavioral Health Management 15(5):8–11, 1995

Schneider P: Moves and countermoves: the strategies driving vendor consolidations. Healthcare Informatics 13(9):56–60, 1996

Schwartz M (ed): Using Computers in Clinical Practice. New York, Hawthorn Press, 1984

Schwartz M: The Perfect Chart User's Manual. North Tonawanda, NY, Multi-Health Systems, 1995

Seidel WT, Joschko M: Assessment of attention in children. Clinical Neuropsychologist 5:53–66, 1991

Spitzer RL, Williams JBW, First MB, et al: Structured Clinical Interview for DSM-IV. Washington, DC, American Psychiatric Press, 1995

Taintor Z: Computers and diagnosis. Am J Psychiatry 137:61–63, 1980

Taintor Z, Bunt G, Mehta R, et al: Fully informed patients make better partners. Presentation at the New York State Office of Mental Health Research Conference, Albany, NY, December 1993

Tireless Tutor: a tireless tutor that "never gets mad at you." Business Week, August 19, 1985, p 77

Visit virtual trade shows on the Web without leaving your office. Health Systems Technology 17(8):34, 1996

Vijay V: Building a key ideal. Infocare [Supplement to Healthcare Informatics], November 1994, pp 24–30

Wakerly R, and First Consulting Group Authors: Community Health Information Networks—Creating the Health Care Data Highway. Chicago, IL, American Hospital Publishing, 1994

Werthman MJ: A managed care approach to psychological testing. Behavioral Health Management 15(5):15–17, 1995

Wheeler M: The healthcare enterprise Web and the culture of clinical information systems. Health Management Technology 18(1):24–26, 1997

White SL, Wingfield CC: The Charter Medical Corporation clinical information system: a preliminary report. The Psychiatric Hospital 23(1):19–23, 1991

Whiting-O'Keefe QE, Simborg DW, Epstein WV: A computerized summary medical record can provide more information than the standard medical record. JAMA 254:1185–1192, 1985

Wong ET, Abendroth TW: Reaping the benefits of medical information systems. Acad Med 71:353–357, 1996

Work M: Integrated delivery systems continue struggle with enterprise automation. Health Care Technology 17(8):50, 1996

Wyatt RJ: Practical Psychiatric Practice: Forms and Protocols for Clinical Use. Washington, DC, American Psychiatric Association, 1994

Zieman G: Designing the computer system, in The Complete Capitation Handbook. Edited by Zieman GL. Tiburon, CA, Centralink, 1995, pp 137–150

Chapter 26

Using the Internet

Bertram Warren, M.D., F.A.P.A., Thomas Kramer, M.D., F.A.P.A., Steven E. Hyler, M.D., and Robert Kennedy, M.A.

Introducing or trying to offer an explanation of the Internet is a little like trying to describe what psychotherapy is. It really is something that needs to be experienced rather than described.

And as psychotherapy is founded on basic communications skills that are refined with scientific process and methods, the World Wide Web (also known as WWW or the Web) can be viewed as a refinement of the science and technology of the Internet.

Essentially, the World Wide Web is an attractive visual facade that resides on top of the Internet. In general, since its inception, the Internet has been an unfriendly system that only the "techies" could negotiate. It is founded in esoteric terminology (Unix based), and even friendly menus do not help the novice traverse places on "the Net." The Web is a true visual and graphic (and thus friendly) way of traveling the world via computers on the Internet. Everything is a mouse click away.

More and more, people are beginning to think of the Web as the Net. The Web is quite prolific. People interestingly enough have started speaking of it anthropomorphically and have given it a life of its own. It has been expanding at the rate of millions of sites per year, and each of these sites can have any number of "Web pages" available on them. Because the Web is easier to travel on, it is much more accessible to the general public than the Net. This is generally because it is not machine specific; that is, it can be accessed by IBM-compatible computers, Macintosh computers, or Unix-based computers. Eventually, people will be able to access the Web through their televisions over cable modems or cable networks.

The Web is structured via computers connected to the Internet that function as Web servers. Any personal computer connected with a typical "university connection" or T1 connection to the Internet can function as a Web server. Many people choose to turn their connected computers into a personal Web server. Individuals with personal Web sites are referred to as having their own home page. Many commercial Internet providers also offer personal Web pages for a nominal fee.

Author note. Writing of this chapter was coordinated among the authors using only the Internet—no calls or letters back and forth!

Computer users elsewhere in the world can connect to any Web page that is available on the WWW as long as they know the proper Web address. The Web functions through pages of information. When you access a site, you are presented with a page. This page is a graphic image that scrolls on your computer screen. It might contain text, pictures, sound, or animation. These Web pages are sent or transferred by a method known as hypertext transfer protocol (HTTP). This HTTP process tells the Internet how to send the pages from the server, or sending computer, across the Internet to your computer. Your computer can view these pages if you use a Web browser, which is a specific type of software that knows how to handle the HTTP information coming across the Net.

Web pages interact with you, the viewer, and with each other with this hypertext protocol. Essentially, hypertext is a jump point on a page that takes you to another page. For example, if you are reading a paragraph on a clinical syndrome, a reference might be presented in a different color. If you clicked on this colored reference with your computer's mouse, your screen would jump to that reference. The amazing aspect of the Web is that the reference that you jump to can be a Web page on the same computer that you are accessing or on another computer elsewhere in the country or even on a computer halfway across the globe. Some Web pages are composed only of references, and all of the documents referenced reside elsewhere in the world.

The concept of clicking to access another Web page also has been extended to other aspects of multimedia on the Internet. Clicking on a button on a Web page could produce sound, play a video clip, produce an animation, or allow you to move through a three-dimensional image such as a room. It also can allow you to download a file from the other computer (known as file transfer protocol or FTP).

Accessing a Web page or finding the address of a Web site is done through a naming convention called *uniform resource locator (URL)*. This is the Web's electronic equivalent of a post office address or e-mail address. Each URL is unique and looks something like the following: http://www.psych.org. This is the unique address of the American Psychiatric Association's Web site. To get to this site to view the various pages of information, announcements, and other items of interest, you would instruct your Web browser software to access the URL. The next thing you would see is the APA logo scrolling on your computer screen.

History of the Internet and the World Wide Web

The World Wide Web was born of two completely separate technologies. Its existence and current state of sophistication are made possible by these originally isolated developmental processes. The first was the development of the Internet by the Department of Defense. The second was the development of easily understood and manipulated programming language and browsing capability.

In 1969, the Department of Defense's Advanced Research Project Agency (ARPA) began the Internet. As the Defense Department became increasingly dependent on technology in general and computers in particular, it felt that any disruption of command links in a nuclear era could be fatal. It was bad enough that an enemy could destroy a powerful and important computer, but it was much worse if an enemy could destroy the connections between computers and cut off the flow of crucial control information. As a result, it was necessary that certain computers always be able to connect to certain other computers without any possibility of failure. The only way to do this was to connect virtually every computer to virtually every other computer. This way, in much the same way telephone systems are organized to route calls away from trouble spots, if a certain computer failed or was destroyed, it would not be difficult to simply make connections between other computers to go around the problem.

The other development in the creation of the World Wide Web was a language in which information could be presented in a way that would facilitate searching and retrieval. In 1965, Ted Nelson first coined the term *hypertext*. Hypertext is nonlinear—it is not necessary with hypertext to read until you find what you are looking for. In hypertext, certain areas of text are connected to certain other areas of text. This connection is similar to secret passageways that allow you to get from one room to another directly, as opposed to having to walk all the way around the house. This text is usually highlighted, such as by a different color or a symbol or picture, which denotes it as being linked to another area. The first efforts to implement hypertext were constrained by 1960s' technology. Ted Nelson's project was to put the entire literary corpus online. By 1992, the project was dropped. In addition to issues of cost, more than 10 languages of hypertext and hypermedia had already been developed, and there was very little agreement as to a standard.

Meanwhile, the Cold War essentially ended in the 1980s. As a result, the Department of Defense lost interest in its network of computers. The ARPANet was dismantled and taken over by the U.S. National Science Foundation. By the end of the 1980s, events were coming together that were making the World Wide Web possible. In 1989, Tim Berners-Lee proposed using the Internet to share research worldwide. He had been influenced by Ted Nelson's project but was unconcerned about copyright issues. It was Berners-Lee who actually first devised the name *World Wide Web*. By the end of 1990, technology was implemented that allowed browsing whole computer libraries effectively and quickly. More importantly, a new hypertext language—hypertext markup language, or HTML—was created. This language was to become the gold standard of the World Wide Web. Anything written in HTML could be transmitted around the Internet in HTTP.

In 1991, a series of conferences around the world announced the World Wide Web to the academic community. In 1993, the final pieces of the puzzle were put into place. The first truly user-friendly and effective browser for the World Wide Web, called *Mosaic,* was released. Mosaic's contributions included aspects that enabled the World Wide Web to have pictures, sounds, basic animations, and videos, making the Web truly multimedia. In 1993, there were 50 World Wide Web servers available.

Another major development was the creation of a unified standard for finding material on the Internet. This standard required addresses that would enable the user to locate anything available on the Internet. These addresses became referred to as URLs. They allow you to access any publicly available data on any machine on the Internet. The basic parts of the URL are 1) the method of communication to be used, technically called the *access protocol;* 2) the machine on which the data reside; 3) the port from which you request the data; 4) the path of that data; and 5) the name of the file containing that data. Once this methodology was agreed on, it was possible to locate information on the World Wide Web in much the same way that street signs, traffic lights, and other traffic regulators make traveling around a city possible.

Currently, it would be functionally impossible to describe the size and breadth of the World Wide Web. Any numbers quoted would be obsolete an hour later. It is fair to say, however, that the World Wide Web is the most rapidly growing communications medium. This is true not only in a general sense but also true for psychiatry in particular. It is also impossible to give a comprehensive list of psychiatric resources on the World Wide Web. What we include here is simply a sample of what is currently available, and readers should understand that this list is expanding on a daily, if not hourly, basis.

Current Perspectives

The Web has become the fastest-growing, most important electronic communication medium since the telephone. Those are strong words, but the proliferation of the World Wide Web has astonished even the experts in the communication industry. Web sites number in the millions, and that number is increasing exponentially each year. The types of Web sites also are as diverse as humans are different.

Those in the education field already are a presence on the Internet, and adapting to the Web has been easy for them. Today, not only colleges and universities are present on the Web, but elementary and high schools have set up and maintain their own Web sites.

Businesses have taken to the Web with great alacrity. Again, the variety of businesses on the Web is as broad as those listed in the yellow pages of the telephone book. Electronic commerce is beginning to take shape, and new definitions of "doing business" are being formed.

Museums and art galleries as well as individual artists have a definite presence on the Web. Because of their graphic nature, artwork and photographs can be presented on a Web page with amazing detail and color.

Publishing is the substance of the Web. Essentially, using the concepts of Web pages and hypertext documents, the World Wide Web is electronic publishing reincarnated. This publishing can be electronic journals, electronic newspapers, full-text electronic books, or simply ideas, thoughts, musings, and poetry posted for the world to see. An important aspect of this new medium is that it is not refereed or censored in any way. So, like public access cable channels, anyone can set up a URL and create Web pages to say or show whatever he or she likes. Censorship will continue to be a hotly debated issue, and software is available to allow parental guidance and censorship of various Web sites or discussion groups on the Internet.

The entertainment business also has adopted the Web as a powerful advertising medium. The music industry, the movie/film industry, television stations, and radio stations all have a tremendous presence on the Web and are generally the most popular and actively accessed Web sites. Countries and cities without access to libraries and textbooks have turned to the Net and the Web to learn. Small towns advertise their existence with descriptions, pictures, and sounds of their locale and invite tourists to visit them electronically and then, they hope, in reality.

In 1937, H. G. Wells wrote:

> There is no practical obstacle whatever now to the creation of an efficient index to all human knowledge, ideas and achievements, to the creation, that is, of a complete planetary memory for all mankind. The whole human memory can be, and probably in a short time will be, made accessible to every individual. And what is also of very great importance in this uncertain world where destruction becomes continually more frequent and unpredictable, is this, that . . . it need not be concentrated in any one single place. It need not be vulnerable as a human head or a human heart is vulnerable. It can be reproduced exactly and fully, in Peru, China, Iceland, Central Africa or wherever else. . . . It can have at once, the concentration of a craniate animal and the diffused vitality of an amoeba.

Psychiatry and Other Web Sites

Not too long ago, a search of psychiatry-related resources might have turned up a dozen or so pages. Searching now will reveal thousands of such pages. These include the good, the bad, and the ugly. There is no real quality assurance on the Web, so cruiser beware of the accuracy of any information posted. The URLs listed below should be good places to start your searches. New pages are turning up all the time, and URLs (and links) rapidly become obsolete. Half of the fun of cruising the Web is finding on your own the pages that interest you. Happy hunting!

Associations, Societies, Institutions, and Organizations

American Academy of Child and Adolescent Psychiatry home page
http://www.psych.med.umich.edu/web/aacap/

American Medical Association home page
http://www.ama-assn.org/

American Psychiatric Association
http://www.psych.org/

American Psychoanalytic Association (APSA)
http://apsa.org/

American Psychological Association PsychNET
http://www.apa.org/

Centers for Disease Control and Prevention home page
http://www.cdc.gov/

HyperDOC: U.S. National Library of Medicine (NLM)
http://www.nlm.nih.gov/

Internet Links to Mental Health Resources
http://www.mentalhealth.com/p13.html#Per/

Milton's InterPsych Page
http://www.psych.med.umich.edu/web/intpsych/

National Alliance for the Mentally Ill (NAMI) home page
http://www.nami.org/

National Alliance for Research on Schizophrenia and Depression
http://www.mhsource.com/narsad.html

National Clearinghouse for Alcohol and Drug Information
http://www.health.org/

National Institute of Mental Health home page
http://www.nimh.nih.gov/

National Mental Health Association
http://www.worldcorp.com/dc-online/nmha/index.html

Online Psych—Psychiatry and Psychopharmacology
http://www.onlinepsych.com/tour/psypharm.htm

Physicians' Online home page (pages of psychiatry-related resources)
http://www.po.com/

Psychiatric Society for Informatics home page
http://www.psych.med.umich.edu/web/psi/

PsychScapes Worldwide—Connections in Mental Health
http://www.mental-health.com/

Society of Biological Psychiatry (SOBP)
http://www.sobp.org/

Society for Computers in Psychology
http://www.lafayette.edu/allanr/scip.html

Welcome to Mental Health Infosource
http://www.mhsource.com/main.html

World Health Organization WWW home page
http://www.who.ch/

Medical University Departments of Psychiatry

Columbia University Department of Psychiatry
http://cpmcnet.columbia.edu/dept/pi/psydep.html

New York State Psychiatric Institute
http://www.nyspi.cpmc.columbia.edu/

New York University Department of Psychiatry
http://www.med.nyu.edu/Psych/NYUPsych.Homepage.html

University of Chicago Department of Psychiatry
http://http.bsd.uchicago.edu:80/psychiatry/home.html

University of Michigan Department of Psychiatry
http://www.psych.med.umich.edu/web/UMpsych/

Specific Mental Disorders

Alzheimer's Web home page
http://werple.mira.net.au/dhs/ad.html

Bipolar disorder
http://www.mentalhealth.com/dis/p20-md02.html

Major depression
http://www.mentalhealth.com/

Mental disorders listing
http://www.mentalhealth.com/p20.html

Mood disorders
http://avocado.pc.helsinki.fi/janne/mood/mood.html

Obsessive-compulsive disorder (OCD)
http://www.fairlite.com/ocd/

The Personality Project—other Web pages
http://fas.psych.nwu.edu/perproj/other.html

Schizophrenia: A Handbook for Families
  http://www.mentalhealth.com/book/p40-sc01.html

Schizophrenia: Questions and Answers
  http://www.mentalhealth.com/book/p40-sc04.html

Schizophrenia: Youth's Greatest Disabler
  http://www.mentalhealth.com/book/p40-sc02.html

Freud and Jung

FreudNet: The A. A. Brill Library
  http://plaza.interport.net/nypsan/

Carl Jung: Anthology
  http://miso.wwa.com/nebcargo/Jung/

Mental Health Software File Transfer Protocol Site

Directory of /pub/psychiatry
  ftp://ftp.iupui.edu/pub/psychiatry/

American Journal of Psychiatry,
American Psychiatric Press, and Psychiatric News

The American Journal of Psychiatry
  http://www.appi.org/ajp/ajptoc.html

American Psychiatric Press
  http://www.appi.org/

Psychiatric News
  http://www.appi.org/pnews/

Other Online Journals

Psychiatry On-Line Priory Lodge Education 1996
  http://www.cityscape.co.uk/users/ad88/psych.htm

Usenet Newsgroups

Newsgroups are a popular resource for those who surf the Web. There are thousands of newsgroups that focus on just about any topic imaginable (e.g., knitting, Legos, and ferrets). Newsgroups can be accessed either through most Web browsers or through special programs called *newsreaders*. Newsgroups can be open (i.e., accessible to anyone on the Internet or Web) or closed (i.e., a person must register and sometimes send specific information such as a curriculum vitae to the person who runs the group). Closed newsgroups are also known as *listservs*, and the messages to the group are generally sent as e-mail to the subscriber.

There are generally two types of open newsgroups on the Web. A newsgroup that has *alt* (for alternative) in the name (e.g., alt.psychology.personality) is unmoderated. This means that all messages addressed to the group are posted, without anyone reviewing the content. Discussion in these groups can get quite heated and often filled with flames and counterflames (i.e., unrestrained series of insults). The other type of newsgroup, without alt in the title, is called a *moderated* newsgroup. In this group, there is a moderator who runs the group and reviews the messages before they are posted. Only messages thought to be of interest and value to the group members are posted.

To find a list of newsgroups or review topics that are posted on the newsgroups, you can use one of the search engines on the World Wide Web that includes newsgroups in its searches. Examples of newsgroups that relate to psychiatry, psychology, and mental health include the following:

- alt.alcohol
- alt.drugs
- alt.psychology.adlerian
- alt.psychology.jung
- alt.psychology.personality
- alt.recovery.panic-anxiety
- alt.recovery.self.help
- alt.support
     alt.society.mental-health
     alt.support.aids.partners
     alt.support.anxiety-panic
     alt.support.attn-deficit
     alt.support.depression
     alt.support.epilepsy
     alt.support.grief
     alt.support.ocd
     alt.support.personality
     alt.support.schizophrenia
     alt.support.social-phobia
- InterPsych
- Psych-pharm
- Psych-therapy
- rec.drugs
- sci.med.psychobiology
- sci.psychology.personality
- sci.psychology.psychotherapy
- sci.psychology.research
- soc.support.depression

Summary

Scientists have begun a global collaboration that has grown to become a worldwide phenomenon. The computer connections that started as scientific collaborations have become the visual telephone lines of a world that has adopted this technology and style of communication for everyday use. Education, commerce, entertainment, and social interaction are the food of the Internet and the world is hungry for more.

Over the centuries, as people traveled the earth, the distances became smaller, and the connections between people became firmer. The global computer network has now connected millions of people who may never have traveled or connected in any other way. The world has truly become more accessible and intimate.

Glossary

@   This symbol is used in a e-mail address to separate the name of the user from the name of the domain (it is pronounced "at").

Address   Referring to an electronic address; a person's e-mail address. It is a series of letters and/or numbers used in combination, e.g., name@organization.com to produce a unique e-mail address.

Anonymous file transfer protocol (FTP)   An FTP file archive that any Internet user can gain access to. *Anonymous* means open to the public or usable by anyone.

Archie   An Internet search program that is used for locating files that are publicly accessible.

ASCII   American Standard Code for Information Interchange. One of the standards for the computer's internal recognition of the letters, numbers, and symbols of the English language.

Asynchronous transmission   Data transmission in which the length of time between transmitted characters may vary. Because the time lapses between transmitted characters are not uniform, the receiving modem must be signaled as to when the data bits of a character begin and when they end. The addition of start and stop bits to each character serves this purpose.

Auto answer   A feature in modems enabling them to answer incoming calls over telephone lines without the use of a telephone receiver.

Auto dial   A feature in modems enabling them to dial telephone numbers over the telephone system without the use of a telephone transmitter.

Backbone   The central portion of a network known for high speed. The central type of connection or wiring structure.

Bandwidth   Refers to the volume of data that can be carried on a transmission line. Telephone lines that are twisted-pair cables have the lowest bandwidth, coaxial cable has higher bandwidth, and fiber optics to date has the highest bandwidth.

Baud   A measure of speed of digital transmission. Baud is usually equal to bits per second (bps).

Baud rate   The number of discrete signal events per second occurring on a communications channel. Although not technically accurate, baud rate is commonly used to mean bit rate.

Binary digit   A 0 or 1, reflecting the use of the binary numbering system (only two digits). Used because the computer recognizes either of two states, off or on. The shortened form of binary digit is bit.

Bit   The smallest piece of information a computer can understand. A bit has the value of "1" or "0."

Bit rate   The number of binary digits, or bits, transmitted per second (bps).

Bits per second (BPS)   The bits (binary digits) per second rate. Thousands of bits per second are expressed as kilobits. Refers to the rate of data transmission.

Browser   A software program that allows the user to navigate through hypertext documents on the World Wide Web, sometimes referred to as a "client." Popular Web browsers are Netscape, Mosaic, or Internet Explorer.

Byte   A grouping of 8 bits. A byte can be represented by two hexadecimal characters or three octal characters.

Carrier   A continuous frequency that can either be modulated or impressed with another information-carrying signal. Carriers are generated and maintained by modems via the transmission lines of the telephone system.

Character   A representation, coded in binary digits, of a letter, number, or other symbol.

Characters per second (cps)   A data transfer rate generally estimated from the bit rate and the character length. For example, at 2,400 bps, 8-bit characters with start and stop bits (for a total of 10 bits per character) will be transmitted at a rate of approximately 240 cps.

Chat   A typed or written "live" conversation that takes place over the Internet between two or more people.

Client   A type of software that makes a demand on a server software, generally in a network environment. The client software is local or runs on a user's computer, and the server software runs a server or network computer.

Cyberspace   A term coined by science fiction author William Gibson in his 1984 novel *Neuromancer,* it describes a society that gathers around the virtual electronic realm of interconnected computers. It could be said that one is in cyberspace when logging onto the Internet or any online service.

Data   Any information the computer processes or stores.

Database   A collection of organized data that can be recalled by some key. (A telephone book is an example of a database, a newspaper is not.)

Dial-up access   A user's type of access to the Internet. A dial-up connection generally uses a telephone line and modem to make a connection.

Dial-up Internet protocol (IP) account   An account that allows the user to connect by modem to an Internet provider to access the Internet.

Domain   The highest subdivision of the Internet. The domain can be a country (*au* for Australia) or an organization or institution (*org* for organization or *edu* for educational institution, etc.).

Domain name   A part of the domain name system naming hierarchy. A domain name consists of a sequence of names or other words separated by periods.

Domain name system (DNS)   A system used by the Internet that translates named domains into numerical addresses that computers recognize.

Download   To transfer a file from a remote computer to your own computer. Upload, on the other hand, means you are sending data from your computer to that remote computer.

Duplex   A communications channel capable of carrying signals in both directions.

E-mail address   The domain-based address that is the English-language equivalent of a user's Internet protocol number through which a user is defined; for example, username@somewhere.com. A user's e-mail address is also referred to as an "Internet address."

Emoticon   Symbols that provide a way for a person to portray a "mood" in computer e-mail and other text communications. More commonly known as "smilies," there are literally hundreds of emoticons, from the obvious to the obscure. This particular example, :) expresses "happiness." If you don't see it, turn the book 90 degrees.

Encryption   Through the use of encryption software, information is coded and thus rendered inaccessible to anyone without the key and decryption software. Encryption is necessary for commerce on the Internet because data, like credit card numbers, passes through a variety of computers, unprotected, before it arrives at its destination.

File transfer protocol (FTP)   The system for transferring files between computers on the Internet. This is the system most commonly used for downloading software.

Firewall   A method of securing a computer connected to the Internet. It is a combination of hardware and software that allows information to go out but limits and implements security on incoming data. Firewalls prevent unauthorized entry into a computer system connected to the Internet.

Flame   Refers to a way of insulting someone in e-mail discussions and frequently carried out as a number of messages posted to a newsgroup demeaning someone.

Flow control   A mechanism that compensates for differences in the flow of data input to and the output from a modem or other device.

Frame   A data communications term for a block of data with header and trailer information attached. Also refers to a style of scrolling boxes used in hypertext markup language (HTML) (the language of the Web).

Frequently asked question (FAQ)   A set of questions that is posted on the Internet at Gopher sites and World Wide Web sites and within Newsgroups. These questions usually address popular topics and provide answers to those topics.

Full-duplex transmission   Transmission in two directions simultaneously. (A telephone call is full-duplex transmission.)

Gopher   A distributed information service that makes hierarchical collections of information available across the Internet. Gopher uses a simple protocol that allows a single gopher client to access information from any accessible gopher server on the entire Internet.

Gopher servers   Gopher allows accessing Internet resources via an easy-to-use hierarchical menu system. When you select a menu item from a gopher menu, the gopher software running on your computer (gopher client software) will either take you to the next menu, display a text document associated with the menu item, or begin to download the image or other digital data to which the menu item points.

Graphic interchange format (GIF)   A graphic format developed by Compuserve that is one of the standards for pictures or graphics on the World Wide Web.

Half-duplex transmission   Transmission in two directions but only in one direction at a time. (Writing a letter is half-duplex.)

Home page   The page of information your browser displays when started is called your "home page." The home page is the root page or starting point to the World Wide Web. Most people configure their home page to provide easy access to the Web resources they use most often. You can configure your browser to automatically load the home page of a any Web site.

Host   Any computer, system, or network that you can connect to with your computer that provides some sort of service. On the Internet, a host computer could provide Gopher, Web, or USENET service, or all three.

Hypertext links   Hypertext allows you to progress or "branch" to other pages of information of interest in nonlinear fashion, allowing you to return the way you progressed through the information originally, or to jump backward and forward along the "path" you have taken in your reading, or "browsing." Hypertext also allows you to easily return to where you started, which is generally referred to as "home."

Hypertext markup language (HTML)   The hypertext document-encoding scheme that is used for resources published on World Wide Web servers. An HTML document is a mixture of ASCII text and special reserved character sequences called *tags* that control formatting of the text. HTML was a subset of standard generalized markup language (SGML).

Hypertext transfer protocol (HTTP)   The protocol for transfer of hypermedia documents that is the foundation of the World Wide Web. In the simplest sense, the protocol consists mainly of "send me this page or file" requests from a Web browser to a Web server, and a "I have it or here it is" or "can't find it" or "try again later" reply from the server to the browser.

Integrated systems digital network (ISDN)   A type of direct connection to the Internet through a high-speed telephone line. ISDN speeds range from 64 kbps to 128 kbps.

Internet   A large network of networks and computers structures that use a specific way of communicating called the Internet protocol (IP). The Internet evolved from the ARPANET (Advanced Research Projects Administration Network), which was run by the U.S. Department of Defense in the 1960s and 1970s.

Internet Explorer   The popular World Wide Web browser application from Microsoft Corporation. It offers many features that facilitate interacting with the World Wide Web.

Internet number   The "dotted-quad" address used to specify a certain computer system. Each computer on the Internet is assigned a unique Internet protocol (IP) number.

Internet protocol (IP)   A specific way of communicating data on the Internet. The IP sends data in packets to another network; then data is reassembled when it reaches its destination.

Internet protocol number Each machine or "host" that participates in any Internet transaction, whether it be a PC or a mainframe computer, is identified by a unique 32-bit value called the *IP number.* The IP number is issued as either a return address or a destination address in all Internet transactions. IP numbers are commonly written out as, for example, 192.203.41.101.

Internet service provider A company that offers a way to access the Internet either through dial-up or direct connections.

Interrupt request (IRQ) IRQs in the computer are used to interrupt hardware and software when there is an event that requires attention, such as data arriving at the serial port.

Joint Photographic Experts Group (JPEG) A graphic image standard used extensively on the World Wide Web.

Listserv A UNIX program that is used to subscribe and unsubscribe people from mailing lists. Listserv can search through old messages for specific information, send out updates of standard files to those who want them, and give information about who else may have subscribed to a particular mailing list.

Local echo A modem feature that enables the modem to display keyboard commands and transmitted data on the screen.

Lurker An electronic voyeur or person who only reads newsgroup entries but does not otherwise participate or respond. Lurking is recommended when first visiting a newsgroup to learn what discussions are taking place and to understand the group.

Lynx A character-based World Wide Web browser program usable through a Telnet connection to almost all UNIX servers on the Internet.

Mail bombing A barrage of angry messages sent via e-mail.

Mail server The system that manages e-mail messages and e-mail addresses to and from a local network.

Mailing lists Any of the tens of thousands of discussion groups pertaining to every imaginable subject that move via the distribution of e-mail from a central computer. Anyone with e-mail capabilities on their computer can subscribe to mailing lists.

Microcom networking protocol (MNP) An asynchronous error-control protocol developed by Microcom, Inc., and now in the public domain. The protocol ensures error-free transmission by modem through error detection (CRC) and retransmission of errored frames.

Modem A device that allows digital information from the computer to be transmitted over analog systems such as the telephone.

Mosaic A World Wide Web browser application available for Windows, Macintosh, and UNIX (Xwindows) platforms, Mosaic was originally developed in 1992 at the National Center for Supercomputing Applications (NCSA) at the University of Illinois at Urbana/Champaign.

Multiuser dimension or dungeon (MUD) An environment that allows participants to interact with each other using different names or by role-playing characters in various situations.

Multipurpose Internet mail extension (MIME) A way of extending electronic mail to allow attachment of messages and nontext files.

National Science Foundation (NSF) The government agency that helped establish the Internet in the United States.

The Net Another name for the Internet.

Netscape The popular World Wide Web browser application from Netscape Communications Corporation. Netscape is one of the most stable and fastest Web browsers on the market and provides data encryption and security functions and many other features.

Newsgroup A type of discussion group on the Internet. Generally organized by topic, individuals post messages or questions and others respond.

Node A computer that is attached to a network; also called a *host*.

Packet A piece of data that is sent across a network.

Parity An error-detection method that checks the validity of a transmitted character. Character checking has been surpassed by more reliable and efficient forms of block checking. The same type of parity must be used by two communicating computers.

Passive mailing list A mailing list where mail originates from a single source, usually the list administrator.

Pine A UNIX-based, menu-driven e-mail program. Initially, Pine offered a limited set of functions geared toward the novice user. Recent versions include optional power-user and personal-preference features.

Point of Presence (POP) The closest location or telephone access number for a network or telephone company.

Point to Point Protocol (PPP) Generally a dial-up protocol that allows a computer to connect to the Internet over a standard telephone line and behave as if it is connected directly to the Internet.

Protocol A system of rules and procedures governing communications between two or more devices. Communicating devices must follow the same protocol to exchange data. The format of the data, readiness to receive or send, error detection, and error correction are some of the operations that may be defined in protocols.

Router A special computer that connects two or more networks and "routes" data from one network to the other.

Serial interface An interface that sends one bit at a time. Modems usually are connected to serial interfaces.

Serial line Internet protocol (SLIP) SLIP and point-to-point protocol (PPP) are two methods for connecting to the Internet over a modem. Internet service providers offer SLIP and PPP access at up to 28,800 bps or more. SLIP is the older protocol; PPP is supposedly more reliable and faster.

Serial transmission The transfer of data characters one bit at a time, sequentially, using a single electrical path.

Server A computer that shares its resources, such as printers and files, with other computers on a network. When a user of the Internet connects to a computer offering Gopher, file transfer protocol (FTP), World Wide Web, or e-mail services, the computer offering these services is in the role of a server.

Simple mail transfer protocol (SMTP) The established standard protocol for the distribution of e-mail on the Internet.

Snail mail Plain, old-fashioned local post office delivery; very slow when compared to the seemingly instantaneous transmission of e-mail.

Special interest group (SIG) A group of people that get together to share a common interest. This can be in an office or online. It is generally moderated by a central leader.

Start/stop bits The signaling bits attached to a character before the character is transmitted during asynchronous transmission.

Subscribe To add your name to a mailing list or newsgroup.

SYSOP Slang acronym for SYStem OPerator; "system" in this use being understood as a bulletin board system (BBS) or e-mail newsgroup, and "operator" being the owner or manager of the system.

TCP/IP This is actually two acronyms, but they are almost always seen together. They stand for transport control protocol and Internet protocol, respectively, and are the two fundamental packet-oriented network communication protocols of the Internet. TCP/IP software is available for nearly every type of central processing unit (CPU) and operating system, and most of them are either built into the operating system itself or available for free. Other Internet protocols for terminal emulation, file transfer, e-mail, news, and information publishing are layered on top of TCP/IP.

Telnet The Internet standard protocol for remote terminal connection service. Telnet allows a user at one site to interact with a remote system as if the user's terminal were directly connected to it.

Terminal   A device whose keyboard and display are used for sending and receiving data over a communications link. Differs from a microcomputer in that it has little or no internal processing capabilities.

Throughput   The amount of actual user data transmitted per second without the overhead of protocol information such as start and stop bits or from headers and trailers.

Transmission rate   The speed at which information is sent from one computer to another.

Unsubscribe   To remove your name from a mailing list or newsgroup.

Uniform resource locator (URL)   A method for specifying the exact location of an Internet resource on the World Wide Web and the network protocol necessary to retrieve and interpret the resource. For example, the URL http://www.psych.org indicates the location of the American Psychiatric Association. It is a unique "address" on the Internet.

Upload   To send a file from your computer to a remote computer. Download, on the other hand, means you are transferring a file from a remote computer to your own computer.

Usenet   A virtual collection of thousands of topically named newsgroups, the computers that run the protocols, and the people who read and submit Usenet news. Some Internet service providers charge a fee to provide newsgroup services.

V.42   A standard for modem communications that defines a two-stage process of detection and negotiation for error control. V.42 also supports error control protocol data compression.

Veronica (Very Easy Rodent-Oriented Index to Computer Architecture)   A database query system providing access to information resources held on most of the world's gopher servers. In addition to gopher data, Veronica includes references to many resources provided by other types of information servers.

The Web   The World Wide Web.

Web browser   A program that can retrieve HTML documents from Web servers using the HTTP protocol and format them for graphic display. A browser also knows how to interpret hyperlinks within the body of an HTML document and use them to navigate from one HTML document to another on the same or another Web server. Mosaic, Netscape Navigator, and Internet Explorer are examples of Web browsers.

Web page   The World Wide Web consists of information organized onto many thousands of pages stored in computers physically located throughout the world. Each "page" is a document with a unique address on the Web, with most containing links to other documents. These links are highlighted words or pictures within the page that, when selected, bring another page of information.

Web server A program that understands the HTTP protocol and responds to requests from Web browsers using that protocol. A Web server program must run on an Internet host that is addressable with an Internet protocol (IP) number/domain name system (DNS) host name. The machine that runs the Web server program is often referred to informally as a Web server as well.

Wide-area information system (WAIS) A database retrieval system on the Internet that supports full-text searches, which are not supported by Veronica in Gopherspace. WAIS gives users the ability to search existing databases of articles, books, references, abstracts, and special information (such as newsgroup archives and file transfer protocol [FTP] site listings).

Wide-area network (WAN) A network spanning hundreds or thousands of miles.

World Wide Web The Web, invented by physicists at the European community's particle physics research center in Switzerland (CERN), is more of a conceptual construct than a physical entity. All the Web servers on the Internet taken together constitute the World Wide Web, but there is no central administration or coordination of servers. Each server is identified by a domain name system (DNS) host name; each document or other resource on a Web server is designated by a uniform resource locator (URL).

WWW A colloquial abbreviation for the World Wide Web.

Xmodem The first of a family of error-control software protocols used to transfer files between modems. These protocols are in the public domain and are available from many services.

Chapter 27

2005: Information Technology Impacts Psychiatry

Norman Alessi, M.D., Milton Huang, M.D., and Paul Quinlan, D.O.

For most psychiatrists, the term *information technology* has little to no meaning. For some, it might conjure up the idea of a computer, a telephone, or a fax machine; for others, the Internet or the World Wide Web (WWW). Obviously, it encompasses far more than technology, including—but not limited to—networking, operating systems, programming languages, hardware of all types, and software applications at all levels. As used today, the term has much farther-reaching consequences than merely dealing with technology. It implies organizational and strategic advantage through process reengineering. It is regarded as the fundamental agent of change that facilitates increases in efficiency, productivity, and quality. The organizational changes as well as the increased information technology will result in the "information-based organization" (Frenzel 1996). The term and the processes that it encompasses have implications that will have far-reaching impact, not only in the business of mental health care, but also in the practice of psychiatry.

In this chapter, we explore the future impact of information technology on psychiatry. First, we review three major trends that are, and will continue to be, fueling the development of our specialty during the next decade; second, we present three scenarios of how the practice of psychiatry might look in the year 2005, given the increased significance of information and information systems and the broad social consequences of information technology; third, we review a model for adapting to information technology; and, finally, we discuss five recommendations for expediting the implementation of information technology in American psychiatry (Aburdene 1994).

Three Fundamental Trends Driving Change

To make predictions about the future, one has to make assumptions. These assumptions then can lead to the development of a broad range of scenarios reflecting the consequences of these factors (Schwartz 1991). There appears to be three major trends that will significantly influence the practice of psychiatry and the delivery of mental health services during the next decade. These are 1) American health care changes, 2) significant advances in information technology that will influence the culture of the world, and 3) increased "consumer" influence in deciding the type of care patients receive as they make greater use of information technology.

In and of themselves, these three trends are each major forces, but the interface of these, as well as their culmination, will result in even greater changes. When they come together, they will form new information resources—fueled by demand—as well as new knowledge sources (Ball and Douglas 1996). These will be used not only by physicians to facilitate the practice of medicine, but also by others to facilitate the process of delivering, receiving, or influencing their care. Given these trends, a physician may or may not be involved in the delivery of care. Physicians must grasp these three major trends and utilize their best judgment in dealing with the business, science, and art of these forces as they drive the practice of psychiatry within our ever-changing culture of information technology.

American Health Care Is Undergoing Radical Changes

Too often when we think about the changes in health care, we too rapidly equate the changes with managed care and, in turn, issues concerning length of hospitalization, types of therapy, and reimbursement. The radical changes that are fueling these paradigm shifts are not just dealing with "care" but, broadly, with the processes involved in the delivery of care. These changes involve the professionals delivering care and the manner in which they operate. They go far beyond just the physician-patient relationship: the context of care is changing.

The Pew Health Professions Commission prophetically discussed these "context" trends in its first report, "Healthy America: Practitioners in 2005" (Shugars et al. 1991). In this report, "core competencies" necessary for a successful professional practice in the future were outlined. These included providing community-centered health care, expanding access to effective care, emphasizing primary care, involving patients and families in the decision-making process, accessing technology appropriately, supporting diversity within the delivery of care, expanding accountability, managing information, and continuing education. These are as relevant today as they were 5 years ago and appear to be growing in relevance. These core competencies increasingly are being perceived as the basic elements of a practice today.

In the commission's 1993 report, "Health Professions Education for the Future: Schools in Service to the Nation," the paradigms of the emerging health care system were characterized as orientation to health, population perspective, intensive use of information, focus on the customer, knowledge of treatment outcomes, constrained resources, coordinated services, reconsideration of human values, increased expectations of accountability, and growing interdependence (O'Neal 1993). In its most recent report, "Critical Challenges: Revitalizing the Health Professions for the Twenty-First Century," the commission lists emerging market trends such as developing purchasing cooperatives; linking primary, specialty, and hospital care; and consolidating health care resources into more integrated systems (O'Neal 1995). These emerging paradigms are taking place in an economic environment that is fueled by competition to gain increasing control over market share. It is our prediction that by 2005, 80%–90% of all care, including mental/behavioral health care, will occur within integrated systems of care in which an economy of scale can be obtained. Competitive advantage will not be based on cost alone but on the previously listed factors. This will be the health care market of the future.

All medical practitioners will be influenced by these market forces. These forces not only will involve pressure to practice in a "corporate" environment, but also will involve increased regulatory control of the practice of psychiatry. This control will be reflected in the development of standards for quality of care. The guidelines being developed by the National Committee for Quality Assurance (NCQA) and the Health Plan Employer Data and Information Set (HEDIS) will have an impact on the practice of medicine and psychiatry in a managed care environment, just as guidelines of the Joint Commission on Accreditation of Healthcare Organizations (JCAHO) did on hospital care. These standards will allow different groups to create benchmarks so that they can compare their products and services with others. Collecting data to meet these standards will become ubiquitous, and every act considered crucial for care will be seen as a potential market advantage.

Advances in Information Technology

Revolutionary changes in the health care arena pale in comparison to the rate of change occurring in information technology. Such changes are happening at both the technical level and the organizational/cultural level. Advances in hardware, software, and networking technologies occur at such an incredible pace that corporations are developing new techniques and strategies that allow them to incorporate these changes. We next review these two levels of information technology.

Table 27–1 describes hardware, software, and networking in greater specificity and describes the advances that each is undergoing. More important than these advances are the implications that they have for psychiatry and the cultural shifts they will produce.

Table 27–1. Advances in information technologies

Information technologies	Information technology components	Parameters of advances	Advances
Hardware	Central processing unit (CPU)	Speed (increasing) Chip size (decreasing) Power consumption (decreasing) Cost (decreasing)	The speeds of CPUs are doubling every 18–24 months. Associated with these increases in speed are decreases in cost. Decreases in chip size and power consumption allow the construction of smaller and more efficient devices.
	Storage	Types of storage media (increasing) Cost per megabyte (decreasing) Durability of storage media (increasing) Access speed (increasing)	The types of storage media available are expanding, as is their volume. Current types include removable magneto-optical and optical. With video and sound becoming increasingly important, there will be ongoing pressure to create cheaper and faster devices that store greater volumes of data.
	Multimedia	Sound-based communication Graphics-based communication Video-based communication Virtual reality	These media are becoming the cornerstone of all computing. The most significant advances are in the areas of video and graphics. Video is becoming more like television (i.e., full frame, full motion). New compression methods are accelerating these changes. In graphics, 3-D is becoming more requested. Advances in this area will lead to greater applications with models of virtual environments and virtual reality.

	Data access	Personal digital assistant Smart cards	The size of the computer can be a barrier to use, yet new types of hardware store and process information in a highly portable fashion.
Software	Business support	Financial Personnel management Credentialing	Business support software that simplifies and manages complex financial guidelines and reports has been developed. Software also has been developed for other managerial tasks such as credentialing and personnel management.
	Clinical operations	Scheduling Flagging and monitoring cases Treatment planning	Clinical operations software moves business support software into the clinical realm, managing clinical information and alerting physicians about cases that need attention or planning that needs to be done.
	Clinical care	Diagnostic interviewing Medication management and review Electronic medical records Patient education Psychotherapy	Clinical care software assists the physician directly in delivering psychiatric care. Interviewing, recording information, educating the patient, and even delivering medications or therapy have been addressed in limited forms with new software. The power of such systems will continue to expand.

(continued)

Table 27–1. Advances in information technologies (*continued*)

Information technologies	Information technology components	Parameters of advances	Advances
Software (*continued*)	Research support	Bibliographic search Research communication Research database	Software that supports clinical research enhances the communications of clinicians. Research databases improve clinicians' ability to find relevant articles and information, simplify the process of data gathering and database analysis, and provide new methods for faster and more complete communication between clinicians.
Networking	Connections	Higher connection speeds Cheaper cost to lay down connections More types of connections available	Network connection speeds continue to climb. This increasing bandwidth allows more information to move more quickly and is essential for moving large amounts of information that are used in video and multimedia software. Part of these changes come from new types of connections, whether based on telephone lines, cable lines, or cellular networks. All are being pushed to their limits of transmission speed.

Routing	Higher speeds to direct messages	Many new types of routing devices are under con-
	Cheaper devices for directing messages	*tinuous development and competition. More routing*
	More types of routing and switching devices	*devices allow more messages to move through a*
	Less network congestion	*network and more locations to be plugged in. Rapid*
		switching also aids in the distribution of information
		from centralized locations.
Communication protocols	More protocols available for different types of communication	New types of messages are moving through these expanding networks. The shared protocols of the
	Higher-speed communications	World Wide Web have created a giant base of people
	Broader use of similar communica-	sending text and graphics communications to one
	tion protocols	another. Further growth will permit the expansion
		of video-based communications or even virtual
		reality–type communications with people meeting in
		virtual rooms.

Hardware.   With advances in computer speed and memory, there will be increased potential for all practitioners to have on their desktops enough power to run advanced programs that incorporate multimedia applications and complex databases. These tools will be inexpensive and widely available, and we all will be expected to use them.

Psychiatrists will need to modify their normal practice and allocate study time to be able to use these tools. We will need to learn how the basic elements of video and nonwritten computer-based communications work (Huang and Alessi 1996b). Those who wish autonomy will have the daunting task of choosing, maintaining, and supporting these advancing systems. Others will rely on corporate decision making for their hardware and will change their practice to fit the company model. In this fashion, practice patterns will fractionate, with growing "universal" practice standards on one hand and independent practitioners on the other who design their own alternative methods of operation.

Software.   With advances in software, more people will be able to do more advanced computing tasks, with fewer technical skills being required to do them. Increased user-friendliness will open the doors for more users and allow more people to feel less intimidated and more empowered by computer programs. The domain of computing will no longer belong to the "techie." It will become a greater expectation that everyone can operate a computer, just as most people today can operate a television set or telephone (Sager 1996).

Psychiatric specialists will need to contribute to these trends by defining their needs and working with software designers to create the psychiatric tools of the future (Alessi and Huang 1996).

Networking.   With improvements in connection speed and cost, more computer hardware is being networked together. Software bridges the gaps, creating easy-to-use communications tools between distant computer-based systems. The growth of newer technologies is creating a meld between traditional telecommunications devices and connections on one hand and computer networks and connections on the other. We will see an increase in the use of "computers" for daily communications, and our daily communications tools such as the telephone will acquire the complex functionality of a computer. These systems will become more mobile and more interconnected with unified communications systems.

Psychiatry will change as we begin to use these communications systems in our daily work. These changes will range from electronic publication and retrieval of research and practice standards to actually seeing patients by using video-based "telemedicine" systems (Bennett et al. 1996).

The Patient as Consumer

The impact of information technology on the practice of psychiatry will affect psychiatrists, but we will not be the only group changed by this revolution. Consumers of mental health services will have greater access to expanding realms of information. They will gain answers concerning their questions about psychiatric disorders, treatment modalities, and alternative medicine theories and applications through their home computers via the Internet.

The Internet is a network of computers spanning the world that provides more than file access (Huang and Alessi 1996a). Through the Internet, individuals can reach distant libraries to examine digital versions of textbooks, journals, and manuscripts. Databases maintained in academic, federal, state, and some private institutions can be accessed for clinical knowledge and treatment modalities. Individuals can communicate via electronic mail (e-mail), voice, and video with anyone on the Internet with an e-mail address. Through simultaneous connections, multiple users can interact with each other in "chat rooms" to exchange information or simply listen to one or more speakers. The Internet can be accessed through commercial Internet providers— which have grown to include major telecommunication corporations, such as AT&T and MCI, and online services, such as CompuServe and America Online—or through academic institutions for individuals attending or working there. A greater ability to access information allows the user to enter and roam the Internet and gain greater knowledge about his or her condition.

The Internet is highly available for a patient or family member; he or she can enter a wide variety of Internet sites based on his or her level of understanding of the disorder. However, this benefit for the patient can create potentially greater complications in the therapeutic alliance. Conflicts in establishing a collaboration between the patient and the practitioner have been addressed over the years and have consistently identified the need for better patient education as a means of facilitating collaboration (Haiman 1995; Schroeder 1973). The future psychiatrist may be faced with the dilemma of being less informed than his or her patient.

Pre-Internet Access to Mental Health Information

Before the Internet, patients had access to information; however, accessing the information had its shortcomings. Obtaining resources required travel to bookstores, libraries, or support groups. In bookstores and libraries, patients needed to rely on one or a few individuals to recommend literature sources. Support groups such as the National

Alliance for the Mentally Ill greatly expanded the number of resources and the number of knowledgeable individuals who could guide someone new to the field. Unfortunately, meeting times were limited and therefore restricted access to the information. Although contact with support groups via telephone was an option, the patient or family was not able to access information consistently.

In the past, the role of the patient and family also was viewed differently by the treating mental health professional. The ability of a patient to understand his or her condition often was limited by the physician's idea that health care technology was too complex for the layperson to comprehend (Meyer 1985). The patient could ask his or her practitioner, therapist, psychiatrist, or other mental health professional questions about his or her condition and treatment. Unfortunately, this was time limited and required the patient to comprehend what was happening to him or her at the time. In addition, family members had limited access to information concerning a relative. Patients and family were given what the treating professional deemed appropriate. No standards existed to identify what was appropriate patient information. This lack of standards left patients with unasked questions and treating professionals with a sense that they had done enough in educating the patient.

Post-Internet Access to Mental Health Information

The evolution of the Internet has led to predictions for better systems in disseminating consumer mental health information. Herzlinger and Freeman (1996) described an Internet-savvy patient who utilizes currently existing technology to interface with a psychiatrist, gatekeeper, and pharmacist to facilitate treatment of agoraphobia from her own home within 2 hours of noticing symptoms. LaPorte (1994) also described methods for long-distance education of health care consumers over the Internet. The means of accessing information and clinical help already exist. Potential also exists to alter dramatically the patient's ability to obtain relevant information and interact with a diverse group of individuals with expertise in dealing with the patient's disorder. Two information servers and e-mail have leveraged mental health consumers into a position that has liberated their reliance on treating professionals. Gopher, derived from *go for*, provides a means of identifying databases listed as menus on a Gopher server. Within the menus, an individual can search for topics of interest. The Gopher search can be initiated from one's home computer utilizing an Internet access. Similarly, WWW can be accessed through the home Internet connection, but a greater variety of sources of information and interactivity exists on the WWW. The WWW serves hypertext documents that link to other related information. The user can follow a flow of ideas rather than searching terms in a catalog or menu. Like Gopher, WWW lacks regulation concerning what information can be disclosed, and no means exist to monitor for inaccurate information. The user is on his or her own to determine what is accurate information. Compounding this problem is the vulnerability that the user communicates blindly to others regarding his or her questions.

Chat rooms allow multiple users to communicate and exchange ideas. Innocently, a user can enter these areas and compromise his or her patient confidentiality to eavesdroppers. Persuasive arguments can be made by individuals in the chat room speaking against traditional treatment standards, potentially compromising the patient's care. These interactions via computer superficially appear to be no different than what a patient may experience during other social interactions. The computer interface, however, hides the subtle signs one sees in person to guide the decision that what is stated is true. E-mail creates a similar scenario, but unlike the traditional postal service, its speed can provide a sense of near real-time conversation.

When a patient or family member approaches the treating professional with newfound knowledge and ideas for treatment, the professional's response can be detrimental to the alliance. The fear of technology and lack of understanding of information databases create a negative countertransference. The professional may dismiss the information as non-peer-reviewed and unacceptable. The schism formed by such a response leaves the patient dependent on the professional's knowledge base, with no reassurance that his or her ideas are useful. The patient will seek a psychiatrist who learns new technology and has new information. In addition, this type of patient will become a partner in his or her own care, reshaping the landscape of mental health care in America.

The Practice of Psychiatry: 2005

The following three scenarios indicate how the practice of psychiatry might look in 10 years, given the forces of information technology. The issue is not the availability of technology, but the forces that will lead to the acceptance and application of technology. The scenarios include a list of assumptions about the particular topic. We hope the assumptions listed will illustrate how these forces of information technology will come together and impact how information is applied in the practice of psychiatry. Several questions that might be elicited by these assumptions then follow.

Scenario 1: Face-to-Face in Cyberspace

Assumptions:

- Computers will be multiform, existing as desktop units, hand-held units, disposable data cards, and identification badges.
- Computers will be ubiquitous, with greater introduction into everyday appliances from telephones to televisions to wristwatches.
- Computers will be easier to use with more intuitive interfaces such as speech recognition, handwriting recognition, or graphic displays.
- All people in society will take these computer systems for granted, expecting the availability of the information these systems represent. People will expect physicians to be able to use these systems in the management of their health care.
- Physicians will gather information on patients using information devices or "appliances." Information could be gathered by taking notes on a data device or by videotaping appointments.
- Psychiatric information will be entered into these ubiquitous computers at the demand of both the new health care industry and the new consumer-patient. A videophone might be used to make appointments, and software programs might be used to automatically check and approve standardized medication and treatment databases.
- Health information will be stored in databases and transmitted through networks to many different people and organizations.
- The ability to obtain patients will be related to the quality of data a physician generates, whether the data are outcome statistics in a database or in online advertising.
- Patients will be evaluated and treated, but the only psychiatrist-patient contact will be "cyber-based" care.
- Disorders will be redefined based on new technologies (i.e., capture and analytic techniques will lead to documentation that is digital).

These assumptions reflect the continuing growth of the "telecosm" (Gilder 1996), where more and more networking power continues to expand, producing a smaller and smaller world tied together by advanced communications instruments.

There are many questions that will be raised about these assumptions:

- Will psychiatry keep up with the rest of society in accepting these devices?
- Will psychiatrists put the necessary effort into determining the impact of these devices on the physician-patient relationship and the quality of care?

- What happens to the physician-patient relationship when the psychiatrist is recording information by computer for his or her databases or when a video recorder is running in the background?
- What does privacy mean in the information era?
- What happens to the physician-patient relationship when the psychiatrist advertises electronically?
- What does *care* mean when contact is only electronic? How will the psychiatrist's responsibilities to his or her patients change?

Scenario 2: Practicing on a Tether

Assumptions:

- Industry standards for almost every facet of health care delivery will evolve.
- A clinician's practice will constantly be monitored by either an employer or a governmental regulatory body.
- An electronic device will be ever present during almost all patient encounters to allow collection of data about many facets of the encounter.
- The data will be entered by one of several modes, including—but not limited to—voice, pen, keyboard, or video.
- All data will be collected in data repositories/warehouses.
- Profiles will be obtainable for a practitioner by diagnosis, severity of illness, treatment regimen, and outcome.
- Profiles will be benchmarked to practitioners across the nation.
- Decisions will be made based on benchmark outcomes, which will determine continued employment by a group, reimbursement, and licensure.
- These data will be available not only to providers, but also to patients.

These assumptions reflect a growing desire to monitor the physician for quality assurance and to guarantee maximum return on investment by the employer of the physician. Advances in database structures, collection devices, and analytical tools will make this possible. The demand to know by both the health care industry and patients will fuel the application and development of these tools.

There are many questions that will be raised about these assumptions:

- Can accurate data be collected in these situations?
- Will there be a scientific basis for the collection and analysis of data?
- Will data be skewed to guarantee that the provider always looks good?

- Will the presence of "devices" make the practice of psychiatry impossible?
- Can patients be trusted to make sense of such data?
- Will anyone be able to practice under this scrutiny?

Scenario 3: The End of the Reign of the Omniscient Psychiatrist

Assumptions:

- Individuals will become increasingly more informed mental health consumers.
- Individuals will be able to access a practitioner's profile from a national database and learn his or her benchmark for treating similar cases.
- Contact with the treating psychiatrist will be made via mail to address prescription renewals, medication side-effect questions, and treatment alternatives.
- Video conferencing will be used in consultation with academic sites to improve the treatment course for patients with complicated psychiatric conditions.
- Patients will become experts concerning their conditions, with knowledge exceeding that of psychiatrists' professional education.
- Patients will review their health rating through a national medical and psychiatric history database for errors, and reports will be generated only at the request of the patient or health care provider.

With the emergence of Internet-based mental health information, the professional is placed in a new position as a "reviewer" of consumer informatics research. It is unrealistic to expect a psychiatrist to be able to review all information on the Internet that would affect his or her patients. However, reviewing information and ideas presented by the patient can prevent dismissing relevant and useful interventions in the treatment course.

Reviewing and discussing information brought to the session also strengthens a partnership between the patient and the psychiatrist. Potential dangers exist for the patient in the advancement of information technology. National databases selling for profit a patient's private mental health history, electronic eavesdroppers willing to sell information about patients to unscrupulous health care providers, and charlatans attempting to undermine treatment standards to propagate their ideas for profit all pose a serious risk to the mental health consumer. Crawshaw et al. (1995) promotes in a patient-physician covenant that, as physicians, we are obligated to be advocates for our patients. In the information age, are we morally responsible for protecting our patients from the abuse of an information-driven economy?

There are many questions that will be raised about the degree of the psychiatrist's responsibility to the patient:

- Are psychiatrists responsible in cautioning patients about disclosing information about themselves over the Internet, which may lead to a compromise in patient confidentiality?
- Should psychiatrists refrain from recording patient history, which could be construed as a liability for a patient when seeking employment, obtaining insurance, or adopting a child?
- How will a psychiatrist respond to the demand by a health care corporation to include his or her patients' records in a national database identifying patients using illegal substances, engaging in sex with multiple partners, or having a past criminal history?
- Will patients seek psychiatrists who are not affiliated with health care corporations and pay out of pocket to avoid having their psychiatric history disclosed to a national database?
- Will patients have adequately informed representatives in Congress to implement federal regulation of mental health care databases?
- Are we, as psychiatrists, capable of instituting moral and ethical guidelines to protect the interests of our patients in the information age through the formation of a task force within our professional organizations, and are we capable of lobbying these guidelines in the federal and state governments?

Adapting to Information Technology

One of the most formidable tasks facing anyone or any organization when deciding that greater information technology is needed is the process of implementation. It is not as easy to implement information technology as one might imagine. The foremost difficulty one encounters is not technology but threat of change. We are all creatures of habit, and certainly the habits we least like to abandon are those concerning the processes of work. We are all process devout, and, depending on our perspective, we are either enslaved by our habits or liberated by them.

Therefore, introducing a new technology almost always implies changing these processes. Although the intent may be positive, there are stages through which the process must progress. One model proposes six stages in introducing and assimilating new technology (Nolan and Gibson 1974). This model is based on introducing technology into an organization, but it also can be viewed as a model for introducing technology into a specialty such as psychiatry.

The six stages of introducing technology are summarized as follows:

- *Stage 1: Initiation.* The technology is introduced into the organization and some user begins to use it. Use is usually slow and is often met with criticism by those who see only its limitations when compared to the previous way of doing business. This stage can last for months to years, as those who have something to lose become increasingly oppositional. Questions often arise about security and the alteration of the physician-patient relationship.
- *Stage 2: Contagion.* More people become aware and acquainted with the technology. Demand and use increase and the utilization grows rapidly. Enthusiasm grows. This is an important step because once it begins, it can be quite surprising and difficult. When the contagion stage begins, it will be obvious, and it will last only for months, but possibly longer. The demand for the resource can grow so rapidly that it outstrips the ability to provide the technology. Early adopters are sometimes criticized and labeled "haves" while all others are "have nots."
- *Stage 3: Control.* If the demand continues, the issue of cost-benefit ratio will become an issue. Due to the demand, the administration has to determine the value of the technology to its overall goals and objectives. If a strategic plan and the placement of this technology were not developed, then it certainly will become necessary to do so at this point. Efficiency, integration, quality, and cost will become four major considerations.
- *Stage 4: Integration.* With the growth of data and systems, the need for systems integration becomes apparent. There are questions concerning database design, data dictionaries, overlap, future growth, and others that become apparent only when some growth has occurred. If different databases were developed by different groups with different tools and on different operating systems, turf wars can erupt with considerable associated rancor.
- *Stage 5: Data administration.* The value of databases becomes a concern. Mechanisms are created to manage and control data, allowing greater efficiency in the use of data for a wide number of efforts.
- *Stage 6: Maturity.* If this stage occurs, then technology and management processes become integrated.

One has to be cognizant that the above staging may apply to only one technology; although this staging certainly will help in understanding a system, it may not necessarily help in the integration of future technology. Each technology will require reassessment to determine its value, and each will have its own timetable. To further complicate matters, multiple technologies might, and more than likely will, be introduced at the same time. Change will be complex and difficult.

Implementing Information Technology in American Psychiatry

Psychiatry must make every effort to prepare its members for the changes that lie ahead. There will be countless opportunities for those prepared for the new era, and there will be countless frustrations for those who are not. Many organizations at many levels will need to make changes to guarantee that such changes occur. From the trainee to the seasoned professional, change and adaptation will be needed.

The following are five recommendations that will help American psychiatrists adapt in these turbulent times:

1. *Assist the leaders in psychiatry to develop a greater appreciation of the significant trends of the day and the implications associated with information technology.* Leaders may include, but are not limited to, executives of the American Psychiatric Association and other major psychiatric organizations, chairs of psychiatry departments, residency training directors, and significant potential future leaders identified during their training.

2. *Make courses concerning information technology and informatics mandatory in all residency training programs.* These will need to cover several major areas, including issues concerning technologies, organizational effects of technology, impact of technology on the physician-patient relationship, and influence of technology on the practice of psychiatry (Huang and Alessi, in press).

3. *Form a national task force or working group that will work toward the development of standards.* Rapidly changing technology challenges the development and deployment of standards at a number of levels, including the technical level, applications level, workstation level, and interface level (W. E. Hammond 1994; J. E. Hammond et al. 1991). Several areas affected by these standards include telemedicine, database development, and interface development for the acquisition of data for clinical care, quality management, and outcomes (Stead and Sittig 1995). Support might be gained from a mix of several sources, including government, nonprofit groups, and vendors.

4. *Develop programs of psychiatric informatics in a number of departments of psychiatry.* Departments of psychiatry should strive to develop curricula emphasizing technology and information management techniques. Such programs should produce future leaders who can promote further education and research in the informatics arena. Obtaining grants and other types of funding should be a major goal of training as well.

5. *Work with the National Institute of Mental Health (NIMH) to establish funding for research regarding the implications of technology in psychia-*

try. The implications would need to be investigated for a number of technologies at both the diagnostic and therapeutic levels.

Summary

This chapter can only be a catalyst in developing future discussions concerning information technology and psychiatry. It does not attempt to deal with the many complex issues that these significant trends will elicit. Undoubtedly, countless papers, presentations, discussions, debates, and frank arguments will occur as a result of these trends and their impact on the practice of psychiatry. It is our belief that the future will be heavily influenced by the advances in information technology and that whoever is a leader in this area will gain significant market advantage that will determine the destiny of psychiatry and the welfare of our patients.

References

Aburdene P: Megatrends for the information age. Bull Med Libr Assoc 82:12–17, 1994

Alessi NE, Huang MP: Riding the third wave: psychiatry in the information era. Psychiatric Times, June 1996, p 20

Ball MJ, Douglas JV: How information technologies are transforming behavioral healthcare, in The Computerization of Behavioral Healthcare. Edited by Trabin T. San Francisco, CA, Jossey-Bass, 1996

Bennett J, Huang MP, Alessi N: Barriers to telemedicine in psychiatry, in Mental Health Computing. Edited by Miller M, Hammond K, Hile M. New York, Springer-Verlag, 1996, pp 415–428

Crawshaw R, Rogers DE, Pellegrino ED, et al: Patient-physician covenant. JAMA 273:1553, 1995

Frenzel CW: Management of Information Technology, 2nd Edition. Danvers, MA, Boyd & Frazer, 1996

Gilder G: Telecosm feasting on the giant peach. Forbes, August 26, 1996, pp 85–96

Haiman S: Dilemmas in professional collaboration with consumers. Psychiatr Serv 46:443–445, 1995

Hammond JE, Berger RG, Carey TS, et al: Making the transition from information systems of the 1970s to medical information systems of the 1990s: the role of the physician's workstation. J Med Syst 15:257–267, 1991

Hammond WE: The role of standards in creating a health information infrastructure. Int J Biomed Comput 34:29–44, 1994

Herzlinger RE, Freeman MA: Reclaiming behavioral healthcare. Behavioral Healthcare Tomorrow, August 1996, pp 99–104

Huang MP, Alessi NE: The Internet and the future of psychiatry. Am J Psychiatry 153:861–869, 1996a

Huang MP, Alessi NE: Tools for developing multimedia in psychiatry, in Mental Health Computing. Edited by Miller M, Hammond K, Hile M. New York, Springer-Verlag, 1996b, pp 322–341

Huang MP, Alessi NE: An informatics curriculum for psychiatry. Academic Psychiatry (in press)

LaPorte RE: Global public health and the information superhighway. BMJ 308:1651–1652, 1994

Meyer LS: Untangling communication lines to connect consumers and providers. Nursing and Healthcare 6:366–368, 1985

Nolan RL, Gibson CF: Managing the four stages of EDP growth. Harvard Business Review, January 1, 1974, pp 1–15

O'Neal EH: Health professions education for the future: schools in service to the nation. San Francisco, CA, The Pew Health Professions Commission, 1993

O'Neal EH: Critical challenges: revitalizing the health professions for the 21st century. San Francisco, CA, The Pew Health Professions Commission, 1995

Sager I: The race is on to simplify. Business Week, June 24, 1996, pp 72–75

Schroeder OC: Health consumers and medical practitioners: is conflict inevitable? Postgrad Med 53:203–205, 1973

Schwartz P: The Art of the Long View. New York, Doubleday, 1991

Shugars DA, O'Neal EH, Bader JD (eds): Health America: practitioners in 2005: an agenda for action for U.S. health professional schools. Durham, NC, The Pew Health Professions Commission, 1991

Stead WW, Sittig DF: Building a data foundation for tomorrow's healthcare information management systems. Int J Biomed Comput 39:127–131, 1995

Afterword to Volume 16

*Leah J. Dickstein, M.D., Michelle B. Riba, M.D., and
John M. Oldham, M.D.*

We hope that in reading this volume you have gained new knowledge and understanding that will enable you to provide patients with the best care possible. We chose to present psychiatric disorders, treatment modalities, and issues for which so much new information is available and that affect so many patients—specifically, the many uses of cognitive therapies for a substantial number of disorders; issues about early traumatic experiences and repressed and recovered memories in adulthood; obsessive-compulsive disorder across the life span; updates on psychopharmacological information, again across the life span; psychological and biological assessment of psychiatric patients; and the increasingly practical and necessary uses of computers in psychiatric practice.

We believe you will refer many times to the extraordinary amount of material these authors have included to assist you in updating and improving your patient care. Consider sharing the volume, as well as previous volumes, with colleagues and health care staff.

Our sincere thanks to the American Psychiatric Press staff and leadership for what we are proud to state is an excellent volume. Finally, we thank you, our readers, for your consistent support in making the Review of Psychiatry series, in 16 annual volumes, such a resounding success and worthwhile effort.

Index

Audiological assessment, of children, V-45

Audiotapes, and feedback in social phobia, I-26–27

Auditory perception, and neuropsychological assessment, V-39–40, V-53

Augmentation strategies, in pharmacotherapy
for antidepressants in bipolar disorder, IV-76
OCD and, III-48, III-62–63
for valproate in bipolar disorder, IV-54

Autism, differential diagnosis of communication disorders, mental retardation, and, V-44–48
OCD in children and adolescents and, III-11
serotonin reuptake inhibitors for OCD in, IV-5

Automatic negative thoughts, and substance abuse disorders, I-49–50, I-57

Automatic process, of voluntary thought suppression, II-110

Automatic speech recognition, VI-24–25

Autonomic symptoms, and hypochondriasis, I-17–18

Avoidance, in generalized anxiety disorder, I-19

Avoidant personality disorder
behavioral strategies in, I-76, I-80
cognitive therapy for, I-91, I-95, I-101
core beliefs in, I-77, I-80
reactions to current situations and, I-83

BABS (Brown Assessment of Beliefs Scale), III-91

Bayley Scales of Infant Intelligence—Revised, V-47

BEAM (brain electrical activity mapping), V-18

Beck Anxiety Inventory, I-56

Beck Depression Inventory, I-56, I-146, IV-132, VI-26–27

Beery Developmental Test of Visual-Motor Integration, V-53

Behavior. See also Behavioral therapy; Safety behaviors
ADHD and, IV-97, V-49
bipolar disorder and, IV-41
chronic or severe depression and deficits of, I-143–145
cognitive therapy for personality disorders and, I-76–77, I-78, I-80–81, I-100
eating disorders and abnormalities of, I-107–108
OCD in children and adolescents, III-9–10
panic disorder and, I-24
posttraumatic stress disorder and exposure therapy, I-30

Behavioral Informatics Tomorrow (Morrissey 1997), VI-38–39

Behavioral MAPS (Master Assessment and Progress Scale), VI-26

Behavioral memories, and traumatic memories, II-24

Behavioral reenactments, and traumatic memories, II-27

Behavioral therapy. See also Cognitive-behavioral therapy
computer technology and, VI-6
for OCD, III-49–50

Beliefs About Substance Use Inventory, I-56, I-57

Beliefs
generalized anxiety disorder and, I-19, I-20
personality disorders and, I-77–78, I-97–101
substance abuse and dysfunctional, I-48–52, I-57–58, I-59–61

Bender Gestalt, V-53

Benton Face Recognition Test, V-39

Benton Line Orientation Test, V-39

Benton Test of Visual Retention, V-38

Benzodiazepines
anxiety in elderly and, IV-158, IV-159
bipolar disorder and, IV-67
brief psychotic disorder and, IV-24

dementia in elderly and, IV-167
mood stabilizers and, IV-66,
IV-73
prenatal exposure to, III-106
sleep disorders in elderly and,
IV-161
substance abuse and, I-53
Benztropine, IV-8
Beta-blockers
anxiety in elderly and, IV-159
clonidine and, IV-108
dementia in elderly and, IV-168
lithium and, IV-52
neuroleptics and, IV-17
Billing, and computer technology,
VI-30–31
Billing Practice Management Software,
VI-31
Binge-eating disorder. *See* Eating
disorders
Biochemical markers, and laboratory
tests, V-12–13
Biological assays, and therapeutic
drug monitoring, V-22
Biological markers, state-dependent
and trait-dependent, V-8
Biological models
cognitive models of anxiety
disorders and, I-21
for traumatic forgetting, II-168
Biopsychosocial perspective, on
OCD in elderly, III-59
Bipolar disorder
antiepileptic drugs for, IV-5
ADHD and, IV-110
cognitive therapy and, I-147–157
OCD and, III-87
psychopharmacological
treatment of across life
span, IV-31–78
Block-cuing, and intentional
forgetting, II-84–88, II-94,
II-95–96, II-98
Blue Cross–Blue Shield, VI-33
Bodily sensations, and panic attacks,
I-11–12, I-13
Body dysmorphic disorder, and
OCD, III-34
Body image, and eating disorders,
I-108, I-120–121

Borderline personality disorder
behavioral strategies in, I-77, **I-81**
cognitive therapy for, I-91, I-96,
I-97–98, I-100
countertransference and, I-103
OCD and, III-90
schemas in, I-78–79
therapeutic relationship and
cognitive therapy for,
I-87–88
Boston Diagnostic Aphasia
Examination, V-40
Boston Naming Test, V-48
BPRS (Brief Psychiatric Rating Scale),
IV-167
BPRS-C (Brief Psychiatric Rating
Scale for Children), IV-10
Brain electrical activity mapping
(BEAM), V-18
Brain imaging techniques, and
laboratory assessment of
psychiatric disorders, V-14–17
Brief Psychiatric Rating Scale (BPRS),
IV-167
Brief Psychiatric Rating Scale for
Children (BPRS-C), IV-10
Brief psychotic disorder, and
psychopharmacology, IV-24
Brief therapy, and cognitive therapy
for panic disorder, I-32–34
Brofaramine, IV-152
Brown Assessment of Beliefs Scale
(BABS), III-91
Budget planners, and
understanding of assessment
instruments, V-73
Bulimia nervosa. *See also* Eating
disorders
outcome research on cognitive
therapy for, I-122–130
target weight ranges and, I-110
Bupropion
ADHD and, **IV-93,** IV-104–105
bipolar disorder and, IV-64, IV-65,
IV-76
depression in elderly and, IV-151
Buspirone
for anxiety in elderly, IV-158–159
as augmenting agent, III-48, III-63
for dementia in elderly, IV-167

Instrument panels, for healthcare delivery systems, V-98, V-101
Insurance. *See* Health insurance
Intake, and computer technology, VI-25
Intellectual abilities, and neuropsychological assessment, V-37
Intelligence, and neuropsychological assessment, V-37, V-51
Intentional forgetting
    adults and emotional or traumatic stimuli, II-88–91
    adults and emotionally neutral materials, II-84–88
    children and, II-91–93
    context and, II-111–112, II-115
    evidence regarding, II-80–84
    future research on, II-114–116
    other factors affecting memory and, II-112–114
    processes of, II-93–98
Internal State Scale (ISS), I-157
Internet
    access to health care information through, VI-77–79
    bulletin boards and information on psychological instruments, V-60
    current perspectives on, VI-52–53
    description of, VI-49–50
    glossary of terms, VI-58–67
    history of, VI-50–52
    patients and, VI-77
    psychiatry-related resources on, VI-53–57
Interpersonal psychotherapy (IPT), for bulimia nervosa, I-127
Interviewing techniques, influence of on memory of traumatic events, II-61–62
Intrusion symptoms, and memory disturbance in posttraumatic conditions, II-23–24
Item-cuing, and intentional forgetting, II-84–88, II-94, II-95–96, II-98
IT'S YOUR CALL (computer-assisted smoking reduction program), VI-32

Joint Commission on Accreditation of Healthcare Organizations (JCAHO), V-84–86, VI-37, VI-39, VI-71
Journals, and software evaluations, VI-19, VI-20–21

Kaiser-Permanente, Inc., VI-33
Kaufman Assessment Battery for Children (K-ABC), V-53
Ketoconazole, III-22
Kidney, and pharmacokinetics
    in children, IV-130
    in elderly, IV-145–146
Korsakoff syndromes, V-38

Laboratory assessments
    bipolar disorder and, IV-45
    computer technology and, VI-8
    general principles for medical, V-7–8, **V-9–10**
    psychiatric disorders and, V-8, V-11–19
    therapeutic drug monitoring and, V-19–27
Lamotrigine, IV-58, IV-69–71, IV-76
Language, neuropsychological assessment of disorders of
    in adults, V-40
    in children, V-47–48, V-52
Late-life bipolar disorder, IV-43–44
Learning disabilities and disorders
    ADHD and, IV-88, IV-98
    memory and, V-38–39
    neuropsychological assessment of children and, V-52
    personality disorders and, I-82
Learning theory, and OCD, III-39
Legal system
    psychological assessment instruments and, V-71
    recovered memories of childhood sexual abuse and, II-147, II-153
Life events, and OCD in elderly, III-68
Life expectancy, in bipolar disorder, IV-31
Life problems, substance abuse and management of, I-62–63

Narcotics Anonymous (NA), I-53
National Alliance for the Mentally Ill
	(NAMI), IV-46
National Committee for Quality
	Assurance (NCQA), V-86, VI-37,
	VI-39, VI-71
National Depressive and
	Manic-Depressive Association
	(NDMDA), IV-46
National Institute of Mental Health
	(NIMH)
	guidelines for selection of
		psychological instruments,
		V-60–61
	software systems for psychiatry,
		VI-19–20
National Managed Health Care
	Congress (1996), VI-35
National Science Foundation, VI-51
Natural language, and computer
	technology, VI-8
Nefazodone
	bipolar disorder and, IV-64, IV-65,
		IV-76
	depression in elderly and,
		IV-151–152
Negative affect, impact of on
	memory, II-16–30
Negative evaluation, testing of
	predictions about in social
	phobia, I-27
Negative symptoms, and cognitive
	therapy for schizophrenia, I-163
Nelson Adult Reading Test, V-37
Networking, and computer
	technology, **VI-74–75,** VI-76
Neuroanatomy
	OCD and, III-37
	traumatic forgetting and, II-168
Neurobiology, of OCD, III-13,
	III-36–37
Neuroendocrine system, laboratory
	tests for disorders of, V-8,
	V-11–12
Neuroleptic malignant syndrome,
	IV-163
Neuroleptics
	anxiety in elderly and, IV-159
	dementia in elderly and, IV-166
	mania in elderly and, IV-154

OCD and, III-22
	schizophrenia in elderly and,
		IV-13–14, IV-162–163
Neuroleptic threshold hypothesis,
	and antipsychotics, IV-8–9
Neurological testing, and laboratory
	assessment of psychiatric
	disorders, V-17–19
Neurological toxicity, of
	carbamazepine, IV-61, IV-62
Neuropsychological assessments
	of adult psychiatric patients,
		V-33–43
	of children, V-43–54
	cost-effectiveness of, V-32–33
	description of, V-31–32
Neurosensory Center
	Comprehensive Examination
	for Aphasia, V-40, V-48
Neurotoxicity, of lithium in elderly,
	IV-155
Neurotransmitters. *See*
	Neuroanatomy; Neurobiology
Newsgroups, on Internet, VI-56–57
New York State Office of Mental
	Health (OMH), VI-23–24
Nightmares, and traumatic
	memories, II-24, II-26
Nimodipine, IV-63
Nocturnal myoclonus, IV-160
Nonsteroidal anti-inflammatory
	agents (NSAID)
	Alzheimer's disease and, IV-166
	lithium and, IV-52, IV-155
Norfluoxetine, V-25
Nortriptyline
	ADHD and, **IV-92,** IV-101, IV-103
	chronic or severe depression and,
		I-146
	depression in children and
		adolescents and, IV-133
	depression in elderly and, IV-150
	prenatal exposure to, III-105
	therapeutic drug monitoring and,
		V-25
Nurse's Observation Scale for
	Inpatient Evaluation (NOSIE),
	VI-28
Nutritional counseling, and eating
	disorders, I-109–112

Pew Health Professions
 Commission, VI-70–71
Pharmacotherapy *See*
 Psychopharmacology
PHARMAKON system (software
 program), VI-9
Phenelzine
 anxiety disorders and, I-9
 ADHD and, **IV-92**
 depression in elderly and, IV-152
 social phobia and, I-35–36
Phenobarbital
 valproate and, IV-57, IV-58
 substance abuse and, I-53
Phenothiazine, IV-13, IV-15
Phenytoin, IV-58, IV-74
Phobias, comorbidity of with OCD,
  III-12. *See also* Simple phobias
Physical disability, and treatment of
 elderly patients, III-65–66
Physiology, and traumatic
 memories, II-130
Pictorial Test of Intelligence, V-47,
 V-52
Pimozide, III-48, IV-23
Plasma medication levels,
 therapeutic monitoring of,
 V-19–27
Policy-makers, and understanding of
 assessment instruments, V-73
Polysomnography, V-18–19
Positron-emission tomography
 (PET), V-14–15, V-16–17
Postpartum period, OCD during
 clinical examples of, III-106–109
 epidemiology of, III-97–101
 etiology and pathophysiology of,
 III-101–103
 treatment of, III-103–106
Posttraumatic stress disorder (PTSD)
 cognitive approach to
  understanding of, I-20–21
 cognitive therapy and treatment
  of, I-30
 dose-response relationship and
  diagnosis of, II-22, II-156
 extreme trauma and, II-79
 information-processing and, II-27
 outcome studies of cognitive
  therapy for, I-37–38

psychodynamic psychotherapy
 for cases of comorbid with
 dissociative disorders, II-167
psychopharmacology for in
 children and adolescents,
 IV-137
sexual abuse and, II-29, II-90–91
Powersecretary (software program),
 VI-25
Practice guidelines. *See* Guidelines
Preconception counseling, and
 OCD, III-103
Preferential encoding, and
 intentional forgetting, II-93–98
Pregnancy, OCD during
 clinical examples of, III-106–109
 epidemiology of, III-97–101
 etiology and pathophysiology of,
 III-101–103
 treatment of, III-103–106
Pressure threshold, measures of, V-40
Prevalence
 of anxiety disorders in elderly,
 IV-156–157
 of ADHD, IV-88
 of bipolar disorder, IV-31
 of depression in children and
 adolescents, IV-131
 of depression in elderly, IV-147
 of OCD
  in children and adolescents,
  III-7, III-10, III-23
  in elderly, III-57
  in general population, III-73,
  III-97
 of panic attacks, I-12–13
 of schizophrenia, I-157, IV-11–12
 of substance abuse disorders, I-45
Primidone, IV-52, IV-74
*Principles of Medical Ethics With
 Annotations Especially Applicable
 to Psychiatry, The,* II-11
Problem-Knowledge Coupler System
 (software program), VI-28
Problem-oriented medical records,
 and computer technology, VI-9
Problem-solving
 eating disorders and, I-121
 generalized anxiety disorder and,
 I-29

DSM-IV criteria for bipolar
disorder and, IV-39
psychopharmacology for in
elderly, IV-162–164
stimulant-associated toxic
psychosis, IV-99
Psychosocial intervention, for OCD
in elderly, III-64–66
Psychostimulants, and bipolar
disorder, IV-72
Psychosurgery, for OCD, III-48–49,
III-63–64
Psychotherapy, and computer
technology, VI-10. *See also*
Cognitive-behavioral therapy;
Psychodynamic psychotherapy
Psychotic depression, I-142–143, I-146
Psychotic disorders. *See also*
Psychosis; Schizophrenia
OCD and, III-35
psychopharmacology across life
span for, IV-7–24
PTSD. *See* Posttraumatic stress disorder
Puberty, and onset of OCD, III-103
Purdue Pegboard, V-42–43, V-53

Quality assurance, and computer
technology, VI-9, VI-31
Quality of care
as performance measure for
healthcare delivery
systems, V-90–91
psychometric quality of
assessment instruments
and, V-69
Quality of life, and maintenance
antipsychotic treatment for
schizophrenia, IV-19–20
Quetiapine, IV-8, IV-11, IV-18
Questioning, influence of postevent
on memory, II-34–35
Quick-Doc (software program), VI-29

Rape
amnesia and dissociative
symptoms in victims of,
II-156
negative affect and memories of,
II-22

posttraumatic stress disorder and,
I-20, I-37, I-38
traumatic memories and, II-62–63,
II-131
voluntary suppression of
memories of, II-81–82
Rapid cycling, and bipolar disorder,
IV-41, IV-76–77
Raskin Depression Scale, IV-132
Rational/emotional role-play, and
cognitive therapy for
personality disorders, I-101–102
Raven Coloured Progressive
Matrices, V-47
Raven Standard Progressive
Matrices, V-41
Reading disabilities, V-48
Recall, impact of negative affect on,
II-16–30
Recognition memory, and
neuropsychological assessment,
V-34–35, V-38–39
Record-keeping, in treatment of
dissociative disorders, II-168.
See also Patient care
Recovered memory. *See also*
Repressed memory
retrieval environment and, II-83
review of studies of, II-156–161
traumatic memory and, II-34–46,
II-60–67
well-being and, II-67–69
Referrals, for neuropsychological
assessment under managed
care, V-34–36, V-44–50
Refugees, posttraumatic amnesia in,
II-156
Regional cerebral blood flow (rCBF)
mapping techniques, V-17
Relapse Prediction Scale, I-56
Relapse and relapse prevention
anxiety disorders after
discontinuation of
medication, I-9
bipolar disorder and, I-155–156
eating disorders and, I-122
elderly schizophrenia patients
and neuroleptic
withdrawal, IV-17
OCD in elderly and, III-69